YEAR BOOK's
MEDICAL LICENSURE REVIEWS
CLINICAL SCIENCES

Internal Medicine/Surgery/
Obstetrics and Gynecology/
Pediatrics/Psychiatry/
Public Health and Community Medicine

anato, bioch, micro, phts/phar, phys
Ped. preven m, obs/mal

$\begin{pmatrix} 1/5 \\ 2/5 \\ 2/5 \end{pmatrix}$ of Comp ① = Fundamental basic science
" : " " = applic" of = = to mech. of disease
" : = " = Clinical tasks related to diseases

Comp1 Fundamental Knowledge of disease + Process encountered
in supervised setting.

400 Pages.

Comp 2 : to assess Knowl;
+ coy ability in
independent setting.

i.e diagnosis
& management.

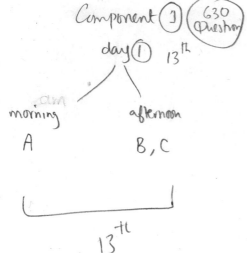

Component ① (630 Question)
day ① 13th
morning — afternoon
A — B, C
13th

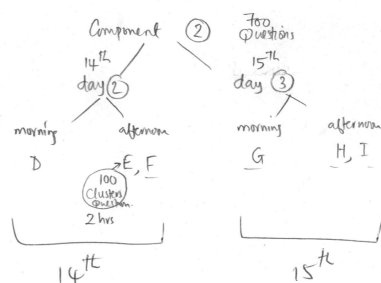

Component ② 700 Questions
14th — 15th
day ② — day ③
morning — afternoon — morning — afternoon
D — E, F — G — H, I
100 Clusters Question. 2 hrs
14th — 15th

YEAR BOOK's MEDICAL LICENSURE REVIEWS

CLINICAL SCIENCES

Internal Medicine/Surgery/
Obstetrics and Gynecology/
Pediatrics/Psychiatry/
Public Health and Community Medicine

Alfred Jay Bollet, M.D.

Clinical Professor of Medicine
Yale University School of Medicine
Chief of Medicine
Danbury Hospital
Danbury, CT

Year Book Medical Publishers, Inc./Fleschner Publishing Co.
Chicago • London • Boca Raton/ Woodbridge, CT

1 2 3 4 5 6 7 8 9 0 M F 92 91 90 89 88

Library of Congress Cataloging-in-Publication Data

Bollet, Alfred J.
    Clinical sciences: internal medicine, surgery, obstetrics and gynecology, pediatrics, psychiatry, public health and community medicine / Alfred Jay Bollet.
        p.   cm. — (Year Book's medical licensure reveiws)
    Includes bibliographies and index.
    ISBN 0-8151-1022-7
    1. Medicine—Examinations, questions, etc. 2. Medicine, Clinical—Examinations, questions, etc.   I. Title.   II. Series.
    [DNLM: 1. Medicine—examination questions. W 18 B691c]
R834.5.B66   1988
610′.76—dc19
DNLM/DLC   88-34
for Library of Congress   CIP

Sponsoring Editor: Richard H. Lampert

CONTRIBUTORS

Hugh R.K. Barber, MD
Chairman, Department of Obstetrics & Gynecology
New York Medical College
Valhalla, NY

Alfred Jay Bollet, MD
Clinical Professor of Medicine
Yale University School of Medicine
New Haven, CT

Audrey Brown, MD
Professor and Vice-Chairman, Department of Pediatrics
SUNY Health Sciences Center
Brooklyn, NY

Robin J.O. Catlin, MD
Professor and Head, Department of Family Medicine
Louisiana State University Medical Center
School of Medicine
New Orleans, LA

David Fields, MD
Associate Attending
Lenox Hill Hospital
New York, NY

Martin S. Kesselman, MD
Professor and Associate Chairman
Department of Psychiatry
SUNY Health Sciences Center
Brooklyn, NY

Richard M. Stillman, MD
Associate Professor of Surgery
SUNY Health Sciences Center
Brooklyn, NY

ABBREVIATIONS

ADP   adenosine diphosphate
ATP   adenosine triphosphate
ATPase   adenosine triphosphatase
b.i.d.   twice daily
bpm   beats per minute
BUN   blood urea nitrogen
CNS   central nervous system
CPR   cardiopulmonary resuscitation
CSF   cerebrospinal fluid
CT   computerized tomography
DNA   deoxyribonucleic acid
DNase   deoxyribonuclease
ECG   electrocardiogram
EDTA   ethylenediaminetetraacetate
EEG   electroencephalogram
GI   gastrointestinal
GU   genitourinary
ICU   intensive care unit
IM   intramuscular(ly)
IV   intravenous(ly)
NPO   nothing by mouth
PCO_2 partial pressure of carbon dioxide
PO   by mouth
PO_2 partial pressure of oxygen
q   every
q.i.d.   four times daily
RNA   ribonucleic acid
SC   subcutaneous(ly)
SGOT   serum glutamic-oxaloacetic transaminase
SGPT   serum glutamic-pyruvic transaminase
t.i.d.   three times daily

INTRODUCTION

Year Book Medical Publishers has prepared a two-volume examination study aid that is intended to assist students and resident physicians to prepare for medical licensure examinations, such as the National Board of Medical Examiners and FLEX examinations. This volume is devoted to the clinical sciences, and the other to the basic sciences. The material covered provides a relatively quick review of essential points in each field, with sufficient depth to be valuable preparation for these licensure examinations, for undergraduate medical school examinations, and for preparation for discussions during teaching rounds. Each chapter contains a group of questions like those on the National Board and FLEX exams to provide experience with the formats used in these examinations as well as assistance in review of subject material.

In preparing these volumes, the authors assumed that readers had a basic familiarity with each subject, and the material is presented concisely since it is primarily intended for review purposes. Although a great deal of factual information is provided in most subjects areas, concentrating on salient points most likely to be covered on examinations, these volumes are not intended to serve as reference texts. Sufficient explanation is given to help in the understanding of the factual material presented, and therefore in its retention in memory, but these aspects are not discussed in the depth to be expected in a standard textbook. At the end of each chapter, a few basic references are provided to aid readers in selecting sources for exploring topics in further depth.

Each chapter on clinical subjects includes sections covering the factual information needed for decisions that candidates must make in answering patient management problems, which are a standard part of such examinations. These decisions cover diagnostic tests and therapeutic principles. Emphasis has been given to the facts in each subject pertinent to these decisions. Such information is important for multiple-choice questions as well, since such decisions are often the point of such questions.

In the clinical subjects, students are expected to bring information from many different basic science and clinical disciplines to bear on clinical problems. Although the examinations no longer divide the time into specific subject areas, mixing the clinical disciplines throughout the test, we have kept these subjects distinct in this volume for ease of review and in order to make the material more useful during undergraduate clerkship experiences. Students should remember, however, that on National Board and FLEX exams questions on these subjects are intermingled.

Some factual material obviously is more appropriate for specialty board examinations, since certified specialists in the field will be dealing with the type of clinical problem requiring application of that information. It is not appropriate to ask primary care physicians or physicians who are just finishing undergraduate training and entering residency programs to be responsible for such information. The authors tried to keep this in mind in preparing the review book. The chapters are aimed at undergraduate students and house officers who are taking licensure exams, not specialists taking advanced certifying board exams.

In selecting subject material for these volumes, the authors had in mind the philosophy of the examining boards regarding the type of information to cover on these exams. In general, this is the type of information that undergraduate medical students and junior house officers will need to function at the next level of their training. Graduates entering the first year of residency training usually have to work in emergency departments as part of their training; they may be faced with patients presenting with a wide variety of clinical problems and must be able to recognize the nature of the problem, take immediate action when necessary to prevent progression of the disease process, and know when to call for help. The committees that make up the National Board examinations have this function in mind; they wish to evaluate whether students are ready for the additional responsibilities that are needed to function in their further training. Thus, questions are directed at the most important points about the clinical problems an intern may face in the emergency department or as sudden developments in sick, hospitalized patients. In addition there is heavy emphasis on primary care problems the candidate is likely to experience in outpatient settings on rotation through various specialties. These subjects should be stressed by candidates in preparing for these examinations.

House officers must also know enough about problems appropriately treated by subspecialists to know when to refer, to be able to advise patients on appropriate courses of action, or to explain to such patients what is likely to happen to them as workup and treatment progress. Knowledge of subspecialty-level medical problems cannot be ignored, therefore, in undergraduate education or in preparation for licensure exams.

Students and house officers, in considering the importance of specific subjects when studying for examinations, should therefore consider whether they might be faced with such a problem as a first-line physician in an emergency room or in an outpatient setting, and what they must know to function properly as an intern or resident. Study for that function and you will be studying for these licensure examinations as well as for your needs in the immediate future.

For example, in evaluating a patient with anemia, house officers and therefore candidates for licensure should know how to distinguish folate for B_{12} deficiency from iron deficiency, appropriate types of therapy for each, how to identify a patient with an autoimmune hemolytic process, and what types of drugs are likely to be used and their major side effects. But such candidates need not be expected to know the appropriate dosage of immunosuppressant agents or choose among them.

With antibiotic choices, candidates are expected to know the types of drugs that should be used but not necessarily the exact ones that are the drugs of choice today, since rapid developments in many fields cause frequent changes in the specific drugs of choice. Remember that these examinations are prepared almost 2 years before they are given, and the subject committees know that much detailed information can become outdated by the time the examination is given.

In general, therefore, details of dosage are rarely asked, but it is expected that candidates will know major principles of drug use, major side effects to watch for, important drug interactions, and pharmacokinetic principles that are related to major categories of drugs. Similarly, for surgical procedures, students are expected to know indications, likely complicaitons, and what the patient is likely to experience, as well as the usual duration of recuperation and disability.

POINTERS TO REMEMBER WHILE TAKING LICENSURE EXAMINATIONS

When taking multiple-choice tests such as those given by National Board of Medical Examiners and FLEX, candidates should bear certain useful principles in mind.

First, be familiar with types of questions used in National Board and FLEX examinations and practice answering them. Examples are provided after each subject in this volume. When taking the examination, read the instructions carefully and be certain you understand them before proceeding; this is especially important for matching questions, where each item may be used once, more than once, or not at all. In these exams, K-type questions are another source of confusion, since the correct response depends on the pattern of the answers rather than an answer to each individual item. Keep instructions in view; you might write them on the front of an exam book so you can have ready reference after each question. The general pattern is as follows:

Answer A if responses 1, 2, and 3 are correct.
Answer B if only 1 and 3 are correct.
Answer C if only 2 and 4 are correct.
Answer D if only 4 is correct.
Answer E if all are correct.

This format allows the answer sheet to have the same response pattern as in the "one best out of five" (A-type) questions; only one response is given, even though four true-false decisions are made.

My advice in taking these questions is to write T or F next to each statement in the exam book, thinking about them individually, then go back and determine the pattern and select the appropriate response. If you are sure one item is true or false, this obviously can help in a decision with another item because of the restricted number of possible patterns, but do not concentrate on getting help from the patterns or you will spend time worrying about patterns and not the correct answers.

Do not look for "tricks" in the questions. They are intended to be straightforward. If a trick or misleading clue inadvertently slips in, it will cause confusion that will be evident when the pattern of responses is checked after the exam is scored. An aberrant pattern of answers to a specific item in comparison to how candidates did on the remainder of the test will result in the item being eliminated from scoring. These examination questions are prepared by experienced committees helped by professionals in evaluation, and a sincere effort is made to avoid ambiguities and statements that might mislead candidates. The obvious answer is the one wanted, not a subtle possible alternative that applies to relatively few instances of the phenomenon. These questions are generally phrased better than questions prepared by individual faculty members, such as undergraduate medical school exams. I am sure, for example, that you will never see the words "never" or "always" in National Board of Medical Examiners or FLEX exams.

Some useful specific pointers follow:

1. If the question starts out with a lot of information (a long stem), skip to the end and start reading the specific answers at the end, then go back and read the long stem. This way you will know what points in the stem are pertinent to the answers that are given and will not have to reread the stem after you know the thrust of the answers.

2. Keep track of the time. Check the total number of questions in the part of the exam you are doing, how long you have, and therefore when you should be one-quarter, one-half, and three-quarters through. Do not get hung up on items you are unsure of, losing time you will need to answer questions you do know near the end. Mark questions you are uncertain about, keeping a list on the front of the exam book, and after you finish all the items you know, go back and reconsider the uncertain ones. That way you will get through the exam at least once and will be sure to get all the credit for the things you do know.

3. If you are unsure of an answer, guess. There is no penalty for guessing wrong, and remember—on true-false items, you have a 50% chance of guessing right.

4. Spot check periodically to be sure you are answering at the correct place on the answer sheet. Be sure you avoid a systematic error, marking all answers at the wrong place.

5. After you finish going through the exam once, go back and recheck the questions you marked for reconsideration during the first run through the exam. Do not go over answers you were sure about the first time; you will be tired at the end and less likely to make the correct decision on these items. Stick with your first choice. Recheck only the questions you did not answer, guessed at, or felt uncertain about, having marked them as you went through the exam the first time.

ADVICE FOR STUDYING FOR EXAMS

1. Keep in mind the level of information that the committee that drew up the question is expecting; they are not seeking a subspecialist's level of information about rare phenomena. Concentrate on the material you will need to function on your next level of training, and you will be preparing for that function and for the examination at the same time.

2. To make exam study books such as this one most useful, mark the pages with a highlighter or a pencil; write key points in the margin. Remember that importance is a personal matter: Mark what is most important to you, generally noting only points that you are not sure you know.

3. If a point is of critical clinical importance but you are sure you know it, do not mark it. You are not preparing a textbook listing important points for someone else to study; you are preparing a guide for review purposes to suit your own needs. If you know a fact, it is not important to review it for preparation for an exam, no matter how important it is clinically.

4. Keep a notebook handy as you study, preferably one with dividers for subjects. When studying, write *questions* or topic headings in the notebook, not factual answers. The questions can be brief, just enough to remind you to think of the point you want to be sure you have learned, such as "Tests for iron deficiency." Write the *location of the answer* next to the question (e.g., the page number) and highlight the answer in this book. Similarly, questions or topics can be written in the margin of this book, with the answers underlined, rather than rewriting the facts that are in the text in your marginal notes or in your notebook.

5. When reviewing, go through the questions in your notebook or those in the marginal notes you marked in this book. Stop and think of the answers or write them down briefly on separate sheets of paper (or another section of your notebook). Then check the answer your highlighted or underlined in the text. If you are satisfied that you know the point, put a check mark through the question (but do not obliterate it, so you can recheck if you want to). Mark in your notebook (e.g., with an asterisk in the margin) items you missed or are still unsure about; return to those points later and repeat the process until you are satisfied that you know the answers to all the points you marked in your notebook. Mark again any that you are still unsure about, so that when you are reviewing for the last time before the exam you can concentrate on those few points.

6. If your style is to write factual points in your notebooks and you do not want to change your habits, write them all on one side of each page, putting the questions or topic heading on the other side. When reviewing, keep the book folded so you only see the questions, think about the answers, and then look at your notes to check yourself. When reviewing, do not just read facts, but always be checking yourself to see if you know them.

7. Keep importance of the material in mind in a negative sense only: Ignore points that are not important enough to spend time on, in view of purpose and expected level of the exam and the facts you are sure you know.

ADDITIONAL INFORMATION

For more information regarding National Board Exams, write to

National Board of Medical Examiners

3930 Chestnut Street

Philadelphia, PA 19104

For FLEX exams, write to

The Federation of State Medical Boards of the United States, Inc.

Attention: Guidelines

2630 West Freeway, Suite 138

Fort Worth, TX 76102–7199;

For ECFMG exams,

3624 Market Street, Philadelphia, PA 19104–2685

Be sure you have read and understand all the informational material sent to you regarding these exams.

The authors and publishers of this study guide feel that the efforts they have expended to make this book useful to you were well spent. We hope that in using it you agree. And good luck on your examinations.

CONTENTS

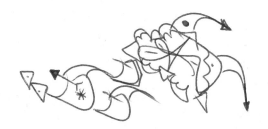

1

INTERNAL MEDICINE
Alfred Jay Bollet

INFECTIOUS DISEASES

USE OF LABORATORY TESTS IN DIAGNOSING INFECTIOUS DISEASES

A variety of lab methods are useful in identifying infecting organisms. **Gram and acid-fast stains** of sputum; of urine; of pleural, peritoneal, or CSF; of any purulent exudate that can be aspirated; or of biopsy material are the most useful procedures. Other microscopic examinations of value include **Wright's stain of thick blood smears** for malaria and babesiosis; **examination of unstained,** warm, unfixed specimens for parasites; **india ink preparations** for *Cryptococcus;* potassium hydroxide **(KOH) preparations** and **silver stains** for fungi and *Pneumocystis carinii;* and **immunofluorescent antibody techniques** for *Legionella* and *Bordetella pertussis.* **Dark-field microscopic exam** can identify *Treponema pallidum,* and electron microscopy can be useful in finding viral particles in cells. **Counterimmunoelectrophoresis** (CIE) or **latex particle agglutination** can be used to identify microbial antigens, especially in CSF, where the procedure can be done in 1 hour and can identify the organism causing meningitis due to pneumococcus, *Hemophilus*, some meningococci, and *Cryptococcus.*

Positive **skin tests** are useful for some infections, especially tuberculosis, but control skin tests must always be performed to be sure that a negative reaction does not mean anergy. Skin tests should not be performed for systemic fungal infections such as histoplasmosis, blastomycosis, and coccidiodomycosis, since they make later antibody titers uninterpretable. **Humoral antibody** responses are frequently useful, but convalescent sera must be compared after an interval of 2 to 4 weeks, and thus these tests are not usually valuable in diagnosing acute disease; a fourfold rise (or fall) in antibody titer is necessary for evidence of a recent infection. Early antibodies are usually of the IgM type; later, IgG predominates.

The histology of infected tissue obtained by biopsy can point to the most likely pathogen. For example, abundant infiltration with polymorphonuclear neutrophils suggests bacterial infection, whereas a lymphocytic infiltrate suggests a chronic process, more compatible with a viral, fungal, or other nonbacterial infection. Eosinophilia points to a parasitic process, whereas a granuloma points to mycobacterial or fungal disease. The histology can be specific in some infections, including syphilis, cat-scratch fever, toxoplasmosis, lymphogranuloma venereum, and some viral diseases.

Positive cultures of an organism from a site that is usually sterile is evidence for infection, but failure to culture an organism is not conclusive. The special media needed, anaerobic conditions, previous incomplete antibiotic therapy, failure to take adequate precautions to preserve delicate specimens, the fastidious nature of some organisms, and obligate intracellular parasitism are among the reasons for negative cultures. In general, the expense of viral cultures and the lack of available therapy make culture for such infections impractical, but antibody studies are worthwhile.

If difficulty in culturing an organism is expected, it is wise to notify the lab beforehand and take proper precautions as soon as the specimen is obtained. Anaerobes must be specially handled, usually in containers that are immediately capped or using special medium; it is not worth culturing sputum for anaerobes if obtained by expectoration, since so many anaerobes are found in the mouth; transtracheal or percutaneous lung aspiration is needed.

IMPORTANT CLINICAL POINTS ABOUT GROUPS OF MICROORGANISMS

Several groups of organisms are obligate intracellular parasites and thus cannot be cultured in cell-free systems; these include viruses, *Chlamydia,* and *Rickettsia*.

Mycoplasmas are free living, can be cultured, but have no cell walls and thus are resistant to agents such as penicillin that affect cell wall synthesis.

Chlamydiae, mycoplasmas, and **rickettsiae** are susceptible to tetracycline; rickettsiae are also susceptible to chloramphenicol, and mycoplasmas to erythromycin.

Gram-positive cocci include streptococci and staphylococci. Group A **streptococci** produce skin and pharyngeal infections, are beta-hemolytic, and are associated with immunologically mediated poststreptococcal diseases such as glomerulonephritis and rheumatic fever. Group D streptococci include the **enterococci,** which are resistant to penicillin. *Streptococci pneumoniae* are alpha-hemolytic (incomplete hemolysis turning the blood agar green) and are especially important as causes of bacterial pneumonia, meningitis, and otitis media. *Streptococcus viridans,* also alpha-hemolytic or gamma-hemolytic (nonhemolytic), comprises common oral and gut flora and is an important cause of bacterial endocarditis, abscesses, and dental infections. **Staphylococci** can infect any organ system, commonly causing sepsis. They are particularly common causes of infections among diabetics, patients on chronic hemodialysis, and intravenous (IV) drug abusers. They colonize the nose and are a frequent cause of hospital-acquired (nosocomial) infections. Most pathogenic staphylococci produce coagulase; one coagulase-negative species can cause urinary tract infection (*Staphylococcus saprophyticus*), and another (*Staphylococcus epidermidis*) is part of the normal skin flora but can produce endocarditis and can infect IV catheters. Positive blood cultures with *S. epidermidis* can be due to contamination or actual infection.

Anaerobic bacteria are mostly commensals that inhabit the skin, gut, and mucosal surfaces but produce infection when introduced into other sites, such as by aspiration into the bronchial tree, by bowel perforation into the peritoneal cavity, or by introduction into tissue with low oxygen tension (PO_2) because of impaired vascularity (such as foot infections in diabetics and perianal pressure sores). They are common around the teeth, where they can produce necrotizing gingivitis, and extend into the jaw to cause osteomyelitis; they also contaminate bite wounds. Anaerobes often cause a foul odor and gas formation in tissues; they should be suspected when Gram stains show abundant gram-positive and negative flora but no growth on ordinary culture. Most anaerobes are sensitive to penicillin. Exceptions include *Bacteroides fragilis,* which is sensitive to metronidazole, clindamycin, and chloramphenicol; and *Clostridium difficile,* a common abdominal pathogen, which is sensitive to metronidazole and vancomycin.

Gram-negative bacteria produce a lipopolysaccharide toxin (endotoxin) that is a potent releaser of endogenous pyrogen (interleukin-1) from monocytes; thus fever is a prominent manifestation, and septic (endotoxin) shock is a common, serious complication. They are important causes of cystitis, pyelonephritis, and sepsis from the urinary tract. One, *Hemophilus influenzae,* is a common cause of community-acquired pneumonia, but the others usually cause nosocomial pneumonias. They rarely cause endocarditis, except for *Pseudomonas* in IV drug abusers. *Salmonella,* which usually causes enteritis, can infect atheromatous plaques or aneurysms. *Proteus* species, which split urea, are associated with staghorn calculi in the kidneys.

Aerobic **gram-positive rods** uncommonly produce infections but are potential pathogens. Diphtheria is now rare, but *Corynebacterium* can infect heart valves and shunts and immunocompromised hosts; *Listeria monocytogenes* causes meningitis, especially in immunocompromised hosts. *Bacillus cereus* causes food poisoning.

Fungi of importance include *Candida,* oval yeasts found in healthy people in the mouth, GI tract, and vagina; it can cause vaginitis and ascending urinary tract infections, especially when there is an indwelling catheter. These organisms also produce **thrush** (candidal stomatitis) in people receiving antibiotics and those with depressed cell-mediated immunity, such as occurs with corticosteroids. *Histoplasma capsulatum* occurs primarily in the main river valleys in the central United States and produces a mild fever with self-limited pneumonia rarely, it causes disseminated disease. *Coccidioides immitis* also produces a mild, self-limited disease in most affected individuals; it occurs primarily in the Southwest, especially in the central valley of California. Erythema nodosum is common early in the course of coccidioides infections; fatal dissemination can occur. *Cryptococcus neoformans* can produce a chronic pneumonia or a chronic meningitis, more frequent in patients on corticosteroid therapy. *Blastomyces dermatitidis* occurs mainly in the mountainous area of the Southeast (e.g., eastern Tennessee and western North Carolina) as well as in river valleys of the central United States and causes chronic, indolent skin lesions, occasionally bone infections or a chronic pneumonia resembling tuberculosis. *Aspergillus* produces an allergic bronchitis due to IgE-mediated allergy following colonization of the respiratory tract, especially in patients with underlying chronic bronchial disease. It can colonize a preexisting cavity and produce a large fungus ball, which can result in severe hemoptysis; it can also cause disseminated infection in a debilitated or immunocompromised host.

FEVER AND FEBRILE STATES

Fever usually is the result of inflammation, as a response to infection or an immunologic reaction. It can occur with certain malignancies, especially lymphoma, renal and hepatic carcinomas, and in hypermetabolic states such as thyrotoxicosis. Fever is usually the result of release of endogenous pyrogen (a component of interleukin-1) from macrophages, acting on the hypothalamus, which alters the temperature-regulating center by means of prostaglandin production. Fever should be controlled, especially if very high, in children susceptible to seizures when febrile, in patients with myocardial disease, and in elderly or frail persons. Inhibitors of prostaglandin synthesis, such as salicylates or acetaminophen, are effective, but aspirin should be avoided in children because of its association with Reye's syndrome.

Hyperthermia, which can be fatal, occurs in heatstroke, in susceptible patients after anesthesia (malignant hyperthermia), as an effect of phenothiazines (neuroleptic hyperthermia), and occasionally with CNS disease. Lower than normal body temperature occurs in uremia, diabetic ketoacidosis, and sometimes in the elderly; a "normal" temperature in such a patient may indicate the presence of infection. Drug fever can occur at any time after institution of therapy but typically begins after 7 to 10 days.

APPROACHES TO THE DIAGNOSIS OF INFECTIONS

Several general principles are useful in the diagnostic approach to patients suspected of having an infectious disease. For example, the apparent site or type of infection triggers immediate diagnostic hypotheses regarding the causative agent. Workup is then planned with those possibilities in mind, and, if necessary, appropriate treatment is begun even if no certain cause can be identified, pending return of laboratory results. This approach is called **the syndromic approach to infections** (Table 1-1).

General aspects of the workup of suspected infection. Special attention should be given in the **history** to such factors as association with school-age children, travel to areas where certain infections are endemic (see section on travel), occupational exposures, intake of foods known to harbor infectious agents (e.g., undercooked shellfish with hepatitis virus or unpasteurized milk for brucellosis), exposure to wild or

Table 1-1. The Syndromic Approach to Infections

Under each type of infection: 1. lists the most important common causative agent, 2. lists relatively common agents, and 3. lists agents that are unusual but important under certain circumstances (noted in parentheses).

Infections of skin and subcutaneous tissues
1. *Staphylococcus aureus*
2. *Streptococcus pyogenes, Candida,* superficial fungi
3. Gram-negative bacteria (esp. with burn wounds)

Paranasal sinus infections
1. *Streptococcus pneumoniae, S. aureus*
2. *S. pyogenes, Hemophilus influenzae*
3. Mucorales (esp. in diabetics)

Pharyngitis
1. *S. pyogenes,* respiratory viruses
2. Gonococcus

Epiglottitis
1. *H. influenzae*

Otitis, mastoiditis
1. *S. pneumoniae, H. influenzae* (esp. in children)
2. *S. aureus, S. pyogenes, Pseudomonas, Proteus*

Pneumonia
1. *S. pneumoniae, Mycoplasma pneumoniae, Mycobacterium tuberculosis*
2. *S. aureus, Klebsiella-Enterobacter, Legionella pneumophila,* respiratory viruses, *S. pyogenes,* gram-negative bacilli, *H. influenzae, Chlamydia psittaci* (psittacosis), systemic fungi
3. *Pneumocystis* (esp. with immunodeficiency)

Lung abscess and empyema
1. *S. aureus,* anaerobic streptococci, *Bacteroides, Fusobacterium, Klebsiella*

Bacterial endocarditis
1. *Streptococcus viridans, S. aureus,* enterococci

2. *S. pneumoniae,* anaerobic streptococci, *Pseudomonas, Candida, Staphylococcus epidermidis, Listeria monocytogenes*

Gastroenteritis
1. *Salmonella, Shigella, Campylobacter jejuni, Escherichia coli,* enteroviruses
2. *Entamoeba histolytica, S. aureus, Giardia, Clostridium*
3. *Vibrio cholerae* (in areas of prevalence)

Peritonitis, cholangitis, intra-abdominal abscess
1. *E. coli, Bacteroides,* enterococcus, anaerobic streptococci, *Fusobacterium*
2. *Klebsiella, Enterobacter, Proteus* species, *Clostridium, S. aureus*

Urethritis
1. Gonoccoccus, *Chlamydia*
2. *Mycoplasma, Treponema pallidum*

Urinary tract infection (e.g., cystitis, pyelonephritis)
1. *E. coli, Klebsiella-Enterobacter, Proteus,* paracolon, enterococcus
2. *Pseudomonas, S. aureus, Staphylococcus saprophyticus*

Pelvic inflammatory disease
1. Gonococcus, *E. coli, Bacteroides, Chlamydia,* anaerobic streptococci
2. *Klebsiella-Enterobacter,* enterococcus, *Fusobacterium*

Osteomyelitis
1. *S. aureus*
2. *Salmonella, S. pyogenes*

Arthritis
1. *S. aureus,* gonococcus, *S. pneumoniae, H. influenzae*
2. *S. pyogenes, Neisseria meningitidis*

Meningitis
1. *S. pneumoniae, H. influenzae, N. meningitidis*
2. *E. coli, Klebsiella-Enterobacter, Proteus, Pseudomonas, S. pyogenes, M. tuberculosis,* enterococcus, *S. aureus, L. monocytogenes*

domestic animals (cats for toxoplasmosis, birds for psittacosis), ticks (Lyme disease, Rocky Mountain spotted fever), alcohol abuse (which can cause hepatic necrosis with fever), and use of illicit drugs, especially intravenously (septic phlebitis, endocarditis).

On the physical exam, certain findings provide diagnostic clues: (1) Conjunctival suffusion is often a clue to viral infection. (2) Fundi can show tubercles or embolic lesions of bacterial endocarditis. (3) Pharyngitis occurs with local bacterial infection or viral disease such as infectious mononucleosis, in which case palatal petechiae may be present. (4) Local lymph node enlargement may occur in an area draining an infection or generalized enlargement with viral infections such as infectious mononucleosis, cytomegalovirus (CMV), or acquired immuunodeficiency syndrome (AIDS) complex. (5) Splenomegaly accompanies many infections, especially subacute bacterial endocarditis (SBE). (6) Skin rashes occur with many

infections (see below). (A general principle to remember is that uncommon presentations of common illnesses are more frequent than typical presentations of rare diseases.)

Fever of unknown origin (FUO) is defined as an undiagnosed febrile state lasting more than 3 weeks. Repeating a detailed history and physical exam is often helpful. Repeat blood cultures, cultures of any suspicious lesions, and biopsies of lesions with examination of stained smears as well as cultures are all worth doing. Bone marrow biopsy may reveal granulomas or malignancy. Often liver biopsy should be considered but is rarely informative in the absence of a clue to disease in that organ, such as enlargement, elevated alkaline phosphatase or gamma-glutamyl transpeptidase (GGT), or defects on liver scan. Exploratory laparotomy is rarely useful without localizing signs in the abdomen, usually revealed by CT scans, which are clearly indicated first. Pyuria with sterile cultures can be a clue to renal tuberculosis.

Blood cultures can be negative in patients with sepsis because of previous administration of antibiotics or difficulty in culturing some organisms. Severe local infections with mixtures of anaerobes and aerobes usually are not associated with positive blood cultures.

The most common intra-abdominal infections that present as FUOs today are peridiverticular abscesses. Other sites to check, especially by CT scan, include pericecal abscess from a ruptured retrocecal appendix and subdiaphragmatic and perisplenic abscesses. Infection in the biliary tract and pelvic abscesses are also relatively common. Abdominal distension with decreased bowel sounds due to ileus is a common (but not specific) finding in patients with intra-abdominal infection.

The most frequent causes of FUO have been infections in about one-third, neoplasms in one-third, and a variety of diseases (connective tissue disease, granulomas, factitious, other) in one-third. The major malignancies to suspect are lymphoma and leukemia; renal and hepatic carcinoma can also cause FUO. The major connective tissue diseases to suspect are giant cell arteritis (older patient, very high erythrocyte sedimentation rate [ESR] if done by the Westergren method), rheumatoid arthritis with febrile onset (Still's disease), which is typical in childhood but can also appear in an adult before evidence of the arthritis, and systemic vasculitis.

SEPSIS AND SHOCK DUE TO BACTERIAL INFECTION

A considerable increase in the frequency of sepsis due to gram-negative rods has occurred with extensive antibiotic use. Frequent predisposing factors include medical instrumentation such as indwelling urinary or IV catheters or arterial lines following invasive procedures or surgery on the urinary tract or abdomen, diabetes mellitus, liver disease, uremia and hemodialysis, advanced malignancies of any site, splenectomy, immunodeficiencies (especially the hypogammaglobulinemias), neutropenia, underlying lymphomas or leukemia, or the use of illicit IV drugs. A sudden deterioration in the status of a patient with one of these predisposing factors should lead to rapid action, since gram-negative bacteremia can progress very quickly.

Bacterial toxins are responsible for the dramatic clinical states in gram-negative sepsis. Shaking chills are common at onset, often with nausea, vomiting and diarrhea, apprehension, lethargy, and obtundation. Hyperventilation is common. The patient may be hypotensive and in "warm shock" (i.e., flushed, dry, and warm to touch) or "cold shock" (clammy, cold skin). Acidosis, a bleeding diathesis due to intravascular consumptive coagulopathy, jaundice, congestive heart failure (CHF), and oliguria may develop. Vesicular, petechial, or necrotic skin lesions may appear; aspiration or biopsy of a skin lesion may reveal the infecting organism. The white blood cell (WBC) count is usually elevated, with a marked increase in band forms ("left shift") and toxic granulations, decreased platelet count and prolonged prothrombin time (PT) and partial thromboplastin time (PTT), and elevated bilirubin and blood urea nitrogen (BUN). Blood cultures are often positive, but Gram stain of the buffy coat may give a faster clue to the nature of the infecting organism.

Skin lesions are often clues to the nature of the infecting organism. Ecythyma gangrenosum, a rounded lesion 1 to 5 cm in diameter, begins with a central vesicle that becomes a necrotic ulcer surrounded by an indurated, erythematous base. It is typical of gram-negative sepsis, especially in a patient with neutropenia. It results from infection of walls of small blood vessels. *Pseudomonas, Aeromonas,* and *Serratia* are the most common causes of these skin lesions.

Treatment consists of removing foci of entry of organisms, appropriate antibiotics, intubation, ventilatory assistance, and hemodynamic stabilization, often requiring a Swan-Ganz catheter since there may be a narrow margin between hypovolemia and fluid overload. Dopamine may be needed as a pressor agent. It is preferable since it tends to increase cerebral, renal, and mesenteric perfusion. Nitroprusside may be needed for afterload reduction. Corticosteroids are controversial but may be valuable to affect neutrophil aggregation and endothelial damage, which contributes to the syndrome. Antibiotic choice usually includes an aminoglycoside plus a penicillinase-resistant penicillin if associated *Staphylococcus* sepsis is suspected, such as in a neutropenic patient when the source is uncertain. If the source is thought to be intra-abdominal, clindamycin or metronidazole should be added to cover anaerobes (e.g., *B. fragilis*). Mortality rates remain high despite all these measures, so prevention and early institution of therapy are most important.

CLUES TO THE DIAGNOSIS OF INFECTIONS WITHOUT AN OBVIOUS PRIMARY SITE

Bacterial infections

The presence of a shunt for hemodialysis or IV access catheter, chronic skin lesions, or IV drug use suggests *S. aureus*. *L. monocytogenes* is encountered primarily in patients with decreased cell-mediated immunity; half the patients develop meningitis.

Enteric infections. *Salmonella typhi* and other salmonellae are acquired by ingestion of food contaminated from human (typhoid) or animal (paratyphoid) sources. Infection requires ingestion of relatively large numbers of organisms. Predisposing risk factors include achlorhydria, malnutrition, underlying malignancy (especially lymphomas, leukemia), sickle cell anemia (salmonella osteomyelitis is a frequent complication), and other defects in host defense mechanisms. The clinical syndrome of typhoid fever begins about 2 weeks after ingestion of the contaminated food or water, with chills, fever, headache, myalgias, and sometimes a change in bowel function (either constipation or diarrhea may occur). Evanescent red macules (rose spots) may appear on the abdomen. The typhoid bacillus penetrates the gut wall, enters intestinal and mesenteric lymphatics, where it can produce ulcerative intestinal lesions in Peyer's patches, and multiplies in macrophages, which produce endogenous pyrogen (interleukin-1). Fever without localizing symptoms is therefore a common phenomenon. Bacteremic spread to other components of the reticuloendothelial system (spleen, liver, bone marrow) is common, and further spread can lead to localization in tumors, aneurysms, bone, and gallbladder (especially in the presence of stones). The disease may resolve, or complications such as bowel perforation or a septic focus may develop. The organisms can be isolated from the blood, stool, or urine, and bone marrow cultures are often positive. Treatment is primarily with chloramphenicol; resistant strains can be treated with ampicillin or trimethoprim-sulfamethoxazole. To avoid bone marrow suppression, ampicillin is preferable for patients with sickle cell anemia.

Fever following exposure to animals

Q fever. *Coxiella burnetii* infects farm animals and then humans by aerosolization from contaminated dusty farm materials or by contact with the placenta or amniotic fluid during delivery of a calf or lamb. There are also wild animal sources. The disease begins explosively and is characterized by severe retrobulbar headache, chills, high fever, myalgias, usually mild pneumonia, and hepatitis. Endocarditis may develop. Hepatomegaly and thrombocytopenia in a patient with the syndrome of culture-negative endocarditis suggest Q fever. Diagnosis requires a fourfold rise in titer of specific complement-fixing antibodies. Treatment is with tetracycline for 2 weeks.

Diagnosis can be confirmed by isolating virus from secretions, such as urine or semen, or by conversion of serology from negative to positive (indirect fluorescent antibody or complement fixation). Viral isolation alone is not conclusive evidence establishing the presence of active infection, especially in male homosexuals.

Toxoplasmosis is usually acquired by ingestion of food (especially meat) containing oocysts, usually acquired by contamination with cat feces. In the United States, about 50% of the population has antibodies. Most infections are asymptomatic, but an infectious mononucleosis-like picture can occur. Maculopapular skin rash, abdominal pain due to mesenteric and retroperitoneal adenitis, and chorioretinitis also occur. Lymph node enlargement may be striking, suggesting lymphoma and requiring biopsy. The pathological examination of a node infected with *Toxoplasma* reveals reactive follicular hyperplasia, with areas of necrosis and sinusoids congested with clusters of macrophages. Acute infection is suggested by conversion of antibody titer to positive or a fourfold increase in titer; usually the IgM titer is >1:1000. Generally, no treatment is needed, except when chorioretinitis develops. In these instances, pyrimethamine plus sulfadiazine may be useful.

CLUES TO THE NATURE OF INFECTION BASED ON IMPAIRED HOST DEFENSES

Often the nature of the infecting organism can be inferred from the nature of the defect in host defense mechanisms.

1. **Abnormal defense of the respiratory tract** predisposes to certain types of infections. The mucociliary blanket of the respiratory tract traps and removes organisms from the lungs; failure of normal movement of the mucociliary blanket (such as occurs with splinting, atelectasis, loss of respiratory muscle function) results in infection with gram-positive and gram-negative bacteria. Infection with anaerobes as well occurs after aspiration of oral flora, most often when there is loss of cough reflex, anesthesia, deep coma or alcoholic stupor or with nervous system disease affecting nasopharyngeal muscles.

2. **Deficiency of secretion of IgA** into tears, saliva, and nasal, bronchial, GI, and GU secretions can predispose to certain infections. IgA contains antibody to specific organisms; the antibody coats them, causing opsoninization, and also affects the ability of organisms to attach to epithelial surfaces and thus to colonize. Abnormal secretory IgA occurs in congenital deficiency and malnutrition; infections with **viruses and bacteria** result, in both the gut and respiratory tract.

3. **Abnormal pulmonary alveolar macrophage phagocytic function**, such as occurs as a result of viral infections or immunosuppressive agents, results in infection with *P. carinii*, *Legionella*, and mycobacteria.

4. **Neutropenia** impairs phagocytosis and inflammatory response; typical infections are with gram-negative bacilli, *S. aureus, Aspergillus, Mucor,* and fungi.

5. **Deficient antibody production by B cells**, which usually require help from T cells, can also predispose to certain infections. The first antibody produced is IgM, followed by IgG, which has greater affinity and usually appears in higher titers. Both IgM and IgG fix complement, which aids in neutralization of infectivity of viruses and can lyse bacteria. Products of complement activation are chemotactic (including C3a, C5a, C567), attracting phagocytic cells and also contributing to the generation of the inflammatory response. Phagocytic cells, including macrophages, neutrophils, and some lymphocytes, have receptors for the Fc fragment of IgG, accounting for the opsonin effect of antibody, facilitating phagocytosis of bacteria. The most frequent infecting organisms seen with the lack of humoral antibody such as occurs in congenital or acquired hypogammaglobulinemia are *S. pneumoniae* and *H. influenzae*.

6. **Complement deficiency**, usually genetic, impairs opsonin effect and phagocytosis. Infections are encountered with all pyogenic bacteria.

7. **Cell-mediated immune responses** are dependent on phagocytic mononuclear cells and T cells and include participation of lymphokines and mediators such as gamma-interferon; this phenomenon includes the differentiation of cytotoxic T cells, which participate in resistance to viral infection. Impaired cellular immunity, such as occurs with immunosuppressive agents, AIDS, and Hodgkin's disease, results in impaired activation of pulmonary macrophages. Infections associated with depressed cell-mediated immune responses include those with herpesviruses, (including varicella-zoster and CMV), various mycobacteria, *P. carinii, Cryptococcus, Nocardia,* and *Legionella*.

8. **Normal flora** produce substances (bacteriocins) toxic to other bacteria. Alterations in this flora can result from antibiotic treatment, leading to infections especially in the gut, where the anaerobe *C. difficile* can grow out, producing necrotizing enterocolitis.

A few additional factors affecting pathogenicity of microorganisms are worth keeping in mind:

The type-specific polysaccharide capsule of *S. pneumoniae* helps defend the organism against phagocytosis; antibodies to capsular polysaccharide diminish the defense of these microorganisms, hence the value of the antipneumococcal vaccine. The organism itself activates complement by the alternative pathway, and bacterial oligopeptides are chemotactic for neutrophils. Antibody is very important in resistance to infection with pneumococci. The "crises" that were seen on days 5 to 9 during attacks of pneumonia before the advent of antibiotics were due to the appearance of antibody. Capsular polysaccharide is also importance in the virulence of the meningococcus. These organisms produce an IgA protease that dissociates the Fc fragment from the Fab portion of the antibody molecule, impairing its function. Bacteriolysis mediated by antibody and complement is critical in host defense against meningococci. As a result, in epidemics, a high percentage of those who become colonized with *N. meningitidis* and who lack serum bactericidal antibodies develop clinical disease.

Host defenses are effective against replication of viruses within cells. When viruses spread between cells by means of intercellular bridges, they escape exposure to circulating antibodies. Destruction of virus by cytotoxic T cells is then essential. Immune mechanisms may attack and destroy cells that have developed viral surface antigens. When viruses destroy host cells and spread by extracellular means, they are exposed to antibody. Resistance to viral infections therefore includes specific IgA, IgM, and IgG antibodies, which combine with proteins in the viral coat and can interfere with penetration of viruses into cells. IgA antibody is important against poliovirus, measles, and rubella, preventing penetration of epithelial surfaces and thus forestalling infection; serum antibody prevents disease. The lack of any increased susceptibility to measles among hypogammaglobulinemic patients points to the relative unimportance of circulating antibody in defense against this organism.

Complement neutralizes some viruses, especially retroviruses, by direct or antibody-dependent changes in conformation or aggregation and also promotes lysis of infected cells expressing viral surface antigens. Opsonization of extracellular viruses facilitates phagocytosis and destruction by macrophages and neutrophils; this process is important in resistance to enteroviruses, but it aids cell penetration by other viruses resistant to destruction (e.g., arboviruses).

Antibody can limit release of propagated influenza virus particles by reacting with a viral enzyme, neuraminidase.

Cellular mechanisms are of particular importance in resistance to spread of viruses by action of cytotoxic T-lymphocytes through antibody-dependent cellular cytotoxicity (ADCC). Infected cells express viral antigens on the surface, are opsonized by IgG antibody reacting with these surface antigens, and then are lysed by killer lymphocytes, macrophages, or neutrophils, which react with the Fc fragments of the antibody by means of their Fc receptors. Interferon activates natural killer (NK) cells to lyse cells infected with virus. Interferons are a family of proteins synthesized by lymphocytes, fibroblasts, epithelial cells, and macrophages early in the course of viral infection, before antibody is formed. Interferon induces cells to synthesize proteins that selectively inhibit production of viral proteins. Gamma-interferon also has immunoregulatory effects. Tubercle bacilli resist intracellular destruction by macrophages because of their surface constituents, which inhibit phagolysosomal fusion. After cellular immunity develops, T-lymphocyte activation of macrophages assists in destruction of tubercle bacilli.

Some of the clinical states that impair cell-mediated immunity and thus compromise defense against intracellular parasites include Hodgkin's disease and other lymphomas, hairy-cell leukemia, sarcoidosis, severe malnutrition, advanced cancer, uremia, inherited disorders seen primarily in childhood, and AIDS. Treatment with corticosteroids, cytotoxic drugs, and radiotherapy may produce a similar effect. Transient impairment can occur during certain infections, such as measles, chicken pox, typhoid fever, tuberculosis, and leprosy. Measles, mumps, and rubella vaccines can also be followed by transient impairment. When the diseases are progressive, a more generalized impairment of immune responses occurs, and secondary bacterial infections with septicemia become common.

Infections in patients with impaired cell-mediated immunity include (1) viruses (varicella-zoster, herpes simplex, CMV); fungi (*Cryptococcus, Candida, Aspergillus,* and Zygomycetes, as well as the usually pathogenic fungi, *Histoplasma* and Coccidiodes); (3) certain bacteria (especially *Listeria, Nocardia, M. tuberculosis, L. pneumophila*); (4) protozoa (*P. carinii, Toxoplasma gondii, Cryptosporidium* sp.); and (5) one particular helminth, *Strongyloides stercoralis.*

Disorders of humoral immunity include common variable immunodeficiency, chronic lymphocytic leukemia, lymphosarcoma, multiple myeloma, and the paraproteinemias, as well as therapy with cytotoxic drugs. Infections that result are with pneumococci, *H. influenzae,* streptococci, and staphylococci. Later in the course of these illnesses, infections with gram-negative rods become more frequent.

In sickle cell anemia, there are multiple reasons for increased susceptibility to infection. Functional asplenia, complement depletion by red blood cell (RBC) stroma, which impairs opsoninization particularly of *Salmonella* and *Staphylococcus,* and infections with those organisms are particularly frequent. Reticuloendothelial (RE) function also is impaired because of preoccupation of RE cells with erythrophagocytosis of damaged RBCs. Antibodies to pneumococci markedly enhance susceptibility to infection with pneumococci, with a high frequency of overwhelming sepsis. This occurs in sicklers (and other aplsenic persons) but improves when antibodies appear spontaneously or as a result of vaccination.

Impaired neutrophil function, such as occurs when there is diminished chemotaxis, also results in bacterial infections. Chemotaxis is decreased with **congenital deficiencies of complement (C3 or C5)** and as an effect of corticosteroid therapy. Demargination (i.e., keeping neutrophils in the vascular tree and thus unavailable to fight infection) as well as defective cell-mediated immunity also contributes to the increased susceptibility to infection accompanying corticosteroid use. Inherited defects in neutrophil function, such as the lack of the killing effect of an oxidative burst in chronic granulomatous disease, also occur. In Chédiak-Higashi disease, there are multiple defects of neutrophil function.

Acquired immunodeficiency syndrome

Infection with the retrovirus known as human immunodeficiency virus (HIV) has become an extremely serious, widespread epidemic. The groups most commonly affected in the United States are male homosexuals, prostitutes of both sexes, IV drug users, hemophiliacs, Haitians, and children of IV drug users. The virus is transmitted by semen during homosexual and heterosexual acts and can also be transmitted from female to male during coitus. The larger the number of sexual partners, the greater the likelihood of infection. It is also transmitted by transfusion of whole blood or component blood products, including Factor VIII and cryoprecipitate, which are given to hemophiliacs. Contaminated needles shared by IV drug users are a major means of transmission, and infants born to mothers who are infected with HIV develop the disease.

The incubation period and attack rates are uncertain. Most cases develop between 1 and 5 years after acquiring the virus, often after a coincidental viral infection that seems to activate HIV, ending a period of latency. Antibody to HIV develops about a month after initial infection and persists during the latent period. It is also present during active infection and is useful as a diagnostic test and a means of screening donated blood. A negative antibody test does not rule out infection, however, since a recently acquired infection can make donated blood infectious before the antibody develops. Many individuals with positive antibody tests seem to be carriers of the virus for long periods without developing the disease; this is especially true of hemophiliacs. Although the virus is present in all body fluids, including saliva and tears, it is very labile, is easily killed by drying or temperature changes, and can be transmitted only inside of cells. There is no evidence that the disease can be transmitted by casual contact, even among household intimates who are not sexual partners. Sexual activity (both heterosexual and male homosexual) and blood products are the only known means of transmission at present.

The virus infects human T-lymphocytes, specifically T-helper cells. Infected patients show a striking decrease in T-helper cells. Clinically, there is diminished skin reactivity to antigens (anergy), decreased ability of T cells to proliferate in vitro in response to stimuli, absence of ability of these cells to kill virus-infected cells and tumor cells in vitro, and lack of ability to produce interleukin-2 and gamma-interferon. Secondarily, B-lymphocyte function becomes abnormal, further impairing resistance to infection, often with an associated polyclonal hyperglobulinemia. Generalized lymph node enlargement is often seen in asymptomatic individuals known to harbor the virus. Episodes of fever, night sweats, weight loss, and diarrhea develop, lasting weeks to months before the first opportunistic infection develops. This phase is sometimes referred to as AIDS-related complex (ARC). When the first opportunistic infection develops, the diagnosis of AIDS is warranted. The infections noted in these patients include **mucocutaneous candidiasis** (such as thrush, which can be treated with clotrimazole troches), or esophageal candidiasis, which requires treatment with ketoconazole or amphotericin B. Chronic oral or perianal **herpes simplex** is frequent, and diagnosis can be made by Wright's stain of a smear or a viral culture; acyclovir therapy is helpful. A very malignant form of **Kaposi's sarcoma** is a common occurrence, at least in homosexual males with known CMV infection). These lesions may appear on the skin, buccal or intestinal mucosa, or in enlarged lymph nodes.

Meningeal infections are common, including cryptococcosis, often associated with crytococcal sepsis; treatment requires amphotericin B. **Toxoplasmosis** of the CNS is also common, presenting as single or multiple brain abscesses. Since serological tests are unreliable, brain biopsy may be necessary; pyrimethamine and sulfadiazine are the recommended treatments. Progressive **dementia** is seen in AIDS patients, perhaps because of the effect of the virus on brain cells or a **progressive multifocal leukoencephalopathy,** a demyelinating disease apparently due to papovavirus. There is no known treatment. Primary lymphoma of the brain is increased in frequency among AIDS patients. Blindness due to chorioretinitis is common, but the cause is not clear; some cases are due to CMV.

P. carinii pneumonia is the most common opportunistic infection in AIDS, usually presenting as gradually increasing nonproductive cough and dyspnea. Arterial hypoxemia is commonly present, and x-ray reveals patchy, widespread, multifocal, mixed alveolar and interstitial infiltrates, in contrast to bacterial infections, which are usually focal. Diagnosis is made by bronchial lavage or transbronchial biopsy. Treatment can be attempted with high doses of trimethoprim-sulfamethoxazole, but side effects, including marrow depression, are frequent; pentamidine is also effective.

Watery diarrhea is a frequent occurrence, and unusual pathogens may be found, including *Cryptosporidium* and CMV; disseminated CMV infection is common, and sepsis from *Mycobacterium avium-intracellulare* is usual; this organism responds very poorly to currently available antituberculous agents. Other infections such as listeriosis, aspergillosis, and nocardiosis, encountered among other types of patients with cell-mediated immune deficiency states, are uncommon among AIDS patients.

The diagnosis of AIDS is based on the clinical syndrome, including membership in one of the high-risk groups, lymphocytopenia with a low ratio of T-helper to T-suppressor cells and anergy to skin test antigens (mumps, candida, etc.), a positive antibody test for HIV, and a typical opportunistic infection with one of the organisms mentioned above, in the absence of any other reasons for impaired immune response. Other convincing evidence is the presence of Kaposi's sarcoma or a CNS lymphoma. Virus detection by culture is possible. The ELISA screening test for antibody has a significant false-positive rate (about 1%); confirmation can be obtained with immunoblotting (Western blot test). The antibody is not protective, as shown by the fact that the virus can be cultured from about 70% of antibody-positive individuals.

Therapy is still experimental but includes treatment of opportunistic infections. Inhibitors of viral reverse transcriptase offer the most hope; other antiviral agents are being studied as well. Immune reconstitution may be helpful in some instances. A vaccine may eventually be developed. Azothymidine (AZT) is of some value in preventing progression of the disease but does not kill the virus, and blood levels must be constantly maintained by dosing every 4 hours.

Prevention of the spread of AIDS is primarily based on (1) screening all blood to be used for transfusion and (2) "safe" sexual practices, both heterosexual and male homosexual. (This primarily means use of condoms.) Isolation precautions with hospitalized known-positive patients involve precautions with blood specimens and equipment plus protection against spread by body secretions, although spread by saliva, tears, etc. has not been established.

CLUES TO THE NATURE OF INFECTION BASED ON TRAVEL HISTORY

A key aspect of the history of any suspected infection is the history of travel, as well as exposure to animals, insect bites, etc. Persons who have traveled are still liable to get the usual illnesses seen in their home community, but the differential diagnosis is heavily influenced by the places visited. Many of the infections likely to be acquired during travel are epizootic in animal reservoirs and transmitted to humans directly or by an insect vector. The diseases suggested by travel are listed below; most are described elsewhere in this section.

Northeast. **Babesiosis** is a malaria-like infection that occurs primarily on Nantucket, Martha's Vineyard, and Long Island. It is tick transitted and has an incubation period of 7 to 14 days. Asplenic patients are more susceptible and have more severe disease. Onset is usually insidious, with fever, rigors, malaise, and myalgias. Hepatosplenomegaly usually develops, with hemolytic anemia, leukopenia, and elevated liver enzymes. Blood smears for malaria reveal the organisms.

Lyme disease occurs in New England, especially in Connecticut, where it was first discovered in this country. It is spreading widely and is common on the islands off Cape Cod, on Long Island, in Wisconsin and Minnesota, as well as on the West Coast (described elsewhere.)

Pneumonic tularemia occurs primarily on Martha's Vineyard. Pneumonia is accompanied by splenomegaly and severe prostration. Rabbits are the main reservoir, with transmission via air but sometimes by the bite of an infected tick, which usually gives a local skin lesion and adenopathy (**ulceroglandula fever**; if near the eye, **oculoglandular fever**.) Diagnosis is aided by finding gram-negative rods on smear obtained from a skin lesion or node aspirate.

Rocky Mountain spotted fever (RMSF) occurs mostly in Appalachian Mountain states. It is transmitted by a tick bite, but most patients do not remember the bite. Clues to the diagnosis include leukopenia, thrombocytopenia, severe illness with disseminated intravascular coagulopathy (DIC), rash occurring on palms and soles, and severe headache. (Other rickettsial diseases such as Q fever and psittacosis do not produce a rash but do produce headache.)

Paralytic shellfish poisoning begins with paresthesias of the mouth, lips, and face. It may progress rapidly to muscle paralysis, including respiratory failure. Shellfish ingest dinoflagellates, which produce a toxin (saxitoxin) that accumulates in their tissues; it is not degraded by gastric juice.

Giardiasis is increasing in frequency because of an increase in the beaver population. The disease is widespread, especially in the Northeast but also in Rocky Mountain states. Ski resort areas are particularly affected. Outbreaks have been reported in Aspen, Colorado, and in European cities such as Leningrad. (The disease process is described under causes of diarrhea, in the section on the GI tract. It is often asymptomatic but can cause abdominal cramps and diarrhea. The main clue is a taste of rotten eggs in the mouth.)

Middle Atlantic and southeastern states. RMSF, tularemia, and histoplasmosis are the main location-specific diseases to consider. (The main manifestation of histoplasmosis is an atypical pneumonia with splenomegaly.)

Naglerial meningoencephalitis is caused by free-living amoebas that are found in stagnant fresh water. The infection is usually acquired during swimming. The organisms penetrate the cribriform plate of the ethmoid nasal sinuses and pass directly into the CNS. A severe neurological defect occurs with CSF pleocytosis; wet prep of CSF and brain biopsy establish the diagnosis, but there is no effective therapy. (This disease is not limited to this geographic area but is widespread.)

South central and Gulf coast. **Typhus** occurs especially in Texas and Arkansas, in areas of production and storage of grain, where the disease is associated with rats and their fleas. Typical manifestations include fever, leukopenia, a truncal rash, and headache— a syndrome resembling RMSF, a similar rickettsial disease. **Blastomycosis** occurs especially in Louisiana and Alabama but also in Minnesota, Wisconsin, and the area around the Great Smoky Mountains in the Southeast (western North Carolina and eastern Tennessee.) The disease is epidemic in dogs, especially beagles, which often transmit it to humans. Presentation is much like pulmonary tuberculosis, but there usually are associated mucous membrane ulcerations in the upper respiratory tract. Systemic dissemination with bone and CNS lesions can occur. One form of the disease is limited to an indolent, chronic skin ulcer. A reservoir for **leprosy** occurs in armadillos, especially in Louisiana.

Southwest. **Plague** occurs especially in New Mexico; it is endemic in prairie dog colonies. The disease may be pneumonic or bubonic (i.e., ulceroglandular, similar to tularemia.) **Coccidioidomycosis** occurs in desert areas, primarily as a pulmonary or meningeal disease. The frequent occurrence of erythema nodosum is a diagnostic clue.

Rocky Mountain states. **Colorado tick fever** is an arbovirus infection, transmitted by a tick. It is endemic and very common after hiking in the area around Estes Park, Colorado (near Rocky Mountain National Park). It causes a saddle-back fever (4 to 5 days of high fever, with a 3- to 4-day interval), severe leukopenia (e.g., total WBC of 400), myalgias, and headache.

Q fever is a rickettsial disease caused by *C. burnetii*, an airborne pathogen. Infection usually presents as an atypical pneumonia, but an FUO is a frequent presentation. A granulomatous hepatitis can occur; there is no rash. The Weil-Felix agglutination reaction is useful in diagnosis.

Pacific northwest. **Relapsing fever** is caused by a tick-transmitted spirochete (*Borrelia recrudescens*). Recurrent episodes of fever occur, with rash, neurological signs, hepatosplenomegaly, and lymphadenopathy.

Central (midwestern) states. **Histoplasmosis, tularemia, leptospirosis,** and **Lyme disease** are the main location-specific diseases to expect.

Foreign travel. The most major diseases encountered are as follows:

1. **Malaria,** which is still endemic in many parts of the world, should be the first consideration in a traveler returning from endemic area who develops a febrile illness. The fever patterns almost never fit the classic descriptions; malaria can present with diarrhea. History of malarial prophylaxis does not rule out the disease, since many people fail to take it properly. Proper prophylactic dosage: Weekly doses of chloroquine for 2 weeks before entry into malarious zone, while there, and for 6 weeks after return. The alternate regimen is primaquine 25 mg/day for 14 days, if the patient has been in a very heavily infected zone. Be sure to screen patients for G6PD deficiency before administering these agents. Fansidar is too toxic for routine prophylaxis, but advise patients to take it along. If malaria develops despite prophylaxis, it is probably chloroquine-resistant falciparum malaria, which occurs mostly in Kenya, and Fansidar in these cases is lifesaving.

2. **Amebiasis** may present as dysentery or as liver abscess (without a history of diarrhea in 75%). It is particularly common in Mexico.
3. **Brucellosis** causes a relapsing fever with lymphadenopathy, hepatosplenomegaly, and leukopenia. The most common site of acquisition is the Middle East, and it is particularly common among workers or visitors to meat-rendering facilities.
4. **Typhoid fever** occurs anywhere, but particularly in Mexico and South America, as does shigellosis.
5. **Cutaneous leishmaniasis** occurs in Mexico and Central and South America and may be encountered in archaeologists and other field workers.

SEXUALLY TRANSMITTED INFECTIONS

Syphilis. Syphilis has increased in frequency in recent years. About 50% of sexual contacts of an infected person develop the disease. Known sexual contacts who cannot be followed with certainty for development of the disease require prophylactic treatment with penicillin.

Primary syphilis usually develops about 3 weeks after exposure, but the incubation period can vary from 10 to 90 days. Typically, a single painless papule appears and ulcerates to form a chancre, with a raised border and a smooth, indurated base. Chancres may be multiple and can appear anywhere infection has occurred; genital and oral or pharyngeal lesions are most common. Healing leaves an atrophic scar.

Secondary syphilis develops 6 to 8 weeks after the chancre appears, affecting skin, mucous membranes, and lymph nodes. A variety of skin lesions are seen, varying from generalized macular and papular lesions to pustules and nodules that are often hyperpigmented, involving the palms and soles. In moist, intertriginous areas, papules coalesce to form plaques, called condylomata, which are full of spirochetes and are particularly infectious. Mucous patches, which are painless red or grayish superficial erosions, are seen in the mouth and vagina. Many patients have a recurrence of the mucocutaneous lesions. Generalized, painless lymphadenopathy is usually present, including epitrochlear nodes. Organ involvement may occur and resolve with treatment, including an erosive gastritis, an immune complex-mediated acute nephritis, or a nephrotic syndrome.

Late or tertiary syphilis appears 1 to 10 years later in 15% of untreated infected patients. Gummas, large areas of necrosis surrounded by chronic inflammation and containing very few spirochetes, can appear almost anywhere. Skin, bone, liver, and brain are common sites. **Cardiovascular syphilis** results from obliterative endarteritis of the vasa vasorum of the aorta, particularly just above the heart, causing intimal thickening and medial necrosis. Calcification appears in the ascending aorta, and aneurysms develop. Obliteration of the coronary ostia can result, causing severe angina. Aortic valve leaflet involvement leads to aortic insufficiency and severe heart failure. **CNS syphilis** appears in 8% of untreated patients 5 to 35 years after infection, resulting in **general paresis, tabes dorsalis** (commonly with Charcot joints), or a combination of the two patterns. Meningovascular syphilis can appear earlier and cause extensive spinal cord or intracerebral functional loss. **Optic atrophy** is also a common manifestation of tertiary syphilis.

The diagnosis of syphilis is aided by finding spirochetes in dark-field examination of material from chancres or moist secondary lesions. Saprophytic spirochetes can confuse the interpretation of smears from oral lesions. Serological tests are essential. If the Venereal Disease Research Laboratories (VDRL) test is positive, titer should be determined for follow-up purposes and fluorescent treponemal antibody after absorption on nontreponemal spirochetes (FTA-ABS) done for confirmation. If the primary infection occurred more than 4 years earlier or the date is unknown, the case is classified as "late latent" and a spinal tap should be performed to check for CNS syphilis. An elevated WBC count and protein with a positive VDRL establish the diagnosis of neurosyphilis. Such a diagnosis, and appropriate treatment, are also warranted in late latent cases if the serum VDRL has become negative but a serum FTA-ABS remains positive and neurological manifestations are present.

Serology should be followed after treatment. Among cases of early syphilis, up to 5% develop a relapse or reinfection; serology usually becomes negative 6 to 12 months after treatment, and failure to convert after 2 years is an indication for retreatment. After treatment, 75% of patients with secondary syphilis become seronegative within 2 years. In any patient, if the VDRL does not become negative or achieve a low, fixed titer (i.e., become "serofast"), the CSF should be examined to check for early, asymptomatic neurosyphilis and the patient should be retreated with penicillin. Patients with late or late latent syphilis should show a decline in antibody titer after treatment, becoming negative or serofast. Every patient should be seronegative or serofast before follow-up is discontinued. If necessary, treatment should be repeated since 2 to 10% of patients with CNS syphilis will relapse after initial treatment.

Therapeutic decisions. Persons with primary, secondary, or early latent syphilis, as well as healthy contacts, should receive 2.4 million units of benzathine penicillin IM once. In the presence of penicillin allergy, tetracycline or erythromycin can be given (2 g/day for 15 days). Late latent or late syphilis should be treated with 3 weekly doses of IM benzathine pencillin. Alternative therapy is not established, but tetracycline or erythromycin for 30 days is recommended. Neurosyphilis should be treated with 10 days of aqueous pencillin G, 20 million units daily for 10 days. Since abrupt release of toxic spirochetal products can occur with treatment, causing an exacerbation of manifestations of tertiary syphilis on an immune basis (Jarisch-Herxheimer reaction), patients with neurosyphilis should be pretreated with corticosteroids.

Gonorrhea. Infection with *Neisseria gonorrhoeae* is particularly common among persons with numerous sexual contacts. The infection rate after sexual contact with an infected partner is about 20% for males and 50% for females. In women, spread to the upper genital tract is increased during menstruation and by intrauterine contraceptive devices but is decreased by oral contraceptives. Overall, about 20% of infected women suffer **pelvic inflammatory disease (PID)**.

Symptoms of urethritis, burning dysuria, and purulent discharge usually appear in men 2 to 7 days after exposure. In women, urethritis may develop, but more commonly cervicitis occurs, manifest only as a yellow vaginal discharge. PID usually begins around the time of menstruation, with endometritis causing midline abdominal pain or salpingitis causing bilateral lower abdominal pain and tenderness or signs of pelvic peritonitis. Gonococcal perihepatitis (Fitz-Hugh–Curtis syndrome) may present as right upper quadrant pain and tenderness. Anorectal gonorrhea may be asymptomatic but frequently causes rectal pain, tenderness, tenesmus, bleeding, and a mucopurulent discharge. Treatment failures are more frequent with anorectal infection, occurring in 7 to 35%. Pharyngeal gonorrhea is frequent after orogenital contact but is rarely the sole site of infection.

Dissemination of gonococcal infection occurs in about 1% of men and 3% of women. Strains of gonococci responsible are penicillin sensitive, have specific nutritional characteristics on culture, and are resistant to normal bactericidal actions of antibody and complement, perhaps because of an affinity for binding of blocking antibody. The "arthritis-dermatitis syndrome" is the most frequent manifestation of dissemination, typically causing arthralgia and several petechial or papular, vesicular, pustular, or hemorrhagic skin lesions, especially on extensor surfaces in distal parts of the extremities. Multiple asymmetric sites of tenosynovitis near the wrists and ankles are frequently associated. Aspiration of vesicular or pustular skin lesions can reveal gonococci on smear or culture, and biopsy can reveal antigens by immunofluorescent staining. Blood cultures are frequently positive. The arthritis usually affects multiple large joints, serially and in a migratory fashion, with sterile effusions. However, septic arthritis can develop, with synovial fluid showing very high neutrophil counts ($>50,000/$mm^3) and occasionally positive cultures. Rarely, disseminated gonococcemia can lead to endocarditis, meningitis, myopericarditis, or a toxic hepatitis.

Diagnosis of gonococcal infection is based on the clinical picture and smears of lesions revealing typical bean-shaped intracellular gram-negative diplococci; smears of urethral discharge in infected males are almost always positive, but smears of cervical exudate are less sensitive. Cultures should routinely be obtained from the urethra, anus, cervix, and pharynx and repeated if necessary. Modified Thayer-Martin medium, containing antibiotics to inhibit growth of other organisms, increases the frequency of positive cultures from areas likely to be contaminated. Such antibiotics are not necessary for cultures from normally sterile areas such as blood, joint fluid, or CSF. Synthetic swabs are preferable for obtaining material for culture, since cotton contains unsaturated fatty acids that can be inhibitory.

Therapeutic decisions. Recommended therapy consists of 4.8 million units of procaine penicillin IM along with 1 g of probenecid; 3 g of amoxicillin PO can be substituted for the penicillin. Tetracycline, 2 g/day PO for 7 days, may be given as well to treat any associated chlamydial infection and may be adequate therapy alone for gonococcal urethritis in males. Acute PID should be treated with procaine penicillin plus tetracycline, but associated severe toxicity requires hospitalization and a broad-spectrum, multiple antibiotic regimen. Surgery may be necessary to drain a pelvic or tubo-ovarian abscess. Disseminated gonococcal disease requires aqueous penicillin G for 3 to 5 days, followed by oral ampicillin to a total of 10 days. Tetracycline may be used for PID in individuals sensitive to penicillin, and cefazolin for disseminated gonorrhea. Cephalosporins are contraindicated if an anaphylactoid, angioedematous, or urticarial reaction suggesting IgE-mediated allergy to penicillin has occurred. Tetracycline or chloram-

phenicol should be substituted. Erythromycin therapy should be avoided, since it is associated with a high frequency of treatment failures. Because of penicillin resistance of gonococci, cultures should be repeated 7 to 14 days after therapy. Anal cultures should be repeated in females and homosexual males, since persistent anorectal carriage is a frequent cause of relapse. Relapse of urethritis in males is frequent after treatment of gonorrhea and is usually the result of infection with another organism, such as *Chlamydia trachomatis.*

A VDRL should be checked in all patients infected with gonococci because of the high incidence of associated infection with syphilis. Penicillin therapy for gonorrhea will also treat early syphilis adequately, but this is not true for the alternate drugs, and in such cases it is recommended to recheck the VDRL serially.

Nongonorrheal urethritis. **Chlamydiae** are obligate intracellular organisms that cannot synthesize ATP and thus require energy from the host cell to survive. They contain both RNA and DNA and divide by binary fission. *Chlamydia psittaci* primarily infects birds but can produce a serious pulmonary disease with systemic manifestations in humans. *C. trachomatis* produces a serious eye disease that has existed since ancient times and is still the most common cause of blindness in the world. *C. trachomatis* is also the most commonly identified cause of nongonorrheal urethritis in men (30 to 50% of cases) and can be found in association with gonorrhea. It also causes epididymitis, proctitis in homosexual males, and cervicitis and PID in females. In the United States, it is now the most frequent infectious cause of sterility. Many women with dysuria, frequency, and pyuria but sterile urine have *C. trachomatis* infection. The distinction between gonorrhea and *C. trachomatis* GU infection is primarily based on the Gram stain of urethral exudate (in males) and culture of urethral or cervical exudate on Thayer-Martin medium. Identification of *N. gonorrhoeae* does not rule out combined infection. Tetracycline is the drug of choice for chlamydial infections.

Herpes simplex virus. Of the herpes simplex viruses (HSV), HSV-2 is the usual cause of genital disease, a common infection in certain population groups. For example, prostitutes show a 70% incidence of genital herpes. Implantation of the virus causes local epithelial cell lysis producing a thin-walled vesicle; multinucleated giant cells appear, displaying characteristic intranuclear inclusions. Tender lymphadenopathy develops regionally. The virus migrates along axons of sensory nerves and becomes latent in sacral ganglion cells, reactivating periodically for unclear reasons in about 60% of patients.

Painful vesicles appear at the site of implantation, usually the penis, vulva, perineum, cervix, anus, or buttocks. Painful inguinal adenopathy, fever, and malaise may be present. A myelitis or radiculitis can occur. Anal or perianal lesions are associated with rectal tenesmus. Reactivation is more common in males, typically occurring in the same location repeatedly and usually preceded by burning or tingling for 18 to 36 hours beforehand. Fever and malaise are less frequent with reactivations.

The diagnosis can be confirmed by Tzank smear, Pap smear, or viral isolation. Serologies are useful only for a primary infection. Treatment with acyclovir shortens the duration of an episode but does not eliminate the latent virus and therefore cannot prevent recurrences. Prophylactic acyclovir decreases the frequency of recurrences. In pregnancy, because of cervical shedding of HSV near the time of delivery, cesarean section is indicated to prevent infection of the baby.

Other venereal diseases.   **Chancroid, lymphogranuloma venereum (LGV)**, and **granuloma inguinale** are much less common. They typically cause perigenital ulcerations, which may or may not be painful, usually with painful regional lymphadenopathy. In LGV, inguinal nodes can develop abscesses and sinus tracts. Diagnosis is made by examining pus from lesions for organisms (e.g., *Hemophilus ducreyi* in chancroid; Donovan bodies in vacuoles in macrophages in granuloma inguinale) or serology in LGV. Treatment with erythromycin or trimethoprim-sulfamethoxazole is effective for chancroid; tetracycline or trimethoprim-sulfmethoxazole is effective for LGV and granuloma iguinale.

Gay bowel syndrome (proctitis or proctocolitis in male homosexuals) can cause anorectal or abdominal pain, tenesmus, and a bloody or mucopurulent discharge. The distal colon infection in these individuals is most frequently caused by *N. gonorrhoeae, C. trachomatis,* and herpesvirus hominis; more proximal sigmoid colitis is most frequently caused by *Shigella, Campylobacter,* and *E. histolytica.* Other organisms that cause this syndrome include *T. pallidum, Salmonella* sp., *Cryptosporidium,* and *S. stercoralis*.

CLINICAL FEATURES OF INFECTIONS OF SPECIFIC ORGAN SYSTEMS

CNS infections

Patients with CNS infections present with fever, headache, usually stiff neck, and some change in mental state. Seizures may occur, but focal neurological changes may not be present.

Bacterial meningitis.   Bacterial infections of the CNS usually develop quickly, and fever, headache, lethargy, and any evidence of neck stiffness are indications for an immediate lumbar puncture. Focal neurological abnormalities and a change in mental status may or may not be present. On the other hand, slower development of illness over week or more, with unilateral headache and neurological findings, suggests a mass lesion. A scanning procedure should be performed before lumbar puncture to avoid the possibility of brain-stem herniation. If the patient is comatose and a distinction between these two possibilities is not possible on clinical grounds, blood and throat cultures should be obtained, antibiotics begun, and an emergency CT scan obtained before lumbar puncture is performed, even though this greatly reduces the likelihood of a positive CSF culture, especially if the organism is a pneumococcus.

Bacterial meningitis is most common in children and adolescents. Pneumococcal meningitis is most frequent and occurs at any age. Meningococcal infections are more common in young adults in closed populations such as schools and camps, in winter and spring. *H. influenzae* is more common in children but has been occurring with increasing frequency in adults.

Meningitis can be a fulminant disease, with fever, headache, lethargy, and stiff neck progressing rapidly to confusion and even coma, often with a petechial or purpuric rash, especially with meningococcal disease. This pattern has a high fatality rate, and treatment is urgent. Slower progression, developing after symptoms of an upper respiratory tract infection, is more

frequent. The CSF typically contains over 1,000 WBC, mostly neutrophils, with glucose under 40 mg/100 ml and protein over 150 mg/100 ml. Early in the course these findings may be lacking, and cell counts can be very low. A repeat lumbar puncture after a few hours may be necessary to confirm the clinical impression. If there has been prior antibiotic therapy, the CSF may contain mostly mononuclear cells; meningitis due to *L. monocytogenes* often produces mononuclear exudate. Gram stain of the fluid can reveal the nature of the infecting organism. If the interpretation of the Gram stain is indefinite, broad-spectrum antibiotics should be given. Viral and even tuberculous meningitis can show predominantly polymorphonuclear leukocytes early in the course; repeat lumbar puncture after a day or more usually shows the more typical mononuclear pleocytosis.

Cultures of CSF, blood, nasopharyngeal secretions, and fluid expressed from skin lesions should be made. If a community-acquired bacterial meningitis seems most likely, therapy should be started before the cultures have revealed the specific organism: Penicillin is followed by chloramphenicol beginning about 1 hour later. This combination will be effective against most common organisms including *H. influenzae,* but third-generation cephalosporins such as cefotaxime are also effective. Such cephalosporins are also indicated for meningitis caused by enteric gram-negative organisms, which are usually not adequately treated by chlormaphenicol.

Household and intimate contacts of patients with meningococcal disease should be treated with rifampin for 2 days, as should hospital personnel who had close contact with respiratory secretions from such patients. In a home with *H. influenzae* infection, children under age 4 should be protected from this organism by administration of rifampin to all members of the household. Workers in child care centers should be handled similarly. (Patients on oral contraceptives receiving rifampin should be warned that their urine will turn orange and that the antiestrogen effect of the drug may render the contraceptive ineffective.)

Effective vaccines are now available for prevention of meningococcal and pneumococcal disease, and one is under development for *H. influenzae.* They should be given to especially susceptible population groups, such as asplenic individuals and those with sickle cell disease.

Tuberculous meningitis can be difficult to diagnose. Onset is gradual; headache, fever, stiff neck, and mental changes, including confusion and disorientation, develop over a few days to a week. If the illness is untreated, coma usually develops within a few weeks and death occurs in 1 to 2 months. CSF cell counts are high, usually with several hundred cells, mixtures of lymphocytes and neutrophils; protein level is elevated, often very high, and glucose low. Smears for acid-fast organisms are positive in only about one-fourth of the cases, and cultures are usually positive but take too long to grow out. Therapy must be started before culture reports are available.

Viral CNS infections.   **Viral meningitis** occurs primarily in children and young adults. Many of the causative agents have a seasonal pattern of incidence. The most common causes of viral meningitis are the **enteroviruses** (including Coxsackie B and echovirus), which occur mainly in the summer or early fall; **lymphocytic choriomeningitis** (LCM), which occurs mainly in the fall or winter; **mumps**, which is mainly a winter or early spring infection; and HSV, which occurs at any time of the year. The usual presentation is headache, which is very severe; fever; and signs of meningeal irritation, which may be mild. The development of seizures, confusion, delerium, or focal neurological changes means that a meningoencephalitis is present. CSF examination should be done immediately, and a pleocytosis of 10 to 1,000 WBC is usually found, with slight elevation of protein. The cells in the CSF may be neutrophils during the first 6 to 8 hours of the illness but rapidly shift to lymphocytes. Glucose is normal but may be low in some cases. The CSF cell count becomes normal in about 2 weeks in most cases. The diagnosis is often established by concomitant findings, such as parotitis or orchitis with mumps, exposure to rodents with LCM, which also has associated severe myalgias and often a rash and orchitis. Viral cultures of the stool are positive in about half the cases; throat and CSF cultures are less frequently positive. Treatment is symptomatic, but acyclovir and vidarabine are useful for severe HSV infections, especially when associated with genital herpes.

Viral encephalitis is also caused by a wide variety of agents, most of which cause subclinical infections. Many have seasonal patterns of incidence, such as the arthropod-spread viruses. California and western equine encephalitis peak in the summer, whereas St. Louis encephalitis peaks somewhat later. Enteroviruses peak in the summer, and mumps in the winter and spring. HSV is the most frequent agent and causes the most devastating form of viral encephalitis; it occurs at any age and all seasons, with no geographic pattern. HSV presumably spreads along peripheral nerves to the CNS. Spread along branches of the trigeminal nerve probably explains the location of the most common focal necrotic CNS lesions, in the inferomedial portions of the temporal and frontal lobes. Patients with HSV encephalitis often have a prodrome of upper respiratory tract infection for a few days, then suddenly develop a severe headache, fever, and personality changes, sometimes with delirium or focal seizures. The CSF shows pleocytosis up to about 1,000 cells, moderate protein elevation (typically to 80 to 90 mg/100 ml). A few patients show decreased glucose levels. In about 5% of cases the CSF is normal. Focal abnormalities are usually seen in the EEG as well as technetium brains scans and CT scans by the third day. Viral cultures of stool, throat, buffy coat, and CSF as well as serology may be positive, but too late to influence therapy; acyclovir should be started immediately. Brain biopsies before starting therapy are no longer considered necessary. Despite acyclovir, there is a high mortality and incidence of residual neurological defects.

Rabies is a form of viral encephalitis with a 100% fatality rate. The disease follows bites of infected animals; domestic dogs and cats who acquire the disease from wild animals are the main source. Nonbite infection can occur if mucous membranes or open wounds are exposed to infected saliva. Bat urine in heavily infested caves is a possible source. The disease spreads along peripheral nerves to the brain, with an incubation period of 20 to 90 days, longer intervals found with more peripheral bites. The disease begins with fever, headache, fatigue, pain at the site of inoculation, confusion, seizures, paralysis, stiff neck, agitation, laryngospasm when drinking is attempted (hence the name "hydrophobia"), followed by paralysis, coma, and death. The hospital staff should be protected from exposure to saliva and other secretions of suspected victims. Pets that have bitten someone and are not known to have been vaccinated against rabies can be observed for 10 days, and if they stay well there is no risk of the bitten person getting rabies. Other animals should be destroyed and the brain immediately examined for inclusion bodies and fluorescent staining for rabies virus. If positive or if the animal escaped, prophylaxis is indicated with human rabies immune globulin locally in the area of the bite as well as IM, and the vaccine should be given IM 5 times over a month. Individuals known to be at high risk, such as cave explorers, should be vaccinated.

Skin infections

There are many types of superficial skin infections. **Folliculitis** is infection around hair follicles. Staphylococci are the usual pathogens; *Pseudomonas* is occasionally responsible. Disseminated candidiasis in neutropenic patients may resemble folliculitis. Subcutaneous abscesses, usually due to staphylococci, are called furuncles or carbuncles. These infections can usually be treated with hot soaks, but antistaphylococcal antibiotics should be used if there is fever or systemic symptoms. **Impetigo** is due to group A streptococcal infection, usually in children; characteristically the lesions start out as small vesicles, which become covered with a dry crust. Penicillin therapy is usually necessary. **Erysipelas** is a superficial streptococcal skin infection, usually on the face; its sharply demarcated markings differentiate it from cellulitis. Penicillin is helpful for these lesions also. **Ecthyma gangrenosum** is a vesicular lesion that develops a necrotic center; it is due to infection with *Pseudomonas* and appears in neutropenic patients.

HSV can cause lesions away from the mouth or genitals, especially on the hands of people who come into contact with the virus frequently, such as dental workers. A **herpetic whitlow** resembling a paronychia is typical, often involving multiple fingers. Gram stain of the lesions shows no bacteria, and incision and drainage should be avoided. Acyclovir is helpful.

Cellulitis usually results from some laceration or other break in the skin surface and is especially common where chronic stasis, edema, or a similar process has decreased local resistance to infection. Local fungal infection, especially between the toes, is a frequent initiating factor. Diabetes is frequently a predisposing factor. Lymphatic spread is common, indicated by streaks of erythema and tenderness plus regional lymph node enlargement. Most cases are due to beta-hemolytic streptococci, but staphylococci are often responsible. Anaerobes and gram-negative bacteria can be introduced through breaks in the skin. Therapy should consist of an antistaphylococcal penicillin. Diabetics may need therapy for anaerobes (e.g., clindamycin or metronidazole) or for gram-negative organisms (e.g., an aminoglycoside). Radiolucent bubbles in soft tissue on x-ray, indicating gas-forming anaerobes, establish the need for extensive surgical removal of necrotic tissues. Subcutaneous infection with little redness of the overlying skin indicates the presence of **fasciitis**; such patients are often much more toxic than expected from the degree of skin change, with tender subcutaneous swelling, often with gas in the tissues. Prompt debridement of all involved tissues, as well as antibiotics (determined by findings on Gram stain), is necessary for these life-threatening infections. Men with diabetes and urethral trauma or obstruction can get a similar necrotizing faciitis of the perineum, called **Fournier's gangrene**.

Osteomyelitis

Bone infections occur primarily in children and in the elderly, in long bones and vertebral bodies. They are particularly common in IV drug abusers and in patients with hemoglobinopathies, since *Salmonella* and *S. aureus* have a predilection for areas of bone infarction. Tubercle bacilli also tend to infect bone, especially the vertebrae. The diagnosis of osteomyelitis is suggested by a history of antecedent trauma or a predisposing disease, fever, pain, swelling, and tenderness over the involved bone. X-rays are usually negative for the first 2 weeks, but technetium or gallium scans are positive earlier. Antibiotic therapy is necessary for 4 to 6 weeks.

Penetrating wounds, including bites and extension from pressure sores or diabetic ulcerations, are also associated with osteomyelitis. Human bites often introduce anaerobic mouth flora; cat bites penetrate deeply because of the sharpness of their teeth and frequently cause osteomyelitis due to *Pasturella multocida*. Penicillin for 4 to 6 weeks is effective for these cases. Anaerobes, streptococci, staphlococci, and gram-negative bacilli may be found in diabetic ulcers; debridement as well as antibiotics is necessary.

Infective endocarditis

IE usually develops on preexisting abnormal heart valves; rheumatic fever was the most common underlying cause in the past, but congenital abnormalities such as bicuspid aortic valves or mitral valve prolapse are currently more frequent. Acute bacterial endocarditis (ABE) due to staphylococci most frequently occurs in intravenous drug users without underlying valvular abnormality; right-sided endocarditis with tricuspid valve is involvement is frequent in such cases. Bacteremia due to dental surgery is a common precipitating cause of subacute bacterial endocarditis (SBE), but bacteremia also occurs with brushing the teeth and sometimes just with chewing.

Fever, usually low grade, with or without chilliness, night sweats, anorexia, and malaise are the usual symptoms of endocarditis. Arthralgias are common. Fever may be absent in elderly patients. Examination usually reveals heart murmurs, often changing under observation, and detectable embolic lesions such as petechiae, fundal hemorrhages, splinter hemorrhages under the fingernails (but these are nonspecific), splenomegaly (in about 50%), and clubbing (in about 20%). Right-sided endocarditis in IV drug users often gives pleuritic pain due to lung infarcts. Serious systemic emboli can occur with all forms of IE. Splenic infarcts can cause left upper quadrant pain and a rub over the spleen; mesenteric infarcts can cause abdominal pain and blood in the stool; and cerebral infarcts can cause loss of major CNS functions. Renal infarcts are also common, causing microscopic hematuria or, if large, flank pain and tenderness. These infected emboli can lead to abscesses at sites of embolization, and if they lodge in a vessel wall, mycotic aneurysms can develop, leading to rupture and massive hemorrhage weeks to months later.

Patients with IE are usually anemic and have an increased ESR, and about half have rheumatoid factor. In the majority of cases, the urine shows protein and microscopic hematuria. Echocardiography can show evidence of vegetations, but their absence definitely does not rule out the diagnosis. When the disease is suspected, three sets of blood cultures should be obtained within the first 24 hours of hospitalization, along with additional cultures if the patient has already received some antibiotics, since the likelihood of positive cultures is reduced. The likelihood that positive blood cultures represents the existence of IE varies with the organism found. For example, *S. aureus* in a blood culture has a 50% likelihood of meaning endocarditis; similar statistics exist for *S. fecalis*. For group B streptococci, the figure would be closer to 1 in 7, whereas for *E. coli* it is 1 in 200; for other streptococci the figure is between these two extremes.

Therapeutic decisions. Choice of antibiotic depends on the organism identified or suspected. *S. viridans* is most common and remains sensitive to penicillin, as are the group D streptococci, such as *S. bovis*; aqueous penicillin G, 12 million units/day for 4 weeks, is the usual course for these organisms. For enterococci, an aminoglycoside must be added to the penicillin. *S. aureus* endocarditis requires 12 g/day of nafcillin; the addition of an aminoglycoside is advisable especially with a severe septic infection, at least until all disease manifestations are controlled. The total duration of therapy should be 6 weeks. In a patient allergic to penicillin, vancomycin can be used. *Pseudomonas* endocarditis is frequent among IV drug users and requires combination therapy, such as tobramycin and ticarcillin. At times, threapy must be instituted without confirming the diagnosis with positive blood cultures; other causes of low-grade fever should be ruled out, including multiple pulmonary emboli or disease in other organ systems such as the biliary tree.

Refractory endocarditis is sometimes an indication for cardiac surgery. More often, surgery is needed for valve replacement because of destruction of a leaflet, causing abrupt hemodynamic changes that precipitate heart failure. Recurrent major embolization from vegetations, even after sterilization with antibiotics, can also be an indication for valve surgery.

Prophylaxis of endocarditis. Patients who have aortic or mitral valve disease or prosthetic heart valves are at high risk for developing IE and should receive antibiotic prophylaxis if bacteremia is likely to occur. When they are undergoing oral surgery, penicillin V orally is recommended (e.g., 2 g/hour before and 1 g every 6 hours after the procedure). Erythromycin can be substituted for patients allergic to penicillin, but in the presence of a prosthetic heart valve, vancomycin is preferable. Prior to GI or urinary tract surgery, ampicillin, 2 g IM or IV plus gentamicin, 1.5 mg/kg, 30 minutes before the procedure is recommended; for penicillin-allergic patients, vancomycin plus gentamicin should be used.

CARDIOVASCULAR DISEASE

SOME KEY CONCEPTS OF THE PHYSIOLOGY AND PATHOPHYSIOLOGY OF THE CIRCULATION

Cardiac output is calculated as stroke volume times heart rate. With heart failure, there is increased sympathetic "tone," which means increased catecholamine effect on the myocardium; catecholamines increase contractility and thus stroke volume, as well as heart rate. The force of contraction of the myocardial fibrils is determined by the **preload**, or stretch (i.e., length); in the intact heart it is equivalent to the ventricular diastolic volume. The **Frank-Starling curve** describes the increase in force of cardiac muscle contraction that results from increased resting length (stretch) of muscle fibrils; an increase in diastolic filling thus increases cardiac output. However, in the diseased myocardium this response curve may be relatively flat, with little or no increase in force of contraction with further stretch (preload).

Afterload is the resistance or impedance to flow against which the heart must push fluid when it contracts. It is approximately equal to the diastolic arterial pressure.

In the normal heart, the force of contraction is increased by increasing preload (stretch) but is decreased by increasing afterload (impedance).

Factors that affect preload include blood volume, venous sympathetic tone, intrathoracic pressure, intrapericardial pressure, atrial contraction, body position, and the pumping action of skeletal muscle.

Peripheral resistance is defined as the difference in pressure across a capillary bed, divided by the flow across that capillary bed ($R = (P_1 - P_2)/flow$).

Factors that affect afterload (impedance) include peripheral vascular resistance, left ventricular volume (i.e., preload) (by affecting ventricular wall tension), elasticity of the arterial tree (compliance), presence of outflow obstruction (e.g., aortic valvular stenosis, hypertrophic subaortic stenosis, or idiopathic ventricular hypertrophy).

Factors that affect contractility (inotropism) (i.e., myocardial performance at a given preload and afterload) include the following: Increased contractility results from sympathetic nerve stimulation, circulating catecholamines, digitalis, calcium, and other inotropic agents. Decreased contractility results from anoxia, acidosis, loss of functional myocardium (as occurs with infarction), and some pharmacologic agents (e.g., beta-blockers).

Factors that affect heart rate include autonomic nervous activity, temperature, and metabolic rate.

The principal substrate for myocardial metabolism is fatty acid, but if insufficient fatty acid is available, carbohydrate is used. However, myocardial metabolism is aerobic, and therefore the heart is unable to develop an "oxygen debt" the way skeletal muscle can. As a result, myocardial anoxia causes symptoms and quickly leads to permanent damage.

PATHOPHYSIOLOGY AND CLINICAL MANIFESTATIONS OF HEART FAILURE

Heart failure is best defined as the inability of the heart to provide sufficient oxygen and nutrients to satisfy the metabolic needs of the body. As heart failure develops, compensatory mechanisms come into play, and many of the symptoms and findings are the result of these adaptations. For example, sympathetic nervous system activity is increased, augmenting contractility (**inotropic effect**) and rhythmicity (**chronotropic effect**). Tachycardia, sweating, and vasoconstriction occur, resulting in cool, cyanotic extremities. The accompanying increase in myocardial oxygen requirements can be deleterious, however, as can the increased peripheral resistance (afterload), resulting in worsening of the heart failure. Sympathetic tone then increases further. The consequence may be progressive deterioration in cardiac function.

Heart failure decreases the effective circulating blood volume, which results in an increase in renin production in the kidneys, leading to increased aldosterone formation. The resulting mineralocorticoid activity causes salt and water retention, augmenting venous return and cardiac dilatation. If it is progressive, edema formation results. The increased sympathetic tone causes venous vasoconstriction, which decreases the capacitance of the venous bed, augmenting venous return.

Although in the normal heart an increase in diastolic filling increases cardiac output, as illustrated by the Frank-Starling curve, a diseased, failing heart may be capable of little or no increase in contractility in response to the increased stretch of the myocardial fibrils. With increasing fluid retention as a result of the heart failure, a progressive increase in left ventricular diastolic volume (preload) occurs, resulting in incomplete emptying of the ventricle and a progressive increase in the pressure at the end of diastole. An increase in the end-diastolic pressure in the left ventricle is reflected by a similar increase in pressure in the left atrium, since the two are in direct communication during diastole, when the mitral valve is open. The pulmonary venous pressure must be higher than the left atrial pressure. Therefore, this pressure change is reflected back into the pulmonary veins and increases the pressure in the pulmonary capillaries (which can be measured as the pulmonary wedge pressure); it leads to pulmonary edema when it exceeds about 20 mm Hg.

Further deterioration in cardiac function can occur if coronary blood cannot increase because cardiac dilatation increases wall tension, which increases oxygen consumption. Increasing work load causes hypertrophy of cardiac muscle, as it does skeletal muscle; both the number and the size of the myocardial cells increase. The increased muscle mass also increases oxygen consumption; in addition, hypertrophied cardiac muscle has lowered contractility. Thus, this compensatory mechanism also can lead to progressive decompensation. Heart failure due to uncorrectable causes has a poor prognosis despite modern treatment; a 50% 5-year mortality rate is usual.

Hypertrophied or ischemic muscles are stiffer than normal (they have decreased **compliance**); this is sometimes referred to as **impaired diastolic function** since it requires a higher enddiastolic pressure to achieve a given degree of stretch (diastolic volume). The increased pressure is also reflected in the pulmonary wedge pressure, increasing the likelihood of development of pulmonary edema. When monitored, the wedge pressure should be maintained at about 15 to 18 mm Hg to avoid pulmonary edema.

Dyspnea, a characteristic manifestation of heart failure, initially is a result of increased stiffness (decreased compliance) of the lungs due to an increase in interstitial water content. Arterial blood gases (ABGs) are usually normal at this stage, but as frank alveolar edema develops, hyperventilation occurs. The impaired diffusion of gases from alveolar air to pulmonary capillaries causes the PO_2 to fall, but initially the increased ventilation decreases the alveolar and arterial PCO_2. As more pulmonary edema accumulates, carbon dioxide (CO_2) diffusion is impaired and CO_2 retention develops. Cardiomegaly becomes detectable on physical examination and by x-ray and echocardiography. The echo can also demonstrate ventricular hypertrophy as well as abnormalities in wall motion. Radionuclide ventriculography can show a decreased ejection fraction. In severe cases, pressure monitoring with a Swan-Ganz catheter is useful.

Therapy for heart failure initially includes decreasing activity to a level that avoids dyspnea. Bed rest is necessary if there are symptoms at rest (class IV heart failure); oxygen may be useful. Low-salt diet is useful to decrease fluid retention, but diuretics are often needed in addition. Water intake should be restricted only if dilutional hyponatremia has developed. **Digitalis** increases contractility; it also increases AV nodal conduction time and refractoriness. Because of this effect on conduction, heart rate will slow if there is atrial fibrillation, but sinus rhythm slows only as a result of improvement in heart failure, decreasing sympathetic tone. Digoxin is the most commonly used form of digitalis because of its rapid clearance if toxicity occurs, but its incomplete absorption can be a problem in patients with intestinal disease (malabsorption states can decrease absorption or inflammatory disease can increase absorption). Digitalis is cleared primarily by the kidneys, and the dose must be adjusted for renal failure. Because it is highly protein bound, it is not cleared by dialysis. Serum levels are useful as guidelines to dosing.

The increased contractility produced by digitalis (or other inotropic agents) shifts the Frank-Starling curve to the left, meaning that it increases ventricular function at a given level of diastolic volume. Increased ventricular emptying causes diuresis and also reduces filling pressure. Although the increased contractility increases oxygen consumption, this may be offset by the decrease in diastolic volume, which reduces wall tension, decreasing oxygen consumption. Digitalis is useful in most forms of heart failure, especially those in which myocardial function is impaired, but it is not helpful when failure is due to obstructive valvular lesions such as mitral stenosis or in states in which there is restriction in venous return to the heart, such as pericardial tamponade or constriction. Digitalis is also very useful in certain arrhythmias, especially atrial fibrillation, flutter, and paroxysmal atrial tachycardia (PAT). Digitalis toxicity can produce arrhythmias, however, especially ventricular premature contractions, by increasing the automaticity of ectopic pacemakers. Hypokalemia increases the toxicity of digitalis. GI symptoms (nausea, vomiting) and vision symptoms (e.g., colored scotomata) occurred more often with the older forms of digitalis but are rare with the digitalis glycosides.

Vasodilators affect both veins and arteries and can decrease the load on the heart muscle (both afterload and preload) and improve myocardial function. Venous dilatation and diuretics decrease ventricular filling (preload), and an overstretched, failing ventricle is benefitted by decreasing ventricular size and wall tension, decreasing oxygen consumption. Since the Frank-Starling curve of the response of the ventricle to increased stretch is relatively flat in heart failure, cardiac output changes little. An excessive decrease in filling pressure can have a deleterious effect if ventricular filling becomes suboptimal, and it may be necessary to monitor filling pressures in severely ill patients, attempting to keep enddiastolic pressure around 15 to 20 mm Hg (normal is about 10).

Arterial vasodilatation decreases the peripheral resistance to systolic emptying by the heart (afterload), improving cardiac performance in the same way as an increase in contractility but without the accompanying increase in oxygen demand. The improved ventricular emptying also decreases ventricular size,

decreasing preload, wall tension, and oxygen demand. Decreasing afterload can improve ventricular function when agents that increase contractility are ineffective. The resulting fall in arterial blood pressure may limit a patient's tolerance for these agents, and therefore the usefulness of arterial vasodilators, but the pressure may not fall significantly since decreasing peripheral resistance may allow a sufficient increase in cardiac output to compensate (blood pressure = cardiac output × resistance). If necessary, blood pressure may be maintained by fluid administration, increasing preload. Vasodilator therapy has been shown to work best in acute heart failure; it may be deleterious to patients with mitral or aortic stenosis. The most commonly used agents are nitroprusside, hydralazine, and captopril; nitroglycerin is primarily a venous dilator.

Sympathomimetic amines are inotropic agents. Dopamine and dobutamine are most useful since they produce less tachycardia and peripheral vascular effects than others, such as epinephrine and norepinephrine and isoproterenol. In low doses (2 μg/kg/minute), dopamine causes vasodilatation in the cerebral, renal, coronary, and mesenteric vascular beds (an action similar to epinephrine). Diuresis can result from increased cardiac output and renal blood flow. Larger doses (5 to 10 μg/kg/minute) are alpha-adrenergic agonists and cause peripheral vasoconstriction. Arterial pressure and heart rate rise. This effect may be desired in hypotensive patients, and the increased oxygen demand caused by the increased heart rate, contractility, and blood pressure may be balanced by the opposite effects of decreased heart size. Dobutamine increases cardiac contractility without the concomitant vasoconstriction caused by dopamine. Other inotropic agents are under development. Aortic balloon-assisted pulsation is a short-term treatment for acute heart failure.

Acute pulmonary edema should be treated with morphine, furosemide, and, if possible, measures to remove the cause of the decompensation. Digitalis is not necessary. Hemodynamic monitoring may be needed, particularly if vasodilating and sympathomimetic inotropic agents are used. If oxygenation becomes a problem, intubation and mechanical ventilation may be instituted.

SHOCK

The first stage or degree of shock, "compensated hypotension," involves a small decrease in cardiac output and compensatory vasoconstriction. Symptoms may be minimal, but if untreated, it can progress to the second stage, in which there is some decrease in tissue perfusion. Decreased function of the brain, kidneys, and myocardium occurs, and increased sympathetic tone is present. In the third stage, there is severe ischemia and tissue damage, including loss of renal function (acute renal insufficiency). Widespread ischemic damage to capillary endothelia occurs, causing increased permeability with fluid transudation and producing extensive tissue edema. The resulting loss of plasma volume (hypovolemia) aggravates the hypotension. Acidosis from release of toxins from peripheral tissue (including lactate) has a further depressive effect on myocardial function.

Shock can result from myocardial damage (**cardiogenic shock**), loss of blood or plasma volume (**hypovolemic shock**), acute adrenal insufficiency, anaphylaxis, acute myocardial infarction (**cardiogenic shock**) and release of endotoxins from gram-negative bacteria (**septic shock**). Fall in blood pressure; tachycardia; tachypnea; cool, pale, moist skin; and oliguria are the usual clinical findings. Other findings specific to the cause of the shock may be present—for example, fever and warm skin with septic shock, flat neck veins with hypovolemic shock, and distended neck veins with cardiogenic shock. Rales will be heard if pulmonary edema is also present.

Therapeutic decisions. Management of shock may require placement of lines to monitor central venous pressure, or a Swan-Ganz catheter may be needed to monitor both pulmonary wedge and arterial pressures. Specific measures aimed at the cause of the shock are essential, including antibiotics for septic shock, epinephrine for anaphylactic shock, corticosteroids for immunologic causes or acute adrenal insufficiency. Cardiogenic shock may require diuretics, inotropic agents, and intra-aortic balloon pumping to assist the circulation. Sometimes, judiciously used vasodilators are valuable. Endotoxin causes a generalized increase in vascular permeability, resulting in transudation of fluid and hypovolemia; large quantities of parenteral fluid may be needed to maintain diastolic filling pressure and should be given despite massive tissue edema. Pressor agents such as dopamine are often needed.

CLINICAL FINDINGS IN PATIENTS WITH HEART DISEASE

Pain of cardiac origin must be distinguished from noncardiac **chest pain**. Ischemic chest pain occurs when myocardial oxygen demand exceeds supply. Angina pectoris is transient ischemic pain that is typically induced by exertion, emotion, or a heavy meal, but it can occur at rest or begin while asleep. Angina due to a fixed degree of coronary artery obstruction recurs repeatedly with a similar degree of exertion. When angina is due to coronary artery spasm (Prinzmetal's angina), the level of activity that induces it varies. Angina is typically relieved within 5 minutes by nitroglycerin. When cardiac pain persists for over 30 minutes, it is probably due to myocardial necrosis, thus indicating myocardial infarction. Ischemic pain is typically retrosternal and can radiate to the left shoulder and arm or to the neck, jaw, or epigastrium. It is usually described as pressing or squeezing and does not vary with respiration. It can be indistinguishable from "indigestion," probably meaning pain of esophageal origin, or gallbladder pain. During an attack, an S4 or paradoxical split of S2 may be heard as a result of myocardial or papillary muscle dysfunction due to the ischemia.

Pericardial pain and pain of unclear etiology that occurs with mitral valve prolapse can be indistinguishable from anginal pain. Pericardial pain is more often described as sharp or knifelike and can vary with respiration.

ISCHEMIC HEART DISEASE

The most common form of cardiac disease today is ischemic heart disease. **Atherosclerosis**, the cause of most ischemic heart disease, has a predisposition to affect coronary arteries, especially in the first 6 cm, as well as at sites of arterial bifurcation, probably because these are sites of maximal turbulence. Blood flow in coronary arteries is reversed by systolic contraction of the myocardium, when intramyocardial pressure is above systolic arterial pressure, creating turbulence in those arteries. Areas of narrowing of the lumen of a coronary artery greater than 50% probably are hemodynamically significant, whereas narrowing greater than 75% definitely is significant. (These measurements are based on arteriography, which looks at the arteries two dimensionally, but they nevertheless are clinically useful.) Temporary narrowing of coronary arteries due to **spasm** can decrease myocardial perfusion sufficiently to cause ischemic pain (Prinzmetal's or variant angina), and **emboli** to coronary arteries can also obstruct blood flow.

Appraisal of **risk factors** for arteriosclerotic coronary artery disease is important both from the standpoint of supporting the diagnosis and as a key aspect of therapy. **Age** and **sex** are relevant in evaluating risk: Incidence increases with advancing age; after menopause, the incidence in females catches up with that in males). **Family history** is important, especially coronary artery disease in a parent or sibling. **Hypertension, hyperlipidemia, smoking,** and **diabetes** are important risk factors because they are modifiable. Elevation of either systolic or diastolic blood pressure is associated with increased risk of stroke or coronary artery disease, without a defined threshold level—the higher either blood pressure, the greater the risk. Similarly, the higher the **serum cholesterol**, the greater the risk of coronary artery disease, without a definable threshold level. Lowering the serum cholesterol with diet or medications slightly decreases risk. Attempts should be made to lower levels of cholesterol to less than 200 mg/100 ml by diet. Drug therapy should be reserved for severe hypercholesterolemia. A high level of high-density lipoproteins (HDL) is protective; the incidence of coronary artery disease is inversely related to level of HDL. Levels of HDL are higher in women at all ages, are increased by exercise, and are reduced in diabetics. On the other hand, serum triglyceride levels are apparently not an independent determinant of risk.

Cigarette smoking is a major independent risk factor for coronary artery disease, and the risk decreases within a year or two after discontinuation. The risk of sudden death is sharpy reduced after cessation of smoking. Glucose intolerance definitely increases the risk of coronary artery disease, and evidence is accumulating that tight control of diabetes decreases the incidence of this complication. Although obesity seems to increase risk, it may not be independent of hypertension, hyperlipidemia, and diabetes. Nevertheless, weight control is advisable. It is still controversial whether level of **physical activity** and **emotional stress** (type A, aggressive, ambitious personality) are risk factors. Although increasing evidence supports a beneficial effect of physical exercise, it may not be independent of other risk factors in the same population. The use of **oral contraceptives** may be another risk factor, especially in combination with smoking. Oral contraceptives can alter blood pressure, coagulation factors, and blood lipids.

Pathophysiology of ischemic heart disease

Ischemia of the myocardium affects contractility and electrical functions of the heart, probably by decreasing generation of high-energy compounds via oxidative phosphorylation. Both systolic and diastolic functions are impaired. The force of systolic contraction is reduced, and diastolic relaxation (compliance) requires increased pressures to achieve a given amount of diastolic filling of the heart and maintain stroke volume. This accounts for the increased enddiastolic filling pressure. Electrophysiological changes result from altered ion transport across myocardial cell membranes. Loss of membrane integrity also allows leakage of intracellular enzymes into the blood, and serum levels of creatine kinase, lactate dehydrogenase, and glutamine-ornithine transaminase increase if there has been sufficient cellular damage during an ischemic episode (myocardial necrosis). The amount of myocardium that can be saved if reperfusion is achieved after such an episode depends on the duration of complete ischemia. Most or all of the affected myocardium can be saved if ischemia lasted less than 15 to 20 minutes, but very little, if any, after 4 to 6 hours.

Angina pectoris, chest discomfort as a result of myocardial ischemia, is considered **stable** if a given degree of physical activity (or emotional stress) produces symptoms. It is **unstable** if increasing frequency, duration, or severity is occurring or if symptoms appear with a degree of exertion that previously was well tolerated, especially if the exertion is minimal. Such pain may represent an impending infarction and is also called **crescendo** or **preinfarction angina**. It requires hospitalization and monitoring because of the possibility of a sudden arrhythmia. The first appearance (onset) of angina is also considered unstable but does not necessarily require hospitalization unless it appeared at rest or while asleep.

Anginal pain is usually described as pressure, heaviness, or tightness over the anterior chest, and classically the patient demonstrates the type of pain by pressing over the substernal area with a clenched fist. The pain reaches a cresendo over a few seconds, lasts half a minute to a few minutes, and is not described as sharp or knifelike or transient. Pain lasting over 20 minutes suggests that myocardial infarction has occurred. Rest or sublingual nitroglycerin relieves the pain. Anginal pain is precipitated by exertion and is usually felt over the midchest; it may radiate to the left shoulder or arm or to the jaw, but rarely is precordial. Some patients develop dyspnea rather than pain when they have myocardial ischemia, a phenomenon called an anginal equivalent. Not infrequently, anginal pain is difficult to distinguish from pain arising from the esophagus, stomach, or gallbladder, and workup for more than one possible cause is necessary. Stress testing for cardiac ischemia should be done first, since it is more life threatening than the other possible explanations.

Physical examination during an attack of angina may reveal an S4 gallop, which is a ventricular filling sound resulting when atrial systole pumps blood into the ventricle because of decreased diastolic compliance. A systolic murmur resulting from papillary muscle dysfunction also may be detected. ECG may show evidence of ischemia but is usually normal at rest in patients with angina. Stress testing can bring out ST- or T-wave changes, and echocardiography or thallium scintigraphy during exercise can reveal areas of ischemia.

Diagnostic decisions. **Treadmill exercise (stress) testing** is indicated for diagnostic evaluation when angina is suspected and to evaluate the new onset of angina, both for diagnosis and to determine functional capacity. The test is valuable for the latter purpose even in cases of chronic, established angina. *Exercise testing should not be performed until an acute myocardial infarction has been ruled out and pain has been relieved by rest and medication. If the pain is severe and occurs at rest, stress testing should be bypassed and* **coronary arteriography** *performed immediately.* The main indications for coronary arteriography are angina refractory to medical management, a high likelihood of high-grade obstruction of the left main coronary artery or severe three-vessel disease (see below for description of this group of patients), patients in the first 4 to 6 hours after a myocardial infarction in whom angioplasty or thrombolytic therapy is contemplated, or patients in whom the diagnosis of the cause of the chest pain remains unclear after other tests have been performed. Some cardiologists recommend coronary arteriography for any patient with known or suspected coronary artery disease in order to determine if the type of lesions that are most likely to benefit from surgery are present. Others also feel that angiography should be done on any patient under 40 years who has significant angina or an acute myocardial infarction, as well as any patient who has been resuscitated after cardiac arrest.

Patients who are most likely to have left main or three-vessel disease include the following: those with unstable angina; those who have recurrent chest pain after a myocardial infarct, especially if it was a nontransmural (subendocardial) infarction; and those who have a markedly positive exercise stress test (positive in the first 6 minutes or first two stages).

Therapeutic decisions. **Treatment of angina** requires increasing the delivery of oxygen to the myocardium or decreasing the oxygen need of the tissue. First, angina can often be prevented by avoidance of experiences known to precipitate it, such as exertion beyond known limits of tolerance, emotional stress, exposure to cold, and ingestion of large meals. The second important principle is correction of aggravating phenomena, such as treatment of heart failure (which increases oxygen demand), avoiding cigarette smoking, and correction of anemia, hypertension, hyperthyroidism, or an infection. Physical conditioning can lower the heart rate and blood pressure for a given amount of exercise and thus decrease oxygen demand. It may also increase collateral coronary vessels.

The most important medications for angina are nitroglycerins, beta-blockers and calcium channel blockers. **Nitroglycerin** is a smooth muscle relaxant that causes venous dilatation, decreasing venous return to the heart and therefore decreasing preload. The accompanying decreased left ventricular volume and wall tension and the fall in arterial pressure (afterload) serve to decrease oxygen demand. Dilatation of larger "conductance" coronary arteries also occurs, increasing oxygen delivery. Sublingual nitroglycerin works in a few minutes and is best for relief of pain or prevention of expected angina when used before a stressful activity. The drug can be given IV for severe angina, applied as a paste for prolonged prophylaxis, or given in a long-acting form (isosorbide dinitrate).

Beta-adrenergic receptor blockers slow heart rate, both at rest and after an exercise stimulus. They decrease oxygen consumption by decreasing myocardial contractility and therefore are contraindicated in the presence of moderate or severe heart failure. They also reduce systemic blood pressure, decreasing afterload (which can benefit heart failure, sometimes sufficiently to counterbalance the effect on contractility). A number of agents are available with varying degrees of selectivity for the beta$_1$ receptors, which mediate the sympathetic effects on the heart, as opposed to the beta$_2$ receptors, which mediate catecholamine effects on glycogenolysis, dilatation of bronchi, and vasodilatation of peripheral arteries. The beta$_2$ effects therefore can cause bronchoconstriction or prevent the response to hypoglycemia mediated by catecholamines, aggravating insulin shock. Drugs with greater beta$_1$ selectivity, such as atenolol and metoprolol, thus may be more useful in patients with a tendency to have diabetes, asthma, chronic obstructive pulmonary disease (COPD), or peripheral vascular disease.

Since calcium ions play a major role in generation of cardiac action potential, as well as myocardial and smooth muscle contraction, **calcium channel blocking agents** are therapeutically useful, dilating coronary vessels and decreasing contractility and thus increasing oxygen supply and decreasing oxygen demand. Of the drugs in this category currently available, verapamil and diltiazem decrease the sinus node discharge rate and atrioventricular (AV) nodal conductivity whereas nifedipine is the most potent vasodilator, with little effect on myocardial contractility or AV nodal conduction. Nifedipine therefore decreases afterload by lowering blood pressure but increases perfusion of the myocardium at the lower blood pressure by causing coronary vasodilation.

The beneficial effects of calcium channel blockers on contractility and heart rate, and thus on oxygen demand, may be reversed by a reflex increase in sympathetic stimulation in response to peripheral vasodilatation. A similar phenomenon can occur as a result of the peripheral vasodilating effect of nitroglycerin. Therefore, in patients with severe angina, combination therapy can be useful (nitroglycerin or a calcium channel blocker, such as nifedipine or verapamil, plus a beta-blocker, or all three types of drugs together).

A typical clinical problem is presented by a patient with a marked increase in the frequency or severity of angina or the appearance of angina at rest or while asleep. Such a patient should be hospitalized and monitored in a coronary care unit. Sedation may be necessary. If sublingual nitroglycerin is inadequate to control the pain, it can be given IV. If the patient is not hypotensive, nifedipine can be added or the other calcium channel blockers can be useful in such patients if they are not in heart failure. Once the patient is stabilized, coronary arteriography is indicated, since these cases are often candidates for bypass grafts. If medical therapy does not control the angina, balloon counterpulsation, if available, may help by improving coronary artery filling in diastole, as well as by decreasing afterload.

Angina due to coronary artery spasm (variant or Prinzmetal's angina) usually occurs at night and rarely leads to infarction but can be associated with arrhythmias and sudden death. Although it is due to spasm, an underlying fixed stenotic lesion may be present and there may be accompanying angina on exertion. Spasm may be seen on coronary arteriography or may be precipitated in the catheterization lab with carefully administered small doses of ergonovine, since these patients show increased sensitivity to vasoconstrictive influences. In such cases, beta-blockers may be detrimental because they can allow unopposed alpha-adrenergic vasoconstriction. Calcium channel blockers and nitrates are usually effective, but bypass surgery is not useful unless significant fixed stenosis is present.

Surgery for coronary artery disease

Coronary artery bypass grafts are now the most common major surgical procedure performed in the United States. The perioperative mortality of coronary artery bypass surgery varies according to the clinical status of the patient, such as the state of left ventricular function. Overall it is about 0.7% if left ventricular function is normal but 1.8% if it is impaired. With left main coronary artery disease, overall mortality is about 2.5%, but with left ventricular function abnormal it is about 4%. Mortality also increases with age and is about 2% overall in patients over age 65.

The results of surgery vary with the location and severity of the vascular lesions. Anginal pain is completely relieved in roughly 65% and improved in an additional 25%. About 3% of patients have a recurrence of angina. Repeat operations carry a higher risk and are less often successful. Patients with one- or two-vessel disease do as well without surgery and can be treated medically unless refractory angina develops. With three-vessel coronary artery disease, data suggest that patients who are asymptomatic or have stable angina do as well with medical therapy; but if they have poor functional capacity in daily activities or on a treadmill stress test, they probably would benefit from bypass grafting. Patients with three-vessel disease and moderate ventricular dysfunction probably also benefit from surgery.

Bypass grafts do not improve left ventricular function sufficiently in patients with pump failure or help with intractable ventricular arrhythmias (the irritable focus must be excised). Patency is more frequently maintained when internal mammary arteries are used in place of saphenous vein grafts.

Percutaneous transluminal coronary angioplasty (PTCA), performed during cardiac catheterization, can relieve obstructing lesions, giving a 25 to 50% increase in arterial luminal diameter in about 80% of cases. In about 5%, immediate rethrombosis occurs, and therefore patients selected for this procedure should be candidates for immediate surgery. Patients with left main coronary artery stenosis are not candidates for PTCA because a new thrombus or dissection of this vessel after angioplasty might impair coronary blood flow too greatly. Mortality from PTCA is about 1%; results of long-term follow-up are not yet available. PTCA can be performed during an emergency situation, such as an acute myocardial infarction, and may decrease the loss of myocardium. This procedure is most useful for proximal discrete stenotic lesions, in the absence of multiple lesions, and is most successful with lesions of the left anterior descending artery.

ACUTE MYOCARDIAL INFARCTION

Transmural myocardial infarction usually results from a fresh thrombus superimposed on an atherosclerotic lesion that was critically stenotic. Most nontransmural infarcts (usually referred to as subendocardial) occur distal to stenotic but not occluded arteries. Thromboses may develop following hemorrhage into a plaque, ulceration of the endothelium over a plaque causing activation of clotting factors or causing platelet thrombi to develop, or as a result of spasm causing closure of a coronary artery at the site of critical narrowing of the lumen by a plaque. The extent of the resulting area of myocardial necrosis is determined by the oxygen demand of the affected tissue, by the size of the area of muscle supplied by the occluded artery, and by the extent of collateral blood flow. Gross pathological changes are not detectable in an area of infarction for at least 6 hours. By 8 to 10 days, the myocardium affected is thinned as debris is removed by phagocytic cells. Granulation tissue extends through the necrotic area by 3 to 4 weeks, and a thin scar forms and becomes firm by 6 weeks.

Diagnostic decisions. Myocardial infarction usually presents with severe chest pain, which resembles anginal pain but lasts until relieved by medication. There are painless, "silent" infarcts, which are usually identified sometime later by ECG changes. They occur primarily in diabetics. During an acute episode, nausea and vomiting can occur. Sweating, weakness, and anxiety are usually present. On examination, there may be tachycardia, elevation of blood pressure, soft heart sounds, an S4 gallop, a fixed or paradoxical split of S2, or a systolic murmur resulting from papillary muscle dysfunction. Pulses may be thready, and the precordial left ventricular impulse may be weakened. Hypotension (cardiogenic shock) can occur, especially if more than 40% of the myocardium is infarcted.

A low-grade fever can develop, usually after about 12 hours. Leukocytosis appears after about a day, usually peaking at 12,000 to 15,000 cells/mm^3. The ESR and other acute-phase reactants rise after about 3 to 4 days. ECG changes (especially in the ST segment and T waves) are present immediately, and cardiac enzymes can appear in the blood in a few hours, peaking on the second day and returning to normal by the fourth day. The creatine kinase (MB fraction) is most sensitive and specific, and a rise to 7 to 8% of the total CPK is significant even without an increase in total enzyme level. Other forms of trauma to myocardium can release CPK, including surgery, as can any form of myocarditis, but *cardioversion and CPR usually do not release this enzyme into the blood.* The serum lactate dehydrogenase (LDH) can be fractionated, and the LDH$_1$ is most specific for the myocardium. It is elevated later than the CPK, peaking at about the fifth day. The SGOT rises a little earlier than the LDH and returns to normal about the fifth day.

Therapeutic decisions. About half the deaths from myocardial infarction occur in the first 4 hours, and therefore lives can be saved by community emergency services with trained medical technicians able to administer CPR and use monitoring and defibrillating equipment. Admission to coronary care unit decreased mortality, primarily deaths that would result from arrhythmias. Immediate therapy consists of sedation as needed, relief of pain and anxiety (primarily with morphine), and use of atropine if necessary to relieve nausea and vomiting resulting from the infarct or as a side effect of morphine. Nitrate therapy can be used for recurrent angina. Oxygen is not needed unless the patient is hypoxemic.

Bed rest is advisable for the first 24 to 36 hours, except for the use of a bedside commode. If the course uncomplicated, patients can usually be transferred out of the coronary care unit after 3 days, since life-threatening arrhythmias rarely appear after that time. Ambulation is usually begun after the fourth or fifth day and progressively increased if the patient is asymptomatic, to include a flight of stairs by discharge. Such condition-

ing avoids unnecessary psychological invalidism as well as thromboembolic complications. Diet can be kept liquid and soft if there is nausea, but otherwise can be normal (but low in fat for educational reasons). Smoking must be avoided. Stool softeners are advisable to prevent straining.

Prophylactic lidocaine IV for the first 48 hours prevents ventricular tachyarrhythmias, but its use is not uniformly agreed on. The dose should be minimized in elderly patients and in those in CHF or with liver disease, and increased if arrhythmias develop. Chronic antiarrhythmic therapy is not necessary after an infarction, even if early ventricular tachyarrhythmias occurred, although episodes of nonsustained ventricular tachycardia should probably receive maintenance therapy with a drug such as quinidine (see the paragraphs below on arrhythmias).

Measures to limit the infarct size are indicated if instituted within the first 4 to 6 hours. Intracoronary streptokinase is currently used, but trials are showing superiority in effect with less hemorrhage, the main side effect, with intravenous human tissue plasminogen activator produced by recombinant DNA technology. Usually a high-grade stenotic lesion exists at the site of the thrombus, and rethrombosis occurs with some frequency. Catheterization and coronary artery angioplasty are useful in such cases, if available.

Use of anticoagulants remains controversial. Early ambulation eliminates the need in most patients. Minidose heparin (5,000 units SC every 8 hours) may reduce the frequency of deep vein thrombosis and embolization if there is no contraindication. The heparin can be discontinued when the patient is ambulatory for 2 to 3 days. Full-dose anticoagulants are advisable in patients at high risk for embolic complicaitons, such as those with ventricular aneurysms or past thromboses or emboli. Pericarditis is a contraindication to anticoagulation because of the risk of hemorrhage into the pericardium.

Most patients can be discharged after 1 to 2 weeks, with instructions to use sublingual nitroglycerin for anginal attacks. Formal rehabilitation programs are advisable. A limited stress test (e.g., up to 70% of predicted maximal heart rate) prior to discharge or a full stress test 6 weeks after infarction can serve as a guide to exercise tolerance and recommendations. Patients considered at high risk for recurrent infarction because of their course or the results of stress testing should be referred for coronary angiography. The use of a beta-blocker prophylactically in doses sufficient to blunt the tachycardia of exercise for 2 years after a myocardial infarct reduces the incidence of sudden death and reinfarction, although such drugs are contraindicated in heart failure patients, who have the highest postinfarction mortality.

Management of other complications. Mild CHF can usually be treated with a diuretic, but severe failure (cardiogenic shock) occurs if the cardiac output falls below 1.8 L/minute/m^2 (normal about 2.5 to 3.6). Swan-Ganz (right-heart) catheterization is indicated in patients with **hypotension** not corrected by IV fluids or treatment of rhythm disturbances, or in the presence of **severe left ventricular failure, suspicion of a ruptured papillary muscle or cardiac tamponade, or ventricular septal defect** (diagnosed by checking for increased oxygen content in the right ventricle due to left-to-right shunting), or when there are unexplained clinical findings (such as unexplained **hypoxia, acidosis, or sinus tachycardia**). Cardiac output can be assisted by administering IV fluid to keep ventricular filling maximal, keeping pulmonary capillary wedge pressure around 14 to 18 mm Hg (normal 10 to 12); higher wedge pressures result in pulmonary edema. If the patient cannot be stabilized, surgery for a correctable cause of cardiogenic shock, such as a ruptured papillary muscle with acute mitral regurgitation or a ventricular septal defect with a large shunt, may be necessary despite the high risk, since otherwise the outlook is extremely poor. If stabilization can be achieved, any necessary surgery should be performed about 4 to 6 weeks postinfarction.

Inotropic agents, diuretics, and vasodilators to reduce afterload can help patients with severe failure. If available, aortic balloon counterpulsation can sustain such patients until surgery can be undertaken. Right ventricular infarction can cause shock because of poor left ventricular filling, and fluid administration to raise the filling pressure is helpful even in the presence of distended neck veins and other evidence of venous congestion. If left ventricular function remains good, most patients with right ventricular infarction do well.

A **ventricular aneurysm** can be asymptomatic or contribute to heart failure by expanding during systole, thus decreasing systolic output; it can be the site of ectopic irritable foci leading to development of ventricular tachyarrhythmias, or mural thrombi can form in an aneurysm and cause systemic arterial emboli. An aneurysm should be suspected when there is a surprisingly strong precordial impulse in a patient with poor heart sounds and evidence of low cardiac output, with suspicious ECG findings (evidence of transmural infraction with persistently elevated ST segments). Echocardiography is usually definitive. Anticoagulants are indicated if emboli have occurred, and aneurysmectomy may become necessary to improve cardiac output or eliminate the source of tachyarrhythmias. A systemic embolus that blocks circulation to a significant area of tissue should be removed surgically if possible.

Rupture of the infarcted ventricular wall usually occurs in the first 5 days after the acute event and is usually rapidly fatal because of cardiac tamponade. Pericarditis occurs in about 10% of patients with an acute myocardial infarct, usually producing a friction rub and precordial pain but no serious sequelae. Anti-inflammatory medication (e.g., a nonsteroidal agent) is usually sufficient therapy; anticoagulant therapy should be avoided because of the danger of hemorrhage into the pericardium. About 5% of patients develop Dressler's syndrome, which is the appearance of pericarditis, pleural effusion, and often fever, weeks to months after a myocardial infarct, apparently on an immune basis. Dressler's syndrome can also develop after cardiac surgery or other causes of acute pericarditis. Therapy with corticosteroids may be necessary.

Arrhythmias that compromise cardiac output, increase myocardial oxygen requirements, or predispose to more malignant rhythm disturbances must be treated. Any reversible cause of arrhythmias, such as excessive digitalis or a metabolic abnormality, should be corrected. Only about half the patients who have premature ventricular contractions (PVCs) develop serious tachyarrhythmias, whereas about half of those who develop ventricular fibrillation have no prior PVCs. Therefore, aggressive therapy for PVCs is not necessarily indicated beyond routine use of lidocaine. Idioventricular rhythms with rates of 60 to 100 beats/minute may not need treatment, since they do not increase the incidence of more severe arrhythmias and rarely cause hemodynamic consequences. More rapid ventricular tachycardias not suppressed by lidocaine should be treated by substitution or addition of IV procainamide or bretylium. A sustained period of tachycardia should be terminated by use of cardioversion if necessary. Development of impaired hemodynamic function requires immediate cardioversion. Ventricular fibrillation develops in 2 to 3% of patients with myocardial infarction who are hospitalized. Prompt cardioversion with 200 to 400 joules is necessary. When such severe ventricular arrhythmias develop in the first 48 hours, chronic antiarrhythmic therapy may not be necessary, since they are due to the acute ischemia. Arrhythmias developing later usually require maintenance therapy (see the paragraphs on arrhythmias.)

Persistent sinus tachycardia not due to anxiety can be difficult to treat. Since it increases myocardial oxygen demand, a cause should be sought and treated if possible. Pericarditis, tamponade, pulmonary emboli, or fever may be responsible. For the same reasons, a rapid ventricular rate caused by atrial fibrillation needs correction. If drugs fail, cardioversion is necessary. First-degree AV block does not need therapy, but second-degree block (Mobitz type I) is usually due to increased vagal tone or ischemia of the AV node. It occurs more often in patients with inferior infarction and is usually temporary, requiring no therapy. Mobitz type II second-degree block usually occurs more commonly with anterior infarctions and requires temporary pacing. Similarly, a prophylactic pacemaker is needed for complete heart block, especially if the infarct is anterior. New intraventricular conduction defects (left or right bundle branch block or hemiblocks) probably are the result of extensive infarction, and the prognosis is poor. Temporary pacing may be helpful, especially in the presence of new bifascicular block. Preexisting bundle branch block with or without axis deviation (hemiblock) is not an indication for pacing.

MYOCARDITIS AND PERICARDITIS

Myocarditis is frequently asymptomatic, detected only on the basis of ECG changes (ST- and T-wave changes, conduction defects). Some patients note fatigue and weakness (symptoms of inadequate cardiac output or "forward failure"), whereas others develop precordial pain and manifestations of severe CHF. Arrhythmias can occur.

Acute rheumatic fever was the most common cause of myocarditis in the past, but more common causes today include viral infections (especially Coxsackie B), rickettsial infections (especially Rocky Mountain spotted fever), protozoal infections (especially trypanosomiasis, e.g., Chagas' disease in Brazil and other parts of South and Central America), and irradiation. Other causes include toxins such as alcohol, lead, cobalt, drugs, especially doxorubicin (Adriamycin); metabolic disorders such as glycogen storage disease, thyrotoxicosis, mxyedema; thiamin deficiency (beriberi); protein starvation; some muscular dystrophies; and a peripartum cardiomyopathy seen especially in older multiparous blacks with poor nutrition.

Although there are a variety of toxic and metabolic causes of cardiomyopathy, the resulting clinical syndromes are similar and often progress to interstitial myocardial fibrosis. Dilatation of the heart is common, heart sounds are poor, gallop sounds are frequent, and an apical systolic murmur may be heard if functional mitral regurgitation develops. When patches of fibrosis appear, Q waves appear that are similar to those seen with myocardial infarction. Echocardiography also reveals evidence of dilatation of the ventricle, poor wall motion, sometimes intraventricular thrombi.

Therapy is supportive, with the usual measures for treatment of heart failure or arrhythmias if necessary. Corticosteroids may be of value, especially for severe, active rheumatic carditis.

A **hypertrophic form of cardiomyopathy** affects the intraventricular septum primarily and causes subvalvular outlet obstruction in the left ventricle. It is also called idiopathic hypertrophic subaortic stenosis (IHSS). The disease is hereditary, transmitted in an autosomal dominant pattern, but sporadic cases occur. A pressure gradient develops in the left ventricle during systole as a result of the development of obstruction as the hypertrophied septum moves close to the outer ventricular wall. There is also stiffness of the ventricle, impairing diastolic filling. Elevation of pulmonary venous and wedge pressures results in dyspnea. Reduced compliance of the right ventricle results in a large jugular venous **a wave**. The development of the obstruction during contraction usually generates a harsh systolic outflow murmur, crescendo-decrescendo, heard best along the left sternal border and the apex with radiation into the base of the heart and axilla but rarely into the neck. The carotid pulse is bifid, with a brisk, rapid upstroke, a midsystolic dip, and a second late systolic rise, reflecting the development of the obstruction to outflow and correlating with the murmur. Arrhythmias such as atrial fibrillation are poorly tolerated, and any phenomenon that decreases ventricular filling increases the degree of outflow obstruction. Ventricular arrhythmias are a cause of sudden death in these patients.

A variety of measures can affect the physical findings. A Valsalva maneuver or amyl nitrite decreases venous return and therefore decreases ventricular size, increasing the degree of obstruction to outflow and increasing the intensity of the murmur. Squatting, elevation of the legs, isometric muscle contraction, and phenylephrine all can increase venous return, dilating the ventricles and decreasing obstruction, thus decreasing the intensity of the murmur.

Diagnostic decisions. ECG shows evidence of left ventricular hypertrophy. Echocardiography can visualize the ventricular septal hypertrophy diagnostically. Cardiac catheterization can be useful but is not usually necessary unless surgery is contemplated.

Therapeutic decisions. The course is variable. Interventions that decrease ventricular volume (e.g., digitalis) aggravate the problem and should be avoided. Diuretics can also be harmful for the same reason. Beta-blockers decrease contractility and therefore can decrease the degree of obstruction to outflow during systole. Calcium channel blockers can have a similar effect, but nifedipine is a potent vasodilator and may be dangerous even though it has a greater negative inotropic effect. Prophylaxis against bacterial endocarditis is indicated in these patients. Surgical septal myotomy may be needed in some patients.

Restrictive cardiomyopathies are much less common; the most frequent cause is systemic amyloidosis, but idiopathic endomyocardial fibrosis, hemochromatosis, sarcoidosis, and other infiltrative processes can cause the same syndrome. The main pathophysiological problem is restriction of ventricular filling in diastole, resulting in findings suggestive of constrictive pericarditis (see below).

PERICARDITIS

Acute pericarditis was most often due to rheumatic fever or tuberculosis. Viral infections and uremia in patients in chronic renal failure are the most common cause at present, as is extension of tumor into the pericardium. Pericarditis causes precordial chest pain, aggravated by lying flat and relieved by sitting or leaning forward, with a pericardial friction rub. The rub can have three components, one corresponding to atrial systole, a second during ventricular systole, and a third during early diastolic ventricular filling. The presence of a rub does not rule out a large effusion. Single-component rubs, limited to systole, must be differentiated from systolic murmurs. Concomitant pleurisy with effusion is common, and a pleural rub may be heard as well. Tachycardia is commonly present, since limited ventricular filling restricts systolic stroke volume and the heart must compensate with increased rate to maintain output; atrial rhythm disturbances are common. ECG shows characteristic changes (ST-segment elevations, later T-wave flattening; if a large effusion is present, voltage may be low). Chest x-ray will show enlargement of the heart if an effusion is present. A pleural effusion may be present. The ESR is usually elevated, but cardiac enzymes are normal.

A large effusion can cause an increase in intrapericardial pressure, since the pericardium is not compliant. Pulmonary and systemic venous pressure increase to maintain cardiac filling, resulting in dyspnea, distended neck veins, and often edema. An increase in heart rate occurs to maintain cardiac output despite the low ventricular filling and low stroke volume. A rapid, thready pulse results. Crackles of pulmonary edema are usually absent. Compression of the left lower lobe posteriorly produces dullness and decreased bronchial breath sounds below the scapula (Ewart's sign). An apical cardiac impulse may be undetectable, and the precordium may be quiet on auscultation.

When cardiac tamponade occurs, a pulsus paradoxus (systolic pressure falling >10 mm Hg on inspiration) develops (but is not specific since it can occur with severe COPD, asthma, and myocardial disease). A large "water-bottle" heart is seen on x-ray, and ECG can show low voltage or electrical alternans. Catheterization reveals equalization of pressures in all four chambers during diastole, with high systemic venous pressure and reduced stroke volume and cardiac output.

Therapeutic decisions. Therapy for acute pericarditis requires first determining the etiology and directing specific treatment if possible. Nonsteroidal anti-inflammatory drugs (NSAIDs) are helpful, but corticosteroids are often needed. If a large effusion with tamponade develops, a tap is useful and a drain may be left in place; examine the fluid for bacteria, cells, cytology, and culture. Surgical removal of a portion of the pericardium (a "window") may be needed. Before surgery, if hypotension is present, give IV fluids to maintain ventricular filling and cardiac output.

Constrictive pericarditis is the result of fibrosis of the pericardium. Tuberculosis was the most common cause in the past, but thickening of the pericardium can result from bacterial, viral, fungal, neoplastic, or uremic pericarditis, as well as from systemic connective tissue diseases. Symptoms include dyspnea, fatigue, and abdominal swelling. On examination there are distended neck veins with exaggerated y descent, corresponding to rapid early ventricular filling. Tachycardia, hepatomegaly, ascites, and peripheral edema are found. Retraction of the chest wall over the cardiac apex may be seen. An early diastolic filling sound similar to an S3 gallop may be heard, ending with a pericardial knock. Pulsus paradoxus is not usually present, but Kussmaul's sign (inspiratory decrease in systemic venous pressure) often is detectable.

Diagnostic decisions. Echocardiography is helpful, and cardiac catheterization reveals the characteristic square root sign during right and left ventricular filling (early diastolic dip in pressure with a subsequent rapid rise to a plateau), and there is equalization of enddiastolic pressures in all four chambers and the pulmonary artery. The right atrial pressure shows sharp x and y descents, resulting in a typical M-shaped contour. CT scan can reveal the thickness of the pericardium.

Therapy includes sodium restriction, diuretics, and pericardiectomy. Surgery should be performed relatively early since atrophy of the underlying myocardium can develop, restricting postoperative improvement.

CONGENITAL HEART DISEASE

Congenital heart diseases are broadly divided into cyanotic and noncyanotic types. Peripheral cyanosis results when there is a shunt of nonoxygenated blood into the left side of the heart (right-to-left shunt), increasing circulating unsaturated venous blood. These forms of heart disease are rare and are seen primarily in infants and children. The most common is **Tetralogy of Fallot**, in which there is an intraventricular septal defect with some degree of pulmonic stenosis and some degree of overriding of the aorta over the right ventricle; right ventricular hypertrophy also is present.

The main forms of congenital heart disease seen in adolescents and adults are the septal defects and coarctation of the aorta. **Atrial septal defect** (ASD) and **ventricular septal defect** (VSD) are most common. Both can cause minimal functional change or can result in CHF. An ASD may cause a systolic flow murmur because of increased flow across the pulmonic valve, with enlargement of the right ventricle. A fixed, widely split second sound (S2) is typical. A VSD usually causes a holosystolic murmur along the left sternal border, often with a thrill, and S2 may be normal or widely split. Both show cardiac enlargement, primarily of the right ventricle on x-ray, and typical echocardiographic findings.

ASD is classified as ostium primum when the defect is low in the atrial septum, ostium secundum when the defect is in the region of the fossa ovalis, or sinus venosus defect when in the upper septum near the entrance of the vena cava. Secundum defects are usually associated with cleft mitral valve or VSD. Sinus venosus lesions are often associated with anomalous drainage of a pulmonary vein into the right atrium, producing a left-to-right shunt. Since the compliance of the right atrium, ventricle, and pulmonary arterial tree is greater than on the left side of the heart, shunting through an ASD is usually from left to right. Echocardiography usually outlines the abnormalities seen with ASD, including the right ventricular dilatation.

With a VSD, shunting is usually left to right, but the hemodynamic consequences of this congenital lesion depend on the size of the lesion. A small defect can have little clinical effect. If large, equal pressures coexist in the two ventricles, and the volume of the shunt depends on the relative resistance of the two arterial trees. As pulmonary vascular resistance increases, flow gradually decreases and may reverse, becoming right to left. There is an increased incidence of aortic insufficiency in patients with ASD, and other congenital defects may occur. Surgical treatment is necessary for ASD and VSD if the hemodynamic effects of the defects are significant.

Coarctation of the aorta is usually not clinically manifest until adolescence or adulthood. Hypertension is found, but it is limited to the upper extremities. Pulses may be weak, and blood pressure is low in the lower part of the body. There is usually evidence of left ventricular hypertrophy, with a heave on palpation and an S4. X-rays show enlargement of the left ventricle and often notching of the underside of the ribs due to the large, tortuous intracostal arteries. Late complications include heart failure and dissecting aneurysm or rupture of the aorta. Associated intracerebral aneurysms are frequent and can also rupture. A bicuspid aortic valve is often associated and is susceptible to SBE. Surgical treatment is essential.

VALVULAR HEART DISEASE

Valvular abnormalities lead to increased myocardial work and ventricular hypertrophy, which increase myocardial oxygen demand. At the same time, the increased intramural pressure decreases coronary blood flow to the myocardium, since blood flow ceases during each cardiac cycle while tissue pressure (myocardial wall tension) is higher than arterial pressure. Some valve abnormalities, such as aortic or mitral valvular insufficiency, cause a volume overload in the ventricle, leading to dilatation and increased oxygen consumption because of the increased wall tension. Mitral or tricuspid regurgitation puts less of a strain on the ventricle than aortic regurgitation, since the abnormal flow is emptying into a chamber of low pressure. Although these valvular abnormalities are relatively well tolerated for long periods, ventricular muscle dysfunction develops with all types of valvular disease. Auscultatory findings are diagnostically useful with valvular lesions. Murmurs are usually heard on physical examination, and often they are characteristic enough to be diagnostic. An S4 gallop is often heard during late diastolic filling of the ventricle when the hypertrophy of the ventricular wall has caused decreased compliance. An S3 gallop develops with the increased early diastolic filling in volume overload states.

Mitral stenosis

Mitral stenosis develops most commonly as a result of rheumatic fever and therefore has decreased in frequency in recent years as rheumatic fever has declined. The other valvular lesions seen in rheumatic fever also occur as a result of degenerative or ill-defined causes and remain common. When fibrosis appears in the mitral valve leaflets as a result of the rheumatic process, they become stiffened, obstructing flow from the left atrium to the ventricle during diastole. Some degree of mitral regurgitation during systole usually occurs concomitantly. As a result, the left atrium enlarges and pressure within it rises. The pressure is transmitted back to the pulmonary venous system (where it must be higher than in the atrium for blood to flow), leading to stiffening of the lungs and causing dyspnea, often with orthopnea and occasionally paroxysmal nocturnal dyspnea. The increased pulmonary vascular resistance causes secondary thickening of the pulmonary vessels. Pressure rises in the pulmonary artery and the right ventricle, which hypertrophies and dilates, and eventually right heart failure appears.

The enlarged left atrium often becomes a source of atrial fibrillation. Since the diminished mitral valve area requires a longer period of diastole for adequate ventricular filling, a rapid heart rate shortens diastole, and cardiac output can decrease markedly. At the same time, pulmonary venous pressure can rise abruptly, and pulmonary edema can develop suddenly. This sequence of events can occur as a result of exercise or when the onset of atrial fibrillation causes a rapid ventricular rate.

Although in the past rheumatic fever usually appeared first in childhood, it required multiple attacks and a long period of gradual valvular fibrosis before mitral stenosis appeared. Functional problems were seen most often in adults in their late 20s to late 40s. Symptoms of dyspnea and findings of right heart failure were most common. Severe hemoptysis could result from the higher venous pressure in dilated and tortuous bronchial veins, which developed because of shunting of pulmonary venous blood into the systemic circulation. Atrial fibrillation because of the poor emptying of the atria led to formation of thrombi. Systemic emboli were major complications in these patients, as they still are in patients with chronic atrial fibrillation, often resulting in hemiplegia or gangrene of an extremity. Late in the course of mitral stenosis, when cardiac output decreased, fatigue, weight loss, and physical wasting became evident.

The classic physical findings of mitral stenosis include an accentuated first heart sound (because of the rapid closure of the valve as left ventricular pressure quickly increases against the high atrial pressure). An opening snap of the mitral valve can be heard if the valve is not heavily calcified. As the process becomes more severe, the interval between S2 and the opening snap shortens, since the higher the left atrial pressure, the shorter the interval before the valve opens. A third heart sound is rarely heard. A low-pitched, diastolic rumbling murmur is heard over the ventricular apex beginning after the opening snap and often extending through all of diastole. A presystolic accentuation of the murmur is characteristic, as flow across the valve increases with atrial contraction. The presystolic accentuation is lost with the onset of atrial fibrillation. The murmur is easiest to hear with the patient lying on the left side (left lateral decubitus position).

Diagnostic decisions. Echocardiography is the preferred method of establishing the diagnosis of mitral stenosis, since it is noninvasive and shows characteristic changes. It can also give an estimate of the cross-sectional area of the valve orifice, probably more accurately than by catheterization. The normal valve area is about 4 cm^2; severe mitral stenosis can decrease the area to less than 1 cm^2.

Therapeutic decisions. Treatment consists of diuretics and salt restriction to decrease the volume overload in the left atrium and digitalis to control the ventricular rate with atrial fibrillation. The inotropic effect of digitalis is of little value in these cases because of the mechanical obstruction to blood flow. Propranolol can be useful to prevent tachycardia with exercise. Systemic emboli require continuous anticoagulation; emboli despite anticoagulation require valve surgery. Functional class III or IV symptoms are also an indication for valve surgery.

Patients with mitral stenosis should receive penicillin prophylaxis to prevent recurrences of rheumatic fever as well as to prevent bacterial endocarditis at the time of dental or other surgery.

Surgery can consist of mitral commissurotomy, valvuloplasty, or replacement with a prosthetic valve. Restenosis usually occurs 8 to 10 years after commissurotomy, but during that period there is no need for anticoagulants. Anticoagulation must be maintained after prosthetic valve replacement. Perioperative mortality is around 2% with commissurotomy and 5% with valve replacement.

Mitral regurgitation

Currently, mitral regurgitation is more often due to a process other than rheumatic fever. However, if combined with aortic valve disease, rheumatic fever is the most likely etiology. Mitral valve prolapse, degenerative changes of the valvular apparatus often with annular calcification, rupture of a chorda tendineae or dysfunction of a papillary muscle after myocardial infarction, and Marfan's syndrome are other known etiologic factors. Mitral regurgitation can occur as a result of marked dilatation of the left ventricle from any cause.

Since the pressure in the left atrium is far below that of the left ventricle, regurgitant flow occurs at a relatively constant rate throughout systole and the murmur of mitral regurgitation is holosystolic and of constant intensity. Left ventricular diastolic volume increases, a large proportion of the outflow during systole going in the wrong direction. Although this diastolic overload can be tolerated for long periods, left ventricular contractility can eventually become irreversibly impaired. The increased diastolic volume leads to a large ventricle that is easily palpable precordially. The increased pressure in the left atrium causes pulmonary hypertension, and right ventricular failure can ensue. Symptoms resemble those seen with mitral stenosis but usually appear at a later age. Atrial fibrillation develops, but not as frequently as in mitral stenosis.

Therapy is also similar to that for mitral stenosis, and surgery is needed when functional class III or IV symptoms develop. Chronic anticoagulation is not usually needed unless emboli occur, but it is needed after valve replacement.

Acute, severe mitral regurgitation appearing after a myocardial infarction results from a ruptured chorda or papillary muscle and is not well tolerated; surgery is usually needed on an emergency basis. Afterload reduction with vasodilating agents can increase the proportion of the ejection fraction that moves forward and can tide a patient over during the interval until surgery can be performed.

Mitral valve prolapse

Mitral valve prolapse, the "floppy valve, click, and murmur syndrome," is a very common condition, especially in women, and is often familial. A variable degree of mitral regurgitation occurs. The manifestations of the regurgitation are similar to those of any other cause. In this condition, the valve leaflets are excessively flaccid and mobile, sometimes due to Marfan's syndrome or other metabolic connective tissue disease but usually without a definable cause. Myxomatous changes can be found on pathological examination. Symptoms are varied, often with chest pain of undefined cause. Ventricular arrhythmias occur, and there is an increased incidence of bacterial endocarditis in these patients. However, the great majority of the patients are asymptomatic and the process discovered only on the basis of the physical findings.

Diagnostic decisions. Echocardiography reveals that during ventricular contraction the mitral leaflets prolapse into the atrium, generating the click and late systolic murmur characteristic of the syndrome. Decreasing the volume of the left ventricle, such as occurs when venous return is decreased by standing or a Valsalva maneuver, causes the prolapse of the valve leaflets to occur earlier in systole, and the click and murmur are heard earlier.

Therapy is usually not needed, except for antibiotic prophylaxis of bacterial endocarditis. Beta-blockers may diminish the frequency of arrhythmias. If severe mitral regurgitation develops, surgical replacement of the valve is necessary.

Aortic stenosis

Congenital bicuspid valves are the most common cause of aortic stenosis today, the valve leaflet gradually thickening, usually with calcification, and becoming stenotic around the sixth decade of life. Aortic stenosis is about three times more common in males. The obstruction to outflow causes elevation of the left ventricular pressure. Hypertrophy of the muscle develops, maintaining stroke volume until late in the course. The thick ventricle is noncompliant, however, and an S4 gallop sound is a common early finding.

Elevated wall tension and hypertrophy increase oxygen demand and decrease coronary blood flow, and angina pectoris commonly develops. Fibrosis appears in the myocardium, and contractility is eventually impaired. Left ventricular enddiastolic pressure becomes elevated. Once the compensatory mechanisms become inadequate, rapid progression is usual, leading to angina, heart failure, syncope, and sudden death if the obstruction is not relieved surgically.

The cardinal symptoms of aortic stenosis are angina, syncope, and symptoms of left ventricular failure, such as dyspnea and orthopnea and paroxysmal nocturnal dyspnea. A systolic ejection murmur is audible, radiating into the neck. Sometimes it is very loud and there is a thrill. The murmur has a crescendo-descrescendo or "diamond-shaped" quality (the latter term is based on its characteristic appearance on a phonocardiogram), reflecting the changes in rate of flow across the valve during systole. The aortic second sound is usually decreased or absent, or there is paradoxical splitting of S2. The precordial impulse is increased, with a left ventricular "heave" or lift. An S4 gallop can often be felt as well as heard. An aortic ejection click is occasionally heard in congenital stenosis. The pulse classically is diminished in volume and rises gradually (pulsus parvus et tardus). There may be accompanying aortic regurgitation, adding a diastolic murmur to the physical findings.

Diagnostic decisions. Echocardiography is diagnostic, although it may not give an accurate estimate of the area of the valve orifice. The degree of left ventricular hypertrophy, however, is a good reflection of the degree of stenosis. Cardiac catheterization is needed to determine the size of the valve orifice and the gradient across the valve. It should be performed as soon as a patient develops syncope, angina, or left ventricular failure.

Therapeutic decisions. Surgical valve replacement is usually necessary and has the best prognosis if left ventricular function is still good. Valve replacement is usually advisable before symptoms appear in children with congenital aortic stenosis. Anticoagulation is necessary after replacement with a mechanical prosthesis. Porcine valves do not require anticoagulation, but their durability is probably less.

Aortic regurgitation

The most common causes of valvular lesions producing aortic regurgitation used to be rheumatic fever and syphilis, but other causes are more common now, including bacterial endocarditis, ankylosing spondylitis, rheumatoid arthritis, and congenital lesions. With aortic regurgitation, the backflow of blood into the left ventricle causes volume overload, increasing the stretch of the myocardial fibrils and strengthening contractility, according to the Frank-Starling mechanism. The volume of each systole increases, but when the volume in the left ventricular exceeds its capacity to dilate, enddiastolic pressure rises and left atrial pressure increases similarly. The backflow of blood into the ventricle decreases diastolic pressure in the aorta, giving the widened pulse pressure characteristic of this syndrome. Coronary blood flow occurs during diastole and therefore is decreased. The increased work performed by the ventricular muscle increases oxygen demand, and therefore anginal pain occurs frequently. These patients may remain asymptomatic for years, but overstretching of the myofibrils can result in irreversible deterioration in cardiac function before symptoms develop.

The adaptive processes in chronic aortic regurgitation slow the progression of the disease, and the course is usually more slowly progressive than that of aortic stenosis. Syncope and sudden death are rare, in contrast to aortic stenosis. Once heart failure appears, it usually responds better to therapy with salt restriction, digitalis, diuretics, and careful afterload reduction, at least at first.

Acute regurgitation, such as occurs with infective endocarditis, can lead to rapidly progressive symptoms, and surgical correction can be required urgently. The rapid progression may result from the fact that increasing the diastolic volume in the left ventricle causes the enddiastolic pressure to rise quickly, probably because the thickened ventricle is relatively noncompliant. This enddiastolic pressure is reflected back into the left atrium and pulmonary vascular bed, and there can be a sudden onset of severe pulmonary edema.

The systemic arterial blood pressure adapts to slow onset of regurgitation by peripheral vasodilatation, decreasing systemic vascular resistance to permit better peripheral runoff. Diastolic arterial pressure therefore falls. This adaptive process does not occur when the regurgitation suddenly appears and becomes severe, aggravating the problem of decreased peripheral flow.

The physical findings in aortic regurgitation include the wide pulse pressure and manifestations of a hyperdynamic circulation, including head bobbing with each systole, pistol shot sounds and to-and-fro murmurs over major arteries with slight compression (Duroziez's sign), pulsating capillaries in the nail beds (Quincke's sign), etc. Various eponyms are applied to these findings. Interestingly, the systolic blood pressure in the legs is considerably higher than in the arms, and this sign is the most dependable. The second heart sound may be decreased. The murmur of aortic regurgitation is usually best heard with the patient upright and leaning forward; it may be faint and heard only in expiration. It is high pitched, beginning shortly after the second sound in early diastole and decreasing in intensity later in diastole (descresendo). If the regurgitation is severe, it can become loud and can extend through most of diastole. The left ventricular impulse is displaced laterally and downward and increased in force and area. In some severe cases, a late diastolic rumble may be heard, resembling the murmur of mitral stenosis— an **Austin Flint murmur** (remember the A for aortic regurgitation). It probably results from early closure of the mitral valve as a result of the increased pressure in the left ventricle in late diastole.

Diagnostic decisions. Echocardiography shows the dilated left ventricle and aortic root, fluttering of the anterior leaflet of the mitral valve caused by the regurgitant jet, and sometimes changes in the mitral valve leaflets documenting multiple valvular lesions as is seen in rheumatic fever. Cardiac catheterization is useful to quantitate the degree of regurgitation, the pressure changes, and the state of left ventricular function.

Therapeutic decisions. Therapy with digitalis, diuretics, and salt restriction is of temporary value only, and surgery is usually necessary, preferably before irreversible changes in ventricular function develop. Prosthetic valves require long-term anti-coagulation.

Right-sided valve lesions

Tricuspid lesions are rare. Regurgitation is usually the result of extreme right ventricular dilatation. Stenosis can occur as a result of rheumatic fever. The findings are predictable from the pressure changes in the right atrium, reflected in the neck veins. Hepatomegaly is common and can show systolic pulsations with tricuspid regurgitation. Echocardiography is the most useful diagnostic test. Stenotic lesions may require surgery, but otherwise, measures directed at the cause of the right ventricular failure are the basis of treatment.

Pulmonary valve lesions are usually congenital, detected in early childhood, and require surgical correction. Acquired pulmonary regurgitation can result from extreme right ventricular enlargement as a result of mitral stenosis. The murmur of pulmonary valvular insufficiency that is heard in these cases resembles that of aortic insufficiency. When it occurs with mitral stenosis, it is called a **Graham Steell's murmur** (remember the S for mitral stenosis.)

IMPORTANT ARRHYTHMIAS

Patients vary greatly in sensitivity to symptoms of arrhythmias, which include palpitations, syncope, and manifestations of heart failure. Patients may sense a slow or sudden of onset of palpitations, slow or rapid heartbeat, and irregularities. Physical exam can detect underlying systemic or cardiac disease, evidence of AV dissociation (variation in jugular venous pulse, canon a waves, and variation on intensity of SI, called bruit de canon) due to variation in ventricular filling as atrial contraction varies in its relation to ventricular systole.

Disturbances of the sinus node

Sinus tachycardia (a regular rhythm >100 beats/minute) occurs with fever, anxiety, hyperthyroidism, anemia, as an effect of drugs including alcohol, catecholamines, and atropine, as well as a result of pulmonary and cardiac disease. Therapy should be aimed at the underlying cause. **Sinus bradycardia** produces a regular rhythm less than 60 beats/minute and occurs in well-trained athletes, increased intracranial pressure, myxedema, hypothermia, and as an effect of vagal stimulation, parasympathomimetic drugs or beta-adrenergic blocking drugs, or amiodarone. Bradycardia can occur during the acute phase of an inferior myocardial infarction. Treatment of bradycardia is usually not necessary, but if cardiac output is low it can be helped by speeding the heart rate with atropine or, if necessary, isoproterenol. No drugs may be effective, and cardiac pacing can be necessary. P waves are normal in these arrhythmias.

Sinus arrhythmia is defined as a variation in sinus rate with variations in respiratory cycle of over 10%. Treatment is not necessary. **Sinus pause** or **sinus arrest** results in P waves with intervals that bear no relationship to the normal interval, whereas **sinoatrial exit block** occurs with P-P intervals that are multiples of the normal interval, implying that an impulse was generated that did not exit the node to cause atrial depolarization and the sinus node kept to its regular rhythmicity. Myocardial infarction, degenerative changes, or excessive vagal tone can produce these changes. An underlying disease should be treated, but the rhythm disturbance usually needs no treatment. However, if symptoms develop, pacing is necessary. **Carotid sinus hypersensitivity** causes sinus arrest or sinoatrial exit block as a result of light pressure over the carotid sinus receptors. AV block can occur. To warrant this diagnosis, by definition, symptoms and ventricular asystole of over 3 seconds must occur with pressure over the carotid sinus. The vasodepressor form of carotid sinus hypersensitivity causes a fall in systolic pressure of 30 to 50 mm Hg. Treatment in symptomatic patients requires ventricular pacing, but the vasodepressor form may not respond adequately to pacing or atropine. Surgical denervation of the carotid sinus may be required.

The term **sick sinus syndrome** refers to a variety of sinus and AV nodal abnormalities, including spontaneous sinus bradycardia, sinus arrest or exit block, combination of sinus node and AV nodal conduction abnormalities, and alternating paroxysms of atrial tachyarrhythmias and bradyarrhythmias (the brady-tachy syndrome). Pacing for symptomatic bradyarrhythmia and drug therapy for tachyarrhythmia may be needed.

Atrial arrhythmias

Premature atrial contractions (PACs) are not usually followed by a compensatory pause, in contrast to PVCs. PACs occur without underlying heart disease in the presence of fever, inflammation, infection, or as a reaction to emotional stress, alcohol, tobacco, or caffeine. They can occur as a result of myocardial ischemia. Ordinarily they do not require therapy but can develop into a form of chronic supraventricular tachycardia.

With **atrial flutter,** the rate of atrial contraction is 250 to 300/minute, but the ventricular rate is usually half that (2:1 block). A greater degree of block in the absence of drugs suggests an underlying abnormality in conduction. The atrial activity is seen on ECG as regular peaked waves occurring without isoelectric intervals between. Ventricular contractions are usually regular with atrial flutter, since there is usually a 2:1 block, allowing half the atrial contractions to be transmitted, but irregular conduction can occur. Chronic atrial flutter is usually associated with underlying heart disease, but paroxysmal atrial flutter occurs with hyperthyroidism, alcoholism, pericarditis, and pulmonary embolism. Patients with flutter have fewer systemic emboli than those with atrial fibrillation.

Carotid sinus massage usually does not terminate atrial flutter, although the increased vagal effect may slow the ventricular response. Verapamil, beta-blockers, or digitalis may slow the ventricular response, and sinus rhythm may resume. Cardioversion (usually requiring less than 50 joules) can restore sinus rhythm, but atrial fibrillation may develop, requiring a second shock of higher energy. Drugs such as quinidine, procainamide, or disopyramide may terminate the atrial flutter and are useful in prevention of recurrences. They should not be administered unless measures are taken to cause increased AV block, such as administration of digitalis, since they may not change the basic atrial rhythm while reducing the atrial rate to around 200. At that rate, 1:1 ventricular conduction can occur, giving a ventricular rate that can cause hemodynamic compromise.

Atrial tachycardia, with rates of 150 to 200, is associated with variable degrees of conduction. The ECG shows periods of isoelectric intervals between atrial contractions, in contrast to atrial flutter. This rhythm disturbance is usually due to digitalis toxicity in patients with significant organic heart disease. Stopping the digitalis is usually sufficient therapy. If the arrhythmia is not due to digitalis, that drug is useful to slow the ventricular rate, and atrial activity can subsequently be corrected with quinidine, procainamide, or disopyramide.

Atrial fibrillation causes totally chaotic, ineffective contractions. Conduction is variable, and therefore the ventricular rhythm is irregularly irregular, usually with a rate between 100 and 160. It is easier to slow the ventricular response in atrial fibrillation than with atrial flutter. Chronic atrial fibrillation is usually associated with underlying heart disease. In the past, rheumatic heart disease with mitral valve abnormalities was the most frequent cause. Hyperthyroidism, pulmonary emboli, cardiomyopathy, and hypertensive or ischemic heart disease may be present. Systemic emboli occur with considerable frequency in patients with atrial fibrillation, and the abnormal rhythm can cause significant deterioration in cardiac function, particularly in patients with valvular disease. Physical examination reveals the irregular rhythm, variation in the intensity of the heart sounds due to differences in ventricular filling. A pulse deficit (ventricular rate exceeds radial pulse rate) is usually present in patients with rapid ventricular rates.

The first principle in **therapy** of atrial fibrillation, as in any

arrhythmia, is to seek and treat any underlying precipitating cause, such as hyperthyroidism or pulmonary emboli. If atrial fibrillation is associated with increased heart failure, DC cardioversion is indicated, usually requiring 100 to 200 joules. If cardiac function is satisfactory, digitalis can be given to increase the degree of AV nodal block, decreasing the ventricular rate to around 60 to 80 beats/minute. Beta-blockers or calcium channel blockers can also be used to decrease the ventricular rate. Quinidine can be used to attempt to convert to sinus rhythm or to maintain sinus rhythm after cardioversion, but patients with chronic atrial fibrillation (especially if over 1 year duration) usually return to atrial fibrillation. Anticoagulants are usually given for 2 weeks prior and 2 weeks after conversion, to decrease the likelihood of emboli at the time atrial contraction is restored.

Ventricular arrhythmias

PVCs appear on the ECG as early, bizarre, prolonged QRS complexes, clearly differing in contour from the normal QRS seen in that lead. The T wave is large and always opposite in direction from the main deflection in the QRS. There is usually no retrograde conduction to the atria and sinus node. Therefore a **compensatory pause** occurs, since the regular sinus beat meets refractoriness at the AV node or below and is not conducted, but the sinus continues at its regular rate and the following regular beat is conducted. Hence the interval between two normal complexes flanking the PVC is at the interval between three normal beats.

Couplets of PVCs occur, but three in a row, with a rate of over 100/minute, is defined as a paroxysm of ventricular tachycardia. If the PVCs have a different shape on the ECG, they are considered multifocal. Although usually asymptomatic, PVCs can cause palpitations and frequently cause hypotension since the early beats occur before there is adequate ventricular filling, decreasing stroke volume. Anemia, ischemia, fever, infection, anesthesia, tobacco, alcohol, caffeine, anesthetics, and emotional stress increase the frequency of PVCs.

Therapy is not necessary for occasional PVCs in a patient without organic heart disease. PVCs are associated with an increased incidence of sudden death in patients with ischemic heart disease, hypertrophic cardiomyopathy, and mitral valve prolapse. Although therapy has not been shown to decrease the frequency of sudden death in these patients, maintenance quinidine, procainamide, or disopyramide is usually given after a period of IV lidocaine if emergency therapy is necessary.

Ventricular tachycardia can be difficult to differentiate from supraventricular tachycardias with bundle branch block or other intraventricular conduction abnormalities, which may appear as a result of the ischemia caused by the tachycardia. There are subtle ECG findings that can help to make the distinction, and the ventricular rate can be slowed with supraventricular tachycardias by increasing vagal tone to increase the degree of AV block (e.g., with carotid sinus stimulation). Similarly, a P-R interval of <100 msec, more atrial impulses than ventricular (e.g., 2:1 conduction), appearance of wide QRS complexes after a long/short cycle, and rsR′ in V1 all favor supraventricular origin. Evidence for alteration of some QRS complexes by conduction of occasional atrial impulses (fusion beats, i.e., partial alteration of the QRS) makes a ventricular origin of the tachyarrhythmia likely. Ventricular flutter causes regular sine wave oscillations on the ECG, at 150 to 300/minute.

Ventricular tachycardia occurring in patients hospitalized for acute myocardial infarction increases the mortality rate during the first year. This rhythm abnormality usually indicates serious underlying heart disease. Patients with episodes associated with symptoms or recurrent sustained ventricular tachycardia should be treated. Some physicians also treat those with asymptomatic, nonsustained tachycardias. Emergency **therapy** consists of IV lidocaine or, if that is unsuccessful, procainamide or bretylium. Hypotension, angina, symptoms of decreased cerebral perfusion, or cardiac decompensation requires immediate therapy with DC cardioversion (10 to 50 joules) synchronized with the QRS to avoid precipitating ventricular fibrillation. It may be necessary to cardiovert ventricular tachycardia induced by digitalis despite the increased risk. Underlying aggravating causes should be treated before starting maintenance drug therapy; quinidine, procainamide, disopyramide, and tocainide are used. Phenytoin can be useful in patients on digitalis; beta-blockers are useful in patients who have angina or excessive catecholamine stimulation. Combinations of drugs may be necessary. Recurrences despite drug therapy may be treated with pacing.

A polymorphic form of ventricular tachycardia with unusual ECG characteristics, **torsades de pointes**, more often leads to ventricular fibrillation, and therapy is more urgent. The ECG shows QRS complexes that change in amplitude and appear to twist around the isoelectric line, with a long Q-T interval. A variety of drugs can induce this syndrome, including the antiarrhythmic agents, psychoactive drugs (phenothiazines, tricyclic antidepressants), and metabolic abnormalities including potassium depletion. Temporary pacing may be needed to control the tachycardia, and isoproterenol, magnesium, and bretylium are reportedly useful.

Congenital ECG abnormalities including prolonged Q-T intervals and the full torsades de pointes occur, and there is increased risk of sudden death, especially when it has occurred earlier in family members. If there is no family history or symptoms, therapy is not recommended. With episodes of syncope, beta-blockers are useful, combined with phenytoin or phenobarbital if necessary. If drugs fail to prevent recurrent syncope, left cervicothoracic sympathetic ganglionectomy is reported to be effective.

Ventricular fibrillation is fatal in 3 to 5 minutes, since no cardiac output occurs. It rarely if ever ceases on its own. There is usually underlying heart disease, such as an acute myocardial ischemic episode, with or without infarction, or a precipitating accidental electric shock. Immediate nonsynchronized DC cardioversion with 200 to 400 joules is necessary. Acidosis and hypoxia develop rapidly and should be treated as quickly as possible. Lidocaine or a similar drug should be given IV after conversion to prevent recurrence.

Therapeutic decisions. Ventricular arrhythmias are the most common cause of sudden cardiac death. About three-fifths of patients resuscitated from ventricular fibrillation have an underlying extensive coronary artery disease, but only 20% have an acute myocardial infarction. Most have previous symptoms of heart disease. Patients with ventricular fibrillation

at the time of an acute MI usually do not need long-term antiarrhythmic therapy, but chronic or late ventricular tachyarrhythmias do require such therapy. Other causes of ventricular tachyarrhythmias associated with sudden cardiac death include mitral valve prolapse, cardiomyopathies, myocarditis, antiarrhythmic drugs, and ECG syndromes including prolonged Q-T interval, Wolff-Parkinson-White syndrome. The occurrence of complex ventricular ectopy, such as multiform PVCs, pairs, and ventricular tachycardias in patients who survive infarction, have an increased incidence of sudden cardiac death. It is not proved that drugs lower this frequency, but prophylactic therapy is probably indicated. Poor left ventricular function definitely increases the incidence of sudden cardiac death in patients with any type of rhythm disturbance. Antiarrhythmic therapy is indicated in patients who have had a cardiac arrest without a myocardial infarct or who have recurrent symptomatic ventricular tachyarrhythmias. Coronary artery bypass surgery alone usually is not sufficient therapy to prevent recurrent ventricular tachyarrhythmias.

Prolonged ECG monitoring (Holter monitor) is useful to determine the frequency and nature of arrhythmias and the effectiveness of a drug regimen. Implantable defibrillators are becoming available for arrhythmias that cannot be controlled with drugs.

HEART BLOCK

A defect in conduction of supraventricular impulses is referred to as heart block. In **first-degree AV block**, there is prolongation of the P-R interval; all beats are conducted. In **type I second-degree block**, there is progressive lengthening of the P-R interval, until a beat is not conducted (the Wenckeback phenomenon). **Type II** refers to occasional block in conduction of an atrial beat without prior changes in the P-R interval and is more serious since it often progresses to syncopal episodes due to **complete AV block** (Stokes-Adams attacks). Type I block is usually benign. It can occur in athletes and is typical of acute rheumatic carditis. In patients with myocardial infarction, type I block usually occurs when the infarct is inferior, and it is transient, not requiring a pacemaker. Type II usually occurs with anterior infarcts, and temporary or permanent pacing may be required. It is associated with a higher mortality, primarily because of extensive tissue damage leading to pump failure. Either type I or type II AV block can occur as a result of drugs that decrease AV nodal conduction (e.g., digitalis, beta-blockers, calcium channel blockers).

In complete AV block, there is no conduction from the atria to the ventricles. The ventricular rate is slow but regular. When the pacemaker is in the AV node, QRS complexes are of normal configuration and the rate is 40 to 60 and is affected by autonomic influences. When the block is lower in the conducting system (bundle of His or Purkinje's fibers), the pacemaker is in a ventricle and there are wide QRS complexes at a slower rate with less autonomic influence. **Congenital AV block** in children is usually asymptomatic. In adults, a wide variety of diseases can cause heart block, including electrolyte abnormalities and drug effects. Therapy for AV block includes atropine (for AV nodal block), isoproterenol, which can affect block at any level, and ventricular pacing.

Therapeutic decisions. Temporary pacing is definitely indicated for any type of complete AV block that is symptomatic, as well as for asymptomatic cases due to surgery and probably all type II cases. **Pacing** is also definitely indicated during acute myocardial infarction, for (1) a newly acquired bifascicular bundle branch block (BBB), (2) newly acquired BBB with transient complete AV block, (3) appearance of type II second-degree AV block, or (4) complete heart block. It is also indicated for the following lesions if symptomatic: (1) atrial fibrillation with a slow ventricular response, (2) sick sinus (brady-tachy) syndrome, and (3) hypersensitive carotid sinus syndrome. In most of these instances, permanent pacing is often necessary (except for newly acquired bifascicular BBB).

AV dissociation, independent electrical activity in the atria and ventricles, can occur as a result of slowing of the sinus node, allowing escape of a ventricular pacemaker or activation of a ventricular focus discharging at a faster rate than the sinus node. Therapy depends on the nature of the underlying abnormality.

Syncope in cardiac disease is usually due to inadequate cerebral perfusion because of low cardiac output. It occurs in severe aortic stenosis, hypertrophic obstructive cardiomyopathy, other obstructive valvular lesions, and massive pulmonary embolus. These episodes usually occur when exercise decreases the systemic vascular resistance and the heart is unable to increase output sufficiently past the obstructing lesion. Both fast and slow arrhythmias can cause syncope, as can the hypersensitive carotid sinus syndrome.

Other causes of syncope include **vasovagal syncope,** which refers to fainting, usually due to stress or pain, probably the result of vagal hyperfunction slowing heart rate. Benign syncope can also occur with **coughing** or urination (**micturition syncope**), probably as a result of similar vagal effects. The **hypersensitive carotid sinus syndrome** is potentially more serious and can require pacing. **Orthostatic hypotension** is a common cause of syncope, especially with volume depletion, after a long period of bed rest. Many drugs, particularly those used in the treatment of hypertension, can cause it. More difficult to manage problems of orthostasis occur with autonomic dysfunction in diabetics and in Parkinson's disease.

Some pointers about **antiarrhythmic drugs** follow:

Lidocaine has extensive first-pass metabolism in the liver and thus is only useful IV. It is useful for a variety of ventricular arrhythmias but is generally ineffective against supraventricular arrhythmias.

Tocainide is an analogue of lidocaine that is effective PO, but it is less effective.

Quinidine is useful PO against atrial and ventricular tachyarrhythmias. It has vagolytic actions as well as alpha-adrenergic blocking effects and may cause significant hypotension. Decreasing vagal effect on AV nodal conduction can increase the ventricular response in patients with atrial flutter, and therefore the patient should be digitalized beforehand. Quinidine increases serum levels of digoxin and digitoxin.

Procainamide is similar to quinidine but has less anticholinergic effect. High doses depress ventricular function. It does not increase digoxin levels but does cause a systemic lupus erythematosus (SLE) syndrome. About 60 to 70% of patients who receive procainamide develop antinuclear antibodies

(ANA), but less than half of them develop symptoms. Manifestations of SLE gradually clear after stopping the drug; therefore, a positive ANA is not a reason to stop the drug.

Disopyramide has a greater anticholinergic effect than either quinidine or lidocaine but has no antiadrenergic effects. It does have marked negative inotropic effects, however, and should rarely be used in patients with poor ventricular function. It does not alter digitalis metabolism.

Phenytoin is useful for treating either atrial or ventricular arrhythmias due to digitalis toxicity but has little value in other types of arrhythmias.

Of the calcium channel blockers, **verapamil** is most useful for arrhythmias. It can decrease the ventricular response in patients with atrial flutter or fibrillation, even if maneuvers that increase vagal activity are ineffective, but it rarely converts them to sinus rhythm.

Before using any antiarrhythmic drugs on a chronic basis, underlying predisposing factors should be corrected. These include thryotoxicosis, digitalis toxicity, hypokalemia, hypomagnesemia, hypoxemia, or any other metabolic abnormalities. CHF should be corrected, as should anemia or infection. Smoking, alcohol intake, caffeine or theophylline intake, and over-the-counter-drugs with cardiostimulants (e.g., nasal decongestants) should be eliminated.

CARDIOVERSION AND CARDIOPULMONARY RESUSCITATION

A note on cardioversion

Before elective cardioversion is performed, the patient should be told about the procedure, a thorough physical examination should be performed including palpation of all pulses, blood gases and electrolytes should be adjusted, and the patient should be fasted for 6 to 8 hours. Digitalis should be withheld the morning of cardioversion. Diazepam or a rapidly acting barbiturate should be used for sedation. An IV should be started and resuscitation equipment should be available. Shocks of 25 to 50 joules are adequate for most tachyarrhythmias; atrial fibrillation usually requires 100 to 200 joules and ventricular fibrillation 100 to 400. If low-energy shocks fail to terminate the arrhythmia, the shocks should be repeated at higher energy. Patients at high risk for emboli (e.g., history of emboli, mitral stenosis, enlarged left atrium or ventricle, prosthetic valve, or significant heart failure) should receive anticoagulants. Most supraventricular and ventricular tachyarrhythmias terminate with DC shock, although rhythms due to increased automaticity (irritability), especially if caused by digitalis, may not.

Basics of cardiopulmonary resuscitation

Remember the ABCs: airway, breathing, and circulation. Be sure that the mouth and pharynx are not obstructed. Tilt the head backward and hyperextend the neck to remove the tongue from the posterior pharynx. If no breathing is noted, give four quick mouth-to-mouth breaths, checking to see if the chest rises with each breath. If so, do not waste time on intubation. If no carotid pulse is detected, start external cardiac compression, over the lower half of the sternum (not the xiphoid process), with the patient on a hard surface. Depress the sternum 3 to 5 cm approximately 60 times a minute, with a ratio of 5 compressions to 1 ventilation with two rescuers, or 15 compressions alternating with 2 ventilations every 15 seconds if alone.

Principles of advanced life support. Defibrillate as soon as possible; it is the single most definitive therapy for most cardiac arrests.

Start oxygen and a fast-running IV infusion.

Administer sodium bicarbonate, 1 mEq/kg IV, to treat metabolic acidosis if there has been any significant period of arrest; repeat every 10 minutes until blood gas measurements are available to serve as a guide.

If asystole or fine ventricular fibrillation of low amplitude is present, epinephrine (5 to 10 ml of a 1:10,000 solution) can be given IV or into the heart every 5 minutes as needed.

Profound bradycardia can be treated with atropine, given IV as 0.5-mg boluses at 5-minute intervals, to a total dose of 2 to 4 mg. If ineffective, isoproterenol can be started as a constant infusion at 2 to 20 μg/minute, titrating the rate of infusion by the heart rate.

If both these measures do not correct the bradycardia, emergency insertion of a pacemaker is necessary.

Other therapeutic decisions. Ventricular tachyarrhythmias can be treated and recurrences prevented with IV lidocaine, procainamide, or bretylium tosylate. Pulmonary edema can be treated with IV furosemide and morphine. Myocardial contractility can be increased with calcium chloride (2.5 to 5.0 ml of a 10% solution), especially if electromechanical dissociation is present, but calcium should be given with caution to a patient known to have excess digitalis effect. Be sure not to give calcium chloride in the same solution as bicarbonate, since a precipitate will form. Electromechanical dissociation can be caused by inadequate cardiac filling due to hypovolemia, pericardial tamponade, or pulmonary embolus. Massive fluid replacement is necessary for hypovolemia. Pericardiocentesis for tamponade and emergency embolectomy might be attempted for a massive embolus blocking flow into the pulmonary circulation.

PERIPHERAL VASCULAR DISEASE

Arterial disease

The most common manifestation of arterial peripheral vascular disease is **intermittent claudication**, pain and fatigue of muscles during use, relieved by rest. The pain is often described as a cramp. Calf muscles are most commonly affected, as a result of femoral artery arteriosclerotic disease, but more proximal disease in the aortoiliac area can cause claudication in the thigh, buttock, or low back, sometimes with impotence (Leriche's syndrome). Rest pain, usually worse at night, occurs with more severe arterial disease and often has a "stocking" distribution, suggesting a neuropathic origin.

The patient may note numbness and coldness, which can be confirmed on examination, revealing diminished pulses and sometimes bruits over narrowed vessels. Pallor, trophic changes as a result of the ischemia (e.g., loss of hair, shininess of the skin, and in more advanced instances muscle atrophy), and delayed venous filling when the limb is made dependent can also be detected. Ulcerations, especially over the malleoli, and areas of gangrene can appear, especially in diabetics, but these symptoms usually remain stable for long periods.

A specific syndrome of upper extremity arteriosclerosis, the **subclavian steal syndrome**, results from obstruction near the origin of the subclavian artery. In these cases, use of the arm, increasing flow into the subclavian artery, can cause reversal of flow in the vertebral artery, resulting in syndromes suggestive of a vertebral-basilar artery transient ischemic attacks such as drowsiness or faintness, vertigo, paresthesias of the face, vision abnormalities, ataxia, or dysarthria. Doppler studies are useful for localizing and quantitating obstructive arterial lesions.

Therapeutic decisions. Therapy for arteriosclerotic peripheral vascular disease consists of exercise to tolerance; avoidance of tobacco, beta-blockers, or other drugs that decrease peripheral flow; meticulous care of the skin and nails to avoid trauma and infection; and avoidance of exposure to cold. Angioplasty or bypass surgery is necessary if the lesions threaten to progress to gangrene or exercise tolerance is so low that it interferes with life-style. Amputation is necessary if gangrene or intractable infection appears. Vasodilating drugs are of little value and may aggravate the ischemia by increasing flow to less-affected areas.

Arterial emboli originate in the atrium, usually as a result of atrial fibrillation, or in the ventricle, usually at the site of an aneurysm resulting from an infarct. A "paradoxical embolus" originates in the venous system and crosses an open foramen ovale (or other right-to-left shunt), settling in the systemic circulation. Emboli tend to deposit at arterial bifurcations (one lodged at the bifurcation of the aorta is called a saddle embolus) and areas of narrowing caused by atherosclerotic plaques. A thrombus usually forms and propagates distally. An arterial embolus usually causes a sudden onset of pain, numbness, paresthesias, and coolness in the affected area, with absent pulses distal to the site of obstruction. The severity of the process depends on the extent of collateral circulation. Therapy consists of keeping the affected area warm to minimize vasospasm, administering heparin to prevent further emboli and thrombus propagation, administering streptokinase or human thromboplastin activator, or surgical removal of the embolus if possible. Amputation is necessary if gangrene develops. The source of the embolus should be eliminated or chronic anticoagulant therapy given, but anticoagulant therapy does not prevent recurrent atheromatous emboli, which typically arise from an atheromatous lesion in the aorta.

An **arteriovenous fistula** can result from a traumatically induced communication between an artery and a vein, or it can be congenital. The area around the fistula becomes warm, while there is coolness more distally. The rapid runoff lowers the diastolic pressure, and a bruit and thrill may be detectable over the lesion. Cardiac output increases, and high-output failure can result. The pulse rate is increased, and compression over the fistula causes a prompt fall in pulse rate (Branham's sign). Traumatic fistulas require surgical treatment, but congenital lesions are usually multiple, and only very large ones are approached surgically.

Raynaud's phenomenon

Raynaud's phenomenon, painful coldness of the fingers and sometimes of the toes, often extending more proximally, is precipitated by exposure to cold or emotional stimuli. It results from vasospasm and can occur without underlying disease (and is then called Raynaud's disease) but usually is associated with arteriosclerosis or a connective tissue disease. Scleroderma, polymyositis, and SLE are the most common underlying connective tissue diseases. Trauma (such as occurs in jackhammer operators), nerve compression syndromes (especially carpal tunnel), other neurological diseases, or frostbite may be initiating factors, as may a hematologic abnormality such as cryoglobulinemia. Drugs that cause vasospasm can induce or aggravate the problem, including ergotamine or beta-blockers. Women are more commonly affected.

During an attack, the fingers typically turn white and later become cyanotic. After the attack they may be red from hyperemia. Minor trophic changes may occur in the skin, resulting in a dry, shiny, atrophic appearance without any fine hairs, but thickening and loss of flexibility indicate underlying scleroderma. Dilated, tortuous, abnormal capillaries can be seen in the nail folds in patients with scleroderma with the aid of an enlarging lens such as an ophthalmoscope. Treatment involves elimination of smoking, avoidance of exposure to cold, and use of vasodilating agents such as calcium channel blockers. Biofeedback is often useful.

Frostbite occurs most often with exposure to cold and dampness, tissue damage probably resulting from freezing and vasoconstriction. Edema and blister formation can occur with thawing. Prolonged immersion in water produces a similar syndrome (immersion or trench foot) without the exposure to cold, because of intense vasoconstriction. Treatment consists of immediate but not excessive rewarming; massage and exercise should be avoided. Care to prevent infection is extremely important. Development of gangrene requires amputation.

Venous disease

Varicose veins and peripheral thrombophlebitis are the most common venous problems. Venous stasis or injury predisposes to phlebitis, and other risk factors include underlying malignancies, use of oral contraceptives, pregnancy, prolonged immobilization, heart disease, or major surgery. Calf veins are the most common sites of thrombophlebitis. The problem may be asymptomatic, but local pain and tenderness, swelling of the calf, and asymmetric edema frequently develop. Tenderness may be detected on compression or by having the patient dorsiflex the foot (Homans' sign). A palpable venous cord is sometimes detectable, especially if the phlebitis is superficial. None of the findings are dependable, since thrombi that are the source of pulmonary emboli often occur without any of these findings. Aids to diagnosis include Doppler exam and venography.

Therapeutic decisions. Management includes elevation of an affected extremity to eliminate the effect of gravity on venous flow, use of NSAIDs, and anticoagulation. Heparin should be given immediately to raise the PTT to 2 to 2.5 times normal while coumarin is started. The heparin can be discontinued as soon as the PT is in a therapeutic range. Ambulation is safe after about a week, and elastic support stockings should be worn. Recurrent thrombophlebitis requires chronic anticoagulation, but if there is a contraindication to anticoagulation (e.g., hypertension or an active peptic ulcer) or if pulmonary emboli occur despite anticoagulation, surgery to introduce a permanent obstruction in the vena cava (such as plication or introduction of an "umbrella") is necessary. Clot-dissolving agents, such as streptokinase, urokinase, or human tissue plasminogen activator, may be useful but are clearly indicated for severe iliofemoral thrombophlebitis. Low-dose (minidose) heparin seems to prevent phlebitis from developing in many situations, including following major surgery or myocardial infarction.

SURGERY IN PATIENTS WITH HEART DISEASE

General anesthetics, especially spinal anesthetics, reduce myocardial contractility and can cause hypotension. There is no overall difference in risk between general and spinal anesthesia. The risk of surgery is determined by the extent of the procedure. Herniorraphy and transurethral prostatectomy have a low risk, but chest and abdominal surgery a much higher risk. Among patients who had an antecedent myocardial infarction, the reinfarction rate is 4 to 8%, and the mortality from perioperative infarction is higher in this group. Patients with stable angina have about the same risk as those with a history of prior myocardial infarction. Elective surgery should not be performed on patients with unstable angina until the cardiac problem is stablized and, if possible, the need for coronary artery surgery evaluated. Following a myocardial infarct, the mortality rate falls off as the time from the infarct increases and becomes level after about 6 months.

Decompensated heart failure should be treated before surgery, any arrhythmias controlled, and pacing instituted for symptomatic heart block. Patients with valvular disease or prosthetic heart valves should receive antibiotic prophylaxis for endocarditis. Mild to moderate hypertension does not alter the risk of surgery, but severe hypertension should be controlled prior to surgery.

HEART DISEASE AND PREGNANCY

The cardiac output increases in pregnancy, peaking at 30 to 50% above basal in the 20th to 24th week. Heart rate is usually increased about 10 beats/minute. Stroke volume increases, as does blood volume (40 to 50%). Systemic and pulmonary vascular resistance are decreased, as is systolic blood pressure. A midsystolic murmur may appear, as can edema, fatigue, dyspnea, and decreased exercise tolerance. Mitral stenosis is aggravated by the increased output and heart rate. The incidence of heart failure increases, as does the risk of complications from atrial fibrillation, emboli, and endocarditis. If pregnancy is expected, a porcine valve should be used for surgical replacement since it avoids need for prophylactic anticoagulation. Heparin does not cross the placenta but coumarin does.

HYPERTENSION

Hypertension can be defined as blood pressure greater than 140/90 mm Hg, but morbidity and mortality rates increase progressively with increasing blood pressure, beginning below that level. No threshold blood pressure level has been defined. Nevertheless, the following standards are in general use:

Diastolic Pressure (mm Hg)

Normal	<85
High normal	85–90
Mild hypertension	90–104
Moderate hypertension	105–119
Severe hypertension	>115

Normal blood pressure levels are lower in children and pregnant women; 120/80 should be considered the maximum normal level. Isolated systolic hypertension also exists, increasing mortality from vascular disease despite a normal diastolic pressure. A systolic pressure of 140 to 159 constitutes borderline systolic hypertension; >160 is isolated systolic hypertension.

Blood pressure is controlled by a variety of mechanisms. One consists of the baroreceptors in the carotid sinuses, which can detect a fall in blood pressure and provoke a response from the brain stem that increases adrenergic outflow. Heart rate, cardiac contractility, and systemic arterial resistance are increased, restoring blood pressure. A second mechanism centers on the kidneys. A fall in perfusion pressure induces secretion of an enzyme, renin, which acts on its substrate in the plasma to form angiotensin I, which is converted to angiotensin II, primarily in the lungs. Angiotensin II is a potent vasoconstrictor and also stimulates the adrenal cortex to release angiotensin, which causes renal retention of salt and water, increasing the plasma volume. Among the factors that stimulate renin release from the juxtaglomerular cells in the kidney are decreased renal perfusion pressure, decreased delivery of sodium to the distal renal tubule, and beta-adrenergic stimuli. Local production of prostaglandin in the kidneys is involved. The third aspect of blood pressure control is the plasma volume, which is regulated by the kidneys. These three physiological mechanisms of blood pressure control can each be affected by pharmacologic measures.

Essential hypertension has no definable cause, but the mechanisms underlying the increased blood pressure probably consist of abnormal "settings" of all three mechanisms of blood pressure control. There is increased sympathetic tone with increased peripheral arterial resistance, an upward "resetting" of the level of plasma volume at which renal natriuresis occurs, and an increase in angiotension II for a given level of peripheral vascular resistance.

Onset of the disease often takes place in the late teens, but there are usually no symptoms, and hypertension is not detected until later in life. Untreated hypertension leads to an increased incidence of arteriosclerosis and its complications, as well as direct damage to the heart, kidneys, and blood vessels. The most frequent causes of death are myocardial infarcts, heart failure, and strokes. Renal failure also occurs, especially in patients who develop an accelerated or malignant phase, which is characterized by markedly elevated blood pressure (diastolics between 120 and 150 mm Hg). With **accelerated hypertension**, necrosis appears in the walls of arteries, with deposition of fibrinoid, and the additional narrowing of the vessels adds to the problems of organ perfusion, especially in the kidneys. Fundal vessels show characteristic necrotic lesions with marked and irregular narrowing, hemorrhages, and exudates. Papilledema often develops. These patients usually have headaches and blurred vision. Microangiopathic hemolytic anemia can develop. Lesions typical of periarteritis nodosa can be found. Heart or renal failure may develop rapidly, and this condition is fatal within a few months if untreated.

Evaluation of a newly diagnosed patient should include determination of the blood pressure on several separate occasions while sitting and lying, examination of optic fundi for evidence of vascular changes, examination of the heart and peripheral vessels, as well as checking for signs of heart failure. Routine laboratory evaluation should include urinalysis, BUN, serum creatinine, electrolytes, cholesterol, triglycerides, and an ECG. A chest x-ray to determine heart size is also useful.

Pheochromocytomas are one of the potentially reversible causes of hypertension, if the tumor can be identified and successfully removed (see the section on endocrinology), as is **aldosterone secreting adrenal tumor**, or **Conn's syndrome**, another potentially correctable cause of hypertension. The hypertension is caused by volume expansion due to mineralocorticoid excess. This syndrome is characterized by hypokalemia and metabolic alkalosis because of the effect of the hormone on renal tubular function. High levels of aldosterone can be demonstrated in the plasma, along with very low levels of renin, since these tumors are secreting the hormone autonomously. Aldosterone antagonists such as spironolactone are useful in medical management of patients with these tumors.

Coarctation of the aorta is another remediable cause of hypertension, usually detected as hypertension in children or young adults. The congenital narrowing of the aorta usually occurs in the arch, at the site of insertion of the ductus arteriosus, and flow below this level is restricted, dependent on collateral vessels. Pulses are weak or absent in the legs, and blood pressure in the legs is much lower than in the arms. The decreased flow to the kidneys stimulates the renin-angiotensin system, contributing to the hypertension. Surgical correction is necessary and is usually successful.

Therapy of hypertension

Lowering the elevated blood pressure decreases the high morbidity and mortality associated with hypertension. Diastolic pressures above 95 should definitely be treated. The goal should be levels below 90 mm Hg unless the patient cannot tolerate the therapy. Nonpharmacologic measures should be used first, including correction of obesity (if possible), sodium restriction, decrease in heavy alcohol consumption, and use of tobacco. Behavior modification is helpful in some tense, anxious patients. A stepped-care approach is usually recommended, each successive step being taken if the prior steps do not adequately control the blood pressure:

Step 1: A diuretic (e.g., thiazide) or a beta-blocker (e.g., propranolol or atenolol).

Step 2: Add a central adrenergic blocker (e.g., clonidine), or the diuretic or beta-blocker not used in step 1, or a peripheral alpha-blocker (e.g., prazosin).

Step 3: Add another drug, either a vasodilator (e.g., hydralazine or prazosin), or an angiotensin converting enzyme (ACE) inhibitor (e.g., captopril), or calcium channel blocker (e.g., nifedipine).

Step 4: Add minoxidil or guanethidine.

Although stepped care is effective, there has been increasing use of agents listed as step 2 or 3 in place of a diuretic, which previously was the most frequent type of drug given as step 1. Specifically, beta-blockers or ACE inhibitors are becoming the first drugs used, with good results and few side effects. With the potent agents now available and the advantages of additive effects of drugs with differing (and thus not additive) side effects, control of blood pressure can almost always be achieved. Hospitalization is rarely needed except for malignant hypertension, in which rapid achievement of control is necessary to avoid a cardiovascular accident or renal failure.

There are differences in the response of various populations of hypertensives to these drugs. For example, blacks in general respond better to diuretics, whites to beta-blockers, as the first drug. Older patients do better with diuretics, younger ones with beta-blockers. Therefore, the following modifications of the stepped care plan are recommended for step 1:

Diuretics work best among patients who are black, elderly, or obese or who have CHF, chronic renal failure, or a contraindication to beta-blockers (e.g., asthma, claudication).

Beta-blockers are best for young patients (especially whites), those with a hyperkinetic circulation (i.e., have tachycardia, palpitations) or symptomatic arteriosclerotic heart disease (especially angina), or those who have had a myocardial infarction or who have associated migraine or gout.

ACE inhibitors work best for young white patients, those with associated CHF, males who develop impotence from beta-blockers, and those with heavy proteinuria, diabetic glomerulosclerosis, or chronic renal failure (i.e., those with decreased capillary filtration pressure).

Calcium channel blockers are best for the elderly, those with angina, blacks, and those with migraine (but they are short-acting and expensive).

Side effects of the antihypertensive agents should be kept in mind. Rapid lowering of blood pressure with any drug can cause weakness and faintness. Postural hypotension is also frequent, especially with alpha-blockers. Marked hypotension after the first dose is also common, especially with alpha-blockers. Impotence is a problem with beta-blockers, which must be avoided in patients with asthma. Rebound hypertension can occur when a drug is withdrawn, especially with central adrenergic inhibitors such as clonidine. Alpha-adrenergic blockers may cause tachyphylaxis (development of tolerance to increasing doses). Diuretics can cause hypokalemia. (If hypokalemia is a problem, K-sparing diuretics, beta-blockers, or ACE inhibitors can be used.)

Several causes of hypertension are potentially reversible by surgery, especially those due to tumors such as pheochromocytomas or adrenal tumors that secrete aldosterone or those due to coarctation of the aorta. Another correctable cause is renovascular hypertension, in which there is stenosis of one or both renal arteries, caused either by fibromuscular hyperplasia, a congenital abnormality that is more common in young women, or an atherosclerotic plaque.

Diagnostic decisions. In this condition there is elevated renin output from the affected kidney and usually suppressed levels on the contralateral side. Renal vein catheterization is necessary to obtain samples for this assay. Renal ultrasonography may reveal a small kidney on the affected side, but renal arteriography is the key step in diagnosis.

Therapeutic decisions. Surgical correction of the obstructive lesion is possible, but the success rate in ending the hypertension is disappointing and treatment with ACE inhibitors and other antihypertensive drugs is usually effective.

DISEASES OF THE KIDNEYS AND URINARY TRACT

Glomerular diseases present as either nephrotic or nephritic glomerulopathies. Nephrotic syndromes include edema and marked proteinuria; nephritic syndromes present with hypertension, hematuria, and milder degrees of proteinuria. Pathologically, the glomeruli show proliferation of mesangial, endothelial, and/or epithelial cells, with infiltration with neutrophils and macrophages. The major causes of nephritic syndromes include postinfectious glomerulonephritis (primarily poststreptococcal, but also seen following staphylococcal, pneumococcal, and several viral infections) and SLE, which show mainly proliferative glomerulopathy. Crescentic glomerulopathy is seen in idiopathic rapidly progressive glomerulonephritis and Goodpasture's syndrome (in which the disease is due to antibasement membrane antibodies).

Regardless of etiology, the severity of the clinical syndrome correlates with the extent and severity of the pathological change in the glomeruli. **Focal nephritis**, affecting foci within some glomeruli, causes moderate proteinuria and microscopic hematuria but little or no fall in glomerular filtration rate (GFR). A **diffuse proliferative glomerulonephritis**, in which most flomeruli show extensive change, causes decreased GFR with azotemia and hypertension as well as proteinuria and hypertension. Extensive crescent formation in the outer walls of the glomeruli is associated with marked and rapid deterioration of renal function. In a given case, the clinical syndrome and corresponding pathology can change with time from one type to another.

BASIC CONSIDERATIONS IN THE WORKUP OF PATIENTS WITH RENAL DISEASE

Maximum tubular concentrating capacity is estimated by restricting water intake until three consecutive urine specimens show no further increase in osmolality (or the patient has lost 5% of body weight).

Fractional excretion: GFR × serum concentration (= total amount filtered) divided by the excretion rate (in g/unit of time). This calculation is actually C_{solute}/C_{Cr}. For example, the fractional excretion rate of sodium can be calculated from a single urine sample in which sodium and creatinine are measured, along with serum sodium and Cr. The formula becomes $[U_{Na} \times P_{Cr}/U_{Cr} \times P_{Na}] \times 100$.

Kidney size is assessed by flat plate and, much more accurately, by ultrasonography. If there is azotemia and the kidneys are small, chronic renal disease is suggested, but the diagnosis is not sure with normal or large kidneys. With chronic renal disease and azotemia, the patient is usually anemic and tends to have higher phosphate levels than with acute renal failure.

Nuclear scans: Technetium 99-DPTA is used to assess renal perfusion; valuable information is obtained if the uptake is asymmetric. ^{131}I-labeled hippuran can assess renal tubular function, since it is excreted by the tubules. Normal perfusion with decreased uptake of hippuran over the kidneys is seen with acute tubular necrosis.

Radiologic and endoscopic procedures: The intravenous pyelogram (IVP) is useful to demonstrate calculi, scars of pyelonephritis, cysts, and tumors. Ultrasonography is also valuable for identifying stones. CT scan demonstrates size, whether masses are solid or cystic. Cytoscopy visualizes bladder lesions. Retrograde pyelography is valuable for obstructing lesions (especially if the kidney does not visualize by IVP). Arteriography is useful primarily if the patient is thought to have renovascular hypertension, before surgery, but also may be useful to determine if a lesion is a tumor by demonstrating neovascularization.

Renal biopsy helps to determine the nature of glomerular pathology before instituting potentially toxic therapy such as prednisone or immunosuppressants.

ACUTE GLOMERULONEPHRITIS

Patients with the syndrome of **acute glomerulonephritis**, whether following a streptococcal infection or other etiology, usually present with some edema that is often facial, grossly bloody or "smoky" urine, oliguria, and frequently hypertension. Moderate proteinuria is common, often with RBC casts. Mild or moderate azotemia is usual; acute renal failure can occur but is rare. Complete recovery is the rule; progression to chronic renal failure is rare. The onset often follows a streptococcal infection, which may be in the throat, skin, or elsewhere, and there usually are antistreptococcal antibodies in the serum. Complement levels are decreased during the active phase of the disease.

Cases following staphylococcal, pneumococcal, varicella, Epstein-Barr virus, and other infections usually run a similarly benign course, but glomerulonephritis due to SLE is not as benign. Pathologically, glomerulonephritis due to SLE usually shows endothelial and mesothelial cell proliferation, some leukocyte infiltration, IgG and C3 deposition in the glomeruli, and electron-dense subepithelial deposits.

Treatment is directed at eliminating any infecting organism if possible, salt and water restriction, and addition of a diuretic if edema and hypertension are present. Use of corticosteroids and immunosuppressants is usually unnecessary.

OTHER TYPES OF ACUTE NEPHRITIS

Anaphylactoid purpura is a disease usually seen in children with palpable purpuric lesions in the skin and episodes of abdominal pain, both suggestive of a vasculitis, and a picture of acute nephritis. Few cases progress to severe renal disease.

Rapidly progressive glomerulonephritis is a disease process affecting young adults primarily, with an initial clinical picture similar to that of other types of acute glomerulonephritis. Biopsy shows crescentic lesions with extensive pathology, and the majority of cases progress to renal failure in about 6 months. Serum complement levels are usually normal in these cases, although IgG and C3 deposition along the glomerular basement membranes is present. **Goodpasture's syndrome** is due to an antibasement membrane antibody, which also affects capillaries in the lung. Hemoptysis is a common accompanying manifestation. Therapy with corticosteroids, plasmapheresis,

and immunosuppressants may succeed in arresting the disease process.

Other types of nephritic syndromes include the **hemolytic-uremic syndrome**, which occurs mainly in children, often following an infection that suggests influenza. It is characterized by sudden onset accompanied by abdominal pain and acute GI symptoms, often with GI bleeding. A microangiopathic hemolytic anemia is common, sometimes with thrombocytopenia. Uremia may appear quickly, and dialysis may be needed to tide the patient over the acute phase. Recovery is usual in children, but chronic renal failure usually develops when the disease appears in adults.

Some cases present with a mixed picture of nephrotic and nephritic manifestations or evolve from one type to the other relatively quickly. These cases are sometimes classified as the **mixed glomerulopathies. Membranoproliferative glomerulopathy** is usually seen in children and young adults. The cause is unknown. Many cases present with a nephrotic syndrome and continue to have marked proteinuria throughout their course. About a third have hematuria, hypertension, and azotemia, thus resembling acute nephritis. The complement levels are usually low. Renal biopsy shows mesangial cell proliferation and thickening of capillary basement membranes. Subendothelial deposits may be seen on electron microscopy, but some cases show dense deposits within the basement membranes. Some cases show a 7S gamma-globulin, called the C3 nephritic factor, which can activate the third component of complement. Although spontaneous remissions do occur, a high proportion of cases go on to chronic renal failure over the course of about 10 years without any evidence of an influence of therapy. In some cases, the nephritis recurs in transplanted kidneys.

Mesangioproliferative glomerulopathy is seen primarily in a disease called **idiopathic IgA nephropathy**. This syndrome usually begins as recurrent gross hematuria in young males with mild proteinuria (<1 g/day), although a small percentage develop frank nephrotic syndrome. Serum complement levels are normal. IgA, IgG, and IgM deposition can be demonstrated along the mesangium in these cases. This disease has turned out to be more serious than originally thought, progressing to renal failure in 10 to 20%, especially those with more marked proteinuria. Corticosteroids and immunosuppressants do not modify the outcome in these cases, and the disease tends to recur in transplanted kidneys.

RENAL FAILURE

Pathophysiology

Loss of kidney function results in loss of ability to regulate composition of body fluids. Abnormal water balance can cause edema, CHF, or hypertension. Abnormal balance of solutes can cause hyperkalemia, hyperphosphatemia, or metabolic acidosis. Loss of ability to excrete nitrogenous wastes results in a rise in BUN and creatinine. Since the amount of creatinine excreted each day is proportional to muscle mass, the rate of accumulation of creatinine varies with the muscle mass of the patient. This is especially notable with a small, frail, elderly patient, who can have significant renal failure with low serum creatinine. The BUN reflects protein intake and protein catabolic rate, as well as renal function. The rate of accumulation of BUN is increased by a greater catabolic rate and can be over 40 mg/100 ml/day in a febrile patient with tissue necrosis. Since urea is absorbed by the renal tubules, hypovolemia, which reduces water presented to the renal tubule, can result in greater urea reabsorption and increased BUN; creatinine is not affected.

Workup of patients with acute renal failure

In **urinalysis,** RBCs and especially RBC casts in the sediment point to glomerular disease. WBCs and WBC casts indicate inflammation but not necessarily infection. WBC clumps are more indicative of infection. Red urine suggests hematuria, but if there are no RBCs, it suggests myoglobinuria, which can cause azotemia by plugging renal tubules. Concomitant muscle swelling would suggest rhabdomyolysis, supporting this diagnostic possibility.

Serum complement, if decreased, suggests immune complex disease and a need for ANA to check for the possibility of SLE. Antibasement membrane antibody determination is used to check for Goodpasture's disease. (The latter is often accompanied by hemoptysis since pulmonary capillaries are also affected.)

Diagnostic decisions.   The following considerations are useful in the diagnosis of the cause of acute renal failure:

Severe acute glomerulonephritis, acute tubular necrosis, immune-mediated interstitial nephritis or vasculitis affecting the kidneys, infection, obstruction, drug toxicity, and hypercalcemia are possible causes. Normal or very sparse urine with acute onset of azotemia suggests obstruction.

Lymphocytes or eosinophils in the urine suggest an immunologically mediated interstitial nephritis.

Acute tubular necrosis usually results in some degree of proteinuria and granular casts. Abnormal tubular function can result in glucosuria without hyperglycemia. Similarly, tubular damage is suggested, in the presence of oliguria, by a urine sodium concentration >40 mEq/L or fractional sodium excretion > than 1% of filtered sodium and urine osmolality close to that of serum.

Prerenal azotemia usually is accompanied by very low urinary sodium concentrations, but exceptions occur if a diuretic has been given, when renal shutdown is due to administration of radiopaque material for an IVP in susceptible individuals (such as in patients with multiple myeloma), during the generation phase of metabolic alkalosis, and if preexisting renal disease has caused salt wasting.

Patients with acute renal failure can be oliguric (defined as urine flow <500 ml/100 ml) or polyuric. Total anuria suggests a vascular catastrophe, such as occlusion of the renal arteries or bilateral cortical necrosis. Total anuria can occur with severe acute glomerulonephritis or tubular necrosis. Ureteral obstruction has to be bilateral to cause anuria.

Sonography is useful to determine kidney size, as well as the presence of stones. Small kidneys and anemia and hyperphosphatemia suggest underlying chronic renal disease with a superimposed acute episode.

ACUTE TUBULAR NECROSIS

Acute tubular necrosis (ATN) is a term that is not an accurate description of the pathology. The condition usually follows a hypovolemic or hypotensive episode or exposure to a nephrotoxic agent (such as an aminoglycoside, which can give characteristic lipid whorls in the cytoplasm of renal tubular cells.)

Prerenal azotemia should be ruled out, since it is reversible. It is suggested by a BUN/Cr >20:1, low urine sodium concentration on a spot urine (<20 mEq/L), and fractional sodium excretion < 1%. Hemodynamic monitoring during administration of fluid may be necessary to rule out prerenal azotemia, especially in the elderly or severely ill individuals. Partial urinary tract obstruction can give findings similar to those seen with prerenal azotemia.

Diagnostic decisions.   The diagnosis of ATN is suggested by proteinuria with granular casts and the presence of tubular epithelial cells in the urine sediment, a BUN/Cr < 20:1, a urinary sodium > 40 mEq/L and fractional excretion > 1%, with a relatively low urine osmolality (usually around 250 to 300 mOsm/kg H_2O).

Therapeutic decisions.   Management includes careful control of fluid administration to avoid overload, oral resins to treat hyperkalemia, use of bicarbonate to treat acidosis, antacids to bind phosphate, and adequate protein intake to avoid protein catabolism (usually 40 g/day is adequate). Serum levels of drugs that are cleared primarily by the kidneys should be carefully monitored. Diuretics, both loop agents (e.g., furosemide) and osmotic diuretics (e.g., mannitol) can be tried and if unsuccessful, discontinued. Sometimes a diuretic can convert an oliguric ATN into a polyuric case, which is easier to manage since fluid overload is less likely to occur. As improvement occurs, patients with ATN tend to become polyuric, often doubling urine output every 24 hours. During the polyuric phase, careful monitoring of fluid balance is necessary to prevent hypovolemia or electrolyte depletion.

Dialysis is indicated for complications of renal failure that cannot be controlled with conservative measures—for example, fluid overload, severe azotemia (e.g., BUN > 70), abnormalities in clotting function, and uncontrollable hyperkalemia. With use of all available measures, the mortality of ATN remains around 50%.

CHRONIC RENAL FAILURE

As chronic renal failure develops, the ability of the kidney to maintain normal concentrations of body fluids with variations in intake is decreased. For example, as GFR falls, the filtered load of sodium decreases. Since the daily excretion of sodium is normally equal to the daily intake, with constant intake, the fractional excretion of sodium has to increase. If intake exceeds the capacity of the tubules to adapt, sodium and water retention occur with edema formation. Similarly, if sodium intake is low, fractional excretion of sodium must fall, and if the capacity of the tubules to conserve sodium is exceeded, "salt wasting" occurs.

As phosphate retention occurs, the serum phosphate rises and the serum calcium falls concomitantly. A rise in parathyroid hormone (PTH) excretion occurs, increasing urinary phosphate excretion and normalizing the serum levels of PO_4 and calcium. As further PO_4 retention occurs, another rise in PTH excretion occurs, ultimately producing the bone disease referred to as renal osteodystrophy. The PTH may contribute to the renal injury by causing calcium deposition in the renal parenchyma. Hypertension resulting from renal disease can accelerate the progression of the renal damage if it is not adequately treated.

Another frequent complication of chronic renal failure is pericarditis, which can be hemorrhagic. The development of CNS dysfunction, varying from confusion and somnolence to coma, is a frequent indication for dialysis. Peripheral neuropathies (e.g., glove and stocking hypesthesia) can develop, as can autonomic neuropathies with GI motility disturbances and labile blood pressure. Such patients may be intolerant of dialysis. Other manifestations of chronic renal failure include anemia, abnormal WBC function with increased susceptibility to infection, a proximal myopathy, arthritis often due to calcium pyrophosphate crystal deposition (pseudogout), pruritus, gastroenteritis and colitis, and uremic osteodystrophy. The bone disease is characterized by bone pain, fractures, and cystic lesions in bone (the term **osteitis fibrosa cystica** is usually used). Alkaline phosphatase levels are elevated. Chronic metabolic acidosis and poor nutritional state are blamed for a concomitant osteoporosis, which often aggravates the uremic bone disease.

Therapeutic decisions.   Management of chronic renal failure includes careful regulation of intake of fluid and electrolytes to avoid depletion or accumulation. Protein intake is limited to minimal requirements (about 40 g/day) of high-quality protein (i.e., rich in essential amino acids and balanced in all amino acids, which means predominantly animal protein) to minimize accumulation of nitrogenous compounds. Bicarbonate can be given for acidosis, and aluminum-based antacids are given to decrease phosphate accumulation. Administration of calcium and vitamin D (or its metabolites) can minimize the bone disease. Sometimes a parathyroidectomy is necessary if marked hypercalcemia and severe bone disease develop. In diabetics, insulin requirement often decreases. RBC transfusions are sometimes needed to maintain adequate hematocrit.

Dialysis is necessary when these measures are inadequate or complications of uremia develop. Chronic peritoneal dialysis, hemodialysis, and transplantation all are options at this stage. Cardiovascular instability is less of a problem with peritoneal dialysis and is safer in diabetics who have retinopathy. The use of heparin, which is needed with hemodialysis, is unnecessary. Death rates with chronic dialysis generally average around 10 to 15%/year. With transplantation, the need for continued use of immunosuppressants is a major consideration since they can increase bone marrow suppression and susceptibility to infection.

DISTURBANCES OF ACID-BASE METABOLISM

A most important initial step in approaching a patient with an acid-base disturbance is to consider the history: How did this abnormality come about? Most often, the nature of the acid-base disturbance can be predicted from the history. For example, vomiting causes loss of gastric HCl, resulting in a metabolic alkalosis (Table 1-2); diarrhea causes predominantly loss of alkaline intestinal fluid, causing metabolic acidosis (Table 1-3); acute respiratory failure causes retention of CO_2, which forms H_2CO_3, resulting in respiratory acidosis.

The first step in the approach to metabolic acidosis is to

Table 1-2. Causes of Metabolic Alkalosis

Continuous administration of alkali.
Examples: chronic HCO_3^- administration, milk-alkali syndrome.

Chloride-responsive forms of alkalosis
1. Vomiting, with gastric fluid loss.
2. Use of diuretics.
3. Loss of acid in stool, as in villous adenoma.

Chloride-resistant alkalosis
1. Hyperaldosteronism, primary or as in Bartter's syndrome, or secondary aldosteronism, as in malignant hypertension and renovascular hypertension or renin-secreting tumors.
2. Mineralocorticoid excess, as occurs with prednisone therapy and in Cushing's syndrome.
3. Others, including parathyroid disease with hypercalcemia and refeeding after starvation.

determine the **anion gap:** Subtract the $[Cl^-] + [HCO_3^-]$ from the $[Na^+]$. The difference is normally 8 to 12 mEq/L. An increase is strongly suggestive of organic anion accumulation (e.g., lactic acid or ketoacids). Typically there is a low $[HCO_3^-]$ and a high $[Cl^-]$ (i.e., a **hyperchloremic acidosis**).

Therapeutic decisions.   First remove the underlying cause whenever possible. Administer alkali (e.g., HCO_3^-) as the condition indicates—definitely give it if the pH has fallen below 7.20. Lactate and citrate can be given for less severe alkalosis. Aim for a HCO_3^- above 10, preferably 12 or more. Estimate HCO_3^- need from fact that HCO_3^- distribution is usually twice the extracellular fluid volume (about 40% of body weight). Thus, if patient weighs 70 kg, to raise $[HCO_3^-]$ from 6 to 12 mEq/L requires about $6 \times (0.4 \times 70) = \sim 170$ mEq of HCO_3^-. Try not to overcompensate. Stopping the cause of overproduction of acid and the fact that bicarbonate penetrates the blood-brain barrier slowly can result in persistence of the hyperventilation. Alkalosis can develop, resulting in alteration of mental status and convulsions.

Milk-alkali syndrome, now rarely seen, is characterized by metabolic alkalosis, hypercalcemia, hypocalciuria, deposition of calcium in abnormal sites (band keratopathy, nephrocalcinosis, and resulting renal failure). It develops in patients who have peptic ulcer disease and who ingest large amounts of absorbable alkali, usually along with milk. The availability of unabsorbable alkali has virtually eliminated this syndrome. Typical findings include plasma HCO_3^- of about 40 and Ca up to 16 mg/100 ml. The hypercalcemia is accentuated by renal functional damage, impairing the ability of the kidneys to excrete the calcium.

Acute alkali administration rarely exceeds the capacity of the kidneys to excrete HCO_3^- more than transiently. When milk-alkali syndrome has caused chronic renal failure, a mixed metabolic acidosis and alkalosis will be present.

Loss of gastric juice through vomiting results in loss of Cl^- as well as acid, hence a marked hypochloremia is usually found. Potassium loss occurs concomitantly, and dehydration can be severe. Alkalosis can appear as a result of vomiting even

Table 1-3. Major Causes of Metabolic Acidosis

Causes of loss of bicarbonate

1. Loss of alkaline intestinal secretions: Diarrhea or drainage of biliary or pancreatic secretions by tube to the outside.
2. Surgical diversion of urine to the intestine (ureterosigmoidostomy), which results in reabsorption of the acid formed by the renal tubules.
3. Dilutional acidosis. (Mild metabolic acidosis can result from marked increase in the volume of distribution of bicarbonate, without a concomitant increase in its production.
4. Bicarbonate-wasting renal diseases (renal tubular acidosis [RTA]) type I.
5. Administration of inhibitors of renal carbonic anhydrases such as Diamox, which causes an iatrogenic type I RTA.

Addition of acid

1. Administration of HCl, NH_4Cl, or cationic amino acids (e.g., parenteral hyperalimentation with arginine mono-HCl).
2. Lactic acidosis. Most frequently due to anoxia, as occurs in shock, acute respiratory distress syndrome, prolonged convulsive seizure, low cardiac output, carbon monoxide poisoning, sepsis. Occasionally seen with severe alcoholism, usually with ketoacidosis. Also seen with salicylate, methanol, ethylene glycol, some other drug poisonings. Some diseases increase the risk of development of lactic acidosis, especially diabetes mellitus.
3. Diabetic keotacidosis. (See the discussion of diabetes in the section on endocrinology.)
4. Other causes of ketoacidosis: Starvation, alcoholic binge, ingestion of ethylene glycol, methanol, or salicylate. (Salicylate effect occurs by increasing alveolar ventilation through stimulation of the respiratory center, making it more responsive to a given level of PCO_2, resulting in decreased PCO_2. This causes a respiratory alkalosis, but the uncoupling of oxidative phosphorylation causes increased peripheral CO_2 production, and the organic acids formed by salicylate metabolism add to the metabolic acidosis. In infants, salicylates usually cause a metabolic acidosis, but in older children and adults, it is a less dominant part of picture. Diagnosis can be confirmed by determination of the salicylate level in blood.)
5. Infantile organic acidosis. Seen in newborns with inborn errors of amino acid metabolism, especially leucine, isoleucine, and valine (maple syrup urine disease, isovaleric acidemia, "sweaty feet syndrome," etc.).

Failure of excretion of acid by the kidney

1. RTA as a single renal abnormality or as part of generalized renal disease. Chronic uremia is characterized by uremic acidosis because of accumulation of SO_4, PO_4, and organic acids.
2. Adrenal insufficiency.

in an achlorhydric patient, since the gastric juice will contain Na and Cl, but proportionately more Cl will be lost, resulting in alkalosis. Gastric alkalosis results in the most marked elevations of plasma HCO_3^- seen. Values of 50 to 60 mEq/L occur, and a level that high suggests this diagnosis. Deficits of several hundred millequivalents of potassium and over 1,000 mEq of Na are also seen. Urinary chloride excretion will be low, and when replacement therapy results in excretion of 60 to 100 mEq of chloride pay day, stores have been repleted.

Treatment of milk-alkali syndrome consists of removing the cause; rarely acid (HCl or NH_4Cl) must be administered. Gastric acid loss can usually be successfully treated with NaCl solutions plus adequate amounts of KCl, monitoring plasma electrolytes. Ordinarily no treatment is needed for the alkalosis that can result from treatment of organic acidosis, since the kidneys are able to excrete the excess alkali.

Diuretics such as furosemide cause alkalosis by increasing renal excretion of acid, causing excretion of fluid with lower HCO_3^- than that of plasma, and by contraction of volume around existing extracellular bicarbonate stores (**contraction alkalosis**). The effect of contraction on the plasma bicarbonate is more marked in edematous patients. Prevention consists of concomitant administration of a distal tubular blocking agent such as spironolactone or triamterene, which inhibit sodium reabsorption at distal sites and thus have less effect on hydrogen and potassium excretion. There is danger of hyperkalemia when these agents are used in patients with renal failure. Replacement is generally with KCl, since Na is usually contraindicated in edematous patients being given diuretics, with or without concomitant distally acting agents.

Villous adenomas can cause daily fluid losses of 1 to 3 L, with severe volume and potassium depletion. Stupor, hypotension, and paralysis can result. Most of these patients become severely hypokalemic and azotemic, with a metabolic acidosis, but some become alkalotic, apparently because of loss of surprisingly large amounts of chloride in the stool. The loss of isotonic fluid with a chloride higher and bicarbonate lower than extracellular fluid would lower plasma Cl^- and raise HCO_3^-. Volume contraction augments the HCO_3^- concentration. Increased urinary K^+ losses in the alkalotic state add to the hypokalemia. Therapy consists primarily of replacement of water, sodium, and potassium. Measures to correct the diarrhea usually fail, and the tumor must be removed.

Syndromes characterized by **increased secretion of aldosterone** lead to sodium retention, volume expansion, moderate degrees of hypertension, and an alkalosis that is resistant to chloride administration. Hypokalemia is characteristically present and is a clue to the diagnosis unless the patient has received diuretics or has another explanation for the development of hypokalemia. Measurement of plasma renin and aldosterone is useful. Sometimes a CT scan is desirable if a primary adrenal tumor is suspected. Response to spironolactone can be diagnostically useful. Therapy consists of correction of the underlying disorder and administration of KCl.

Respiratory acidosis results from alveolar hypoventilation of any cause, local causes (airway obstruction), central causes (oversedation or anesthesia), cardiac arrest, neuromuscular abnormalities, or restrictions in lung volume (such as pneumothorax or flail chest). Chronic hypercapnia results from COPD, chronic depression of the respiratory center, chronic neuro-muscular defects (polio, amyotrophic lateral sclerosis), and restrictive lung diseases (pulmonary fibrosis, kyphoscoliosis, etc.). Diagnosis of the cause and nature of the acid-base defect is usually obvious, although it may be necessary to establish that the elevated $PaCO_2$ is not due to a metabolic alkalosis. Treatment consists of measures to correct the hypoventilation. Administration of bicarbonate is rarely useful; most of it will be excreted in the urine.

Respiratory alkalosis results from increased alveolar venti-lation decreasing arterial PCO_2. It occurs as result of high altitude or other conditions of low oxygen tensions; severe anemia; voluntary hyperventilation; intracerebral disease; stim-ulation of the central respiratory center, which can occur on a pharmacologic basis (such as with salicylates); anxiety; or disease such as acute gram-negative septicemia, interstitial lung disease, and occasionally other pulmonary diseases such as pulmonary embolism. Clinically, light-headedness and occasionally seizures occur. A decrease in cerebral blood flow results from hyopcapnia causing vasoconstriction of the cere-bral vasculature. Diagnosis is made by checking the arterial pH (>7.40) and $PaCO_2$ (<40). HCO_3^- is usually only slightly decreased, one reason for the rapid increase in pH. Treatment is primarily directed at the cause.

Mixed acid-base disturbances are common. Analysis of the clinical state may be more informative than simple analysis of laboratory observations. For example, during gram-negative sepsis, a metabolic acidosis combined with a respiratory alkalosis is usual. In COPD, a chronic respiratory acidosis is usually combined with diuretic-induced metabolic alkalosis. With cardiopulmonary arrest, respiratory acidosis combined with a metabolic acidosis is usual. Whenever the laboratory findings do not conform to the pattern seen in a primary disorder, a mixed disorder is very likely. Mixed disorders can be missed by solely analyzing the lab findings. For example, a metabolic acidosis superimposed on a metabolic alkalosis have opposite effects on pH and bicarbonate. Another example is salicylate intoxication, which causes a mixture of respiratory alkalosis and metabolic acidosis. Another factor confusing interpretation of lab values is the lag time for compensatory adjustments to occur. Acute respiratory acidosis may require 2 to 3 days for full adjustment.

TUBULOINTERSTITIAL DISEASE

Tubulointerstitial disease is a process that primarily affects the renal tubules but can extend and cause secondary glomeru-lar destruction. Diseases that originate in the interstitial portion of the kidney include hereditary polycystic disease and chronic interstitial nephritis, which is usually due to drugs (lead, analgesics). Primary diseases of the renal tubules cause loss of the regulation of the extracellular fluid by the renal tubules, and changes in acid-base (RTA), fluid balance (diabetes insipidus, salt-losing nephropathy), or mineral regulation (phosphaturia) occur.

Polycystic disease

Most cases are asymptomatic until the fourth or fifth decade of life, but a separate genetic form of the disease affects infants, usually with concomitant hepatic fibrosis, and death occurs in the first year. Lumbar pain is often the first symptom in adults, and large palpable kidneys are detectable. Sharp pain can occur from rupture of a cyst; hematuria, gross or microscopic, is frequent. Hypertension can develop early, and urinary tract infections are common. Loss of concentrating capacity results in polyuria and nocturia. These patients may have associated hepatic cysts or intracranial cerebral aneurysms.

Diagnostic decisions. Diagnosis is established by ultrason-ography or IVP, and screening tests for genetic counseling should be performed on teenage members of affected families. Therapy consists of treatment of complications, especially the hypertension. Nephrectomy may be necessary for hematuria or recurrent infection of a cyst. Transplants are often successful.

Medullary disease

Medullary cystic disease is a rare hereditary disease, often associated with retinitis pigmentosa. It causes renal failure in early adulthood, even during adolescence. **Medullary sponge kidney** results from passage of renal stones, giving characteristic changes on IVP with contrast-filled medullary cysts. It is a benign disease; treatment should be directed at the stone problem.

Chronic interstitial nephritis

No cause is found in about half the cases. Others are due to abuse of analgesic drugs, heavy metals such as lead or gold, or radiation. Patients may be asymptomatic when azotemia or hypertension is found. Secondary infection with pyelonephritis is a common initial finding. Phenacetin, the analgesic agent known to cause this syndrome, has been taken off the market in the United States, and new cases seem to have stopped occurring. Acute interstitial nephritis follows use of some of the newer NSAIDs, most frequently fenoprofen (Nalfon). The medullary tubular lesion causes decreased urinary concentrat-ing capacity. Actual necrosis of renal papillae can occur, causing gross hematuria, appearance of necrotic tissue in the urinary sediment, and characteristic changes in the IVP.

Lead nephropathy follows use of lead paint or ingestion of contaminated illegal alcohol (moonshine). The syndrome includes neuropathy, anemia, gout, and an interstitial nephritis with azotemia. Secondary pyelonephritis is frequent. Increased urinary lead following a test dose of EDTA is a useful diagnostic test but is not effective as therapy.

Disorders primarily affecting tubular function

Fanconi's syndrome results from loss of proximal tubular functions. Failure of normal reabosrptive mechanisms results in glycosuria with normal or low blood sugars—the result of a low "renal threshold," aminoaciduria, phosphaturia, uricos-uria, and loss of bicarbonate in the urine. The GFR is not decreased, and azotemia does not result unless there is other pathology. The hereditary form of Fanconi's syndrome is usually seen in association with cystinosis. In **Wilson's disease**, which results from excess accumulation of copper in the body, the copper poisons the renal tubular cells, resulting in this syndrome. The syndrome can also result from **myeloma, amyloidosis,** and **Sjögren's syndrome.**

The amino acids that appear in the urine with proximal tubular defects include the dibasic amino acids (lysine, ornithine, arginine, and cystine). Cystine tends to form calculi because of its low solubility at mildly acid pH. In **cystinuria**, the result of a defect in cellular transport of the amino acid, accumulation of cystine in the tissues does not occur. In **cystinosis**, there is an intracellular defect in the metabolism of the amino acid, resulting in its accumulation. Daily excretion of over 400 mg of cystine per gram of creatinine occurs in both states. Intake of large amounts of fluid ($>$ 5 L/day) to keep the urine dilute is the most important aspect of treatment.

Hypophosphatemia results from the tubular defect. The familial form of this entity has also been called **vitamin D-resistant rickets**. The serum PO_4 is below 2.5 mg/100 ml, and the urinary phosphate is inappropriately high (PO_4/Cr ratio >2.5). Serum Ca and PTH are normal. Bone disease with biopsy findings characteristic of osteomalacia (rickets) occurs, and treatment requires huge doses of vitamin D as well as oral phosphate.

Nephrogenic diabetes insipidus is a hereditary disorder in which the collecting tubules fail to respond to antidiuretic hormone (ADH). A similar, reversible acquired disorder can result from lithium or demeclocyline. Symptoms include excretion of huge volumes of urine, 10 to 20 L/day in adults, with concomitant thirst. Resulting hypertonic states can cause encephalopathy, and neurological defects can result. Diagnosis is established by demonstrating failure to raise the urine osmolality above that of plasma after 12 to 18 hours of dehydration or administration of exogenous ADH. Treatment includes maintenance of high fluid intake and salt restriction plus thiazide diuretics, which cause modest reduction in extracellular fluid (ECF) volume. This results in an increase in the amount of glomerular filtrate reabsorbed isotonically in the proximal tubules, thereby reducing the volume of fluid delivered to the ADH-insensitive collecting ducts.

Bartter's syndrome, a rare disease primarily affecting females, causes stunted growth, polyuria, and recurrent episodes of muscle weakness. Patients show severe hypokalemia (<2.5 mEq/L) and a hyperchloremic alkalosis. There is also hyperreninemia and, therefore, hyperaldosteronism. Pathologically, the distinctive lesion is hyperplasia of the juxtaglomerular apparatus. There is increased production of prostaglandin E_2 (PGE_2), which increases renin secretion, leading to the increased formation of aldosterone, which causes the electrolyte changes. However, the PGE_2 blocks the vasoconstrictive action of angiotensin II, and these patients do not become hypertensive. Treatment with NSAIDs that inhibit the production of PGE_2 helps but does not completely correct the electrolyte changes, leading to the concept that the primary defect is in tubular function, causing a secondary increase in prostaglandin formation.

RENAL TUBULAR ACIDOSIS

RTA comprises a group of disorders in which there is a defect in tubular hydrogen ion transport, leading to systemic acidosis. In **type I**, or **distal RTA**, the collecting tubules are unable to maintain a gradient of H^+ between the tubular fluid and the plasma because of either the inability to prevent back-diffusion of H^+ or a defect in the secretory mechanism for H^+. As a result, there is inability to lower the urine pH in the face of an acid challenge.

In **type II**, or **proximal RTA**, there is a defect in rate of secretion of H^+ in the proximal tubule. As a result, the reabsorption of HCO_3^- is decreased. Bicarbonate wasting occurs until the plasma HCO_3^- is low enough to allow complete reabsorption of that which is filtered. A chronic state of hyperchloremic acidosis results.

There is no type III RTA. In **type IV RTA**, there is a failure of the collecting system to respond to aldosterone and the linked secretion of H^+ and K^+ is impaired. The serum K^+ is increased. This syndrome is primarily the result of interstitial renal disease, such as nephrocalcinosis, hypergammaglobulinemic states, amyloidosis, sickle cell disease, and Sjögren's syndrome. Bone disease often results because of mobilization of bone mineral to buffer the retained H^+. Bone calcium loss and hypercalciuria occur. Osteomalacia (rickets in children), nephrocalcinosis, and nephrolithiasis occur frequently.

Diagnostic decisions. The diagnosis is supported by the finding of a hyperchloremic acidosis with hyperkalemia and urinary pH above 6.0 even in the face of acid load (e.g., oral NH_4Cl).

Therapeutic decisions. Treatment of distal RTA, type I or type IV, consists of oral bicarbonate; larger amounts are needed in type IV. In type I, which sometimes occurs as part of more varied proximal tubular defect such as in Fanconi's syndrome, the HCO_3 loss is modest and bone loss for buffering effect does not occur. There is no resulting bone disease and nephrocalcinosis. In type II, the proximal tubular defect cannot be corrected with HCO_3; modest salt restriction helps. In type IV, the distal tubular defect may result from a lack of adrenal production of aldosterone. In these patients, plasma renin levels are increased. When the decreased aldosterone is due to a tubulointerstitial defect, renin levels are decreased (**hyporeninemic hypoaldosteronism**). The defect may be unresponsiveness of the distal tubule to aldosterone despite high levels of both renin and aldosterone, such as occurs with tubulointerstitial disease affecting the distal nephron. A similar phenomenon occurs with spironolactone, which blocks aldosterone effect on the collecting tubule, and with the diuretics triamterene and amiloride. These diuretics thus do not cause potassium loss (potassium-sparing effect).

URINARY TRACT OBSTRUCTION

Urinary tract obstruction is the most common cause of anuria, but in most cases obstruction is partial and causes polyuria due to progressive dilatation of the upper urinary tract (hydronephrosis) and tubular damage, which impairs concentrating capacity. Loss of urinary acidification also occurs as a result of loss of distal tubular function. With unilateral ureteral obstruction there is usually no change in apparent urine flow, and azotemia does not develop.

Diagnostic decisions. Urinary tract obstruction can produce pain and a palpable flank mass due to the hydronephrosis. Renal sonography can demonstrate the hydronephrosis and presence of a calculus. The IVP is often useful and may be positive earlier than a sonogram, showing a delay in excretion on the affected side. Contrast material may still be demonstrable 24 or 48 hours later.

Prolonged obstruction can lead to progressive dilatation of the renal pelvis (hydronephrosis), with destruction of renal tubules, glomerular sclerosis, and eventually marked thinning of the renal cortex.

Therapeutic decisions. Therapy consists of identification of the cause of the obstruction and its correction, usually by means of surgery. Relief of obstruction often leads to **postobstructive diuresis**, partly because of the impaired distal tubular function and loss of concentrating capacity and partly because of the osmotic effect of retained solutes on urine flow.

Intrarenal tubular obstruction can occur with **uric acid nephropathy**, amyloidosis, and multiple myeloma. Urate excretion following tumor lysis with chemotherapy may be so marked that extensive deposition of crystals of uric acid (which are very insoluble in dilute acid) may occur within the kidney. Therapy consists of water diuresis and alkalinization of the urine to increase urate solubility. Prevention involves use of allopurinol.

URINARY TRACT INFECTION

Lower urinary tract infection (UTI) (cystitis and urethritis) is discussed under infectious diseases.

Pyelonephritis usually results from ascending infection of the urinary tract, and therefore symptoms of lower UTI (frequency, urgency, burning on urination) are usually present. Chronic pyelonephritis causes interstitial scarring and can cause renal failure, but this outcome is usually limited to susceptible hosts, such as patients with diabetes mellitus, chronic obstructive lesions of the urinary tract, or other underlying chronic renal disease. Symptoms of lower UTI are primarily the result of cystitis, with irritation of the trigonal portion of the bladder. Fever may be present, but high, spiking fever, especially when accompanied by chills, means infection of the upper urinary tract (i.e., pyelonephritis).

Diagnostic decisions. With either type of infection, urinalysis reveals pyuria, often with WBC clumps, stainable bacteria, and positive cultures with colonies in excess of 10^5/ml from urine obtained as a midstream catch. An IVP should usually be obtained in a male to determine if an obstructive lesion is present, but UTI is so frequent in females that further workup is not necessary unless there is some special indication, such as recurrences.

Therapeutic decisions. Treatment can usually be started as soon as a culture is obtained. Since coliform organisms are the most frequent pathogens, ampicillin, a sulfa compound, or tetracycline is usually appropriate. Infection resulting from chronic obstruction or acquired in the hospital may be due to a less common pathogen, and other agents, such as an aminoglycoside, may be needed.

RENAL CALCULI

Pathogenesis. **Calcium stones**, as the oxalate or phosphate, are the most common renal stones. Other frequent stone constituents are **uric acid, cystine,** and **magnesium**. Most stones are idiopathic. About 5% of calcium stones are due to hyperparathyroidism. **Hypercalciuria**, defined as the excretion of more than 400 mg/day on a low calcium intake, occurs without hypercalcemia in most idiopathic stone formers. The underlying mechanism may be excessive calcium absorption in the gut or increased fractional calcium excretion by the renal tubules. In either case, supersaturation of the urine occurs, and

in the presence of a nidus or "seed," stone formation can occur. Increased urinary uric acid, with formation of uric acid crystals in the urine, may be responsible for the seeding of the calcium stone in many cases.

Elevated serum calcium, with increased calcium excretion and stone formation, can occur due to hyperparathyroidism, sarcoidosis, distal RTA, and hypervitaminosis D.

Chronic UTI with *Proteus* sp, urea-splitting organisms, leads to formation of stones containing calcium, triple phosphate, and magnesium (struvite). These stones can grow large, filling the calyces (**staghorn calculi**). It is extremely difficult to eradicate the infection in the presence of stones.

Diagnostic decisions. Stones may be asymptomatic, present as UTI or as acute renal colic due to passage of a stone into the ureter, causing severe flank or generalized abdominal pain, often with radiation into the groin and usually with hematuria. Flat plate of the abdomen may visualize the stone if it is radiopaque, but pure urate stones are radiolucent. An IVP can show evidence of obstruction, such as dilatation of the ureter, and when the stones are radiolucent, filling defects may be seen. Workup of stone formers should include 24-hour urine evaluation for calcium and urate, serum calcium, urate, phosphate, and alkaline phosphatase. If an elevated serum calcium is found, serum PTH should be determined. Serum $1,25(OH)_2$ vitamin D_3 can be obtained to confirm the mechanism of hypercalcemia in sarcoidosis. Other workup for sarcoidosis can include serum protein electrophoresis and node biopsy. A radionuclide scan is useful to seek a parathyroid adenoma.

Therapeutic decisions. The first aim of treatment is maintenance of diuresis to dilute the urine; surgery may be required for an obstructing stone. Antibiotic therapy is necessary for any infection. Idiopathic hypercalciuria can be reduced with a thiazide diuretic and salt restriction. Allopurinol prevents urate stones and may be useful even without excess urate excretion to prevent recurrent calcium stones.

RENAL PROBLEMS IN PATIENTS WITH OTHER DISEASES

(See also discussions of these diseases in other sections of this chapter.)

Renal disease is a common complication of inadequately controlled **diabetes mellitus**. It may be manifest as a defect in distal tubular function (type IV RTA) or as glomerulosclerosis, which can cause chronic renal failure. The metabolic alterations in renal function can present as hyporeninemic hypoaldosteronism with hyperchloremic acidosis and hyperkalemia, usually with hypertension. This syndrome can antedate significant decrease in GFR.

The lesions probably begin as basement membrane alteration due to binding of carbohydrate to the collagen, leading to thickening and alterations in permeability. Diabetic glomerular disease occurs most frequently in type I diabetes, usually after 15 to 20 years. The initial manifestation is asymptomatic proteinuria. Diabetics who have no proteinuria after 20 years rarely develop glomerulopathy. Once significant proteinuria begins, rapid progression is the rule. The GFR falls progressively, and renal failure is present after 5 years. Concomitant retinopathy occurs—the process is often called diabetic retinorenal syndrome. When proteinuria appears without retinopathy or within 10 years of onset of the diabetes, a different cause should be sought.

The glomerular lesion is called **Kimmelstiel-Wilson nodular glomerulosclerosis.** Typically, hyalin nodules are seen within capillary loops, but most cases show diffuse glomerulosclerosis with basement membrane thickening and arteriosclerotic lesions of both afferent and efferent arterioles. Interstitial atrophy also occurs.

Diabetics in renal failure do not survive as long on hemodialysis as do nondiabetics, and the same lesions can develop in transplanted kidneys, but renal failure infrequently develops.

Another renal lesion seen in diabetics is **papillary necrosis,** in which sloughing of the renal papillary tissue causes hematuria and sometimes renal colic. Necrotic papillary tissue may be observed in the urine sediment. Characteristic alteration in the calyces are seen on IVP.

Multiple myeloma causes renal disease, primarily due to deposition of Bence Jones protein (kappa or lambda immunoglobulin light chains) within the lumen of renal tubules, causing obstruction. Amyloid deposits within glomeruli are also seen, and hypercalcemia secondary to bone lesions can also cause functional changes (loss of concentrating capacity and polyuria). Patients with myeloma tend to develop renal failure secondary to contrast materials used for x-ray, and these should be avoided or patients should be very well hydrated beforehand to keep the urine maximally dilute.

Amyloidosis can cause renal failure or functional changes such as tubular dysfunction (Fanconi's syndrome). Deposition of amyloid in glomerular vessels causes a nephrotic syndrome. Amyloid deposition elsewhere (tongue, liver, spleen) can cause organ enlargement and provide a clue to diagnosis, as can the appearance of cardiomyopathy, peripheral neuropathy, or intestinal malabsorption. Biopsy of rectal mucosa is useful to establish the diagnosis, with Congo red staining demonstration of green birefringence under polarized light and electron-microscopic demonstration of characteristic fibrils. Once nephrotic syndrome appears, renal failure is usually rapidly progressive. Therapy is ineffective. (Also see the sections on sickle cell disease and the hepatorenal syndrome.)

RENAL TUMORS

Most renal tumors arise from tubular cells. The most frequent presenting manifestations are hematuria, flank pain, and a palpable mass. Kidney size can be evaluated by IVP. An ultrasound examination or CT scan can reveal whether the enlargement is cystic or solid. If solid, it should be removed surgically since most are malignant (renal cell carcinoma). If cystic, it should be aspirated for cytologic examination or culture. Arteriography sometimes is useful, since tumors are usually highly vascular whereas cysts or abscesses are not.

Patients with renal cell carcinoma may present with only weight loss, fever, anemia (sometimes polycythemia), and ectopic hormone production (especially PTH or prostaglandins causing activation of osteoclasts, resulting in hypercalcemia, or ectopic ACTH producing Cushing's syndrome). Metastases can also cause hypercalcemia, since the tumor tends to go to bone as well as to the lungs and liver.

DRUGS AND THE KIDNEY

Alterations in drug dosage with renal failure

Dosage of drugs that are excreted primarily by the kidney must be adjusted in the presence of renal failure. Those cleared mainly by the liver do not require such adjustment. Table 1-4 is a partial listing of some of the more important drugs in each category.

Drug dosage can be adjusted by lowering the amount given or by increasing the interval between doses. Characteristics of each drug determine the preferable method. For example, gentamicin should be given in full initial dosage in order to achieve sufficient concentration for antibiotic effect. Subsequent doses should be lower or less frequent than usual in order to avoid accumulation. Although nomograms exist to serve as a guide in dosage for most drugs, assay of drug concentration in plasma is of great help in determining dosage schedules because of individual variation.

Renal toxicity of drugs

Renal function may be impaired by drug effects in a variety of manners:

Changes in renal perfusion can cause prerenal azotemia, as occurs with drugs that cause marked lowering of blood pressure (vasodilators) or changes intrarenal perfusion (aspirin, NSAIDs).

Retroperitoneal fibrosis reported to be caused by some drugs can alter renal function by causing ureteral obstruction (methysergide, practolol).

Intrarenal obstruction can occur as a result of precipitation of insoluble drug or from metabolic products resulting from

Table 1-4. Considerations in Use of Drugs in Patients With Renal Failure

Cleared by liver (no adjustment needed)	Cleared by kidney (adjust dosage)	Toxicity a major problem (avoid use)
General		
Acetazolamide	Hypoglycemics	Procainamide
Aspirin	(oral)	Propranolol
Benzodiazepines	Lidocaine	Quinidine
Cimetidine	Lithium carbonate	Spironolactone
Clonidine	Morphine	Theophylline
Codeine	Phenytoin	Triamterene
Digoxin	Prazosin	
Hydrazine		
Antibiotics		
Aminoglycosides	Cloxacillin	Penicillin
Amphotercin B	Erythromycin	Penicillin G
Carbenicillin	Isonaizid	Rifampin
Cephalosporins	Nafcillin	Sulfonamides
Chloramphenicol	Nalidixic acid	Tetracycline
Clindamycin	Nitrofurantoin	Vancomycin

drug administration within renal tubules (older sulfonamides, ethylene glycol, uric acid following chemotherapy).

Direct glomerular injury occurs with gold and penicillamine; the histology is a membranous glomerulonephritis.

Immune-mediated glomerular injury can result in vasculitis or proliferative glomerulonephritis. Penicillins, sulfonamides, phenytoin, allopurinol (all cause glomerular injury) and fenoprofen are drugs responsible.

Immune-mediated interstitial disease (acute interstitial nephritis) is caused by penicillins, especially methcillin, allopurinol, cimetidine, phenytoin, rifampin, sulfonamides, fenoprofen, others. Pathology includes interstitial infiltration with eosinophils. In some patients, a rash, fever, and peripheral eosinophilia may be associated. Steroid therapy may be useful. NSAIDs can also cause an interstitial nephritis; the infiltrating cells are usually lymphocytes rather than eosinophils. Fenoprofen has been the agent most frequently implicated, but a small number of cases have been reported with almost all the other NSAIDs. These lesions are usually reversible after stopping the drug without steroid therapy.

Direct tubular injury occurs with aminoglycosides and some agents used in cancer chemotherapy. Specific alterations in tubular function occur with some drugs. **Proximal tubular functions** are affected by heavy metals and outdated tetracycline, causing manifestations of Fanconi's syndrome (glycosuria, phosphaturia, RTA). **Impaired concentrating capacity** (the syndrome of renal diabetes insipidus) can occur following lithium, demethylchlortetracycline, and amphotericin B. **Loss of diluting capacity** and therefore of ability to excrete a large water load can occur following administration of vincristine, cyclophosphamide, or chlorpropamide. **Distal RTA** (type IV) with hyperkalemia can occur following amphotericin B, beta-adrenergic blocking agents, and NSAIDs.

Chronic renal failure occurs following use of several types of drugs. Analgesic nephropathy was common when phenacetin-aspirin combinations were marketed over the counter. These preparations have been almost totally removed from the market in the United States. The disease process probably resulted from a combination of the effects of aspirin decreasing renal medullary perfusion through its effect on renal prostaglandin production and accumulation of metabolites of phenacetin in the renal papillae and interstitium, reaching toxic concentrations after large amounts of the drug were ingested over a period of years. Renal papillary necrosis occurred in these patients.

Aminoglycosides can also cause permanent renal failure. These drugs are excreted unchanged and accumulate in renal tubular cells because they can be transported across both the luminal and antiluminal borders of the tubular cells. The altered lipid metabolism can cause the appearance of lipid cytosegrosomes in the cytoplasm. Toxicity is related to total dosage of these drugs and is increased by preexisting renal disease, decreased ECF volume or other causes of decreased renal perfusion, hypokalemia, and concomitant use of other nephrotoxic drugs. It is therefore important to monitor aminoglycoside levels in patients who have any impairment of renal function and who are receiving these agents. The renal toxicity is usually reversible if the drug is stopped early, but it can become permanent, requiring maintenance hemodialysis.

NSAIDs cause a reversible form of azotemia in susceptible individuals because of their effect on intrarenal prostaglandin production. In patients with decreased renal perfusion, such as hypervolemic states, or in patients with intrinsic renal disease or those using diuretics, autoregulation of renal perfusion includes increased synthesis of vasodilating prostaglandins, which also increase renin production and thus aldosterone formation. Inhibition of the cyclooxygenase involved in this pathway by the NSAIDs alters this compensatory pathway, and the decrease in GFR that results can cause azotemia, sodium and fluid retention, and a hyperkalemic hyperchloremic acidosis. These phenomena are reversible when the drug is stopped.

Treatment of drug-induced renal toxicity

The first aim of treatment is the removal of the offending drug. The means needed vary with the characteristics of the individual drug and are summarized in Table 1-5. The indications for the performance of such procedures are listed in Table 1-6.

PULMONARY DISEASES

WORKUP OF PATIENTS WITH PULMONARY DISEASES

In the workup of patients with pulmonary diseases, the following are important clues to seek in the history and physical examination:

Symptoms

Cough is the most frequent manifestation of pulmonary disease. It can arise from any irritation of the bronchial mucosa, such as the presence of excessive amounts of secretions, irritation of the epithelium by infection or irritant,

Table 1-5. Removal of Drugs Causing Toxicity

1. **Drugs removed by hemodialysis:** Aminoglycosides, aspirin, ethanol, glycol, lithium, methanol, phenytoin.

2. **Drugs removed by hemoperfusion against activated charcoal:** Benzodiazepines, digoxin, ethychlorvinyl, glutethimide, meprobromate, methaqualone, phenobarbital, theophylline.

Table 1-6. Indications for Hemodialysis for Treatment of Drug Intoxication

1. Potentially lethal levels of drug.

2. Severe intoxication with coma, hypotension, hypoventilation, hypothermia.

3. Presence of severe renal or hepatic dysfunction, making it unlikely that normal routes of elimination will work at a sufficiently fast rate.

4. Presence of toxic substance or the likelihood of its metabolism to a toxic substance with direct tissue-damaging effect (e.g., ethylene glycol, methanol).

stimulation of parenchymal receptors such as occurs with excess fluid (pulmonary edema), or physical stresses such as fibrosis of interstitial lung disease. Nighttime cough can be due to aspiration of secretions from the nasal sinuses (postnasal drip) or esophagus (with gastroesophageal reflux). Chronic irritative bronchitis from inhalation of tobacco smoke (smoker's cough) is common, but cough indicating the presence of serious pulmonary disease is often ignored because it is attributed to smoking.

Hemoptysis can result from an infection eroding the surface epithelium, as occurs in bronchitis, bronchiectasis, and pneumonia. Tuberculosis was formerly a common cause of hemoptysis in the United States but is rare now. If no infection is evident, hemoptysis should always suggest tumor at the present time, since carcinoma of the lung is epidemic. Thorough workup is indicated.

Episodic **dyspnea** can be due to bronchospasm; dyspnea with exercise can be due to cardiac or pulmonary disease.

Chest pain is "pleuritic" if exacerbated by inspiration or coughing, but similar pain can be due to disease in the chest wall or pericardium.

Other factors in the history of patients with pulmonary disease include occupational exposures, smoking history, exposure to animals, presence of similar disease in family members (such as occurs in inherited disorders like immotile cilia syndrome, cystic fibrosis, and alpha$_1$-antitrypsin deficiency.)

Physical findings

Respiratory rate above 22/minute suggests underlying pulmonary disease.

Retraction of neck and intercostal muscles during breathing points to generation of excessive negative pressure in the chest during inspiration. It can occur in any severe form of dyspnea but when persistent suggests obstructive airway disease.

A **downward tug on the trachea** is also a sign of obstructive pulmonary disease.

Inward motion of the abdominal wall during inspiration suggests diaphragmatic paralysis. Impending fatigue of respiratory muscles may be signaled by chaotic movement of the abdominal wall during breathing.

Patients with COPD often **exhale through pursed lips,** apparently to increase resistance to air flow and thus allow generation of higher intrathoracic pressures to help force air movement.

Increased anteroposterior dimension of the thorax (barrel chest) occurs with emphysema. Other deformities of the chest wall, such as occur with kyphoscoliosis, can restrict ventilatory movement, leading to recurrent pulmonary infections and COPD.

Splinting, reduction in movement of one side of the chest, usually due to muscle spasm, prevents pleuritic pain by preventing motion. It can be so successful that the patient feels no pain, and the presence of pleurisy can be missed if the splinting is not detected. It is best observed by placing both hands extended over the ribs, with the thumbs maximally extended and meeting in the midline. This allows lateral movement of each thumb from the spinous processes to be seen.

Deviation of the trachea from the midline helps detect change in volume of one hemithorax. For example, pleuritic chest pain with splinting on one side, hyperresonance of that side, and deviation of the trachea to the other side would suggest a tension pneumothorax. If the splinted side is dull, a large pleural effusion is likely, probably inflammatory in view of the evidence of pleural irritation.

Percussion can delineate the extent of an area of consolidation or effusion, mediastinal shifting or widening, and location of the diaphragms. Whether heart size can be detected with reasonable accuracy is debated, but considerable cardiac enlargement can be observed, as can dextrocardia. Palpation of the precordial impulse is a better way of checking for cardiac dilatation and hypertrophy.

Loudness of **breath sounds** depends on rate of flow through large airways, the source of the sounds, and transmission of the sounds to the chest wall. Movement of air can be decreased by splinting, overdistension (emphysema), or bronchial obstruction, and transmission can be dampened by fluid or accentuated if the lung tissue has become relatively solid (consolidation). Compression of lung tissue, such as occurs immediately over a pleural effusion, also increases transmission of breath sounds. Increased transmission of the breath sounds generated in larger airways is called **bronchial breathing**. It is accompanied by increased transmission of voice sounds and often a change in their character, especially whispered sounds (pectoriloquy) and the sound of "e" spoken to sound like "a" (egophony).

Adventitial sounds can arise in the bronchial passages (wheezes or rhonchi), especially when air passes over an area of narrowing and when extra amounts of secretions are present. Wheezes are more common during expiration, since airways are narrower than during inspiration due to the lower negative pressure in the thorax. Generalized wheezing occurs with the bronchospasm of asthma, but a localized wheeze can occur over a single, partially obstructed bronchus, such as occurs with a tumor or a foreign body.

Rales, now more generally called **crackles**, are probably caused by the popping sounds made by the opening of small airways that are coated by a membrane of moisture. Areas of decreased lung volume will have such closed small airways during expiration, and hence such crackles (or fine, moist rales) can be heard at the lung bases when patients who have not been breathing deeply (such as occurs postoperatively after abdominal surgery) take a deep breath on command. They also occur when pulmonary vascular engorgement has occurred during CHF, increasing the amount of fluid in alveoli and small airways. When larger airways are affected by the same process, coarser sounds are heard.

An adventitial sound arising from the pleura, such as a **friction rub**, is a harsh, leathery noise probably due to movement of fibrinous exudate on the surface of inflamed pleura during breathing. Splinting of a hemithorax can prevent a rub from being heard and can prevent rales from appearing. Relieving pain with a narcotic, by ending the splinting, can result in the appearance of such physical findings.

Extrathoracic findings are often helpful in the diagnosis of pulmonary disease but are nonspecific. **Cyanosis** of the skin or nail beds was thought to require 5 g/100 ml of unsaturated hemoglobin but probably requires only 3 g/100 ml. Sensitivity of cyanosis as a sign of unsaturated hemoglobin diminishes with anemia or decreased peripheral perfusion. **Clubbing** (i.e., thickening of peripheral tissues of the fingers), especially the nail beds, with straightening (loss of the angle between the skin and the nail immediately over the nail beds) and subsequently more marked changes can result from any disease that leads to circulation of unsaturated hemoglobin (such as cyanotic congenital heart disease, as well as pulmonary diseases) and also occurs in chronic pulmonary infection, especially bronchiectasis (but is rare in tuberculosis), chronic liver disease, inflammatory bowel disease, and bacterial endocarditis. The most common cause of clubbing in the United States today is carcinoma of the lung. A congenital form of clubbing also occurs, but the history is unreliable since most patients with acquired clubbing are unaware of the development of the nail changes and will say that their nails have always been that way. Only definite familial occurrence is convincing that it is a congenital process.

DIAGNOSTIC PROCEDURES IN PULMONARY DISEASE

Chest x-rays remain the initial step in the workup of pulmonary disease and can reveal abnormalities when the physical findings are normal. Fluoroscopy can detect abnormalities in diaphragmatic movement. Lateral decubitus films can aid in detecting pleural fluid, since it will alter the distribution of the density caused by fluid. Comparison of x-rays taken on inspiration and expiration can detect radiolucent obstructing lesions, since the side with a narrowed bronchus will not decrease in volume normally during expiration and the mediastinum will shift toward the opposite side. Instillation of radiopaque material into the bronchial tree can reveal the presence of bronchiectasis. CT scans aid in detection of certain types of disease, especially small densities like nodules not seen on standard chest x-rays, but specificity is low. CT scans are very helpful in revealing the presence of calcification in lesions, as well as in delineating hilar and mediastinal abnormalities. Ultrasonography is occasionally useful in determining whether a pulmonary lesion is solid or fluid filled (i.e., cystic). Angiography is especially helpful in detecting congenital abnormalities of the vasculature and obstructing arterial lesions, such as pulmonary emboli. Magnetic resonance (MR) imaging and digital subtraction angiography are becoming additional useful procedures.

Pulmonary function studies

Routine spirometry detects vital capacity (VC), forced vital capacity (FVC), forced expired volume in 1 second (FEV$_1$), and the forced midexpiratory flow rate (FEF$_{25-75}$) (the difference in volume per second between 25 and 75% of total expiration). Residual volume (RV), the air left in the lung after full expiration, is difficult to measure accurately. The functional residual capacity (FRC) is the volume left after a normal expiration and is easier to determine. FRC is usually measured by the washout of a gas, usually nitrogen or helium. Body plethysmography is more accurate and can also determine total airway resistance. Airflow can be observed dynamically by a flow-volume loop (a record of the change in volume versus time). Characteristic changes are seen, for example, in obstructive lung disease, restrictive lung disease, and upper airway obstruction.

Diffusion capacity of the alveolocapillary membrane for carbon monoxide (DL$_{CO}$) helps delineate a restrictive process, which has a normal diffusion capacity, from parenchymal disease with decreased DL$_{CO}$.

Other diagnostic procedures

Arterial blood gases (ABGs) reveal partial pressures of oxygen (PaO$_2$) and carbon dioxide (PaCO$_2$) and pH. Alveolar-arterial oxygen differences and venous admixture (Q$_S$/Q$_T$) are useful indicators of pulmonary function. When interpreting the results, the normal PO$_2$ at the patient's age must be taken into account, as must a history of smoking and other factors that can lower the PO$_2$.

Sputum exams for cytology and culture are valuable initial tests. It is important to obtain a true sputum specimen, not just saliva. Alveolar phagocytes (dust cells) or bronchial epithelial cells should be present, not just squamous cells from the mouth. If the patient has difficulty producing a specimen, try first to obtain one on arising in morning. If unsuccessful, a fiberoptic bronchoscopy may be needed to obtain a satisfactory specimen. Neutrophils usually indicate the presence of infection. Gram stain and examination of morphological characteristics of microorganisms are often helpful, especially if bacteria are detected in pus cells.

Fiberoptic bronchoscopy can be indicated to ascertain the cause of a cough, hemoptysis, a persistent localized wheeze, or other evidence of bronchial obstruction or to investigate atelectasis suspected of being due to a tumor or other type of bronchial obstruction. Paralysis of a recurrent laryngeal nerve of unknown etiology also is an indication for bronchoscopy because of the likelihood that the cause is bronchogenic carcinoma. The need to evaluate a patient with diffuse interstitial or parenchymal disease is also an indication for this procedure; a transbronchial biopsy is usually obtained. Bronchoscopy is therapeutically useful to remove thick, obstructing secretions or a foreign body or to arrest an accessible cause of hemorrhage. At times the procedure is valuable in the preoperative assessment of a patient with a lung abscess, carcinoma, tuberculosis, or bronchiectasis.

A transbronchial parenchymal lung biopsy is indicated when bronchoscopy is performed for assessment of a lung infiltrate of unknown cause, especially when interstitial disease or infection of unclear etiology is suspected. Specimens can be obtained for smear and culture, often using special staining and culture techniques (e.g., for *Legionella*), as well as for histological examination.

Open (surgical) lung biopsy is usually indicated only when other procedures have been unsuccessful in establishing a diagnosis; procedures that usually should be performed first include assessment of exposure to various dusts and toxins, careful examination of the sputum for microorganisms and malignant cells, and sometimes a therapeutic trial, such as antibiotic therapy or intensive treatment for CHF.

Pleural biopsy can be indicated in exudative pleural disease to establish a diagnosis of a granulomatous disease such as tuberculosis, a malignant tumor, or rheumatoid pleuritis. Cytological examination of aspirated pleural fluid and culture should be performed first (with incubation of the culture for an adequate period if tuberculosis is suspected).

Mediastinoscopy is useful for diagnosis of mediastinal disease of unknown cause when it is not possible to obtain a biopsy from some other site. Usual indications are consideration of sarcoidosis (if no involved peripheral or scalene node is available) or lung cancer (when bronchoscopy is negative and no supraclavicular node is available for biopsy). The procedure is sometimes indicated for evaluation of the extent of spread of a lung cancer before resective surgery, radiation, or chemotherapy.

As a general rule, invasive procedures with biopsies should not be performed unless there is a reasonable likelihood of obtaining information that will modify the therapeutic program or to obtain baseline data to evaluate the effectiveness of therapy at a later date.

PNEUMONIAS

Clinical picture.   Cough, fever, and malaise are the usual presenting symptoms of pneumonia, at times with blood-streaked sputum and pleuritic chest pain. Physical findings include crackles and signs of consolidation. X-ray will show a pulmonary infiltrate, in contrast to simple bronchitis. The patterns of radiological findings are rarely diagnostically useful.

Diagnostic decisions.   Making a specific diagnosis of the infecting organism may be difficult. Sputum Gram stains are a useful initial step in workup but are often unrevealing. It is important to obtain sputum, not saliva. The presence of polymorphonuclear neutrophils establishes that an infection is present. Intracellular organisms should be sought since they are the most significant. Cultures of blood or pleural fluid are more often helpful than sputum cultures, since overgrowth with oral flora is not a problem, but cultures take several days and are often negative. Serological studies can take up to 5 weeks to demonstrate a change in titer but can be useful in retrospect, especially for *Mycoplasma* and *Legionella*, as well as viruses.

Choice of initial antibiotic therapy is based on the most likely etiologic agent, and often this choice is necessary before bacteriologic information is obtained. The microbial agents that cause pneumonia tend to follow certain patterns that are useful in the initial choice of antibiotic therapy:

In the usual community-acquired pneumonias, over 95% are due to viruses, *Mycoplasma*, pneumococci (*S. pneumoniae*), or *Legionella*, with the first two accounting for over 50%.

Following influenza, *S. pneumoniae, S. aureus,* and *H. influenzae* are usually found.

The most frequent causes of pneumonia in patients with underlying chronic bronchitis are *S. pneumoniae* and *H. influenzae.*

When pneumonia follows aspiration of material from the mouth and pharynx, anaerobes are important pathogens. Gram-negative organisms are rarely responsible for community-acquired pneumonias.

A dry cough and young age without underlying illness suggest a viral etiology. Bacterial etiology is more likely with frank rigors, productive cough, purulent sputum, chest pain, and leukocytosis.

Another approach to consideration of the likely etiologic agent is to consider the component of resistance to infection impairment that led to the pneumonia, as outlined in Table 1-7.

Table 1-7. Types of Pulmonary Pathogens Usually Seen With Impairment of Specific Components of Resistance to Infection

Component of resistance	Usual pathogens
Mucociliary apparatus	Mostly bacteria
Pulmonary alveolar macrophages	Mycobacteria, *Legionella, Pneumocystis carinii*
Polymorphonuclear neutrophils	*S. aureus,* gram-negative organisms, *Candida, Aspergillus, Mucor,* other fungi
Antibodies*	*S. pneumoniae, H. influenzae*
Cellular immunity*	Herpesviruses, facultative intracellular bacteria, and most systemic fungi, including mycobacteria, *P. carinii, Cryptococcus, Nocardia, Legionella,* and *Listeria*
Complement*	Pyogenic bacteria

*Depend on previous exposure to become active.

Therapeutic decisions.   The initial antibiotic chosen for community-acquired pneumonias is often erythromycin since it will cover mycoplasmas and *Legionella* (the erythromycin-sensitive pneumonias), as well as the other usual community-acquired agents. Whether or not hospitalization is indicated depends on the general state of the patient; most can be treated at home.

Pneumonia acquired in the hospital (nosocomial pneumonia) is generally more serious and continues to have a high fatality rate. A majority are due to gram-negative bacteria aspirated from the oropharynx or via an endotracheal tube. Prior antibiotics reduce the amount of competitive normal flora, and gram-negative colonization of the oropharynx is much more frequent in ICU patients than in normal individuals (> 50% versus 2 to 18%). Such colonization makes interpretation of smears and cultures difficult, and identification of the organism is vitally important since appropriate antibiotic therapy must be tailored to its sensitivities. Therefore, in the presence of fever, leukocytosis, new infiltrates on x-ray, and clinical deterioration, transtracheal or bronchoscopic aspiration and even open lung biopsy may be necessary to help in antibiotic choice.

Specific types of pneumonia

Pneumonia in the immunocompromised host is a very common, serious clinical problem. The nature of the underlying disease influences the frequency of certain types of infection. The specific functional defect is an important clue, as summarized in Table 1-7. The clinical picture can also provide diagnostic clues. For example, 1 to 4 months following renal transplants, CMV is a common cause of pneumonia.

Rapid progression suggests *P. carinii*, gram-negative bacteria, tuberculosis, and cryptococcosis. CMV, *Aspergillus*, and *Mucor* usually cause a slower rate of progression, whereas *Nocardia* is generally the slowest.

Skin lesions may be found with bacteremic states, *Cryptococcus*, and *Nocardia*.

Eye lesions are seen with *Candida, Aspergillus, Toxoplasma,* and CMV.

Mucor causes necrotic lesions in the nasal passages.

Meningitis is most frequently caused by tuberculosis and *Cryptococcus* in these patients, whereas encephalitis is more frequent with herpes simplex (HSV) and *Toxoplasma*. In these immunocompromised patients, aggressive steps may have to be taken to identify the infecting organism, including transtracheal and bronchial aspiration and, if necessary, open lung biopsy.

Aspiration pneumonias primarily occur in patients with impaired cough reflex, after heavy sedation such as surgical anesthesia or even an alcoholic binge, and in the presence of neurological disease. Anaerobic bacteria are the most frequent pathogens, especially if the aspiration pneumonia was acquired outside of the hospital. *S. aureus, S. pyogenes,* and gram-negative bacteria are more frequent in nosocomial aspiration pneumonias. Dependent areas of the lung (bases of the lower lobes, apical segment of the upper lobes) are most frequently affected, and the sputum and breath may have a characteristic putrid odor. Abscess formation is common. Invasive aspiration may be necessary to obtain an etiologic diagnosis, but empiric therapy is often adequate. Penicillin G is useful for the oropharyngeal organisms, including *B. fragilis*, and clindamycin or metronidazole may be necessary as well. Surgical drainage may be needed, especially if an empyema develops.

Additional comments about specific etiologic agents:

Viruses are common and usually occur as community epidemics, with symptoms developing 1 to 2 days after exposure. The clinical picture is usually a dry cough with dyspnea, normal findings on physical examination, and mild interstitial infiltration on chest x-ray. Influenza is the organism most frequently identified. It is particularly risky for the elderly and patients with underlying heart or kidney disease. CMV in posttransplant and AIDS patients has recently come into prominence. In these settings, it can have a 50% mortality rate. Varicella developing in adults has a 10 to 20% incidence of pneumonia and may leave a pattern of diffuse, tiny calcifications over both lung fields. Serological findings with convalescent sera can be diagnostic, but the information is rarely useful, particularly in the absence of effective antibiotic therapy for these agents. Serological confirmation is useful, however, for establishing a pattern helpful in diagnosing future cases.

S. pneumoniae, the pneumococcus, is still a common pathogen, with about 25% of the adult population carrying it in the nasopharynx. Increased frequency of pneumococcal infection occurs in people without a functional spleen (postsplenectomy, sickle cell disease) and in people with diabetes mellitus, renal failure, lymphomas, and chronic pulmonary disease. Patients typically present with symptoms of upper respiratory tract infection, followed by cough, chills, fever, dyspnea, often pleuritic chest pain, and sometimes mental confusion. Typical findings include crackles and sometimes consolidation over part of one lung, as well as the appearance of labial HSV. Chest

x-ray can show extensive, even lobar consolidation, but less extensive infiltration is more frequent today, sometimes with only air bronchograms pointing to the site of the lesion. Pleural effusions without identifiable organisms are common, and blood cultures are positive in about 25% of the cases. Sputum Gram stains are often helpful, but cultures are not dependable since there is a high carrier rate in normal people and difficulties in growing the organisms result in a high false-negative rate in people with the disease. Progression to abscess or cavity formation is extremely rare with pneumococcal pneumonia. Penicillin G remains the primary form of treatment, although erythromycin is useful in penicillin-sensitive individuals and vancomycin is needed in some patients.

S. aureus is an uncommon cause of community-acquired pneumonia but is common following a viral pneumonia, since most adults have intermittent or persistent nasal colonization with this organism. The onset resembles pneumococcal pneumonia, but progression to necrosis of pulmonary parenchyma with abscess formation and occasionally empyema can occur. When the pneumonia has developed following spread via the bloodstream, hematogenous skin lesions are common and positive blood cultures are the rule. A diagnosis of infective endocarditis is usually warranted. Sputum Gram stains are usually helpful, and in contrast to pneumococcal infection, the organism can usually be grown when the sputum is purulent. A negative culture would militate strongly against infection with *S. aureus*. Therapy requires a penicillinase-resistant form of penicillin, such as nafcillin. *S. pyogenes* causes a similar clinical picture but is a rare cause of pneumonia.

Gram-negative bacilli are more frequent in hospital-acquired pneumonias, especially in seriously ill patients in ICUs, probably because they are ubiquitous on the hands of hospital personnel and on instruments. *Klebsiella pneumoniae* is more frequent among alcoholics, *E. coli* among patients with intestinal or urinary tract sepsis, *Pseudomonas* among patients with cystic fibrosis. Therapy of these cases usually requires a penicillinase-resistant penicillin or cephalosporin and an aminoglycoside. *H. influenzae* is a very common commensal, and evidence for its being the cause of infection requires isolation from blood, from pleural fluid, or directly from the lung. Sputum culture alone is not convincing. Ampicillin is usually the appropriate antibiotic.

M. pneumoniae produces many extrapulmonary problems as well as pneumonia. The lung findings resemble those seen in viral pneumonia, but myalgias, arthralgias, rashes (erythema nodosum, Stevens-Johnson syndrome) and neurological complications (meningitis, encephalitis, myelitis, neuropathies) also occur. Diagnostic aid is obtained from cold agglutinin titers, which are positive in about 50% of cases after 1 to 2 weeks of infection. This test is not specific, however. Confirmatory specific serological tests require acute as well as convalescent serum obtained at least a month after onset of the infection. Tetracycline and erythromycin shorten the period of illness.

Legionella organisms are widely distributed, found in water in cooling towers and other industrial and home sites. Outbreaks of infection occur, but sporadic infections are more common. In patients with serious underlying disease, there is a significant mortality. The illness usually starts with a dry cough, dyspnea, chills, fever, and malaise. GI symptoms, headache, and confusion are common. Crackles are usually heard on physical examination, but signs of consolidation are rare. Chest x-ray usually shows patchy infiltration, occasionally with a lobar distribution. The diagnosis of *Legionella* infection should be strongly considered in a patient with a patchy pneumonia and involvement of the GI tract and CNS. Examination of sputum or other secretions by direct immunofluorescence can reveal the presence of the organism, and a special stain (Giminez, which is more sensitive than the previously used silver stain) can detect the organism in biopsied tissues. Special charcoal yeast extract medium must be used to culture the organisms, but their slow growth can require up to 10 days. Serological tests require 4 to 8 weeks for confirmation. Therapy must therefore be started without bacteriologic confirmation. Erythromycin usually gives definite improvement within 4 days and reduces the mortality, which is reported to be as high as 20% in previously healthy patients and up to 80% in immuno-compromised hosts.

OTHER PULMONARY INFECTIONS

Tuberculosis is now an infrequent disease in the United States. It usually begins by infection from aerosolized infectious secretions that localize in the lungs, causing a mild process that may involve regional lymph nodes. Arrest of the disease usually occurs, with conversion of skin test to positive after 2 to 10 weeks. A small percentage can develop progressive pulmonary disease or spread to another organ via the bloodstream. At any time later, the initial lesion may reactivate and cause progressive pulmonary disease, with or without new spread to nodes and distant organs. Impaired resistance makes such an outcome more likely and is seen in diabetics and in patients who are immunocompromised, are malnourished, are exposed to silica dust, or are on maintenance hemodialysis.

Reactivated disease most commonly progresses in the apical segments of either upper or lower lobes and may progress to cavitation and spread transbronchially to cause extensive pneumonia. Calcification may appear in old lesions in which there are areas of caseation necrosis. The pleura may be affected early during the initial (primary) infection or later with reactivation. Other organs most frequently affected include the bone, GU tract, peritoneum, pericardium, brain, and meninges. Massive spread into the bloodstream can give widespread, tiny, millet-seed sized foci (miliary tuberculosis) in the lungs and in most other organs.

A negative skin test (done by intradermal injection of 0.1 ml of purified protein derivative [PPD]) in a patient who clearly has had time to develop this phenomenon and has other positive skin tests (intact T-cell functions) points strongly against this diagnosis. A positive test requires at least 10 mm of induration 48 hours after injection. Definitive diagnosis requires demonstration of the organism by acid-fast staining of sputum or culture from sputum. If expectorated sputum is unavailable, swallowed sputum can be obtained by early morning gastric aspiration. On smears, the organism must be differentiated from other acid-fast bacteria and *Nocardia*.

Therapy of active tuberculosis today includes use of more than one drug. Most regimens employ two or three drugs given simultaneously to prevent development of antibiotic resistance. Isoniazid, rifampin, and ethambutol are usually used. Nine months to a year of therapy are usually given.

A person known to have a negative tuberculin skin test that converts to positive should be given a course of antibiotic therapy even if examination and x-rays reveal no evidence of active disease. The most common regimen used today is isoniazid for 9 months, but in people over 35, liver toxicity is common and may require switching to another antituberculous drug.

An increasing percentage of patients are being found to have infection with different mycobacteria than *M. tuberculosis,* particularly those with underlying COPD or silicosis. *M. kansasii* and *M. avium-intracellulare* are most frequent, the latter especially so in patient with AIDS. The disease is usually confined to the lung, except in AIDS patients, who commonly have positive blood cultures and widespread disease. These other acid-fast bacilli are very resistant to antibiotic therapy.

It is helpful to divide **fungal infections** into two groups, those that occur in hosts with impaired defense mechanisms, such as *Candida, Mucor,* and *Aspergillus,* and those that occur in otherwise healthy individuals, such as *Histoplasma, Coccidioides,* and *Blastomycosis. C. neoformans* infects both types and is especially common after prolonged therapy with corticosteroids.

Histoplasmosis occurs especially after exposure to bird droppings and is most common in the main river valleys of the eastern half of the United States. **Coccidioidomycosis** occurs primarily in the southwestern United States and the valleys of California, whereas **blastomycosis** is usually seen in the mountainous areas of the southeastern United States. Blastomycosis typically causes skin lesions and occasionally affects the lungs or GU tract. Coccidioidomycosis commonly causes skin lesions (erythema nodosum) during the early phase of infection, and histoplasmosis typically causes multiple small lung nodules that can appear later as many tiny calcified foci.

Candidal infections may be limited to the oropharynx, may extend down the esophagus, or may spread into the lung. Since the organism is ubiquitous, positive smears and cultures are of little value. Culture from a tissue biopsy is usually necessary, especially if pneumonia is suspected. **Aspergillosis** occurs primarily in patients with prior chronic lung disease. It can cause a large mass (aspergilloma) in a lung cavity that typically is surrounded by a crescent of air or an invasive, widespread disease. Allergic reactions to colonization of chronic bronchitis with *Aspergillus* cause aggravation of the underlying asthma, fleeting shadows on chest x-ray, eosinophils in sputum and blood, and a positive skin test. Symptoms respond to corticosteroids. **Mucor infections** occur primarily in diabetics and resemble invasive aspergillosis, usually with rhinocerebral involvement.

Therapeutic decisions. Therapy of these fungus infections usually requires amphotericin B, although topical antifungal agents may be more appropriate for oral or esophageal candidiasis (thrush).

OBSTRUCTIVE LUNG DISEASES

Pathophysiology and clinical findings. Narrowing of an airway causes more resistance to airflow in expiration than in inspiration. Any narrowing is aggravated by the intrathoracic pressure, which is higher during expiration, decreasing the size of bronchi. Since the elastic recoil pressure of the lung tissue exerts traction on the airways, tending to keep them open wider, reduction in elasticity such as occurs in emphysema further narrows bronchi during expiration. Active bronchoconstriction adds further to obstruction to airflow. Constriction results from cholinergic stimuli to bronchial smooth muscle via vagal nerves, resulting from stimulation to irritant receptors just beneath the mucosa of the upper respiratory tract. Prostaglandins and leukotrienes derived from arachidonic acid are also bronchoconstrictive, as is histamine. These pathways are hyperreactive in patients with obstructive lung disease. Bronchial secretions are more abundant and thicker in patients with chronic inflammation, further narrowing airways. Chronic inflammation can lead to loss of ciliated epithelium, diminishing ability to move secretions, as well as to peribronchial fibrosis, contributing still more to the narrowing.

The pulmonary diseases characterized by obstruction of airflow during expiration include acute airway narrowing, such as occurs in asthma, permanent overdistension of the lung, as in emphysema, and chronic processes affecting the bronchi, including chronic bronchitis with or without bronchiectasis.

In obstructive lung disease, pulmonary function tests show an increase in RV and FRC, although total lung capacity (TLC) is normal or increased. VC is decreased, since the RV takes up a higher proportion of TLC. One of the main factors responsible for the increase in RV and FRC is the tendency of abnormal small airways to collapse and close during expiration, trapping air.

Patients with active bronchoconstriction, such as occurs during an attack of asthma, tend to have dyssynchronous control of respiratory muscle function, with active contraction of inspiratory muscles during expiration, tending to maintain a higher FRC. The work of breathing is increased in these patients, adding to the sense of dyspnea and to their functional problems. The work of breathing is high because of the increased airway resistance. Breathing at a higher lung volume means that a greater pressure change is necessary for a given change in volume, further increasing the work of breathing. The higher volume of the thorax stretches the inspiratory muscles, moving them to a suboptimal position in their length-tension curve. These factors bring about fatigue of the respiratory muscles, impairing their function. Overdistension of the lungs as a result of airway trapping tends to dilate airways, and thus hyperinflation diminishes the symptoms of asthma.

The abnormality in gas exchange is aggravated by disturbances in the matching of ventilation and perfusion. As the PO_2 tends to decrease, most patients increase minute ventilation, keeping PCO_2 normal or even below normal. As the process worsens, further increases in ventilation become impossible because of the high energy requirements of the work of breathing or muscle fatigue, and hypercapnia develops. Increasing the PCO_2 increases the efficiency of its elimination, since the pressure gradient is increased. Acute exacerbations, such as infection (producing exudate in alveoli interfering with gas exchange) or heart failure (causing changes in blood flow distribution), may increase the ventilation-perfusion mismatch, resulting in a sudden worsening of the gas exchange abnormalities. Hypercapnia and hypoxemia may worsen during the night because of the decrease in minute ventilation that occurs with sleep.

Cigarette smoking is currently the most important factor in the genesis of **emphysema**, perhaps because irritants cause mobilization of macrophages and neutrophils into the lungs,

resulting in protease activity in excess of inhibitory antiproteases. Genetic factors probably play a role, since only about 10 to 15% of smokers develop emphysema, and the genetically inherited abnormality in control of proteases, alpha₁-antitrypsin inhibitor deficiency, results in severe emphysema in early adulthood.

Pathologically, there is destruction of alveolar walls and enlargement of air spaces distal to the terminal bronchioles, enlarging the total lung volume. The destructive changes cause a decrease in elastic recoil and therefore a decrease in lung compliance (meaning that there is an increase in the pressure that must be generated to produce a given change in volume of the lung). Clinically, patients with emphysema have dyspnea, at first with exercise, then at rest, with or without cough and sputum. Examination shows increased volume of the thorax, decreased breath sounds, and increased use of accessory muscles for breathing. These patients tend to be thin, perhaps losing weight because of the high caloric expenditure of the extra work of breathing.

X-rays show evidence of hyperinflation, changes in vasculature, and sometimes evidence of bullae. Routine pulmonary function studies usually show decrease in the VC, FEV_1, and flow rates and increased RV, FRC, and TLC. Some improvement in function may occur with bronchodilators.

Chronic bronchitis, defined as cough with sputum production for 3 months each year for 3 or more years, often is the result of cigarette smoking or exposure to other environmental irritants, but climate also plays a role, judging by the frequency in different geographic areas. Bacterial infection is a common secondary development, aggravating the underlying disease and leading to progression, as well as to acute exacerbations. Airway obstruction commonly occurs, and the findings depend on the degree of emphysema that results. Marked obstruction leads to significant degrees of hypoxemia, which in turn causes pulmonary arterial vasoconstriction. Pulmonary hypertension and cor pulmonale can result. Secondary polycythemia is a common associated finding.

Bronchiectasis, dilatation of segments of bronchi due to destruction of the musculoelastic layer of the bronchial wall, can develop following necrotizing infection or exposure to corrosive gas. Much less common than in the past, it is usually seen in patients with recurrent lung infections due to hypogammaglobulinemia or some other cause of decreased resistance to infection. Congenital causes include the **immotile cilia syndrome**, resulting from abnormal microtubules in the epithelial cells and often accompanied by sinusitis and dextrocardia or situs inversus.

In patients with bronchiectasis, there is failure to clear secretions normally, resulting from loss of ciliated epithelium, dilated segments, and loss of normal muscular peristaltic action. As a consequence, episodes of secondary infection are common, causing further destruction of bronchial walls. Chronic cough is usual, with abundant, purulent, even foul sputum, often with hemoptysis during exacerbations of infection; examination reveals localized crackles and wheezes, often with clubbing.

Chest x-ray may be surprisingly normal or may reveal extensive fibrosis and infiltrations (which increase during exacerbations of infection). Evidence of emphysema may be present. Bronchography demonstrates the lesions, but CT scan can also be definitive. Pulmonary function studies show variable findings, depending on the degree of bronchial obstruction and emphysema. Pulmonary fibrosis may cause restrictive changes in lung volumes.

Cystic fibrosis is an autosomal recessive genetic disorder that occurs in about 1 in 2,000 births among whites. Thick, viscous, tenacious mucus is secreted, leading to pulmonary infections, and usually bronchiectasis develops in childhood. Clubbing and cor pulmonale frequently develop. Similar changes in GI secretions lead to neonatal meconium ileus, and comparable problems can develop later in life. Plugging of pancreatic ducts leads to steatorrhea and malnutrition, and often there is accompanying hepatic cirrhosis, diabetes mellitus, and sterility. Recurrent pulmonary infections usually are the biggest problem, often with mucoid strains of *Pseudomonas aeruginosa.* Milder cases are often overlooked or misdiagnosed as asthma or chronic bronchitis. A diagnostic finding is the presence of high Na or Cl in sweat (>60 mEq/L in children, >80 in adults). Therapy of infections and correction of malnutrition have improved the prognosis.

Asthma is characterized by episodic bronchoconstriction, causing dyspnea with wheezing. Extrinsic, allergic mechanisms cause release of bronchoconstrictive mediators from mast cells sensitized by IgE antibodies on exposure to specific antigens. Other causes in sensitive people include exposure to cold, aspirin and other NSAIDs, and a wide variety of environmental and especially occupational stimulants. In many cases of adult onset, there are no known precipitating factors.

Diagnostic decisions. Workup during an acute attack reveals hyperinflation of the lungs on physical examination and x-ray, decreased FEV_1 that improves with administration of a bronchodilator, and, in appropriate cases of unclear nature, confirmation of the diagnosis by challenge with the suspected stimulant (or methacholine or histamine) during an asymptomatic period, under careful observation. Skin tests are rarely of value (except in diagnosis of aspergillosis.) The blood may show increased eosinophils and IgE levels. In severe attacks, ABGs must be monitored. Hypoxemia is common, with decreased PCO_2 initially, but in severe cases hypercapnia may develop, with a mixed respiratory acidosis (due to retention of CO_2) and metabolic acidosis (due to anoxemia with increased oxygen demand because of the greatly increased work of breathing, causing lactic acidosis). If hypercapnia appears and the patient does not respond to therapy, intubation and mechanical ventilation may become necessary and can be lifesaving.

Therapeutic decisions. The most important measures in the therapy of obstructive lung disease are those directed at decreasing airway obstruction. Hydration is important to keep secretions thin. Measures such as inhaled mucolytics, iodides, etc. are of questionable value. Avoiding inhaled irritants, cigarette smoke in particular, is vital. (Smokers with COPD lose an average of 80 ml of FEV_1 per year; those who quit lose 30 ml/year, the same as nonsmokers). Bronchodilators such as subcutaneous epinephrine and nebulized isoproterenol are useful, but side effects occur as a result of stimulation of both $alpha_1$ and $alpha_2$ receptors. Beta$_2$-specific noncatecholamine agents, such as terbutaline and albuterol, are effective by mouth and have longer duration of action. Methylxanthines (e.g., theophylline) are also very useful bronchodilators, but serum levels >20 μg/lml have considerable toxicity. Anticho-

linergic agents are also useful. Corticosteroids are necessary for severe exacerbations, and sometimes for maintenance. Inhaled agents such as beclomethasone have reduced toxicity. Sodium cromolyn can prevent exacerbations and reduce steroid need. Intermittent positive-pressure breathing is not useful.

Oxygen is useful when hypoxemia is significant (e.g., saturation <90%). Sometimes small amounts (such as a flow rate <4 L/minute) can be sufficient, since desaturation is usually due to ventilation-perfusion mismatch rather than impaired diffusion. When oxygen is administered, care must be taken to see that patients with hypercapnia, in whom the hypoxic drive to breathe is essential, do not develop decreased ventilation with further retention of CO_2, leading to somnolence and coma (CO_2 narcosis). If this occurs, mechanical ventilation is usually necessary. In patients with hypoxemic vasoconstriction, the resulting cor pulmonale may respond to long-term 24-hour oxygen administration, and home oxygen can be arranged.

Antibiotics are often necessary and are chosen according to the organisms isolated when specific pathogens are found. Usually, no specific flora is identified. Broad-spectrum drugs (ampicillin, triple sulfa, tetracycline) can be useful, and sometimes is beneficial when administered prophylactically several weeks each month. Other useful measures include attention to nutritional status and, perhaps, chest physiotherapy.

A recommended sequence of choice of therapeutic agents is shown in the box below.

Therapeutic Agents in Obstructive Lung Diseases

Emergency therapy of bronchospasm
1. Subcutaneous epinephrine or alpha$_2$ agent
2. IV aminophylline
3. Corticosteroids
4. Admit to hospital

Chronic outpatient treatment of bronchospasm
1. Inhalation of alpha$_2$ agent
2. Long-acting theophylline
3. For COPD
   a. Inhaled anticholinergic agents
   b. Corticosteroids

   For asthma
   a. Inhaled steroids or cromolyn
   b. Oral steroids or anticholinergic agent

DIFFUSE PULMONARY FIBROSIS

A variety of stimuli can cause a chronic process characterized by infiltration of lung tissue by inflammatory cells in the alveolar spaces and the lung interstitium, with progression to deposition of fibrous tissue. Clinically these diseases are characterized by dyspnea, nonproductive cough, tachypnea, and the presence of crackles diffusely in the lungs. As fibrosis develops, functional tests show decrease in lung volumes, compliance, and diffusion capacity. Replacement of alveoli by fibrosis and interference with gas diffusion by collagen deposited between alveolar spaces and capillaries lead to ventilation-perfusion imbalance and arterial hypoxemia. Hypercapnia is uncommon, since CO_2 diffuses much more readily than oxygen, but the hypoxemia leads to pulmonary hypertension and cor pulmonale can be a late development.

A variety of basic disease processes can lead to diffuse pulmonary fibrosis. At times the diagnosis is suggested by extrapulmonary findings, such as node or skin lesions in sarcoidosis or joint findings and rheumatoid factor in rheumatoid arthritis, but fiberoptic bronchoscopy and transbronchial biopsy are frequently indicated to establish the nature of the pulmonary pathology.

Pneumoconioses are an important cause of this syndrome. Silica, coal dust, talc, fiberglass, asbestos, and metal dusts, especially those containing beryllium, are major industrial causes of pulmonary fibrosis. Coal dust deposited around first- and second-order bronchioles causes black lung, which infrequently causes functional or clinical abnormalities. About 5% of coal workers develop cough and show a fine reticular pattern on chest x-ray. Nodular densities may appear, and in less than <0.5% they become larger than 1 cm and can progress to massive areas of fibrosis. Silica dust is much more fibrogenic, and diffuse fibrosis develops in most people exposed to such dust for 20 years or more. Intensive exposure to finer dusts can cause severe disease with less than 5 years of exposure. X-rays show evidence of fibrosis, varying from small nodules diffusely distributed, predominantly in the upper lobes, to large nodules, varying from 1 cm to large masses of fibrosis, which can be lobar. Hilar node enlargement is common and can lead to peripherally located calcium deposition (eggshell calcification); silicosis is characterized by increased susceptibility to infection with mycobacteria; and *M. tuberculosis, M. kanasii,* or *M. intracellularis* infections may be superimposed.

Asbestosis causes a dose-dependent pulmonary fibrosis, and often calcified plaques may appear in the pleura. Mesotheliomas of the pleura and peritoneum develop. There is also a marked increase in the incidence of carcinoma of the lung (about 5-fold in nonsmokers and 60- to 90-fold in smokers). A long latent period of 20 to 40 years usually occurs between exposure to asbestos and the appearance of these tumors.

Treatment of pneumoconioses consists of removal from further exposure to dusts and cigarette smoke, treatment of any superimposed infection, and use of bronchodilators and oxygen as needed.

Idiopathic pulmonary fibrosis, sometimes called the Hamman-Rich syndrome or cryptogenic pulmonary fibrosis, can be a rapidly progressive process. Its cause is unknown. **Pulmonary alveolar proteinosis** is a rare disease of unknown cause. The alveoli become filled with an exudate rich in protein and lipid, which can cause severe hypoxemia. Pulmonary lavage is reported to help some cases. Other rare lung diseases include **pulmonary hemosiderosis,** characterized by hemoptysis and occurring primarily in young girls, and **pulmonary histiocytosis X,** or eosinophilic granuloma of the lung, which is characterized by reticulonodular lesions of the mid and upper lung areas with hilar adenopathy and often with a honeycomb appearance. It occurs mainly in young adults, and pneumothorax is a common complication.

Hypersensitivity pneumonitis can appear following development of sensitivity to some inhaled organic substance. Typically, a few hours following exposure the sensitized patient develops cough, fever, and dyspnea. Crackles are heard diffusely over both lungs, and chest x-ray reveals nodular and reticular infiltrates. Symptoms resolve but recur with renewed exposure. Repeated exacerbations gradually lead to diffuse

fibrosis and restrictive changes in pulmonary function. Among the causes of this syndrome are thermophilic actinomycetes found in moldy hay (**Farmer's lung**) and in humidifiers, bacteria found in water (e.g., *Bacillus subtilis*), fungi in moldy organic material (Maple-bark-stripper's lung, sequoiosis), protein antigens from animals such as in bird droppings or dander (**pigeon-breeder's lung, rodent-handler's disease**) and amoeba found in warm water (**humidifier's lung**). Precipitins that react with the specific antigen may be demonstrable in the serum of affected patients, but asymptomatic individuals may show such precipitins. Treatment is mainly removal from further exposure and use of corticosteroids for acute exacerbations. The value of steroids for the chronic fibrotic phase is not certain.

Other causes of pulmonary fibrosis include radiation (exposure to > 5,000 rads during a 4- to 6-week period causes fibrosis, which appears in 6 to 12 months); drugs (some, such as methotrexate, do so by a hypersensitivity reaction, whereas others, such as chlorambucil, are dose related); and noxious gases, including chlorine and ammonia. Other cancer chemotherapeutic agents that can cause pulmonary fibrosis are bleomycin and busulfan; some analgesics are thought to produce this syndrome, including NSAIDs and opiates, as well as antibiotics, including nitrofurantoin and sulfonamides.

Systemic connective tissue diseases can cause pulmonary disease. **Rheumatoid arthritis** can cause a pleural effusion, which characteristically has a low glucose level because of an abnormal transport of the sugar, and pulmonary nodules, which can be a problem to distinguish from tumor nodules. These findings occur primarily in seropositive patients (with circulating rheumatoid factor). In addition, there is increased reactivity of these patients when subject to dusts. As a result, coal workers get a severe form of pneumoconiosis (Caplan's syndrome). Diffuse pulmonary fibrosis or a pulmonary vasculitis, SLE, polymositis, Sjögrens syndrome, or scleroderma. **Wegener's syndrome** causes granulomatous lesions in the upper respiratory passages, including the sinuses and lung parenchyma, as well as a vasculitis, including a glomerulonephritis. The lung lesions typically cavitate. Wegener's responds well to cyclophosphamide. **Lymphomatoid granulomatosis** resembles Wegener's but has a high frequency of CNS involvement and the development of malignant lymphomas.

Pulmonary infiltrates with eosinophilia (PIE) occurs as **Löffler's syndrome,** transient pulmonary infiltrates anywhere in the lungs with peripheral eosinophilia, sometimes due to a parasitic infestation. A more persistent process is called **chronic eosinophilic pneumonia,** which typically involves peripheral areas of the lung. PIE often occurs in patients with asthma who have allergic bronchopulmonary aspergillosis, which can cause necrotic lesions of the bronchi, leading to bronchiectasis. A form of hypersensitivity vasculitis with granulomatous lesions in many organs (allergic granulomatous vasculitis) also causes PIE with asthma.

SARCOIDOSIS

Sarcoidosis is a disease characterized by granulomas in lymph nodes and a variety of organs. Its cause is unknown. In the United States, it is much more common in blacks. The main defect known is in T-cell function, resulting in negative skin test responses, increased levels of serum IgG, and stimulation of macrophages to form granulomas containing giant cells. Lesions occur in the skin, lung, liver, spleen, eyes, CNS, joints, and muscle. About half the patients have pulmonary lesions.

Diagnostic decisions. The diagnosis is usually made by obtaining a lymph node or a transbronchial pulmonary biopsy showing granulomas, in the absence of another cause such as tuberculosis or a fungal infection. Chest x-rays may show only hilar adenopathy (strongly suggestive of sarcoidosis when found in combination with skin lesions characteristic of erythema nodosum), with or without parenchymal infiltrates. Metabolic abnormalities seen include hypergammaglobulinemia, increased conversion of vitamin D to very active intermediates (e.g., the 1,25 dihydroxy form) with resulting hypercalcemia, and increased serum levels of angiotensin-converting enzyme.

Therapeutic decisions. Most patients recover without therapy. Progression to pulmonary fibrosis occurs in about 10%, and corticosteroid therapy can be helpful. Eye and CNS lesions can cause serious functional problems, and steroid therapy is indicated for these cases early in the course.

ADULT RESPIRATORY DISTRESS SYNDROME

Severe pulmonary failure can develop in acutely ill people, such as postoperatively, following severe trauma, or during severe sepsis. The syndrome resembles the respiratory distress syndrome of the newborn and thus has been named the adult respiratory distress syndrome (ARDS). It is characterized by an increase in extravascular lung water, which accumulates in interstitial areas, around airways and arteries, and in alveolar walls. As it progresses, fluid appears in the alveoli. As a result, the lung is stiffened (decreases in compliance) and impaired gas exchange results in severe hypoxemia. In effect, there is pulmonary arteriovenous shunting. An alteration in alveolar capillary membrane permeability seems to be the fundamental defect in this disease process, and the exudate that forms has high protein content. Some cases follow aspiration of gastric acid or other chemical injury, whereas others follow an extensive viral pneumonia. Often the etiologic mechanism is obscure but may involve complement activation, prostaglandin formation, or formation of toxic oxygen radicals. DIC often accompanies ARDS.

Clinically the process begins as dyspnea, hyperventilation, and the appearance of bilateral pulmonary infiltrates on chest x-ray. There is rapid progression, with severe arterial hypoxemia and rapid fall in lung compliance, aggravating the functional problem. Usually the syndrome appears about 24 hours after the initial insult and progresses to severe pulmonary failure by 72 hours. X-ray can show progression of the areas of density to involve all of both lungs.

Therapeutic decisions. Therapy includes treatment of the underlying condition, fluid management, and ventilatory support. Corticosteroids are of questionable value. Antibiotics are chosen according to bacteriologic findings, but prophylactic therapy is indicated. Despite these measures, the mortality rate remains above 50%. High levels of inspired oxygen are often needed but are relatively ineffective because of the extensive shunting; levels of FiO_2 above 0.60 are toxic after about 72 hours, especially in susceptible patients such as these, and if maintained at that level can contribute to the lung damage.

Development of hypercapnia requires assisted ventilation, and intubation or tracheostomy is usually needed early in these cases. Ventilatory support is usually best given with volume control, such as intermittent mandatory ventilation or assisted-control ventilation. This allows greater control than pressure-cycled ventilators, which may reach a preset pressure level without introducing an adequate volume in these patients because of the decreased lung compliance. Positive end-expiratory pressure (PEEP) can prevent collapse of airways during the expiratory phase. Excessive pressures in the lung (pulmonary barotrauma) can cause pneumomediastinum, subcutaneous emphysema, and pneumothorax.

Flow-directed (Swan-Ganz) catheters in the pulmonary circulation are valuable in monitoring fluid need, to avoid inducing CHF, aggravating pulmonary edema on that basis, and because it is valuable to follow the effects of variation in ventilator controls on cardiac output. Decreased cardiac output can develop, partly because of impaired venous return when intrathoracic pressures are maintained at a high level, and increased oxygen extraction peripherally can result in lower venous oxygen content. The very high level of shunting occurring in the lungs thus can give rise to lower arterial PO_2 on this basis, and if this value is misinterpreted, excessive administration of oxygen may be given, aggravating the problem of pulmonary toxicity. Lactic acidosis is another complication of this syndrome, but it is not a sensitive indicator of inadequate oxygen delivery to the tissues since it can be removed very effectively by the liver, if that organ is well perfused.

MISCELLANEOUS IMPORTANT PULMONARY DISEASES

Drowning

Drowning people inhale a variable amount of fluid, sometimes none at all because of a closed glottis. In near-drowning, the aspirated water can lead to hypovolemia if it is salt water or hypervolemia if fresh water. Survivors usually have severe metabolic acidosis, mostly due to lactate, and some develop acute tubular necrosis. Immersion in very cold water has a better prognosis since it decreases oxygen demand. Therapy should consist of CPR, with mouth-to-mouth resuscitation, without wasting time trying to drain water from the lung since there may be very little there. Oxygen should be administered as soon as possible. Bicarbonate is needed, and bronchodilators are necessary for the bronchospasm that usually is present. If the patient survives, ARDS usually develops, and intubation with mechanical ventilation is often required, as well as correction of electrolyte and renal function abnormalities.

Pleural effusions

About 5 to 10 L of fluid are filtered by the parietal pleura each day and absorbed by the visceral pleura, primarily into the lymphatics. Effusions result from changes in hydrostatic pressure or osmotic pressure, favoring increased movement of fluid from the parietal surface, or inflammatory processes, increases in capillary permeability, or lymphatic abnormalities.

Diagnostic decisions. Characteristics of pleural fluid that are of diagnostic value are described in the box that follows:

Examination of Pleural Fluid

Blood is suggestive of malignancy, but small amounts can give a red tinge. (True hemothorax, such as follows trauma, is defined as a hematocrit above 20).

A **transudate**, such as occurs with CHF or nephrotic syndrome with anasarca, has a protein concentration below 3 g/100 ml, a ratio of pleural fluid protein to serum protein below 0.5, LDH below 200 IU/L, and a ratio of pleural fluid to serum LDH below 0.6. **Exudates** have higher levels of protein and LDH.

In rheumatoid arthritis, the pleural fluid **glucose** is low, often below 20 mg/100 ml.

Pleural fluid amylase levels are elevated in esophageal perforation as well as in pancreatitis.

A high **eosinophil count** in pleural fluid can occur with a chronic effusion or with the presence of air or blood in the pleural space.

A high relative **lymphocyte count** (>50%) suggests tuberculosis or a malignancy.

Cytological examination is useful for seeking evidence of malignancy and is more often positive than a pleural biopsy, and a biopsy should not be performed unless cytology is negative or tuberculosis suspected, since smears and cultures of a biopsy have a higher percentage of positives for tubercle bacilli than such examination of the pleural fluid.

Therapeutic decisions. Although diagnostic taps should be performed whenever the diagnosis is in doubt, especially if infection is suspected, repeated taps are generally unnecessary and repeated removal of large amounts of fluid can cause significant protein loss. However, infected fluid should be drained repeatedly, and a tube inserted for drainage is usually needed.

Similarly, pneumothorax often needs insertion of a tube for drainage, since formation of a one-way valve allowing buildup of air and pressure (tension pneumothorax) is common. Symptoms of pneumothorax usually are chest pain and dyspnea. Physical findings may be normal, or hyperresonance and shift of the mediastinum away from the side of the air leak (e.g., tracheal shift) may be detected if a tension pneumothorax has developed.

Obesity, pickwickian syndrome, and sleep apnea

The drive for respiration is controlled by two main centers, a central chemoreceptor that is located in the medulla and is responsive to CO_2 and H^+, and peripheral chemoreceptors in the aortic arch and carotid arteries, which are primarily responsive to hypoxia. The peripheral receptors respond exponentially, meaning that very little change in ventilation occurs until the PO_2 reaches about 60 mm Hg, but lower levels of oxygen tension cause marked increases in ventilation. The central receptors respond in linear fashion to the PCO_2, meaning that any increase causes some response in ventilation, averaging 2 L/minute/mm Hg increase in PCO_2. This response is blunted in obesity-hypoventilation syndrome and in idiopathic hypoventilation, neurological disorders, narcotic ingestion, and hypothyroidism. The exact mechanism responsible

for the hypoventilation in some patients with obesity is unclear. It can cause somnolence, significant hypoxemia with polycythemia, pulmonary hypertension, and cor pulmonale. This complex is usually referred as the pickwickian syndrome.

The **sleep apnea syndrome** can be due to a decreased sensitivity of the central respiratory center or obstruction of the upper airway due to enlarged tonsils, adenoids, macroglossia, myxedema, nasal surgery, or fat deposition. These patients usually snore loudly and often become very restless during sleep, thrashing wildly. Daytime somnolence is usual, probably because of repeated awakenings at night. Headache, morning hypertension, and deterioration in mental acuity are common. Monitoring of the EEG during sleep, electro-oculography, and ABG determinations are helpful in making the diagnosis. Treatment consists of weight loss, removing any airway obstruction if possible, insertion of tracheostomy if necessary, and use of continuous positive-airway pressure to the nose. A stimulant to the respiratory center such as methylprogesterone can be useful.

Carbon monoxide inhalation does not produce pulmonary changes, since it is odorless, colorless, tasteless, and not locally irritating. Because it has a much greater affinity for hemoglobin than oxygen (210:1), it decreases the oxygen-carrying capacity of the blood, as well as shifting the oxygen dissociation curve of hemoglobin to the left (decreasing the dissociation of oxygen to the tissues). A cherry red lip color is characteristic.

Smoke inhalation is often accompanied by burns of the upper airway, which can produce stridor, hoarseness, and dyspnea, requiring intubation. Lower-airway damage, usually due to irritating gases in smoke, can produce ARDS. The chest x-ray can initially be misleadingly normal. It is important to listen for crackles over the lungs, observe for evidence of hypoxia (headache, fatigue, behavioral change), monitor the ABGs, and check for carbon monoxyhemoglobin (COHb). Oxygen saturation may be misleading in CO poisoning, and COHb should be measured (normal <2%, up to 10% in smokers, occasionally 50% in fire victims). Management requires oxygen to speed the elimination of CO, ventilatory assistance as needed, bronchodilators, corticosteroids, and sometimes hyperbaric oxygen for severe CO poisoning. Late development of tracheal stenosis or bronchiolitis obliterans is possible.

LUNG TUMORS

Carcinoma of the lung is now the most common cause of death from cancer in both sexes. It is 10 to 30 times more common in smokers. About 4% of those who have smoked for at least 40 years develop the disease. Exposure to asbestos greatly increases the incidence. Other industrial agents cause some increase. Carcinomas can appear in old scars or granulomatous lesions in the lung.

The most common benign lung tumors are (1) **bronchial adenoma**, which is usually central, bleeds, and can obstruct a bronchus and (2) **hamartoma**, which is usually peripheral and has a typical popcorn appearance on x-ray due to calcification within it. Currently, **squamous cell** and **adenocarcinomas** each account for about one-third of the primary malignant tumors of the lung, with the remainder divided about evenly between **large and small cell (undifferentiated or oat cell) cancers**. Squamous and oat cell lesions tend to be central, commonly causing perihilar masses, whereas adenocarcinomas and large cell lesions tend to be peripheral and not infrequently cavitate. Oat cell has the shortest average doubling time and tends to metastasize early. It has the worst prognosis. Adenocarcinomas also tend to metastasize early.

Other tumors frequently cause **metastases** to the lung, especially kidney, thyroid, bone, and testicular tumors. Malignancies arising in other structures in the thorax often spread to the lung or pleura by direct extension. Some tumors tend to spread into the lungs along the lymphatics (**lymphangitic spread**), including breast, stomach, pancreas, ovary, prostate, as well as primary tumors of the lung. These cases typically develop severe dyspnea with minimal ray changes of reticular or diffuse infiltrates on x-ray.

Carcinomas of the lung cause a variety of clinical syndromes. Cough is the most frequent symptom (about three-fourths of cases), often with some hemoptysis (about one-half of cases). Dyspnea and chest pain are also common. Bronchoalveolar carcinomas tend to produce a lot of sputum. Tumors arising in the apex of the lung (**Pancoast tumors**) can spread into the chest wall and cause loss of function of the inferior cervical sympathetic ganglion. The resulting **Horner's syndrome** typically includes unilateral mydriasis, partial ptosis, and loss of sweating on that side of the face. Extension of the tumor into the mediastinum can cause compression and obstruction of the vena cava, with edema of the face and arms, severe dyspnea with stridor, and headache. A localized wheeze can be heard over a partial bronchial obstruction. Direct extension of the tumor to the pleura can give a large effusion that is often hemorrhagic, with involvement of the pericardium. Phrenic nerve involvement can cause diaphragmatic paralysis. The most common sites of metastases of lung tumors are the brain, liver, bone, lymph nodes, and adrenal glands.

A variety of paraneoplastic syndromes also occur, including polymyositis, the syndrome of inappropriate secretion of ADH (SIADH), clubbing with painful extremities (hypertrophic pulmonary osteoarthropathy), gynecomastia, secretion of PTH with hypercalcemia, the secretion of ACTH with Cushing's syndrome, and other neuromuscular and hematologic abnormalities. The usual associations are shown in Table 1-8.

Diagnostic decisions. Workup for carcinoma of the lung should be triggered by any suspicious lesion, in view of the epidemic nature of the disease at present. The availability of a previous chest x-ray is very valuable in providing guidance regarding the necessity for extensive investigation. A hilar mass is typical of small cell carcinoma, especially with mediastinal widening. A peripheral mass is typical of adenocarcinoma if under 4 cm, but squamous is also possible if it is larger. Apical tumors are usually squamous, and decreased volume of a lobe or segment (atelectasis) usually indicates an endobronchial lesion, typical of squamous cell. A cavitary lesion suggests squamous cell but can be any type except small cell. Routine lab tests can be useful, especially the alkaline phosphatase to screen for bone or liver metastases and serum calcium for bone lesions or a paraneoplastic syndrome with excessive PTH secretion. Bronchoscopy with biopsy of any visualized lesion or cytology should be done quickly. Mediastinoscopy is usually done preoperatively to determine resectability.

A new solitary pulmonary nodule is suggestive of carcinoma of the lung until proved otherwise. Close to 40% are malignant, especially those with indistinct margins. Calcification usually indicates it is benign, unless the calcium is eccentrically placed. A calcified nodule can be followed at 6-month intervals, as can one known to be stable for at least 2 years. Uncalcified lesions that are growing (doubling in volume in between 20 days and 450 days) should be resected.

Therapeutic decisions. Treatment is surgical resection, except with small cell lesions, which can be considered metastatic when first diagnosed. Radiation and chemotherapy are of questionable value but are tried in small cell lesions and with brain metastases. Prognosis is poor.

DISEASES OF THE GI TRACT

DIAGNOSTIC GI PROCEDURES

Useful points about the history and physical examination are included in discussion of each disease process. However, before discussing individual diseases, a general review of the use of radiological and endoscopic procedures in GI tract disease is given since it is of special importance in preparation for board examinations.

Plain films of the abdomen (flat plates) are useful for examining gas patterns, to detect radiopaque lesions such as calculi, or when seeking free air (such as occurs following perforation of a viscus). Films must be made in upright or in lateral decubitus positions to detect free air or air-fluid levels. **Barium** is introduced to examine mucosal patterns, to visualize ulcers, or find mass lesions. Small mucosal lesions may be missed with barium. **Double contrast** with air and barium is more sensitive. **Endoscopic procedures** are more sensitive and dependable for visualization of small mucosal lesions such as Mallory-Weiss tears of the esophagus, erosive gastritis, or colonic polyps. They can visualize sites of bleeding, and a biopsy can be obtained. Endoscopy thus is the preferable procedure for upper GI bleeding and suspected upper GI malignancy, but it can miss submucosal and compressive lesions, which might be seen with barium studies. Endoscopic instrumentation can also be therapeutic, particularly for injection of bleeding esophageal varices. The radiological approach also gives information about transit times, but barium should be avoided if an obstruction is suspected. Barium and air enemas are useful for detection of small lesions of the colon,

Table 1-8. Tumor Types and Their Associated Syndromes

Type of tumor	Paraneoplastic syndrome
Small cell	Cushing's syndrome, Eaton-Lambert syndrome
Large cell	Gynecomastia
Squamous	Hypercalcemia
All types	Thrombophlebitis, clubbing (not small cell), SIADH (especially small cell)

including polyps. However, endoscopic procedures are much more sensitive, especially for rectal lesions, and have the advantage of obtaining tissue by biopsy anywhere in the colon. Sigmoidoscopy and colonoscopy, now done with flexible instruments with little discomfort to the patient, are indicated for investigation of bloody diarrhea, for the evaluation of inflammatory bowel disease and suspected neoplastic disease. They are especially useful for surveillance for malignancy in ulcerative colitis and polyposis of the colon. The colonoscope can be used for removal of polyps.

Ultrasonography (echo) is useful to detect the location and size of masses and organs, determining if a lesion is solid or cystic, to detect gallstones and dilated bile ducts, and to examine vascular structures such as aneurysms. CT is effective for detecting mass lesions, delineating the size of some structures such as the pancreas, and detecting dilated bile ducts. Liver tumors can often but not always be visualized by CT (some are "isodense," i.e., of the same density to x-rays as the surrounding normal tissue). Pancreatic tumors and retro-peritoneal masses are often best visualized by CT, as are small collections of fluid, such as ascites, and subphrenic or peridi-verticular abscesses.

Radionuclide imaging such as technetium-containing sulfur colloid that enters reticuloendothelial cells can visualize the liver and spleen, often outlining primary or metastatic hepatic neoplasms, and ^{99m}Tc-HIDA, which is secreted into the bile, can visualize biliary tract disorders. ^{99}Tc-pertechnetate has an affinity for gastric mucosa and thus can visualize a Meckel's diverticulum, since 99% contain ectopic gastric mucosa. ^{99m}Tc-labeled RBCs can delineate sites of intestinal bleeding. In skilled hands, selective visceral angiographic procedures are also useful for detecting bleeding sites.

Oral cholecystograms can identify gallstones, but nonvisu-alization occurs when gallbladders are nonfunctioning (as in most cases of chronic cholecystitis) and also when there is jaundice (bilirubin levels >2 mg/100 ml). As a result, ultraso-nography has largely replaced cholecystography for detection of gallstones. Enlarged biliary radicals in cases of obstructive jaundice can be visualized by inserting a fine needle with contrast material into the liver (percutaneous transhepatic cholangiography, or **PTC**), but ultrasonography and **CT scans** usually visualize these abnormalities without the risk of an invasive procedure. Extraheptic bile ducts are best visualized with endoscopic retrograde cholangiopancreatography (**ERCP**), an endoscopic procedure in which a scope is passed into the ampulla of Vater. ERCP is indicated for investigation of obstructive jaundice, diagnosis of pancreatic cancer, and therapeutic procedures such as sphincterotomy. ERCP is preferable to transhepatic cholangiography if intrahepatic bile duct dilatation is not present, making insertion of a needle much more difficult, and if a coagulation defect has developed or if there might be a pancreatic or duodenal lesion that can be visualized and biopsied, such as a carcinoma of the ampulla of Vater.

PTC is better than ERCP for visualization of intrahepatic ductal lesions. It can be repeated, allowing examination of the entire ductal system. It also provides opportunity for therapeu-tic drainage of obstructed ducts, but it does not visualize the left lobe of the liver and is invasive, with a risk of bleeding or infection. ERCP is better than PTC for extrahepatic ductal

lesions as well as ampullary and pancreatic lesions. It permits biopsy and sphincterotomy but cannot visualize lesions proxi-mal to an obstruction and carries the risk of perforation of the bile duct, induction of pancreatitis, or infection.

Laparoscopy is a rarely used procedure of most value for visualization and biopsy of suspected tumor nodules on the surface of the liver or peritoneum.

DISEASES OF THE ESOPHAGUS

Gastroesophageal reflux causes "heartburn," substernal burning pain, and is usually due to reflux of acid gastric juice into the esophagus. It may be accompanied by regurgitation of sour material into the mouth, with aspiration causing nocturnal wheezing and pneumonia. Bleeding may occur from erosions of the esophageal mucosa and dysphagia from narrowing of the lumen due to scarring. Smoking, alcohol, caffeine, and pregnancy all can aggravate the problem by decreasing lower esophageal sphincter tone. The diagnosis can be established by the characteristic history, especially if positional changes (such as recumbency after meals) influence symptoms, by barium swallow or radionuclide scan with ^{99}Tc sulfur colloid in the stomach. Esophageal pH can be monitored after instillation of acid into the stomach (Tuttle test) or by dripping HCl into the esophagus to see if symptoms are reproduced (Bernstein test). **Barrett's esophagus**, the presence of gastric columnar epithe-lium as a result of chronic reflux, has a risk of malignant transformation. This diagnosis is best made by esophagoscopy with biopsy. Reflux can be treated by raising the head of the bed, avoidance of food or liquid immediately before bedtime, antacids between meals and at bedtime, and avoidance of cigarettes and alcohol. More resistant cases may require H$_2$-receptor blockers, anticholinergic agents to decrease gastric acidity, or a surgical procedure.

Motility disorders of the esophagus include smooth muscle pathology, as occurs in scleroderma, and loss of normal innervation, such as degeneration of ganglion cells of Auer-bach's plexus in achalasia. Diffuse esophageal spasm can occur for unclear reasons. Barium swallow, sometimes with cine-esophagram and motility studies, can establish the diagnosis. Manometric findings reveal high lower esophageal pressure in achalasia, normal pressure in diffuse spasm, and low pressure with scleroderma of the esophagus. Barium swallow reveals a dilated fluid-filled esophagus with achalasia, noncoordinated contractions with spasm, and dilatation with lack of peristalsis in scleroderma. Achalasia can be treated by forceful dilatation of the lower esophageal sphincter with a balloon or by surgical myotomy. Diffuse lower esophageal spasm can be treated with nitroglycerin, anticholinergic agents, or calcium channel blockers.

Congenital rings and webs can occur in the esophagus, and the Plummer-Vinson syndrome is the association of such a web with dysphagia and iron deficiency anemia. The most common traumatic lesion of the esophagus is a mucosal tear (Mallory-Weiss syndrome) due to strenuous vomiting; bleeding can be severe. A full-thickness tear of the eosphagus (Boerhaave's syndrome) can occur, usually just above the gastroesophageal junction, and requires immediate surgical repair. The most common infections of the esophagus are due to herpesvirus or *Candida*. They cause severe dysphagia and occur particularly in immunosuppressed patients, including elderly people with serious underlying disease.

PEPTIC ULCER DISEASE

Pathophysiology.   Normal secretion of HCl is stimulated by three endogenous chemical agents: gastrin (released by G cells in the antrum of the stomach and duodenum, stimulated by products of protein digestion and alkalinization), acetylcholine (released by vagus nerves, stimulated by stretch of stomach and cephalic stimuli), and histamine released from mast-like cells in the gastric wall in proximity to chief cells. Pepsinogen secretion is stimulated by acetylcholine and possibly by other mechanisms. Normal defense against autodigestion includes the mucus, local secretion of HCO_3 under the mucin layer, local prostaglandin formation, active blood flow, and constant renewal of mucosal epithelial cells. Patients with duodenal ulcers generally have high basal and maximal acid output, but those with gastric ulcers generally have normal levels of acid output. Genetic factors may play a role in the etiology of peptic ulcer disease (PUD), judging by familial occurrences. Cigarette smoking definitely increases the incidence, as do uremia, COPD, alcoholic cirrhosis, hyperparathyroidism (possibly due to hypercalcemia), mastocytosis (which increases production of histamine), cluster (Horton's) headaches, and polycythemia vera. Emotional factors can increase gastric acid secretion and may play a role in some cases. Use of anti-inflammatory drugs (NSAIDs and steroids) can cause gastric erosions and possibly increase ulcer formation. Duodenal ulcers are more frequent than gastric ulcers. Men and women have the same incidence of gastric ulcers, but duodenal ulcers are more common in men.

Clinical features.   The most frequent symptom is burning or gnawing epigastric pain, usually appearing after gastric emptying, such as 1 to 3 hours after meals or at night. The pain is relieved by food or antacids but may be atypical in character, location or timing. A variety of other symptoms may occur, such as bloating or excessive gas. Penetration into the pancreas can cause intractable, severe pain radiating to the back. The physical examination is usually negative in the absence of complications.

Diagnostic decisions.   The diagnosis of peptic ulcer can usually be established by upper GI series, which is less expensive than endoscopy, but the latter is more sensitive. About one-fifth of ulcers are missed radiologically. If the ulcer is gastric, it is important to establish that it is benign, although the incidence of gastric malignancy has diminished markedly in the United States in recent decades. Prepyloric location, small size of the ulcer, young age of the patient, and negative gastric cytology all favor benignity, but biopsy is the most definitive test and requires endoscopy.

Therapeutic decisions.   Medical therapy of PUD is directed toward reducing the secretion of gastric acid and bolstering the defense of the mucosa against autodigestion. The primary agents for reducing gastric acid at the present time are the H_2-receptor antagonists, such as cimetidine and ranitidine. The latter is less likely to cause mental confusion in elderly people, is less antiandrogenic, and has fewer drug interactions resulting from interference with metabolism of other drugs by the cytochrome P450 system in the liver. Oral antacids are still very useful but must be given frequently. Antacids containing calcium are no longer recommended because Ca^{2+} stimulates gastrin secretion, causing a rebound in acid secretion. Antacids containing sodium should also be avoided because their action is too brief and they can cause edema, hypertension, or metabolic alkalosis. Antacids containing aluminum can cause constipation, and those containing magnesium cause diarrhea, but mixtures can be used. They should be taken 1 to 3 hours after meals and at bedtime, as well as at any time symptoms develop. Sucralfate, a sulfated aluminum hydroxide salt of sucrose, is not absorbed and protects against injury to the gastric mucosa by HCl with few side effects. It is effective, as are oral prostglandins, which are under development. The old standby, anticholinergic agents, are still useful. Removal of aggravating factors is an important aspect of therapy. Avoidance of cigarettes, alcohol, and drugs that irritate the stomach (e.g., aspirin) is essential. Attention to aggravating emotional problems is also of vital importance in many patients. Surgical therapy is discussed in the chapter on surgery, as are postsurgical complications such as dumping, diarrhea, afferent loop syndrome, anemia, weight loss due to early satiety, and malabsorption.

Healing rates with medical therapy are high. If 95% of the area of a gastric ulcer has not healed in 3 months, malignancy should be suspected and surgery performed. After healing of an ulcer, in patients over age 60 with underlying heart or pulmonary disease, prophylactic therapy to prevent recurrences is recommended.

Other therapeutic problems.   Many patients with PUD present with a complication as the initial manifestation. Bleeding, which is the most common complication, has a significant mortality. Immediate replacement of RBCs and volume is usually necessary, and many cases require emergency surgery. Penetration of an ulcer into an adjacent organ such as the pancreas causes severe, intractable pain, or acute pancreatitis can develop suddenly. Perforation into the peritoneal cavity can occur, resulting in sudden development of an acute abdomen (severe pain, board-like rigidity with rebound tenderness). Free air in the peritoneal cavity, which can be observed radiologically with the patient upright or lying on one side, is diagnostic of a perforated hollow viscus. Such a patient would be febrile and hypotensive and have a marked leukocytosis with a left shift. IV fluids and emergency surgery are essential. The other common complication of PUD is gastric outlet obstruction. It is caused by inflammation, spasm, or scarring around an ulcer in the pyloric channel and results in intractable vomiting. Examination may reveal dehydration and a succession splash due to the fluid-filled, dilated stomach. There is metabolic alkalosis with hypochloremia and often hypokalemia, resulting from loss of gastric juice. Aspiration of the stomach through a nasogastric tube yields more than 200 ml of fluid, or over 400 ml of a test load of 750 ml of saline can be recovered 30 minutes after placing it into an empty stomach through such a tube (positive saline load test). Endoscopy or upper GI x-rays can confirm the presence of obstruction and rule out a tumor or other cause. Medical therapy usually successfully relieves pyloric obstruction due to PUD.

The **Zollinger-Ellison syndrome**, usually caused by a gastrin-secreting islet cell tumor of the pancreas, is a rare cause of PUD. Gastrinomas are often malignant, and metastases to the liver can be functional. They are often part of the syndrome of multiple endocrine neoplasia type II (MEN II), in which adenomas occur in islet cells, parathyroid, thyroid, and pituitary glands. A gastrinoma should be considered when ulcers appear in unusual places (such as the second or third portion of the duodenum or the jejunum) or are multiple; when the disease is unusually severe and is refractory to treatment, especially if it recurs after surgery; when there is simultaneous watery, secretory diarrhea or malabsorption (which can precede the ulcer); when there is association with hypercalcemia or other endocrine neoplasia (type I); when there is a strong family history of peptic ulcer disease or other endocrine tumors; or when enlarged mucosal folds are seen in the stomach on x-ray.

Increased basal secretion of gastric acid supports the diagnosis of a gastrinoma. Stimulation of the stomach with IV pentagastrin may be used to demonstrate that basal acid secretion is greater than 40% of that possible under maximal stimulation. Measurement of serum gastrin levels is indicated if a gastrinoma is suspected. High levels confirm the diagnosis. Treatment includes attempt at surgical resection and use of large doses of H_2-receptor antagonists.

GASTRITIS

In **acute gastritis**, there are multiple superficial gastric erosions and infiltration of the gastric mucosa with inflammatory cells. It is usually due to drugs (such as aspirin and other NSAIDs), alcohol, ingestion of caustic agents such as lye, irradiation, or emotional stress. Acute medical illness or surgery is often accompanied by a similar process, probably as a result of ischemia. Increased secretion of adrenal hormones may be a contributory factor. Disruption of the barrier to back-diffusion of acid is thought to be an underlying mechanism in acute gastritis of all causes. Mild nausea and epigastric discomfort may be the only manifestations, but vomiting and severe hemorrhage can occur. Radiological procedures are not very useful in diagnosis. Endoscopy can demonstrate reddened edematous mucosa and superficial erosions. Therapy consists of withdrawing any offending agent, especially aspirin, plus use of antacids and H_2-receptor blockade.

Chronic gastritis may be due to same causes as acute gastritis. When it mainly affects the fundus and the body of the stomach, there usually are circulating autoantibodies against parietal cells and atrophy of the gastric mucosa. Pernicious anemia may be associated. When chronic gastritis primarily affects the antrum, there usually are antibodies against gastrin-producing cells. Chronic gastritis is associated with an increased incidence of gastric cancer.

DIARRHEA

Pathophysiology. Evaluation of the patient with diarrhea requires knowledge of the pertinent physiology. Normally the gut receives 8 to 10 L of fluid per day, mostly from secretion; 90% is reabsorbed in the small bowel, and about 1 L reaches the colon, where 90% is absorbed. Solutes are absorbed by specific means, and water follows passively as a result of osmotic gradients. The presence of osmotically active solutes in gut lumen keeps water in the lumen (or attracts it from cells), causing osmotic diarrhea.

The sodium pump creates a gradient that provides the energy for most of the absorptive processes. HCO_3 secretion is driven by Na^+/H^+ exchanges and the alkalinity of GI secretions. In the colon, Na absorption occurs via a specific sodium channel, generating an electrical potential that drives Cl^- absorption and K^+ secretion. Colonic fluid typically contains Na^+, 40; K^+, 90; Cl^-, 15; HCO_3^-, 30; and organic anions, 85 (mostly produced by colonic bacteria from unabsorbed food) (all figures are millimolar).

Osmotic diarrhea is the result of the presence of osmotically active solutes attracting water into the gut. Indirect evidence of the presence of such solutes can be established by the calculation of the osmotic gap following determination of the stool electrolyte concentrations (expressed in mEq/L).

$$Osmotic\ gap = 290 - 2[Na + K]$$

If the gap is over 20, osmotic diarrhea is likely. Osmotic diarrhea results from ingestion of solutes that are undigested and not absorbed, such as occurs with lactulose, mannitol, and certain cathartics (e.g., those containing Mg^{2+}, SO_4^{2-}, PO_4^-, or citrate), from malabsorption of food, or from failure to digest specific dietary components such as occurs in lactase insufficiency. In these cases, there is a large solute gap—that is, estimation of stool osmolality reveals a gap of over 20 mOsm/L higher than can be accounted for by calculation from the formula $2[Na^+ + K^+]$. (When diarrhea is due to PO_4^- or SO_4^+, the measured osmolality will not be much higher than the calculated level and these ions must be measured directly.) Due to fermentation, diarrhea due to undigested carbohydrate usually results in acidity of the stool. Thus, in the presence of an osmotic gap, if the stool pH is under 5.5, carbohydrate malabsorption is highly likely. As a **therapeutic test**, osmotic diarrhea typically stops when the patient fasts or stops ingesting the specific offending solute.

Secretory diarrhea is the result of increased levels of cellular cyclic adenosine monophosphate (cAMP), which inhibits neutral NaCl absorption and stimulates Cl^+ secretion. The classic cause of secretory diarrhea is cholera, in which a toxin produced by the bacteria binds to the mucosal cells and stimulates increased production of cAMP. Since other transport mechanisms coupled with sodium function normally, hydration can be maintained by oral administration of adequate amounts of sodium-glucose solutions. Other bacterial enterotoxins, including the toxin of *Salmonella*, that of some strains of *E. coli* (which produce traveler's diarrhea), vasoactive intestinal peptide (VIP), and prostaglandins act in the same fashion, and nonabsorbed bile acids may stimulate secretion of ions by mucosal cells in the colon through this mechanism. Other agents produce secretory diarrhea through different mechanisms, including a heat-stable toxin produced by *E. coli*, serotonin, castor oil, and phenolphthalein. Small bowel disorders that produce villus atrophy (as in celiac disease) also cause secretory diarrhea.

Diarrhea also can result from disordered intestinal motility, since rapid movement of intestinal contents can decrease time for absorption, such as occurs with irritable bowel syndrome or thyrotoxicosis. Similar phenomena occur following vagotomy, gastrectomy, or with diabetic autonomic neuropathy and as a result of bacterial overgrowth in areas of gut such as a blind loop.

Diagnostic decisions. Symptoms provide valuable clues. Frequent small stools with lower abdominal pain before or during defecation generally mean irritation of the left colon or rectum. Large, voluminous stools generally mean disease of the small bowel or right colon. Blood suggests mucosal inflammation or ischemic disease. Froth and flatus suggest carbohydrate malabsorption. Greasy, foul-smelling stools suggest malabsorption of fat (steatorrhea). Other points in the history can be important, such as intake of drugs such as cathartics, antacids, colchicine, or antibiotics; duration of the diarrhea (acute or chronic); presence of systemic symptoms, e.g., fever (suggest inflammatory bowel disease or infections such as amebiasis); prior surgery (especially gastrectomy, small bowel resection, creation of a blind loop); travel history, homosexuality (in males), flushing (suggests carcinoid syndrome), and presence of similar illnesses in the family (suggest ingestion of toxin in food).

Associated illnesses also provide clues. Arthritis suggests ulcerative colitis or ileitis. Diabetes suggests autonomic neuropathy. Proteinuria suggests amyloidosis. Peptic ulcer disease suggests a gastrin-producing tumor (Zollinger-Ellison syndrome). Chronic frequent lung infections and COPD suggest cystic fibrosis. Generalized arteriosclerosis suggests ischemic disease of the gut. Hyperpigmentation suggests Whipple's disease or Addison's disease.

Laboratory tests. In all patients, stool should be examined for volume and consistency, blood, and pus. With acute diarrhea, WBCs in stool suggest an infection with an invasive organism (e.g., *Shigella, Salmonella,* amoebas, or antibiotic-associated colitis). With chronic diarrhea, WBCs suggest inflammatory bowel disease. Blood generally suggests inflammation and has the same significance as pus. (Culture and examination of the stool for WBCs, blood, and parasites should always precede radiological or endoscopic procedures, since bowel preparations (especially enemas) and barium may alter findings.) A stool culture should be obtained, and stools should be examined for ova and parasites, fat, and phenolphthalein (by alkalinization). When secretory diarrhea is suspected, determination of Na, K, Cl, pH, reducing substances, Mg, PO_4, and SO_4 can be useful. Malabsorption can be established by a Sudan stain for fat, quantitative fecal fat (on 100-g/day fat diet), and measurement of xylose absorption. Hormone assays (VIP, prostaglandins, calcitonin, gastrin, etc.) are likely to be of value only in patients with chronic secretory diarrhea and in whom laxative use and other GI disease have been ruled out.

Therapeutic trials. Diagnostic information can be obtained from fasting (with parenteral fluid replacement) for suspected osmotic diarrhea, effectiveness of antibiotics in bacterial overgrowth (blind loop) syndromes, pancreatic enzymes for exocrine pancreatic insufficiency causing malabsorption, metronidazole for giardiasis, cholestyramine for bile acid malabsorption, and elimination diets, e.g., lactose free.

Therapeutic decisions. First, replace fluid and electrolytes. Second, treat the specific cause, if identifiable. Chronic diarrhea may be treated with opiates (codeine, loperamide) that reduce gut motility, but these should not be used in inflammatory bowel disease if toxic megacolon is impending,

and they can prolong infectious diarrhea. Bismuth subsalicylate (Pepto-Bismol) is particularly useful for traveler's diarrhea; antibiotics can cause pseudomembranous colitis.

Important points regarding individual diarrheal diseases

Food poisoning results from toxins that are either made by contaminating bacteria, developed by spoilage, or naturally occurring in certain plants or animals. The most serious forms of food poisoning occur from preformed toxins made by bacteria, such as occurs with the neurotoxin produced by *Clostridium botulinum,* which usually develops from inadequate heating during the canning process, and *S. aureus* and *Bacillus cereus,* which grow in inadequately refrigerated food. These types of food poisoning are short-lived but violent and generally affect whole groups of people who ingested the same food item. Vomiting, cramps, and diarrhea can be explosive, and fluid replacement is the main form of therapy needed. Similar toxins are produced by *Clostridium perfringens* and *Vibrio parahaemolyticus.* Contaminated fish or shellfish can contain neurotoxins that can produce muscle paralysis. **Mushroom poisoning** produces hepatic and renal failure and has a mortality rate generally over 50%. The **Chinese restaurant syndrome** is due to monosodium glutamate (MSG), which causes a burning sensation in the skin, headache, and chest pressure, usually in minutes to a few hours after eating.

Viral gastroenteritis, the most common cause of **infectious diarrhea** in the United States, generally affects multiple members of the same family. Enterotoxin-producing *E. coli* and *Campylobacter fetus* also are frequent causes, especially in travelers or in focal outbreaks. Bacterial agents such as *Salmonella, Shigella,* and *Yersinia* are less frequent and can cause watery, secretory diarrhea or, if sufficient mucosal invasion occurs, the syndrome of dysentery with chills, fever, cramps, and bloody diarrhea. *Giardia lamblia* is the most common parasitic cause of infectious diarrhea. Previously, it was seen primarily among travelers to certain endemic foci (e.g., Rocky Mountain areas, Leningrad), but in recent years it has become increasingly common all over the United States. It usually is noninvasive, producing minimal symptoms, but may cause a chronic diarrheal syndrome with malabsorption. *E. histolytica* can invade the mucosa, producing a secretory, inflammatory, bloody diarrhea and a clinical picture resembling ulcerative colitis. Hepatic abscesses can occur.

Antibiotic-associated diarrhea is usually due to an enterotoxin-producing strain of *C. difficile.* Culture of this organism from the stool is diagnostic. It is common after use of broad-spectrum agents, especially ampicillin, clindamycin, lincomycin, and cephalosporins, but it can occur after any antibiotic. It can be very severe, with the production of pseudomembranes in the colon, giving a characteristic appearance on sigmoidoscopy. Therapy with oral metronidazole is effective and inexpensive. Oral vancomycin also is effective. Cholestyramine can bind the toxin.

Sexually transmitted diarrheal syndromes occur especially in homosexual males, 40% of whom are reported to harbor multiple pathogens in the colon, including *Chlamydia,* herpesvirus, gonoccocci, *Campylobacter, Shigella, Salmonella, E. histolytica,* and *Giardia,* as well as syphilis. All these organisms should be sought by appropriate examination of the anus for ulcerations, smear and Gram stain, exam for parasites, cultures, and serological tests.

Abdominal cramps and diarrhea are the usual manifestation of **giardiasis**. The main clue is a taste of rotten eggs in the mouth. It is often asymptomatic, but severe symptoms can occur, especially in debilitated individuals.

INFLAMMATORY BOWEL DISEASE

Ulcerative colitis and **regional enteritis (Crohn's disease)** are more common in whites, about equal in incidence between the two sexes and usually begin in early adulthood. The cause is unknown; environmental factors, infectious or antigenic, are likely. Family grouping suggests a genetic factor, but no genetic markers have been identified. Immunologic phenomena occur, including antibody to colonic epithelial cells and cytotoxic T cells, but these could be secondary phenomena. Psychological factors can cause exacerbations.

Clinical picture.   **Ulcerative colitis** causes a diffuse disease without skipping areas of bowel. It involves the rectum in over 95% of cases and may extend proximally to include the terminal ileum. The epithelium is inflamed, appearing red, granular, and friable, and usually contains superficial ulcerations. Microabscesses may be present in the bowel wall. Severe inflammation can cause atony of the muscular layer of the colon, with marked dilatation (**toxic megacolon**). Bacteria can penetrate through the wall of the colon, producing diffuse peritonitis. Scarring beneath the mucosa can lead to narrowing and shortening of the colon, causing loss of haustral markings on x-ray, giving the appearance of lead-pipe colon. Thickened mucosa between areas of ulceration can resemble polyps (pseudopolyps), but prolonged disease can lead to true neoplasia, developing into carcinoma of the colon. Fistula formation and mechanical obstructive lesions rarely develop. Remissions of months or years are common.

Regional enteritis causes inflammation of the entire wall of the gut, mucosa to serosa. It can leave segments of uninvolved gut (skip areas) and involves the rectum in only about half the cases. It can affect the small bowel alone (usually the ileum), the colon alone, or both. Proximal intestine can also be involved. Inflamed loops of bowel can become adherent to each other or to other structures. Fistulas can develop through these areas of adherence, and obstructive lesions can develop. The bowel wall is thickened because of the granulomatous inflammation, and the mucosa typically has a cobblestone appearance. Mesenteric nodes are often affected. Neoplastic change is very rare.

The cardinal clinical manifestations of ulcerative colitis are diarrhea, usually with blood in the stool, and abdominal pain with fever and weight loss. Although it is usually gradually progressive, in some patients an explosive onset occurs, requiring immediate hospitalization because of the danger of toxic megacolon, colonic perforation with peritonitis, or shock or marked hypokalemia due to intestinal fluid loss. Marked weakness, tachycardia, hypotension, leukocytosis, anemia, and electrolyte abnormalities occur in these patients. Abdominal findings vary from diffuse tenderness to marked distension, with absent bowel sounds. The development of toxic megacolon may be heralded by a decrease in diarrhea because of loss of intestinal motility or an increase in toxicity of the patient, with

fever and leukocytosis. Hypokalemia and hypoalbuminemia may develop rapidly. Toxic megacolon can be induced by drugs to reduce the diarrhea (e.g., narcotic derivatives) or by use of barium for a radiological procedure. In these patients, plain film of the abdomen shows a dilated colon with a diameter over 6 cm.

Regional enteritis usually begins insidiously and sometimes presents with a complication such as fistula formation or obstruction. A common form of onset of symptoms is the development of crampy abdominal pain due to low-grade ileal obstruction. Occult blood in the stool is common, but gross rectal bleeding is rare. Onset with symptoms of acute appendicitis is not unusual. When there is colonic involvement, symptoms resemble those seen in ulcerative colitis, but development of rectal fissures and perirectal abscesses suggests regional enteritis. Thickening of the bowel wall and adhesions between adherent, inflamed loops of bowel make obstruction and fistula formation a more common complication than in ulcerative colitis, but hemorrhage, perforation, and toxic megacolon develop much less commonly.

Extraintestinal complications develop commonly with both forms of inflammatory bowel disease. Nutritional deficiency states are common, as are forms of arthritis that can affect large peripheral joints and resemble rheumatoid arthritis (although serological test for rheumatoid factor is usually negative) or the sacroiliac joints and spine, especially in those patients who have the HLA-B27 antigen, thus resembling ankylosing spondylitis and other spondyloarthropathies (such as Reiter's syndrome and psoriatic arthritis). These complications tend to wax and wane with the severity of the bowel disease. Liver disease can occur, typically a fatty liver and pericholangitis manifested primarily by an elevated alkaline phosphatase. However, a sclerosing cholangitis can develop, leading to obstruction of extrahepatic ducts and cirrhosis because of involvement of intrahepatic radicals. There is an increased incidence of cholelithiasis in regional enteritis, perhaps as a result of decreased absorption of bile salts in the ileum. Eye disease can develop, including iritis, uveitis, or episcleritis. Skin lesions occur. Erythema nodosum is common, especially in women, and pyoderma gangrenosum is a severe complication, especially seen with ulcerative colitis. Aphthous ulcers of the mouth are common. Kidney stones may develop, especially in regional enteritis due to absorptive hyperoxaluria. Urinary tract obstruction or fistula formation into the urinary tract may develop in regional enteritis. Amyloidosis has also been reported in regional enteritis. At times, these extraintestinal complications precede the manifestations of the inflammatory bowel disease. Most remit when the bowel disease improves, with the exception of the spondylitis and irreversible, sclerosing cholangitis.

Diagnostic decisions.   The diagnosis is usually suggested by the symptoms, although a long list of other diseases must be differentiated, including bacterial or amoebic dysentery, irritable bowel syndrome, pseudomembranous colitis, and neoplasms. Endoscopy is usually very helpful, as is barium study of the colon and/or small bowel, which should be performed after endoscopy to avoid changes induced by the barium. Stool cultures and examination for parasites are mandatory. The two types of inflammatory bowel disease can usually be distinguished by the appearance and distribution of the lesions and by biopsy.

Therapeutic decisions.   Treatment is directed at suppressing the inflammatory process, maintenance of nutritional status and at psychological problems. Ulcerative colitis sometimes responds to sulfasalazine, an antibiotic combined with a salicylate. Prednisone is often needed, orally or by enema. For severe cases, maintenance of fluid and electrolytes, replacement of blood losses, and broad-spectrum antibiotics are usually needed. A surgical consultation is usually wise. Toxic megacolon may require emergency colectomy. Ulcerative colitis that is intractable and progressive despite all medical measures can be an indication for total colectomy and permanent ileostomy, as is concern about development of carcinoma, which is most frequent with longstanding, unremitting disease of the entire colon. Most patients with ulcerative colitis respond to medical therapy, but relapses are common months or years later.

The treatment of regional enteritis is generally similar to that of ulcerative colitis, but response to therapy is often less satisfactory. The main threats to life in this disease are malnutrition and sepsis. Resting the bowel completely through use of parenteral hyperalimentation can be helpful. Surgery should be avoided whenever possible because of the tendency of the disease to recur proximal to resected areas and for fistulas to form along postoperative adhesions. Surgery can be unavoidably necessary because of intestinal obstruction, fistula, or abscess formation.

ISCHEMIC COLITIS

Generalized arteriosclerosis may cause ischemic injury to the colon, primarily occurring at sites of junction of the areas supplied by different major arteries, the "watershed areas" such as the splenic flexure and the rectosigmoid. Areas with collateral blood supply such as the rectum are usually spared. **Acute ischemic colitis** can present with the sudden onset of abdominal pain, localized tenderness, and blood in the stool, sometimes with fever and signs of peritoneal irritation. Shock may develop. Colonoscopy may show small areas of ulceration; barium enema is dangerous during the acute episode but examination subsequently can show characteristic findings including areas of narrowing with mucosal changes due to hemorrhage and edema described as "thumbprinting." Conservative management is usually successful. Surgery is indicated only for perforation or definite infarction of the bowel. **Chronic ischemic colitis** causes recurrent vague abdominal pain with or without bleeding; scarring of injured areas leads to narrowing of the colon and may cause obstruction.

DIVERTICULAR DISEASE

Colonic diverticula, sac-like herniations of mucosa covered by serosa without a muscular layer, are most common in the sigmoid area and left colon. Usually asymptomatic, they can cause bleeding that can be severe or they can become infected, sometimes as a result of obstruction by a fecalith. Diverticulitis may progress to perforation with localized or even generalized peritonitis. The clinical picture may suggest "left-sided appendicitis" in an older person, with pain, tenderness, fever, and leukocytosis. A tender mass may be felt through the abdominal

wall or on rectal examination. Colonoscopy may show inflammation of the mucosa and narrowing. Barium studies are contraindicated during the acute phase, but CT scan of the abdomen may show a pericolonic inflammatory mass. Treatment consists of withholding solid food and administering broad-spectrum antibiotics active against anaerobes. Surgery is necessary for a large, localized abscess that needs drainage, acute perforation that must be sealed, or later for relief of obstruction. High-fiber diet helps prevent recurrences by keeping stool bulk larger and avoiding high intraluminal pressure. Bowel resection may be necessary for recurrent attacks of diverticulitis.

TUMORS OF THE GI TRACT

Esophagus

Squamous cell carcinoma is the most common tumor of the esophagus. The incidence of carcinoma of the esophagus is higher in some groups (blacks four times higher than whites in the United States) and very high in some areas (such as northern China). The incidence is increased by the combination of heavy smoking and high alcohol intake and following the ingestion of caustic substances such as lye. Adenocarcinoma is increased by the presence of columnar (Barrett's) epithelium as a result of chronic gastric reflux.

Diagnostic decisions.   Pain or difficulty in swallowing solid foods is the most common early symptom and can progress to involve liquids also. Substernal pain usually indicates extension into the mediastinum. The dysphagia can lead to regurgitation and aspiration pneumonia, or extension can lead to development of a bronchopleural fistula with severe pulmonary infection. Dysphagia developing after age 40 must be investigated for carcinoma of the esophagus by barium swallow, and if a suspicious lesion is seen, by esophagoscopy with brush cytology or biopsy. CT can delineate extension, and distant metastases (most frequently to the liver) can be sought by ultrasonography, ^{99}Tc liver or CT scan. ^{67}Ga is picked up by some tumors and their metastases.

Stomach

Adenocarcinomas are the most common malignant gastric tumors. Lymphomas account for about 5%, and leiomyosarcomas are rare. Benign tumors rarely cause symptoms. The incidence of gastric cancer in the United States has declined dramatically since about 1940, but it remains very high in some areas, especially in the Far East and in Orientals who have emigrated to the United States. Among native Americans, it is more common in men, blacks, people with a positive family history, those with blood group A, and in association with gastric achlorhydria, such as after partial gastrectomy for peptic ulcer. Most gastric carcinomas arise from mucosal cells, not parietal or chief cells, in the distal stomach. They may have a stalk or may infiltrate the wall and may become ulcerated.

Symptoms are variable. Epigastric pain is common; it may resemble the pain of peptic ulcer but is usually atypical. Nausea, anorexia, early satiety, and weight loss are other frequent symptoms. Vomiting may occur, especially if the tumor is near the gastric outlet and obstructs. A tumor near the gastroesophageal junction can cause dysphagia. Occult bleeding is common, and iron deficiency anemia usual. The first symptoms may be those of extension or metastases such as obstructive jaundice or ascites, thrombophlebitis, or paraneoplastic syndromes such as dermatomyositis or acanthosis nigricans. Physical examination may reveal an epigastric mass, a Virchow's node (a metastasis to a left supraclavicular node via extension through the lymphatics and thoracic duct), a Blumer's shelf (a perirectal mass at the peritoneal reflection on rectal exam), or an ovarian metastatic mass (Kruckenberg's tumor).

Diagnostic decisions. Workup begins with x-rays, using barium and air, with endoscopy if a suspicious lesion is found. Brush cytology and/or multiple biopsies should be obtained, especially if an ulcerated lesion is present, since it may be very difficult to tell whether an ulcer is benign. Staging is aided by CT scan, with or without ultrasonography of the liver, and by biopsy of suspicious nodes. Evidence of liver metastases can be found chemically with the alkaline phosphatase or GGT, or by CT scan. The carcinoembryonic antigen is too nonspecific to be of diagnostic value but is useful for following patients to detect early evidence of recurrence.

Treatment is surgical, and palliation can be valuable even if cure is not possible. Radiation and chemotherapy are beginning to show some success.

Colon

Adenocarcinoma of the colon is currently the third most common cancer in the United States. Diets low in fiber but high in animal protein and fats have been blamed. A positive family history and conditions associated with increased turnover of mucosal cells increase the risk, including ulcerative colitis and familial polyposis. The left colon is more commonly affected.

Symptoms are usually vague. A change in bowel habits (i.e., the development of constipation or diarrhea) or a change in the caliber of the stool may appear early, especially with left-sided lesions, and can progress to intestinal obstruction. Pain can occur with obstruction of the left colon, but it usually means invasion through the bowel wall on the right side. Blood in the stool may be obvious but is usually occult with lesions of the right colon, and iron deficiency anemia is a common presenting manifestation. Bright red blood in the stool should not be attributed to hemorrhoids or diverticular disease in people over 40 without investigation for malignancy. Weight loss is usually a late manifestation, representing liver metastases.

Diagnostic decisions. Workup includes rectal exam since many carcinomas are palpable, stool for blood, proctoscopy, and sigmoidoscopy. If suspicion still exists, double-contrast barium enema and colonscopy with biopsy and/or brush cytology are indicated.

Therapeutic decisions. Treatment is surgical, sometimes requiring permanent colostomy for lesions too close to the anus. Radiation and chemotherapy are of a little value for metastases.

Screening should include annual testing of the stool for occult blood and periodic proctosigmoidoscopy for people over 40. After two negative annual endoscopic procedures, repeat every 3 to 5 years is recommended, but checkups should be performed more often with positive family history or other risk factors.

INTESTINAL POLYPS

Most neoplastic intestinal polyps occur in the colon. They increase in frequency with increasing age. Most carcinomas of the colon develop in preexisting benign polyps, but only a minority of benign polyps become malignant. Symptoms are diverse. Bleeding is common and usually occult, abdominal pain occurs if there is partial obstruction, and a change in bowel habits can occur. Large **villous adenomas** can cause watery diarrhea with sufficient potassium loss to cause symptomatic hypokalemia. Double-contrast barium enemas can detect polyps, but colonoscopy is more dependable and can include a biopsy or polypectomy, especially for lesions under 2 cm.

The lesions of **familial intestinal polyposis** develop in childhood and can carpet the entire colon. Bleeding and diarrhea are the most common symptoms, and a syndrome resembling ulcerative colitis can develop. These polyps tend to become malignant, and virtually all affected individuals develop carcinoma of the colon by age 40. Because the disease is inherited as an autosomal dominant trait, every member of an affected family should be checked frequently by endoscopy. Total colectomy may be needed prophylactically for multiple polyposis, especially if there is a family history of colon cancer.

Peutz-Jeghers syndrome includes widespread intestinal polyps associated with mucocutaneous pigmentation, especially around the lips. The polyps are hamartomas rather than adenomas and occur in the stomach, small and large intestine, and occasionally in the bronchi or bladder. Malignant transformation is much less common than in the other forms of intestinal polyposis. Surgery is necessary only for complications, such as bleeding or obstruction.

DISEASES OF THE LIVER

Hepatitis

Inflammation of the liver, accompanied by necrosis of hepatic parenchymal cells, may be caused by viral infection, toxins, drugs, immune processes, or ischemia. Many cases are mild and clinically inapparent, but severe liver damage with jaundice can progress to death. The most important toxins producing acute hepatitis are a drug (acetoaminophen) and the toxin of mushroom poisoning (*Amanita phalloides*).

Acute viral hepatitis can be caused by several hepatitis viruses (A, B, and non-A/non-B, a group of at least two agents), Epstein-Barr virus, CMV, and an incomplete RNA virus called the delta agent, which affects only individuals already infected with the hepatitis B virus. The B virus has been well characterized. Each of its main components is antigenic, and serum antibodies provide a way of determining the nature of an infection with this agent. B virus consists of a surface coat (hepatitis B surface antigen, HBsAg), a core of DNA, DNA polymerase, a core antigen (HBcAg), and the e antigen (HBeAg).

Hepatitis A is transmitted almost exclusively by the fecal-oral route. Spread within families, by contaminated shellfish, and within institutions is common. By contrast, spread of hepatitis B is primarily percutaneous, especially by blood or blood products and contaminated needles. The virus is also present in various body fluids, including semen, saliva, and breast milk, but rarely in urine or feces. Spread therefore is mostly to recipients of blood products, among IV drug abusers, and among spouses and sexual partners, especially male homosexuals. Spread within institutions is also common. Recipients of pooled blood products such as Factor VIII were at greatest risk, but screening of donated blood for HBsAg has markedly reduced the incidence of posttransfusion hepatitis. Heating and chemical treatment of plasma eliminate active virus, hence there is no risk for recipients of albumin and immune and hyperimmune serum globulin.

Non-A/non-B hepatitis is similar to hepatitis B in that it is primarily transmitted parenterally. Since there is yet no way of screening blood for the presence of this agent, it is the main cause of transfusion hepatitis at present.

Clinically, acute viral hepatitis begins with a prodromal period of malaise, anorexia, nausea, vomiting, myalgias, and fatigue. Mild flu-like symptoms may be present. For unknown reasons, smokers may develop an aversion to tobacco. Arthritis and urticaria may result from immune complex deposition in vessels of the synovia and skin (most common with hepatitis B), which may be accompanied by a severe form of generalized periarteritis nodosa. Jaundice may appear, but most cases are mild and anicteric. The liver may be enlarged and tender. Fewer than 20% of the cases have splenomegaly.

The prime laboratory manifestation of hepatitis is an elevation of the serum transaminases (ALT and AST, also known as SGOT and SGPT), which can be very marked. Bilirubinemia, a mixture of direct and indirect, is usual, with some bile in the urine and pale stools. Elevated alkaline phosphatase is frequent but usually not marked. The WBC count is usually normal.

Resolution of the jaundice usually occurs in a few days to weeks, and enzymes gradually return to normal over a few weeks. In some instances, symptoms and laboratory findings may persist for months before finally resolving completely. Hepatitis B may continue to be present without evidence of liver disease, reflecting a carrier state that may persist indefinitely. In some patients, the laboratory findings suggest biliary tract obstruction, and the bilirubinemia is mostly direct (conjugated). This form of hepatitis, called cholestatic jaundice, must be differentiated from extrahepatic bile duct obstruction. In a tiny fraction of cases (<1%) hepatic function deteriorates progressively, the liver shrinks in size, and death occurs. This condition is called fulminant hepatitis or acute yellow atrophy. Other rare complications include pancreatitis, aplastic anemia, and a widespread vasculitis resembling periarteritis nodosa, developing at any time in the course of the illness, usually with concomitant cryoglobulinemia and glomerulonephritis.

Serological diagnosis is possible with several types of viral hepatitis. HBsAg may persist for 3 to 6 months but then disappears and is replaced after a brief interval by anti-HBsAg, which is associated with immunity. Anti-HBcAg and anti-HBeAg appear in the acute phase of the illness. They do not confer immunity and may the only markers of infection present during the "window" period before anti-HBsAg is present. IgM antibodies to Epstein-Barr virus or CMV can be detected in some cases. There are no tests yet for non-A/non-B viruses.

Therapeutic decisions. Treatment of hepatitis is nonspecific, consisting primarily of rest and diet as tolerated. Alcohol should be totally eliminated, at least until enzyme levels return to normal. Precautions to prevent spread are necessary. Hepatitis A is usually infectious for only a few weeks, but B should be considered infectious as long as any signs of disease remain, and preferably until it can be shown that HBsAg is no longer present in the blood.

Chronic hepatitis may follow hepatitis B, non-A, non-B, or infection with the delta agent but does not occur after hepatitis A infection. Drugs can also produce a chronic hepatitis. Pathologically, chronic hepatitis is divided into several subgroups:

1. **Chronic persistent hepatitis,** which is most often due to hepatitis B infection. The inflammatory infiltrate is limited to the periportal regions. The prognosis is excellent, and complete recovery the rule.
2. **Chronic lobular hepatitis** is rare and usually viral. There are scattered areas of necrosis throughout the liver lobule.
3. **Chronic active hepatitis** is the most serious problem and may progress to cirrhosis. Portal areas are enlarged, with infiltrating lymphocytes and plasma cells, and piecemeal necrosis, bridging necrosis, and fibrosis characteristic of cirrhosis can develop. About one-fifth of the cases follow hepatitis B infection, and the rest are due to non-A/non-B hepatitis or concomitant infection with the delta agent. Features of immune complex disease (Sjögren's syndrome, thyroiditis, positive ANA, hyperglobulinemia) led to some of these cases being labeled "lupoid hepatitis," but they are not a manifestation of SLE. Signs of severe liver disease, with hepatosplenomegaly, can develop, along with laboratory evidence of severe liver failure. Liver biopsy is valuable in these cases, especially if treatment with immunosuppressive agents is considered. Azathioprine is the agent generally employed along with corticosteroids, but results are generally disappointing (especially in cases due to non-A/non-B viruses), and the prognosis is poor in severe cases.

Toxic hepatitis

Ethanol is hepatotoxic. Fatty liver results from the increase in the reduced form of nicotinamide-adenine dinucleotide (NADH) generated by the metabolism of alcohol, increasing fatty acid and triglyceride synthesis. Individuals vary in their susceptibility to the hepatotoxicity of alcohol, and malnutrition may contribute to this susceptibility. Heptomegaly is the main finding in these patients. Splenomegaly is not unusual. Laboratory studies show mild elevation of transaminases, but rarely other liver functional abnormalities. The AST is increased more than the ALT (the ratio exceeds 2), in contrast to viral hepatitis, in which the transaminases are increased in parallel. Biopsy of an early lesion shows diffuse or centrilobular fatty change in the liver lobule, but more severe cases show the characteristic triad of alcoholic hepatitis: eosinophilic hyalin around the cell nuclei, infiltration with neutrophils, and a network of connective tissue in the lobule surrounding hepatocytes and central veins.

Patients with advanced disease are seriously ill, and characteristic findings of cirrhosis may appear, including jaundice, ascites, and hepatic encephalopathy. More severe abnormalities in liver function are found in these patients, including hypoalbuminemia and prolonged prothrombin time. Fever may occur, probably as a result of hepatic necrosis, but infection must be ruled out since these patients also show increased susceptibility to infection, especially pneumonia.

Hepatitis due to drug toxicity.   Some drugs produce hepatotoxicity in all people who ingest sufficient quantities. Examples are acetaminophen and CCl_4, both of which produce a centrilobular necrosis. Other drugs produce idiosyncratic reactions that are not dose dependent and thus are not predictable. These include halothane, isoniazide, and chlorpromazine, which can cause generalized hepatic necrosis; allopurinol, which can cause a granulomatous hepatitis; and sex steroids, which produce cholestasis without other pathological changes in the liver.

Acetaminophen depletes available glutathione, and a single dose of over 10 g is generally hepatotoxic. The reaction can be fatal, but early treatment with acetylcysteine seems to be protective. Isoniazide produces transaminase elevations in about 20% of people, but about 1% get a severe hepatitis that can be fatal. Severe reactions from isoniazid are more frequent with increasing age, and the drug should be discontinued in anyone over age 35 who develops a significant elevation of transaminase. The hepatotoxicity seen with chlorpromazine generally results in cholestatic jaundice resembling biliary tract obstruction, but a rash, pruritus, and eosinophilia are common. Erythromycin can produce a similar picture but usually with findings suggestive of acute cholecystitis.

Hepatic encephalopathy results from a severe form of hepatic failure. It occurs in severe cases of viral or toxic hepatitis but is most common in advanced cirrhosis of the liver. It is described below.

Inherited functional abnormality

Gilbert's disease is an inherited abnormality in bilirubin transport in which a mild unconjugated hyperbilirubinemia occurs and persists throughout life. Often these cases are detected because an unrelated illness leads to tests of liver function. No other pathology is associated. Other liver function tests, inlcuding the transaminases, are normal, and no treatment is needed.

Cirrhosis of the liver

Cirrhosis results from fibrosis irregularly altering hepatic architecture, intersecting lobules, and foci of hepatic regeneration. The scarring distorts the hepatic vasculature, leading to portal hypertension and disturbed metabolism of the hepatocytes. There are many causes of cirrhosis, but the most common are toxic hepatitis due to alcohol and viral hepatitis due to hepatitis B or non-A/non-B. HBsAg is usually persistently present in the serum of patients with cirrhosis due to hepatitis B virus. **Schistosomiasis** is the most important cause in many areas of the world (although sometimes the hepatic fibrosis in this disease is not classified as cirrhosis because the hepatic lobular pattern is preserved).

Primary biliary cirrhosis is an autoimmune process, whereas **secondary biliary cirrhosis** results from disease in the biliary ducts. Both can give severe hepatic dysfunction similar to that seen in other forms of cirrhosis. In these cases there is evidence of bile duct obstruction (pruritus, jaundice, hyper-

bilirubinemia, elevated alkaline phosphatase and cholesterol) and antimitochondrial antibodies, which may be present for long periods, whereas patients with alcoholic cirrhosis usually show evidence of hepatocellular dysfunction (especially ALT and AST elevation) before such complications of the cirrhosis appear. Primary biliary cirrhosis is mainly a disease affecting women between the ages of 30 and 65.

The most important congenital diseases that cause cirrhosis are **Wilson's disease** and **alpha$_1$-antitrypsin deficiency**. In the former, the Kayser-Fleischer ring around the cornea, tremor of extrapyramidal tract dysfunction, and increased urinary copper are important clues. **Hemochromatosis**, resulting from excess iron deposition in the liver, shows other changes resulting from the iron deposition, including skin pigmentation, diabetes, heart failure, hypogonadism, and joint pain.

Diagnostic decisions.   Cirrhosis of the liver may be asymptomatic and may be detected only at autopsy. Clues include a history of an etiologic factor (especially alcoholism), altered liver size (usually enlarged in alcoholic cirrhosis but often shrunken and irregular in chronic hepatitis B infection), and signs of portal hypertension such as distended abdominal veins with reversal of flow. The stigmata of cirrhosis seen on physical examination include palmar erythema, spider angiomas, and gynecomastia due to incomplete estrogen detoxification.

Therapeutic decisions.   The main complications of cirrhosis are related to the portal hypertension, ascites, and the manifestations of liver cell failure. Bleeding from **esophageal or gastric varices** is usually copious and has a high mortality rate. Therapy includes the use of IV vasopressin to constrict splanchnic arterioles, use of inflatable esophageal and gastric balloons, injection of varices with sclerosing solutions, and operative placement of shunts between the portal and caval systems.

Other clinical problems

Splenomegaly results from the portal hypertension and can result in hypersplenism. Thrombocytopenia is the most common manifestation, and serious bleeding can result since there can also be a deficiency of clotting factors because of impaired hepatic function. Splenectomy is rarely indicated, however.

Ascites results from the portal hypertension, increased lymph production in the splanchnic area, decreased serum albumin due to impaired hepatic function, increased sodium and water retention due to hyperaldosteronism, and other factors. The peritoneal fluid is usually a transudate, with a protein concentration less than 3 g/100 ml, very few cells, and low LDH. Shifting dullness and a fluid wave are usually detectable on physical examination, and ultrasonography can be used to confirm the presence of increased peritoneal fluid. Treatment consists of restriction of sodium intake, with restricted fluid intake if hyponatremia develops; aldosterone antagonists (such as spironolactone) and loop diuretics (such as furosemide) are often useful, but diuresis should be initiated gradually to avoid hypovolemia, which can precipitate renal or hepatic failure. In intractable cases, a shunt (LeVeen shunt) can be implanted between the vena cava and the peritoneal cavity.

The peritoneal fluid can become infected (**spontaneous

bacterial peritonitis), usually with coliform organisms. Fever, abdominal pain, and tenderness may signal the infection, which can be confirmed by tap of the ascitic fluid for Gram stain, culture, and cell count (>500 cells/mm^3, mostly neutrophils). Antibiotic therapy is urgently indicated, but the mortality rate remains high.

Hepatic encephalopathy, another important complication of cirrhosis, probably results from toxins absorbed from the GI tract that are normally detoxified by the liver, possibly aromatic amino acids, which produce alterations in neurotransmitter metabolism. Disturbances of neurological function occur, including apathy, restlessness, and impaired ability to calculate, which can progress to drowsiness, disorientation, stupor, and coma. Disturbances in neuromuscular control cause asterixis, hyperreflexia, and myoclonus. Drug overdose, hypoglycemia, meningitis, or a subdural hematoma must be ruled out.

In patients with cirrhosis of the liver, precipitating causes can often be found, and removal of such factors is the most important aspect of therapy. The most common precipitating factors are GI bleeding, infection, excessive dietary protein intake, constipation, and CNS-depressant drugs. Deterioration in hepatic function due to an alcoholic binge is a frequent precipitating factor. Electrolyte disturbances and azotemia induced by diuretics can also precipitate encephalopathy.

Other aspects of treatment include the following:
1. Removal of protein from the diet; give IV glucose (hypoglycemia is a common accompaniment, perhaps because of failure of the liver to degrade glycogen sufficiently to maintain blood glucose levels).
2. Correction of electrolyte disturbances such as hyponatremia, hypokalemia, respiratory alkalosis, or metabolic acidosis.
3. Treatment of complications, such as infection (often with overwhelming sepsis), disseminated intravascular coagulation (DIC), GI bleeding from stress ulcers, and renal insufficiency (the hepatorenal syndrome). Suppression of gastric acid production (e.g., with IV cimetidine) and correction of clotting abnormalities therefore are important. Vitamin K is usually needed, but occasionally whole plasma is required to replace all the clotting factors. If renal failure develops, it is often irreversible. Every effort should be made to avoid it by preventing development of hypovolemia.

Severe hepatic failure has about a 20% survival rate.

Hepatorenal syndrome is a severe form of renal failure occurring in patients with advanced liver disease. This syndrome occurs primarily in patients with severe ascites and may be due to hypovolemia, which seems to precipitate renal failure by aggravating renal hypoperfusion. The syndrome may be precipitated by aspirin or other NSAIDs, which inhibit synthesis of prostaglandins in the kidney, and such drugs should be avoided in susceptible patients. Renal histology is normal, but renal blood flow and urine flow are very low. The syndrome is characterized by low urine sodium (<10 mEq/L) and azotemia in the presence of hepatic failure, and the prognosis is generally quite poor.

Other liver diseases

Pyogenic liver abscess is rare in the United States. Most cases result from seeding of the portal circulation by bacteria from an infection somewhere in the area draining into the portal vein, such as cholecystitis, diverticulitis, or appendicitis. Anaerobes and enteric flora are the usual organisms found. Pleural irritation with effusion and pulmonary rales are common. Fever, leukocytosis and right upper quadrant pain are common. Localization can usually be obtained with ultrasonography, radionuclide scan, or CT scan. Surgical aspiration as well as antibiotics is usually needed. **Amoebic liver abscess** has increased in frequency as a result of the increase in amebiasis among male homosexuals and travelers to affected areas. Aspiration is necessary to establish the diagnosis, but the organisms may be present only in the wall of the abscess, and therefore it is important to examine the last drops of any aspirated material. Therapy consists of metronidazole and diiodohydroxyquin or similar drugs, along with surgical drainage.

Granulomatous disease of the liver can result from a variety of infections (tuberculosis, atypical mycobacteria, fungal infections such as histoplasmosis, coccidioidomycosis, and nocardiosis and parasitic infections such as shistosomiasis), as well as sarcoidosis, inflammatory bowel disease, and lymphomas. Other causes include primary biliary cirrhosis and a variety of drugs. Workup depends on the associated manifestations, and biopsy of the liver is a key step.

Neoplastic disease of the liver is usually metastatic, but primary hepatocellular carcinoma, although rare in the United States, is very common in the Far East and Africa. It usually arises in patients with underlying hepatic cirrhosis secondary to hepatitis B infection, less often in patients with other types of cirrhosis. It is often multifocal. It occurs more often in males than in females and usually presents with abdominal pain and weight loss, with hepatomegaly and deteriorating liver function. Jaundice, bloody ascites, or portal vein obstruction may develop. Therapy has very limited effect. Other types of primary liver cancer are seen in relation to environmental exposure, such as angiosarcoma following vinyl chloride, arsenic, or Thorotrast (an agent formerly used in radiological procedures). Cholangiocarcinoma can occur in patients with underlying biliary tract disease.

DISEASES OF THE PANCREAS

Acute pancreatitis

The mechanisms that cause acute pancreatitis are unclear but involve intrapancreatic activation of enzymes, resulting in autodigestion. The most important risk factors for development of acute pancreatitis are alcohol abuse and biliary tract disease. Other factors include abdominal trauma, virus infection (especially mumps, hepatitis, and Coxsackie), hyperlipoproteinemias, hypercalcemia, posterior penetration of a duodenal ulcer, complication of endoscopic retrograde pancreatography, and use of certain drugs (especially corticosteroids, diuretics, immunosuppressives, isoniazid). These factors are important in suggesting the diagnosis and measures to prevent recurrences.

The major symptom of pancreatitis is abdominal pain, usually severe, epigastric, persistent, often with radiation to the back and relieved somewhat by leaning forward. There is severe abdominal tenderness without marked signs of peritoneal irritation, but bowel distension (ileus) occurs frequently. Fever, dehydration, and shock can occur. Other possible findings include tender, red subcutaneous nodules resulting from widespread fat necrosis; an epigastric mass resulting from a pseudocyst (a collection of liquefied, necrotic tissue surrounded by a rim of normal pancreatic or other tissue); and formation of hemorrhagic ascites, which can produce discoloration of the flanks (Grey Turner's sign) or around the umbilicus (Cullen's sign). Other major complications that can develop include phlegmon (a massive inflammation producing a solid pancreas), abscess formation, involvement of contiguous organs (e.g., thrombosis of the splenic vein), obstruction of the common bile duct causing jaundice, or necrosis of the bowel). Secondarily, elevation of the diaphragm can cause atelectasis; inflammation can extend through the diaphragm to produce a left pleural effusion; and ARDS, acute renal failure, or DIC may develop.

Diagnostic decisions. The diagnosis of acute pancreatitis is suggested by the severe pain, an enlarged pancreas seen on ultrasonography or CT scan, and elevation of serum amylase or urinary amylase clearance (>4% of creatinine clearance). The serum amylase usually rises within 2 to 12 hours of the onset of the pain and remains elevated for 3 to 5 days. Other laboratory changes include leukocytosis, hypocalcemia, and hyperglycemia. A perforated peptic ulcer, acute cholecystitis, bowel infarction, and other causes of an acute abdomen must be ruled out.

Therapeutic decisions. Treatment includes nasogastric suction at least in severe cases, fluid replacement, relief of pain, and treatment of complications. Small pseudocysts can disappear, but large ones usually persist and may require surgical drainage because of pain, bleeding, erosion into an adjacent organ, or development of infection.

Chronic pancreatitis

Slow, progressive destruction of the pancreas with varying amounts of inflammation, fibrosis, and distortion of the ducts may result from recurrent episodes of acute pancreatitis, particularly in alcoholics or in association with cystic fibrosis. The most common symptom is the occurrence of repeated attacks of severe epigastric pain unresponsive to any therapy except narcotics, often radiating through to the back and relieved by leaning forward. The pain may be aggravated by eating and can be mild or atypical. Weight loss is common because of the associated anorexia and malabsorption, which results from the lack of pancreatic digestive enzymes. Fibrosis may compress the common bile duct and produce jaundice. Destruction of the islets of Langerhans can produce insulin-requiring diabetes mellitus. Rarely a pseudocyst can give rise to a palpable abdominal mass. Gastritis is often a common accompaniment because of the associated use of alcohol or aspirin taken to relieve the pain.

Diagnostic decisions. The diagnosis of chronic pancreatitis is supported by the occurrence of painful episodes, the presence of risk factors, evidence of malabsorption and steatorrhea, and by plain x-ray or CT scan showing calcifications in the region of the pancreas. The serum amylase is usually normal in chronic pancreatitis except transiently during exacerbations. Supporting evidence that can be obtained includes demonstration of distorted pancreatic ducts by ERCP and pseudocyst formation by ultrasonography. Aspiration of duodenal fluid after pancreatic stimulation with secretin shows

reductions in pancreatic juice volume, HCO_3^-, amylase, and trypsin. Pancreatic or other abdominal malignancy, biliary tract disease, and mesenteric vascular disease must be ruled out.

Therapeutic decisions. Treatment requires prevention of injurious stimuli (especially alcohol and large meals), replacement of lost pancreatic digestive secretions, and pain relief, which is difficult to accomplish without producing narcotic addiction. Surgery may be needed to relieve duct obstruction or to drain a pseudocyst.

Carcinoma of the pancreas

Most pancreatic cancers are adenocarcinomas arising in ductal cells. Risk factors that have been suggested are smoking, diabetes mellitus, and increased consumption of animal fats and coffee, but none are certain. Symptoms are usually vague and nonspecific until the disease is advanced. Persistent epigastric pain radiation to the back is common, as are anorexia and weight loss. An aversion to eating meat is reported by many patients. The most characteristic finding is obstructive jaundice, often painless, developing as a result of obstruction of the common bile duct by a lesion in the head of the pancreas. Migratory thrombophlebitis (Trousseau's sign), paraneoplastic syndromes (especially Cushing's syndrome or hypercalcemia), and gastric bleeding from erosion into the stomach are among the more common complications that develop. An epigastric mass may be palpable.

Diagnostic decisions. Workup includes demonstration of an enlarged pancreas by ultrasonography or CT scan and ERCP to demonstrate ductal distortion or to insert a tube to relieve biliary duct obstruction. Laboratory findings such as serum tumor markers (carcinoembryonic antigen, alpha-fetoprotein) are often positive but too nonspecific to be diagnostically useful. (They can be useful prognostically, to follow therapy, or to signal a recurrence.) A needle biopsy can be performed under guidance from an imaging procedure. Surgery is rarely curative, but palliative biliary drainage may be useful. Radiation and chemotherapy have some value. The investigation of possible disease in the pancreas has been greatly aided by the development of ultrasonography, CT scan, and MR imaging, procedures that can visualize enlargement of the organ, stones, and cysts. ERCP can visualize pancreatic ducts, demonstrate obstruction, and sample pancreatic secretions. Selective angiography can also help delineate neoplastic lesions.

HEMATOLOGY

Pathophysiology of the blood and blood-forming organs

The average life span in the circulation for RBCs is 120 days, for platelets about 7 to 10 days, and for polymorphonuclear leukocytes about 6 hours. Because of the relative amounts in the peripheral blood, approximately equal quantities of each component must be released each day from the marrow. Erythropoiesis is controlled by the hormone erythropoietin, which is released by the kidney in response to anoxia. It is also produced in the liver.

Colony-stimulating factors are produced by monocytes and lymphocytes in response to stimuli such as bacterial toxins, and they stimulate granulocyte precursors. Promyelocytes are the largest cells in the marrow except for megakaryocytes. They contain lysosomes and give rise to neutrophilic, basophilic, and eosinophilic myelocytes. Myelocytes are the most abundant myeloid cells in the marrow and are the last cells in the maturation series that proliferate. Bands and neutrophils do not proliferate but show increasing functional activity concomitant with maturation of membrane functions such as chemotaxis, phagocytosis, and bactericidal action. The normal bone marrow has the capacity to increase production 8- to 10-fold in response to humoral signals, such as erythropoietin and colony-stimulating factors. PGE_2 inhibits granulocyte production.

After release from the marrow, granulocytes exist in a circulating pool and a marginated pool of cells adherent to vessel walls. The two pools are of roughly equal size.

Normal RBC mass in males after puberty is 2 to 4 g/100 ml higher and hematocrit 5 to 7% higher than in adult females. Healthy elderly persons have no decline in hemoglobin or hematocrit. Lower levels commonly found are due to chronic diseases common in this age-group. People who live more than 4,000 feet above sea level have an adaptive increase in hematocrit.

ANEMIA

Symptoms of anemia vary with the age and level of activity of the patient, as well as rapidity of onset of the anemia and therefore the time available for adaptation. Rapid bleeding causes hypovolemia and cardiovascular reaction, with hypotension, vasoconstriction, and faintness. With slowly developing anemias, adjustments allow replacement of plasma volume and cardiac output can be above normal. Exertional dyspnea may develop, as may angina if there is coronary artery disease. Pallor is seen with all types of anemia.

Diagnostic decisions.   Anemia can be defined as a decrease in RBC mass or hemoglobin content of the blood below the level needed to supply tissue oxygen demands. Workup should be approached with three basic questions in mind:

1. What is the mechanism for the decreased RBC or hemoglobin mass—e.g., is it bleeding, lack of RBC production, or excessive destruction of RBCs?
2. Are there associated diseases that can cause anemia?
3. What is the morphology of the RBC on smear of the peripheral blood?

Give special consideration to the following aspects of the history and physical examination in the workup of a patient with anemia:

1. Is the patient truly anemic or is there an increase in plasma volume diluting the RBC mass, such as occurs with pregnancy?
2. Is the anemia inherited or acquired? The family history may reveal anemia, jaundice, gallstones, or splenomegaly. Ethnic background is important in view of the distribution of inherited anemias in certain population groups (blacks, Mediterranean, or Far Eastern populations).
3. Is there evidence of a type of blood loss, such as menstrual bleeding?
4. Has there been exposure to toxins (food, drug, or environmental) that could cause hemolysis or bone marrow depression?
5. Are there physical findings relative to anemia such as pallor, jaundice as evidence of rapid hemolysis, beefy red tongue, fissures at the corners of the mouth (cheilosis) indicating nutritional deficiencies (B vitamins or folic acid), or spoon-shaped nails (koilonychia) seen with iron deficiency?

The size and morphology of the RBC and the reticulocyte count should receive the following special considerations:

Start workup with a complete hemogram, including RBC indices—mean corpuscular volume (MCV), mean corpuscular hemoglobin (MCH), and mean corpuscular hemoglobin concentration (MCHC)—checking the **morphology on smear** for microcytosis, macrocytosis, abnormal shape of RBCs, inclusions in RBCs, and hypersegmented polymorphonuclear leukocytes. A large standard deviation of the MCV indicates population heterogeneity, which can be confirmed on the smear. The MCV is the most useful of the RBC indices; microcytosis (<80 μm^3) is seen in iron deficiency, thalassemia, and chronic renal failure; normocytosis (80 to 100) is found in the anemia of **acute** blood loss; macrocytosis (>100) occurs with a marked reticulocytosis in response to blood loss or hemolysis, refractory anemias associated with myelodysplasia, and the macrocytic anemias of folate and vitamin B_{12} deficiency. The MCH is low in iron deficiency and thalassemia; the MCHC can be high in spherocytosis. On inspection of the smear, the small cells of iron deficiency are seen to be uniform, but in thalassemia, variation in size and shape are seen. Further, sickle cells, inclusions (e.g., nuclear remnants, Howell-Jolly bodies), basophilic stippling (RNA remnants in reticulocytes), parasites (malaria, babesiosis), and schistocytes (in DIC) can be seen.

The reticulocyte count normally is 1%. The low RBC mass in anemia with a normal rate of release of reticulocytes from the bone marrow gives a higher percentage of reticulocytes in the circulation. Adjustment to a normal hematocrit must be made for considering the meaning of a given count. The adjustment is calculated as follows:

Corrected reticulocyte count =
determined reticulocyte count $\times$ (patient's Hct/45)

(All references below to reticulocyte counts assume correction has been made.) Reticulocytes normally circulate for 24 hours. During severe anemia, they may remain in the circulation for longer, and this should also be taken into account in interpreting the reticulocyte count. A high count is seen with normal marrow response to bleeding or hemolysis and after therapy of iron, B_{12}, or folate deficiency. A low count is seen after transfusion or in states with depressed marrow function.

(Bone marrow examination and other laboratory tests are discussed under individual disease entities.)

IRON DEFICIENCY ANEMIA

Iron deficiency is by far the most common cause of hypochromic anemia. Other important causes include poor iron utilization in chronic disease, defects in globin synthesis (the thalassemic syndromes), and defects in heme synthesis or porphyrin synthesis (as occurs in lead poisoning or the porphyrias).

The metabolism of iron.   There are 3 to 4 g of iron in the human body, two-thirds existing in circulating hemoglobin, one-fourth in iron stores, and the remainder in myoglobin, iron-containing enzymes such as the cytochromes, and the plasma. Gastric acid releases iron from food and reduces it. About 1 to 2 mg of iron is absorbed as ferrous iron from the diet each day, representing about 5 to 10% of the total ingested. When there is iron deficiency, 20 to 30% of the dietary iron may be absorbed, but many foods interfere with iron absorption, including phytates in cereals and vegetables, casein in milk, clay (ingested by some people), and the drug tetracycline.

Since elemental iron is insoluble, it must be bound to protein carriers. It is transported from the gut bound to transferrin and is stored in reticuloendothelial cells as ferritin. It is released to erythroblasts and incorporated into protoporphyrin. About 25 mg of iron is needed each day for RBC production. Most of it is supplied by recycling from aged RBCs removed from the circulation, primarily in the spleen. Transferrin concentration in the blood varies widely during the day; it is decreased in chronic inflammatory states and increased but unsaturated in iron deficiency. Iron-transferrin complex is incorporated into developing RBCs by micropinocytosis. Iron is released from the resulting acidic vacuoles, and the apotransferrin complex is recycled to the cell surface and the apotransferrin liberated. The freed iron then enters mitochondria and is enzymatically incorporated into protoporphyrin to form heme; the heme is bound to globin in the cytoplasm. The level of free heme regulates the uptake of iron by normoblasts and reticulocytes.

(Clinical note: the weakness of iron deficiency often responds rapidly to iron therapy, before the hemoglobin rises. This is apparently due to incorporation of iron into other enzymes, such as the cytochromes in the mitochondria first. The other iron-containing enzymes have a greater affinity for iron than hemoglobin and require very small amounts by comparison.)

Iron is stored as ferritin or hemosiderin. Aggregates of ferritin can be detected in marrow smears by staining with ferrocyanide. Circulating ferritin concentrations reflect iron stores; normal is 12 to 325 ng/ml (mean 125 for men, 55 for women). In iron deficiency, ferritin is less than 10; in iron overload it reaches over 1,000. Infection lowers ferritin level; hepatitis or other liver disease raises it. Hemosiderin is an insoluble derivative of ferritin. The iron in it is less accessible for erythropoiesis than that in ferritin. Fixed tissue macrophages also contain stores of iron in ferritin, derived from normal breakdown of RBCs. These stores are rapidly released after hemorrhage but are poorly available in the presence of infection, inflammation, and malignancy, accounting for the anemia of chronic infection and other chronic diseases.

Iron deficiency in adults is usually due to blood loss. In growing children and pregnant women, dietary deficiency is more common. Each fetus removes about 400 mg of iron. (See the section in Chapter 4 for additional details.) Following gastrectomy, lack of HCl to convert Fe^{3+} to Fe^{2+} can lead to malabsorption of iron, as can small bowel malabsorption syndromes. GI bleeding is the most common cause of iron deficiency anemia in men, as gynecologic bleeding is in women. Symptoms include fatigue, dyspnea, and weakness on exertion. Physical examination shows little but pallor (and may reveal the bleeding lesion); koilonychia and cheilosis may be found. Blood smear reveals small RBCs with central pallor. The RBCs vary in shape and size (poikilocytosis and anisocy-

tosis). Serum iron is low and transferrin high ($>350 \mu g/100$ ml) with a transferrin saturation under 15%. Plasma ferritin is low, less than 10 ng/100 ml. Free protoporphyrin in RBCs is high, representing synthesis of precursors of heme without the necessary iron to complete the synthesis of the heme. The reticulocyte count is normal (which can be interpreted as lack of the expected normal response to anemia), and the bone marrow shows erythroid hyperplasia with no stainable iron stores.

As iron deficiency develops, the decrease in stainable iron in the marrow is the first parameter to change. Later, iron-binding protein increases, plasma iron concentration falls, and transferrin becomes desaturated. Hemoglobin level falls, and subsequently a normocytic anemia becomes hypochromic and microcytic.

Therapeutic decisions. Therapy consists first in finding the cause of the iron deficiency and correcting it. Restoration of iron stores can be achieved with a variety of iron preparations; ferrous sulfate or gluconate is most frequently used. Slow-release and coated preparations may not be absorbed because the main site of iron absorption is the duodenum. Although iron is better absorbed during fasting, administration with meals is usually necessary because of gastric irritation by iron preparations. Concomitant ascorbic acid enhances absorption by reducing the iron to Fe^{2+}. Because of limited absorption, 6 to 12 months of therapy is usually necessary, and the supplemental iron should not be discontinued until serum iron and transferrin levels are normal.

Weakness responds to therapy within a few days, but it takes about 2 weeks before a reticulocytosis appears and hemoglobin levels begin to rise. Parenteral iron should rarely be used. Indications include inability to tolerate oral iron, severe malabsorption, or active blood loss requiring more replacement than can be obtained orally. If necessary, iron-dextran complex can be given IM after a test for hypersensitivity.

MEGALOBLASTIC ANEMIAS

When DNA synthesis is impaired, slowing in the rate of division of rapidly proliferating cells leads to accumulation in the marrow of cells, with relatively large nuclei containing more than the usual amount of chromatin. Such cells are called megaloblasts. Reduced proliferation of marrow cells results in pancytopenia. Since the cells that are released into the periphery have undergone fewer than the normal number of divisions, the RBCs are larger than normal (macrocytes) and there is hypersegmentation of the nuclei of polymorphonuclear leukocytes since they contain more chromatin in each cell than normal.

Megaloblastic anemias result from folate or vitamin B_{12} deficiency. Reduced tetrahydrofolate is a carrier for one-carbon fragments in the synthesis of thymidine from desoxyuridine. Vitamin B_{12} is a cofactor in the regeneration of the active form of tetrahydrofolate. B_{12} is also a coenzyme in conversion of methylmalonyl CoA to succinyl CoA, a step in the synthesis of myelin. As a result, CNS changes occur with deficiency of that vitamin but do not occur with folate deficiency since folate has no role in CNS myelin metabolism. Demyelination of large fibers in peripheral nerves occurs first, affecting the dorsal columns of the spinal cord later, and sometimes there is pathology in the cerebrum. Nerve cell damage can become irreversible. Earliest symptoms reflect the peripheral nerve damage with glove and stocking paresthesias, then position and vibration sense are lost and deep tendon reflexes increased (dorsolateral column disease). Late changes that can be seen include spastic ataxia, motor weakness, and then dementia (megaloblastic madness). Autoimmune processes may develop, affecting other organ systems, including early graying of hair and vitiligo.

Impaired cell proliferation, as well as shortened life span of RBCs, leads to anemia, leukopenia, and thrombocytopenia. The slowly developing anemia can become very severe. The circulating RBCs are macrocytic, and there is hypersegmentation of the nuclei of polymorphonuclear leukocytes. Hemolysis occurring in the marrow and in extramedullary sites results in elevated serum bilirubin. The marrow is hypercellular, with megaloblasts and giant band forms. Iron stores in the marrow are increased. There is also gigantism of epithelial cells in the mouth and intestine, but atrophy of gastric and intestinal mucosa develops, leading to achlorhydria and further malabsorption of folate.

Folate nutrition.   The daily requirement is 50 to 200 μg. Body stores average 5 to 20 mg and thus can last a few months unless utilization is increased by more rapid turnover of cells, such as occurs in hemolytic anemias (e.g., sickle cell anemia) or exfoliative dermatitis (e.g., extensive psoriasis), as well as in pregnancy. Folate is present in leafy vegetables (hence the name). It is heat labile and in a form linked with glutamic acid units that must be depolymerized. The intestinal conjugases that remove the glutamates are inhibited by phenytoin, oral contraceptives, and alcohol. Intestinal diseases can interfere with absorption. Dietary deficiency is a common cause of megaloblastic anemia as a result of inadequate folate, especially when fresh, uncooked salads and vegetables are not ingested and when requirements are increased. Many drugs interfere with folate metabolism, blocking the regeneration of tetrahydrofolate, including anticancer/immunosuppressant agents such as methotrexate, antibacterials such as Bactrim, and the antimalarial pyrimethamine. The toxicity of these agents can be reversed by giving folinic acid, which bypasses the metabolic block by supplying reduced folate.

Diagnostic decisions.   The diagnosis of megaloblastic anemia is usually made from the RBC morphology, the MCV, the finding of megaloblasts in the bone marrow, and measurement of blood levels of folate and B_{12}. Plasma levels of folate fall quickly with inadequate intake. The RBC folate level is a better reflection of body stores. The underlying cause of the deficiency must be established. Diet, drug, and alcohol history and workup for malabsorption usually reveal the reason for folate deficiency.

Vitamin B_{12} deficiency usually results from pernicious anemia, a state with atrophic gastritis and inadequate intrinsic factor production, which leads to the failure to absorb vitamin B_{12}. The process usually results from autoantibody production, and finding serum antibodies against intrinsic factor is diagnostic, but antigastric parietal cell antibodies are more commonly detected. The process responsible for impaired absorption of vitamin B_{12} can be detected with the **Schilling test**, in which a tracer of radiolabeled B_{12} is given PO with a chaser of a large dose of unlabeled vitamin IV to saturate body stores. The urinary excretion of the labeled vitamin is measured (normally

>7% of the administered dose in 48 hours). If less than 5%, poor absorption has occurred. The diagnosis of pernicious anemia is established by repeating the test with a PO dose of intrinsic factor, which should correct the malabsorption. Sometimes the test has to be repeated after 2 to 3 months of therapy to restore the intestinal mucosa, since the atrophy that exists during florid disease can prevent absorption even with the intrinsic factor. A therapeutic trial of vitamin B_{12} is also useful; 1 to 5 μg IM of the vitamin daily should give a reticulocytosis within 3 to 4 days, and continued therapy should correct the anemia in about a month. Administration of 200 μg of folate per day will lead to a reticulocytosis in folate deficiency but not if there is B_{12} deficiency. Larger amounts of folate can induce a reticulocytosis with B_{12} deficiency but may aggravate the neurological disease, leading to permanent CNS damage.

Therapeutic decisions.   Specific therapy of megaloblastic anemia should reverse the bone marrow abnormalities in 1 to 2 days. Leukopenia and thrombocytopenia reverse within 10 days. Reticulocytosis appears in 3 to 4 days and peaks at 10 days, often reaching as high as 25%. Serum vitamin K can fall, and LDH and bilirubin, which are elevated because of the hemolysis, fall within 1 to 3 weeks. Anemia may be corrected within 1 to 2 months, but often improvement plateaus when the patient runs out of iron, which must then be added to the regimen. Neurological deficits may improve over 6 to 12 months, but long tract abnormalities may be permanent.

APLASTIC ANEMIA

Peripheral pancytopenia with markedly depressed hematopoietic activity in the bone marrow is termed aplastic anemia. In severe states, the reticulocyte count is below 1%, platelets below 20,000 mm³, neutrophil count under 500, and cells occupy less than 25% of the marrow space on biopsy. Aplastic anemias can be inherited (Fanconi's syndrome) or due to a viral infection (especially hepatitis, Epstein-Barr virus). Most cases are due to drugs, such as the dose-dependent effect of cytotoxins used in cancer therapy, which is usually reversible when the drug is stopped. (Cycle-specific agents such as methotrexate spare the early pleuripotential marrow cells, affecting mainly dividing, more mature stem cells. This allows marrow recovery after the drug is stopped.) Other drugs (e.g., chloramphenicol and phenylbutazone) cause an idiosyncratic reaction less related to dose and less often reversible. A variety of environmental toxins such as benzene and radiation exposure can cause aplastic anemia.

Preleukemia can present as marrow aplasia and then evolve into full-blown leukemia. The incidence of acute leukemia is increased in patients who have recovered from aplastic anemia.

Some aplastic states are a result of immunologic suppression of marrow function. Suppressor T cells and immunoglobulins have been demonstrated to inhibit erythropoietin or block differentiation of hematopoietic cells. Immunosuppressives may be of value in some of these cases.

The most successful therapy for severe cases, when possible, is transplantation of HLA-matched bone marrow. In others, prednisone in low doses, androgens, and etiocholanolone have been useful. Antithymocyte globulin is also being used successfully.

HEMOLYTIC ANEMIAS

A wide variety of processes can lead to accelerated destruction of RBCs in excess of the capacity for marrow replacement, despite the capacity of the marrow to increase RBC production up to eightfold. Hemolytic processes result from abnormalities in RBC membrane or enzymes, antibody reactions with the RBC membrane, toxins or bacterial products, heat or mechanical trauma, and genetic abnormalities in RBC metabolism, especially those affecting hemoglobin synthesis. Affected patients are pale, and jaundice may be detectable. In many chronic hemolytic states, there is splenomegaly and hepatomegaly. The morphology of the RBC may be normal or abnormal. Reticulocytes are usually increased, reflecting the attempt by the marrow to keep up with the accelerated rate of destruction. Marrow smears show erythroid hyperplasia. Nucleated RBCs may appear in the peripheral blood because of the rapid release of cells from the marrow. Bilirubin and LDH levels are increased, and urine urobilinogen is increased, reflecting the accelerated RBC breakdown. The increased daily production of bilirubin can lead to gallstone formation.

Intravascular hemolysis, destruction of RBCs in the circulation, is rare, occurring primarily as a result of transfusion reactions or the presence of cold agglutinins. Hemoglobin released into the plasma becomes complexed to proteins, especially haptoglobin, hemopexin, or albumin. These complexes are rapidly cleared by the liver, lowering the levels of haptoglobin and hemopexin in the plasma, but the combination of hemoglobin and albumin, methemalbumin, circulates for days. If the binding capacity of these proteins is exceeded, hemoglobin appears in the urine. The hemoglobin itself is not toxic to the kidney, but the accumulation of RBC stroma in renal vessels can lead to renal failure.

ACQUIRED HEMOLYTIC ANEMIAS

Extravascular hemolysis generally results from antibodies or toxins and occasionally from inherited disorders that lead to a RBC membrane defect (e.g., paroxysmal nocturnal hemoglobinemia). The destruction of the RBC takes place mostly in the spleen rather than in the circulation.

Antibody-mediated hemolytic anemias

Antibodies that arise from sensitization to components of RBCs by transfusion or exposure to foreign antigens are termed **alloantibodies**. Antibodies that arise without such external sensitization are called **autoantibodies**. They usually result from sensitization by haptens (usually drugs) or as a component of a systemic disease such as SLE, inflammatory bowel disease, leukemia, or lymphoma. Only a minority of these autoantibodies to RBCs cause hemolysis.

When antibodies react with the membrane of RBC, they make the cells less deformable and more susceptible to damage while moving in capillaries. They are also susceptible to phagocytosis by macrophages, which react with the Fc component of the antibodies on the surface of the RBC through their Fc receptors. This phenomenon occurs primarily in the spleen.

"Warm antibodies" react at body temperature and occur primarily as autoantibodies arising in systemic disease. At times the development of hemolytic anemia is the first manifestation that such a disease process is occurring. Clinically,

the manifestations depend on the rate of hemolysis that occurs, since the bone marrow can increase output of RBCs by up to eightfold. Mild hemolysis results in no anemia, but with severe hemolysis a profound anemia can develop. These cases have a positive direct **Coombs' test** (done by adding an antibody to gamma-globulin, which reacts with the IgG or occasionally IgM coating the surface of the RBC). Complement is also demonstrable coating the RBC, especially derivatives of the third component of complement (C3), C3b or C3d. There may be an accompanying autoimmune thrombocytopenia (Evan's syndrome). Excessive bilirubin production from the increased destruction of hemoglobin can result in mild jaundice. The hyperbilirubinemia is indirect reacting, unconjugated bilirubin. Splenomegaly is common. The peripheral blood smear may show spherocytosis. The RBCs are normochromic and normocytic. The increased production of RBCs by the marrow, to compensate for the hemolysis, results in reticulocytosis.

Therapeutic decisions. Therapy for hemolytic anemia consists primarily of corticosteroids, such as prednisone, in large doses. They decrease the rate of RBC destruction without much decrease in autoantibody production. If an inadequate response is obtained, splenectomy can be useful. Transfusion should be avoided if possible, since the accelerated RBC destruction results in little response. Supplemental oral folic acid may be necessary since the increased RBC production increases turnover of this vitamin.

"Cold antibody" is much less common, usually IgM, reacting with RBC over a wide range of temperatures, including temperatures as low as 4°C. Cold-reacting antibodies are seen in infectious mononucleosis, CMV infection, *Mycoplasma* pneumonias (in which they are usually polyclonal), and occasionally with lymphomas and Waldenstrom's macroglobulinemia (in which they are typically monoclonal). As with warm antibodies, binding of complement leads to increased removal of RBCs by macrophages, especially in the spleen, and the clinical picture is similar to that described above.

Drug-induced autoimmune hemolysis

A large number of drugs can cause hemolysis, some as a result of hapten formation resulting from binding of the drug to RBC membranes, forming neoantigens. Once this has occurred, readministration of the drug causes hemolysis. Penicillins and cephalosporins are common causes of this type of hemolysis. In the "innocent bystander" type of hemolysis, drugs bound to plasma proteins form neoantigens. RBCs are affected secondarily by complement activation in the plasma and thus are innocent bystanders. This mechanism is responsible for hemolysis caused by most drugs. Common examples are phenothiazines, sulfonamides, isoniazide, and quinine. A positive direct Coombs' test (from IgG coating the RBC) results with some drugs and is most commonly seen with alphamethyldopa (Aldomet) and levodopa. These antibodies show Rh specificity, and the Coombs' test may remain positive for many months after the drug is discontinued.

Hypersplenism

Excessive sequestration of blood cells in the spleen usually results in pancytopenia. The compensatory increased production of cells in the marrow has led to this syndrome being characterized as "empty blood, full marrow," contrasting with the "empty marrow" in aplastic anemia. Hypersplenism can occur with any cause of an enlarged spleen but is most commonly encountered in lymphomas, including Hodgkin's disease, chronic leukemias, some chronic infections, and in rheumatoid arthritis, when leukopenia is the most common result (**Felty's syndrome**).

Chemical and toxic causes of hemolysis

Chloramine, generated from chlorine (which is present in most water supplies) and alum, can cause hemolysis in patients undergoing hemodialysis. Other types of hemolysis occur in various systemic diseases. For example, a spur cell deformity is seen in RBCs, along with increased destruction, in cirrhosis of the liver as a result of altered lipid metabolism and therefore changes in the RBC membrane. Drugs including amphotericin can also cause changes in the RBC membrane, as can snake venom because of its content of lysolecithinase. Heavy metals, including arsenic and copper, can cause hemolysis by binding to sulfhydryl groups on RBC membranes.

HEMOGLOBINOPATHIES

Each hemoglobin molecule consists of two alpha-globin chains and two other chains (in adults mainly beta-globin). Two genes for alpha are on chromosome 16, a series of nonalpha-chain genes are on 11. Normally, synthesis of both types of chains is balanced. If an excess of globin is made, the chains are unstable and precipitate at the RBC membrane to form Heinz bodies, shortening the life span of the RBCs. Hemoglobin F is made in utero and consists of two alpha chains plus two gamma chains. Synthesis of hemoglobin F usually stops shortly after birth as beta-chain synthesis is turned on.

Oxygen is transported by hemoglobin. It is picked up at a PO_2 of 100 in the lungs and delivered to the tissues where the PO_2 is 40. Oxygen unloading is facilitated by binding to hemoglobin of 2,3-diphosphoglycerate (DPG), acidic pH of tissues, and the binding of CO_2. Changes in the structure of the globin chains or in the heme can affect affinity of hemoglobin for oxygen. Mutations in the genes controlling globin synthesis can produce structurally abnormal hemoglobins (the hemoglobinopathies). Amino acid substitutions can affect the solubility of the hemoglobin (e.g., hemoglobin S) or render it unstable (e.g., hemoglobin Koln) or decrease oxygen affinity (e.g., hemoglobin Kansas); or the mutations can decrease the rate of globin synthesis and therefore hemoglobin formation (e.g., the thalassemias). Mutations that affect the normal expression of the beta-chain genes usually result in persistence of hemoglobin F synthesis after birth.

Sickle cell anemia

Substitution of a valine for a glutamic acid at the sixth position of the beta chain of globin results in formation of sickle hemoglobin (hemoglobin S). Hemoglobin S is insoluble when unoxygenated and polymerizes within the RBCs, distorting the shape and altering the RBC membrane, decreasing deformability. These sickle cells tend to occlude small vessels and have a markedly shortened life span. The micro-occlusions cause microinfarcts of organs, including painful bony infarcts and scarring and atrophy of the spleen.

The hemoglobin S gene is present in 10% of the American blacks and in up to 25% of the populations of parts of western Africa, where the heterozygote (hemoglobin SA) shows increased resistance to falciparum malaria. In the heterozygote, there is both hemoglobin S and A in each RBC. About 60% of the hemoglobin is A. Concurrent thalassemia and S ameliorates the effect of the S gene, since there is decreased synthesis of the beta-S chain (and more synthesis of hemoglobin F).

Patients with sickle cell anemia are usually weak and show pallor of the mucous membranes, but they adapt reasonably well to the continuously low hemoglobin concentration. However, heart failure can appear. A major manifestation of sickle cell disease is the occurrence of painful crises due to microinfarcts, especially in bones, which cause local swelling and tenderness, usually in the extremities. The findings can be confused with osteomyelitis or arthritis. Pulmonary infections are common, as are cerebrovascular accidents. Intrahepatic sickling can cause hepatomegaly. Intrarenal sickling produces loss of concentrating capacity, even in sickle trait. Renal papillary necrosis and hematuria can occur. Cutaneous sickling produces skin ulcerations, especially around the ankles and feet. Retinal changes can occur. Growth is often impaired, and the chronic anemia usually results in delayed puberty. Cardiomyopathy is common. The chronic hemolysis not only causes hyperbilirubinemia but also bilirubin-containing gallstones. Folic acid deficiency is common because of the RBC turnover. Loss of the spleen results in poor IgM production and an increased tendency to infections, particularly with pneumococci and *Salmonella*.

The hemoglobin in sickle cell disease is usually between 6 and 8 g/100 ml (Hct 18 to 24%). The cells are normochromic and normocytic (unless folate deficiency has developed). Sickle-shaped cells can be seen on peripheral smear, especially if the blood is deoxygenated while still wet by adding sodium metabisulfite. If positive, a hemoglobin electrophoresis should be performed; it will reveal 90 to 95% hemoglobin S. Bilirubin is elevated, basically as a result of the increased production because of the hemolysis, but the serum bilirubin may be largely direct reacting because of the hepatic damage. The haptoglobin level is low and LDH high.

Sickle cell trait is usually asymptomatic. Usually 55 to 60% of the hemoglobin is A, 40 to 45% S. The total hemoglobin is almost normal, and the only abnormality on workup will be a failure of urine-concentrating capacity because of the infarcts that occur in the renal medulla, where PO_2 is normally low enough to produce sickling. If severe generalized anoxemia occurs, a typical sickle crisis can be precipitated.

Patients with concomitant sickle cell disease and thalassemia have a more benign course, with less severe anemia, and may present with splenomegaly instead of the functionally absent spleen seen in ordinary sicklers. Similarly, patients with a combination of hemoglobin C and S can have splenomegaly. Sickle-thalassemia patients have microcytosis and hypochromia, but the percentage of hemoglobin S is under 80% and the rest is mostly hemoglobin F but distributed unhomogeneously in different RBCs. If hemoglobin F is present, it is usually distributed homogeneously.

Therapeutic decisions. Management of sickle cell disease consists largely of analgesics and oxygen for painful crises, pneumococcal vaccine in early childhood to decrease pneumococcal infections, and early treatment of any infection that occurs. Fever in sickle cell crises represents infection or tissue necrosis. Transfusions should be avoided as much as possible to avoid iron overload. However, transfusion of RBCs may be needed before a surgical procedure. During surgery, it is important to avoid anoxia and hypothermia. Transfusions are also given in the late stages of pregnancy to avoid placental infarcts. Genetic counseling is important, and prenatal diagnosis is possible using amniocentesis samples and restriction enzyme techniques.

Thalassemias

The thalassemias are inherited abnormalities of hemoglobin metabolism in which synthesis of one of the globin chains is decreased, resulting in ineffective erythropoiesis, but qualitatively the hemoglobin that is synthesized is normal. There is increased destruction of RBCs (hemolysis) both in the marrow and in the circulation. As a result, the RBCs that are produced are small and lacking in hemoglobin content (microcytic and hypochromic) and have a shortened life span. Either alpha- or beta-chain synthesis can be affected. The disease processes vary in severity. There are asymptomatic heterozygotic carriers for alpha-thalassemia or mild beta-chain disease (beta-thalassemia minor). On the other hand, the genetic abnormality can cause severe anemia (beta-thalassemia major) or even death in utero from severe heart failure producing hydrops fetalis (homozygotic alpha-thalassemia).

A variety of different mutations have been identified that impair the synthesis of the beta gene of globin and result in different syndromes. **Heterozygotic thalassemia minor** causes mild anemia, usually with hemoglobin levels of 10 to 12 g, and microcytosis (MCV usually in the 60s). The peripheral smear shows anisocytosis, and target cells can be seen. Serum iron and transferrin are normal as opposed to the findings in the hypochromic microcytic anemia of iron deficiency. Electrophoresis reveals 3 to 5% hemoglobin A2 and 2 to 3% hemoglobin F. The rest is hemoglobin A. No therapy is indicated.

Homozygotic thalassemia major is a severe disease causing early death. Both beta genes are abnormal, and very little beta chain synthesis occurs. The excess alpha-globin chains precipitate in the cells, producing Heinz bodies. There is an expansion of the active bone marrow into the skull and facial bones, affecting appearance, as well as the development of extramedullary hematopoiesis in the spleen and liver. Growth is impaired and puberty delayed. The expansion of the marrow in the long bones results in an increased fragility and frequent fractures. The peripheral smear shows microcytosis, hypochromia, and frequent nucleated RBCs. Untransfused, the hemoglobin level would be between 3 and 6 g/100 ml, with practically no hemoglobin A. The major hemoglobin is F with variable amounts of A2. Without transfusion, death by age 2 was common. Present practice is to maintain the hemoglobin around 8 to 10 with frequent transfusions of RBCs. As a result of the transfusions and the excess GI absorption of iron that occurs in this syndrome, iron overload eventually develops, resembling the syndrome of **hemochromatosis**, with diabetes mellitus, cardiomyopathy, and hypofunction of multiple endocrine glands, including the thyroid, adrenal, and parathyroid. There is increased susceptibility to infection, usually worsened

when splenectomy is done late in childhood to decrease the rate of RBC removal and thus lessen the transfusion requirement. Chelation of the excess iron with desferoxamine beginning early in childhood lessens the problem of iron deposition.

Thalassemia intermedia is a state with double heterozygosity for two genes affecting synthesis of beta-globin chains (thalassemia traits), usually resulting in hemoglobin levels of 8 to 10 g/100 ml. Affected persons have normal growth, mature sexually at a normal rate, and have few clinical manifestations of thalassemia, but iron overload can occur because of the increased iron absorption.

The syndromes that occur in **alpha-thalassemia** depend on the specific mutations present at four gene loci and vary from an asymptomatic state with no anemia but low MCV and MCH to a mild hypochromic anemia. **Hemoglobin H disease**, a mild, variable degree of hemolytic anemia with inclusions of precipitated hemoglobin in the RBCs, is another variant, as is **hydrops fetalis**, which results from absence of all alpha-globin production, leading to death in utero from anoxia and heart failure.

A high incidence of thalassemia trait occurs in American blacks. When combined with the sickle cell gene, it ameliorates the severity of the sickle cell disease.

POLYCYTHEMIA VERA

Polycythemia vera is a neoplastic myeloproliferative disorder characterized by autonomous proliferation of all marrow constituents but predominantly affecting RBCs. A hematocrit above 54% in a man or above 50% in a woman requires evaluation for polycythemia. Relative polycythemia can occur as a result of decreased plasma volume (Gaisböck's polycythemia); this occurs predominantly in hypertensive, obese men. In absolute polycythemia, the RBC mass is elevated (>36 ml/kg in men, >32 ml/kg in women), but this may be a response to hypoxemia (secondary polycythemia), and workup must distinguish between this process and polycythemia vera.

Diagnostic decisions. Initial workup of polycythemia consists of inquiry and examination for causes of anoxia, including evidence for COPD. Splenomegaly is characteristic of polycythemia vera. Elevated WBC and platelet count also favor polycythemia vera, whereas a low PO_2 favors secondary polycythemia. Rarely, polycythemia results from an erythropoietin-secreting renal cyst or hepatocellular carcinoma or tissue anoxia due to abnormalities in hemoglobin affinity for oxygen, such as congenital methemoglobinemia.

Clinical features. Patients with polycythemia vera can be asymptomatic or can develop problems related to hyperviscosity, hypervolemia, or platelet dysfunction. These problems vary from tinnitus or light-headedness to symptoms suggestive of transient ischemic attacks (TIA) and even stroke. CHF, myocardial infarction, and venous thromboembolic disease or hemorrhages can occur. The increased cellular turnover leads to elevated uric acid levels, and gouty arthritis can develop. The increased production of basophils in the bone marrow can lead to generalized itching.

The diagnosis of polycythemia vera is based on a family history of the disease, the finding of splenomegaly or manifestations of one of the common complications, and absence of a cause of arterial desaturation, including the determination of

ABGs if there is any question. There is usually an elevated WBC (>12,000) and platelet count (>400,000) and an elevated leukocyte alkaline phosphatase as well as an elevated serum vitamin B_{12} level (>900). ^{51}Cr-labeled RBCs are injected, and the dilution of this label provides a measure of the RBC mass. If it is increased and arterial PO_2 is normal, other causes of polycythemia (renal cyst, hepatoma, cerebellar tumor) can be ruled out with a liver-spleen scan, renal sonogram, and CT scan of the head. A serum erythropoietin level can be determined if any question remains; it should be zero in polycythemia vera, since the marrow is functioning autonomously, independent of the usual stimulus. If the patient is a smoker, determination of carboxyhemoglobin is necessary to rule out a change in oxygen-carrying capacity of the hemoglobin. A rare hemoglobinopathy with high oxygen affinity, failing to release the oxygen to the tissues (Chesapeake hemoglobin), may have to be ruled out also.

Therapeutic decisions. Treatment consists of repeated phlebotomy to keep the hematocrit below levels that lead to hyperviscosity and thrombi, preferably to 45 or less. Depletion of iron stores with chelating agents such as desferoxamine can retard RBC production. Phlebotomy may lead to an increase in platelet count, increasing the likelihood of a thromboembolic complication; antimetabolite therapy may be preferable. Hydroxyurea is the favored antimetabolite at present.

The course is prolonged, usually 10 years or more; most patients die of thrombotic complications, a few evolve into an acute leukemia. If complications do not develop, the disease usually evolves into **myelofibrosis and myeloid metaplasia**, a syndrome characterized by pancytopenia with young forms of WBC and nucleated RBC in the peripheral blood, "dry tap" of the marrow, and marrow biopsy showing fibrosis and little hematopoiesis, but there is abundant extramedullary hematopoiesis with hepatosplenomegaly. Some patients present with the picture of myeloid metaplasia without a clinical history of the phase of polycythemia vera.

TRANSFUSION OF BLOOD PRODUCTS

A unit of blood for transfusion contains 450 ml of blood mixed with 63 ml of citrate, plus glucose, phosphate, and adenine to prolong RBC survival. The shelf life is 35 days. However, it is rarely necessary to give whole blood; separation of the donated blood into components can yield therapy for five different recipients.

The components of whole blood include RBCs, platelets, granulocytes, and plasma and its separate protein constituents (e.g., Factor VIII or antihemophiliac factor [AHF], albumin, gamma-globulin, and other coagulation factors). **RBCs** can be transfused as packed RBCs (after removal of most of the plasma), leukocyte-poor RBCs (including buffy coat-poor RBCs, from which about 80% of the WBCs are removed), or frozen RBCs, which have about 90% of the leukocytes removed. A unit of RBCs is expected to raise the hematocrit by 3 to 5%.

Platelets are usually transfused in amounts equivalent to four or more units of blood; from four to six units of platelets would give a rise in platelet count of about 50,000/mm^3, which can be expected to last about 1 to 3 days unless there is fever or immune platelet destruction, which shortens survival. After repeated platelet transfusions, alloimmunization can occur,

requiring HLA matching of platelet types before transfusion. Platelet transfusions are usually restricted to patients with severe thrombocytopenia who are actively bleeding, but they are also used during chemotherapy of leukemia.

Granulocyte transfusions have transitory effect, usually with a half-life of about 6 hours. Thus such transfusions are rarely used and are reserved for life-threatening, severely neutropenic states.

Coagulation factors are given as fresh-frozen plasma, which supplies all factors including the labile ones. Fibrinogen and Factor VIII (AHF) are stable and can be given concentrated in cryoprecipitate prepared from plasma.

Compatibility testing of blood involves typing and checking for compatibility of the donor blood in the recipient's plasma (cross-matching). People who are type A (40% of the population) usually have antibodies to blood group B; those who are type B (95) have antibodies to A; type AB (3%) will not have antibodies to either A or B. About 45% of the population is blood group O.

Therapeutic decisions. In an emergency, packed O cells can be given to a patient of any ABO type. Rh+ cells can be given to an Rh− individual if the recipient has no anti-D, but there is a 70% likelihood of immunization and thus this emergency procedure cannot be repeated after there has been time to develop antibodies. It may be preferable to give plasma expanders such as saline or albumin until cross-matching can be performed.

Rh system

The Rh system is defined by three loci, Cc, D, and Ee. D is most important, and "Rh negative" means the absence of D. Transfusion of Rh+ (D+) blood to someone who is Rh− (D−) and is sensitized to D will result in hemolysis. Sensitization usually results from a pregnancy in which the mother is D− and the fetus is D+. The transfer of such anti-D antibodies across the placenta during a future pregnancy with a D+ fetus can result in severe disease, including **erythroblastosis fetalis**. Maternal sensitization can be prevented by treating Rh− mothers immediately after an event that can cause fetal cells to enter the maternal circulation (e.g., delivery, amniocentesis, abortion) with Rh immune globulin (RhoGAM), which removes cells with D antigen. If disease does develop in the fetus on the basis of transfer of antibodies from a previously sensitized mother, intrauterine transfusions can be given to the fetus to prevent erythroblastosis fetalis.

LEUKOCYTES

Pathophysiology of polymorphonuclear neutrophils

A main function of polymorphonuclear neutrophils (polys) is defense against bacterial invasion. There are three phases in the attack on bacteria by neutrophils: chemotaxis, phagocytosis, and microbial killing. Killing results from the release of the contents of granules into phagosomes (bactericidal proteins, myeloperoxidase, and cathepsins) and the formation of oxygen free radicals including superoxide and OH$^-$. Microbicidal substances are also generated from halides, such as the hypochlorite ion (OCl$^-$) from chloride.

The primary or azurophilic granules in neutrophils, which fuse with the phagosomes, contain lysozyme, acid hydrolases, neutral and acid proteases (including cathespin G), elastase, and myeloperoxidases. Other, specific, granules contain lysozyme, transcobolamin III, apolactoferrin, collagenase, and C5-cleaving protease. Specific granules fuse with the membrane of both phagosomes and the outer cell membrane, and therefore some of their contents are released outside the cells. In addition to dissolving bacterial cell wall, they degrade connective tissue, digest cellular debris, and bind substances such as iron, which is needed for bacterial metabolism. (This is probably the mechanism responsible for the altered iron metabolism of infection.)

Neutrophil kinetics. Maturation in bone marrow ordinarily takes 7 to 10 days but can be shortened to about 5 days during acute stress. The cells circulate for 6 to 10 hours, then spend 4 to 5 days in tissues. In view of the kinetics, the neutropenic effect of a bone marrow suppressant would be expected to become apparent 7 to 10 days after administration.

Normal circulating neutrophil concentration is 2,000 (1,500 in blacks, due to a larger marginated pool). **Neutropenia** can be caused by radiation or drugs, and occasionally by an immune mechanism. A variety of diseases cause neutropenia, including viral infections (especially hepatitis, infectious mononucleosis), some bacterial infections, and acute effects of alcohol ingestion. **Cyclic neutropenia** occurs intermittently on a familial basis. Vitamin B_{12} and folate deficiencies can cause neutropenia, as can any form of hypersplenism. Counts below 1,000 are life threatening and require "reverse precautions," including isolation, careful oral and anal hygiene, use of stool softeners, immediate investigation of any cause of fever, and rapid institution of broad-spectrum antibiotic therapy pending identification of a causative organism and selection of a more specific agent. WBC transfusion is of little benefit.

LEUKEMIA

Chronic myelogenous leukemia

Chronic myelogenous leukemia (CML) is characterized by proliferation of all marrow cell lines, all of which express a marker chromosome, the Philadelphia chromosome. This fact is interpreted as indicating a mutation in a pluripotent stem cell, translocating the long arm of chromosome 22 to chromosome 9, probably representing activation of an oncogene (human DNA sequences analogous to viral DNA known to cause cancer in other species). CML is most frequent in adults between the ages of 40 and 50. Causes of CML are uncertain except for the known increase in the disease beginning 7 years after the atomic bomb attacks on Japan.

Clinical features. Patients are often asymptomatic, the disease being discovered accidentally on routine blood count, which shows increases in total WBC (often >100,000) with early myeloid precursors and thrombocytosis. The WBCs show decreased alkaline phosphatase levels, and the Philadelphia chromosome can be demonstrated in about 90%. Splenomegaly is usually present by the time of diagnosis and can become a major cause of symptoms. As the disease progresses, anemia, fever, and weakness develop. Thrombocytopenia appears, and increasing numbers of immature WBCs are seen in the peripheral blood. Preterminally, a "blast phase" is usual, and these very immature cells often show new chromosome

abnormalities and sometimes the appearance of lymphoid cell markers.

Treatment of CML is still unsatisfactory, relying mainly on chemotherapy. Bone marrow transplantation is being tried increasingly.

Chronic lymphatic leukemia

Chronic lymphatic leukemia (CLL) is a disease of older people, less than 10% of cases appearing before age 50. It is twice as common in men. The diagnosis is often made by an unsuspected finding of a high lymphocyte count in the peripheral blood (>15,000), made up of small, well-differentiated cells. The marrow is hypercellular, and over 40% are lymphocytes. Peripheral lymph nodes enlarge, as do the liver and spleen, because of accumulation of the neoplastic lymphs. These cells often fail to produce normal amounts of immune globulins, and hypogammaglobulinemia with increased susceptibility to bacterial infection frequently develops. Sometimes autoimmune phenomena appear, including a positive Coombs' test, but hemolysis is rare. Immune thrombocytopenia can develop. In some cases, there is a monoclonal hypergammaglobulinemia, which can be IgG or IgM.

Clinically, CLL can be staged as follows: Stage 0 represents lymphocytosis with marrow findings alone; progression involves the enlargement of nodes in stage I, liver and spleen in stages II; anemia develops in stage III and thrombocytopenia in stage IV. Prognosis depends on the stage of the disease, varying from a median of about 2 years for stage IV to over 18 years for stage I, and still longer for stage 0.

Therapeutic decisions. Treatment is usually withheld until symptoms develop and then kept to a minimum. Chemotherapy can be given for generalized adenopathy, radiation to local areas of bulky adenopathy or splenomegaly; chemotherapy and prednisone may temporarily help the anemia or thrombocytopenia.

Acute leukemias

Acute leukemias are known to appear after exposure to ionizing radiation and to some chemotherapeutic agents and viruses. There is sometimes a familial incidence, suggesting genetic predisposition (an identical twin of a case has a 20% likelihood of developing the disease). Lymphoblastic (ALL) and myeloblastic (AML) types occur, the former primarily in children. The two types can be distinguished on morphological and immunochemical grounds; surface markers for B or T cells may be found in some cases of ALL. The diagnosis is usually obvious since the patients are so sick; they have granulocytopenia with infections, thrombocytopenia with hemorrhages, and anemia. Bone marrow pain, splenomegaly, and adenopathy are common. Peripheral blood smears show an abundance of blast cells with few mature polys, but the total WBC count can be very high (>100,000) or below normal. Hyperuricemia is common and urate nephropathy can occur, but acute gout is rare. Cerebral hemorrhage is common, perhaps initiated by plugging of small vessels by rigid blast cells. Therapy, including chemotherapy, leukaphoresis, allopurinol (to prevent complications from hyperuricemia), transfusions, and radiotherapy, is relatively ineffective in adults, but a cure rate of over 60% is being achieved in children. About 30% of adults with ALL achieve a long-term remission, but the success rate with AML is much lower. Bone marrow transplantation is being tried increasingly often in these cases.

DISEASES CHARACTERIZED BY LYMPHADENOPATHY

Localized lymphadenopathy is usually due to infection. For example, enlarged cervical nodes are usually the result of streptococcal pharyngitis, infectious mononucleosis, or occasionally toxoplasmosis. Enlarged inguinal nodes are usually the result of skin infections or anogenital lesions, often venereal infections. Axillary nodes, on the other hand, if not obviously the result of an infection in the hand or arm, point to the need for careful breast examination for cancer. Mediastinal adenopathy can be the result of tuberculosis or fungal infection, but lymphomas commonly present in this fashion. More generalized adenopathy suggests sarcoidosis, immune reactions (such as a serum sickness-like drug reaction), secondary syphilis, or an early stage of AIDS. If the cause of an enlarged node is not clear, biopsy is indicated to investigate the possibility of a lymphoma.

LYMPHOMAS

Hodgkin's disease

Hodgkin's disease appears primarily in young adults, occasionally in the elderly or in children. It is often detected in asymptomatic patients when routine x-ray reveals mediastinal adenopathy. Fever, night sweats, and weight loss are common early complaints.

Hodgkin's disease is divided into four subgroups, as outlined in Table 1-9. All types show the characteristic binculeate Reed-Sternberg cells.

Staging of Hodgkin's disease is important as a guide to appropriate therapy. Staging is done on the basis of a history and physical, CBC, platelet count, urinalysis, standard screening blood chemistries, chest x-ray, CT scan (of chest, abdomen, and pelvis), and bone marrow aspirate and biopsy. Lymphangiogram and gallium scan may be needed. Rarely, an exploratory laparotomy and splenectomy are necessary for accurate staging.

Table 1-9. Hodgkin's Disease Subgroups

Type	Frequency	Typical case
Lymphocyte predominance	5–15%	Asymptomatic cervical node in young men
Nodular sclerosis	40–75%	Asymptomatic mediastinal mass, especially in young women
Mixed cellularity	20–40%	Young and middle-aged men
Lymphocyte depletion	5–15%	Fever, night sweats, weight loss in older patients (poorest prognosis)

Stage I: Single node region (I) or a single extralymphatic site (IE).

Stage II: Two or more nodal regions on the same side of the diaphragm (II) or a solitary extralymphatic site and one or more lymph node areas on the same side of the diaphragm (IIE).

Stage III: Nodes on both sides of diaphragm (III), accompanied by spleen involvement (IIIS) or a solitary extralymphatic organ site (IIIE) or both (IIISE).

Stage IV: Diffuse involvement of extralymphatic sites (with or without node enlargement).

Additional points in staging depend on symptoms (fever, sweats, weight loss of 10% or more): (A) if absent, (B) if present.

Therapy is often curative, and careful staging is therefore necessary to make the appropriate therapeutic decisions, such as the following:

Stage IA:	Radiotherapy.
Stage IIA, IIB, IIIA:	Consider exploratory laparatomy. Debulking may be needed with chemotherapy before radiotherapy.
Stage IIIB, IV:	Combination chemotherapy.

Non-Hodgkin's lymphoma

Non-Hodgkin's lymphoma includes a variety of disease processes. At one extreme is **Burkitt's lymphoma**, a rare, very malignant monoclonal B-cell neoplasm most common in a malarial belt in Africa and associated with Epstein-Barr virus. It has a specific chromosomal abnormality involving genes that code for immunoglobulins. In the usual cases of non-Hodgkin's lymphoma, malignant cells replace the normal lymph node cells diffusely or in a nodular (follicular) pattern. The predominant cell type varies, consisting of small well-differentiated lymphocytes, larger poorly differentiated cells with a cleaved nucleus, or large cells resembling histiocytes. A variety of classifications have been adopted based on these characteristics. Most of the lymphomas are of B-cell origin. Some consist of T-cells, and a few are of indeterminate origin.

Staging is similar to that for Hodgkin's disease, but these lymphomas are more likely to present with extranodal lesions (such as a gastric or CNS tumor) and are much less often in stage I or II at the time of diagnosis. Radiotherapy alone is the appropriate therapy for stage I or II, but the cure rate is less than 50%. Patients with stage II or IV are treated with chemotherapy, and cure rates vary with the cell type.

MULTIPLE MYELOMA

Neoplastic cells can arise at any stage of B-cell maturation. For example, a pre-B cell causes common ALL; an intermediate B-cell causes CLL; and a mature B cell causes hairy cell leukemia (HLL). If the neoplasm arises from more differentiated cells, such as mature plasma cells, the clinical result is multiple myeloma; plasmacytoid lymphocytes give rise to Waldenström's macroglobulinemia.

The basic structure of all immunoglobulins involves two heavy (H) polypeptide chains and two light (L) chains, linked by disulfide bonds. Both the H and L chains have constant regions of amino acid sequences and variable regions that determine antibody specificity. There are five subclasses based on differences in the constant regions of the H chains: IgG, IgM, IgA, IgD, and IgE. The L chains are either kappa or lambda, and each antibody molecule has two H chains and two L chains of the same type; hybrid molecules are not synthesized. About 10% of patients with CLL have monoclonal IgG or IgM spikes in their serum by electrophoresis, and such spikes are occasionally found with no underlying disease, especially in older people (benign monoclonal gammaopathy), but about 10% evolve into a full-blown disease, usually multiple myeloma.

Clinical features. In multiple myeloma, a malignant proliferation of plasma cells occurs and monoclonal immunoglobulin production is identifiable. Focal proliferation of plasma cells produces plasmacytomas, which can cause lytic bone lesions and pathological fractures, including collapse of vertebrae. Patients are usually older than 50 and often present with back pain, anemia, and an elevated ESR. They may also develop hypercalcemia, renal disease, or infections because of functional hypogammaglobulinemia and thus failure to make normal antibodies. Thus a variety of clinical presentations is encountered.

Diagnostic decisions. Diagnosis is confirmed by finding a monoclonal spike on serum protein electrophoresis, which is found to be a single type of immunoglobulin by counterimmunoelectrophoresis; concentrations of other immunoglobulins are decreased. Free light chains (kappa or lambda) are excreted in the urine in most patients (**Bence Jones proteinuria**). About 20% of patients have Bence Jones proteinuria without a detectable monoclonal protein spike in the serum (**light-chain disease**), and a rare patient has a nonsecretory myeloma without either light chains or a monoclonal spike. The diagnosis is established by serum electrophoresis, urinalysis (preferably using sulfosalicyclic acid to precipitate protein since Bence Jones proteins are soluble at 100°C and can be missed with older methods of detecting urine protein such as heat and acetic acid), and bone marrow aspiration demonstrating over 20% plasma cells (normal is <5%). Sheets of plasma cells or bizarre, multinucleate, malignant-looking plasma cells may be seen on occasion.

The prognosis depends on the tumor cell burden, with survival usually between 2 and 5 years. Therapy is not satisfactory, depending mainly on chemotherapy (alkylating agents and corticosteroids), local radiotherapy for a focal plasmocytoma or to minimize the likelihood of a pathological fracture. Renal failure can result from deposition of light chains in the renal tubules (Bence Jones nephropathy), calcium or urate nephropathy, or the development of amyloidosis. Use of radiopaque materials to perform an IVP can precipitate renal shutdown. Adequate hydration is important to minimize the likelihood of these causes of nephropathy. Pneumococcal vaccine is a valuable prophylactic measure, and early detection and therapy of all types of infections are important.

Waldenström's macroglobulinemia also affects older people primarily, most commonly presenting as anemia along with symptoms resulting from the hyperviscosity syndrome that is caused by the high levels of macroglobulin in the serum. This syndrome can cause nosebleeds, retinal hemorrhages, mental confusion, and CHF. Some IgMs are precipitated by cold, and patients with this type of macroglobulin may have Raynaud's phenomenon (painful blanching of fingers and toes on exposure to cold, followed by cyanosis). More serious arterial occlusions can occur, with leg ulcers and even gangrene. Skin lesions that on biopsy reveal a leukocytoclastic vasculitis can appear. Some IgMs are antibodies directed against a rare RBC antigen (I) and can cause hemolysis. Bone pain, hypercalcemia, splenomegaly, and lymphadenopathy can occur. Therapy may require chemotherapy with alkylating agents and plasmapheresis to remove the large amounts of macroglobulin; the average survival with therapy is only 3 years.

Heavy-chain disease is a rare variant of these syndromes. It clinically behaves more like a lymphoma, but the serum contains large amounts of the heavy chains of one of the immunoglobulins (IgG, IgM, or IgA). **Gamma-chain disease** (IgG heavy chains) is associated with lymphadenopathy and edema of the soft palate. **Alpha-chain disease** (IgA) ("Mediterranean lymphoma") is characterized by intestinal infiltration by lymphoma, and **mu-chain (IgM) disease** is associated with CLL.

BLEEDING DISORDERS

Primary hemostasis is the aspect of coagulation that involves the vessel wall. It consists of aggregation of platelets and adhesion to the damaged surface, forming the hemostatic plug, and participation of von Willebrand factor (Factor VIII), which mediates platelet adhesion and release of substances that augment aggregation. This aspect of clotting is assessed by the bleeding time, which is a general measure of the adequacy of platelet function. Secondary hemostasis is the formation of a clot based on fibrin formation at the site of the initial primary hemostatic plug. The surface membranes of the activated platelets catalyze the formation of thrombin utilizing the prothrombinase complex and calcium, which is released on activation of platelets. Thrombin catalyzes conversion of fibrinogen to fibrin, stimulates further platelet activation, which in turn catalyzes further thrombin formation, and activates Factor XIII, fibrin-stabilizing factor, which results in development of covalent cross-linkages in the fibrin, consolidating the fibrin clot. The third stage in coagulation is clot retraction, resulting from compression of the clot by contraction of the smooth muscle protein derived from platelets (thrombosthenin), producing a smaller, firmer clot.

Evaluation of a patient for a bleeding tendency is necessary during screening before surgery, when there is a history of prior episodes of spontaneous bleeding or excessive bleeding with trauma, as well as when there is active bleeding that is not responding to usual measures.

Diagnostic decisions. A family history of excessive bleeding suggests a form of hemophilia, which comprises 95% of congenital bleeding disorders. Acquired disorders are most often due to drugs, including aspirin and other NSAIDs, antibiotics, alcohol ingestion, liver disease, hematologic malignancy, or uremia, and these causes should be sought in the history. Physical examination includes seeking petechiae, ecchymoses, or hematomas in the skin, mucous membranes, and retina. Sites of increased pressure (e.g., buttocks) should be carefully inspected. Hepatomegaly and splenomegaly should be sought.

With platelet disorders, bleeding is usually from mucous membranes or into the skin (bleeding after dental extraction, epistaxis, and bruising) and is usually immediate and of short duration after minor trauma. Petechiae and purpura are common, and splenomegaly is often encountered in association with thrombocytopenia. In contrast, disorders of the coagulation mechanism tend to produce delayed and prolonged bleeding after trauma or surgery or bleeding into joints or muscles, and eccchymoses or hematomas are common.

Initial laboratory tests necessary in the evaluation of bleeding disorders include platelet count, bleeding time, PT, and PTT. If normal, a serious bleeding defect is very unlikely. If further workup is necessary, assay of individual coagulation factors, tests for anticoagulants, and tests of platelet function can be done and evidence of intravascular consumption of coagulation factors sought.

ABNORMALITIES IN BLOOD COAGULATION

The coagulation mechanism

The blood clotting mechanism is a complex system of enzymes and cofactors that interact to cause a firm fibrin clot to appear, stopping bleeding. The intrinsic pathway is initiated by the activation of Factor XII (Hageman factor) by an altered surface endothelium or by another negatively charged surface such as glass. Cofactors involved in activation of Factor XII include prekallikrein, high-molecular-weight kininogen, and Factor XI. Activated Factor XII, called Factor XIIa (in each instance mentioned below, the factor number with the additional notation "a" indicates its activated form), in turn activates prekallikrein to kallikrein and cleaves high-molecular-weight kininogen to bradykinin and also activates Factor XI to Factor XIa. Factor XIa, with Ca^{2+}, activates Factor IX to IXa, which binds to antihemophiliac factor (VIII). The combination activates Factor VII in the extrinsic coagulation pathway, activates Factor X to Xa, and also converts plasminogen to plasmin, thus it initiates fibrinolysis as well as promoting coagulation. Activation of Factor X takes place on the surface of the platelet or on vascular endothelium.

In the extrinsic pathway, factors released from damaged tissues activate Factor VII directly, and in the presence of Ca^{2+}, Factor VII activates X to Xa; tissue factor plus Ca^{2+} and Factor VIII also can activate Factor XI.

The third main component of the coagulation pathway is the prothrombinase complex, which is assembled on the surface of the platelet membrane and results in the formation of thrombin. This group of enzymes, all serine proteases, includes Factors II (prothrombin), VII, IX (Christmas factor), X, and protein C plus protein S, which has an unknown mechanism of action. Thrombin, in turn, acts on fibrinogen.

Fibrinogen is a high-molecular-weight soluble protein consisting of three pairs of polypeptide chains (A' [alpha], Ba, Gb). Thrombin cleaves small peptides of the A' chain of fibrinogen, forming fibrin I, which polymerizes end to end. Thrombin cleaves small peptides from the Ba chain, forming fibrin II, which polymerizes side to side. Cross-links are formed in fibrin II by the action of plasma glutaminase (Factor XIII). The result is an insoluble fibrin meshwork, the clot.

Thrombin also acts on platelets and the surface endothelium of vessels; its effect on platelets exposes binding sites for the

prothrombinase complex and causes release of substances that promote platelet aggregation, including thromboxane, Ca^{2+}, ADP, von Willebrand factor, fibronectin, and fibrospondin. The thrombin acts on surface endothelium by binding the protein thrombomodulin to activate protein C, which is a potent activator of Factors Va and VIIIa; protein C also activates fibrinolysis. Thrombin also causes endothelial cell contraction, which has a hemostatic effect, but it stimulates endothelial cells to make another prostaglandin, prostacyclin, which is vasodilating.

Finally, the fate of the fibrin clot determines the final stage of the coagulation mechanism. Fibrinolysis is stimulated by thrombin activating plasminogen and stimulating release of other plasminogen activators from vessel walls. Protein C, along with a substance that promotes its action, protein S, inhibits the procoagulant activity of Factors Va and VIIIa. Plasminogen activators result in the formation of plasmin, which is the enzyme that digests fibrin. Both plasminogen and its activators are bound to fibrin in the formation of the clot. Thus activation to plasmin occurs within the clot, providing maximum efficiency of fibrinolysis. Any serine proteases that reach the general circulation, as well as thrombin and plasmin, all are rapidly inactivated by inhibitors in the plasma, including alpha$_1$-antitrypsin, alpha$_2$-plasmin inhibitor, and alpha$_2$-macroglobulin. Antithrombin III also binds circulating serine proteases such as Factor Xa and thrombin; its action is augmented by heparin and complexes of antithrombin III, with proteases rapidly cleared by tissue macrophages (reticuloendothelial cells).

Key clinical points regarding deficiencies of clotting proteins

Most of the proteins involved in the coagulation mechanism are synthesized in the liver, and vitamin K is necessary for the synthesis of many of them (Factors II, VII, IX, and X, as well as proteins C and S). When a deficiency of vitamin K exists, these proteins lack the gamma-carboxyglutamate sites necessary for binding Ca^{2+}. Fibrinogen, Factor V, and the protease inhibitors are also produced in the liver; their levels are reduced in patients with liver disease. The site of synthesis of Factor VIII is uncertain; it is probably the liver. The vascular endothelium synthesizes von Willebrand factor and tissue plasminogen activator.

The proteins most likely to be deficient are those undergoing the most rapid turnover (the shortest half-lives). Among the prothrombin group, Factor VII has a half-life of only 3 to 5 hours, IX 24 hours and X 40 hours, whereas prothrombin has a half-life of 72 hours. In the fibrinogen group, Factor VIII has a half-life of 3 to 6 hours, V 15 to 30 hours, and fibrinogen (Factor I) and XIII over 72 hours.

Deficiency of the contact factors (Hageman or XII, or XI, etc.) does not produce a bleeding tendency; as a group they do not require Ca^{2+} or vitamin K. The prothrombin group all are vitamin K dependent, require Ca^{2+}, and are not consumed during clotting and thus are present in serum (except prothrombin itself). Fibrinogen is removed from plasma during clotting and is thus absent from serum. Fibrinogen is an "acute phase reactant"—that is, it increases in concentration during inflammation and is also increased in pregnancy and with use of oral contraceptives.

Diagnostic decisions. Workup for a possible coagulation disorder is indicated in anyone with a history of excessive bleeding after trauma, dental or other surgery, development of huge ecchymoses, severe nosebleeds, or bleeding into muscles or joints. A family history is also important. If only males are affected, hemophilia is likely, whereas others are autosomal recessive traits that are not sex linked. The workup of coagulation abnormalities should include the following:

1. PT, which measures activity of Factors II, VII, IX, and X.
2. Activated PTT (APTT), which measures activity of Factors VIII, IX, X, XI, and XII.
   (Both PT and APTT measure Factors I (fibrinogen), II (prothrombin), and V.)
3. Bleeding time, which is abnormal only if platelet function is affected. Among the plasma clotting disorders, bleeding time is abnormal only in von Willebrand's disease, which secondarily affects platelet function and prolongs bleeding time.
4. Test for stability of the fibrin clot (in 8 M urea) is indicated with a history of rebleeding after initial clotting or with delayed bleeding after trauma.
5. Finally, the ability of normal plasma to correct defects can be checked and assays for specific factors can be performed.

CLINICAL FEATURES OF SPECIFIC BLEEDING DISORDERS

Thrombocytopenia

Platelet counts below 100,000 signal concern for development of a bleeding disorder, but counts above 50,000 rarely are associated with bleeding. Counts below 20,000 are frequently associated with spontaneous bleeding, especially if the count is falling rapidly; bleeding occurs less often with stable counts, even if low.

Decreased platelet production occurs with many systemic infections, especially viral infections, as well as with deficiencies of folate or vitamin B_{12}, radiation, chemotherapy, or marrow replacement by tumor or fibrosis. Many drugs can inhibit platelet formation, including alcohol, thiazides, and anticonvulsants. Marrow aplasia causes thrombocytopenia. Increased platelet destruction can be caused by many drugs, including digitalis, quinidine, thiazides, phenothiazines, imipramine, gold salts, sulfonamides, and antibiotics (especially penicillin and cephalosporins). Some drugs produce an immune process in which drug-antibody or drug-plasma protein complex adsorbs passively to the surface of the platelet via the Fc receptor on the membrane, resulting in rapid removal of the platelets from the circulation (the "innocent bystander" concept). Other drugs adsorb to the surface of the platelet directly, producing a neoantigen that is the target of antibody. Tests for the role of drugs in these thrombocytopenic states are difficult to perform and unreliable. Stopping any suspected drug and substituting one of entirely different chemical composition is necessary.

Idiopathic thrombocytopenic purpura (ITP)

ITP is an autoimmune disease in which antiplatelet antibodies are produced. Platelet-associated IgG can be demonstrated. Platelet survival is short, and there are increased megakaryocytes in the marrow; the spleen is typically not enlarged. Acute ITP occurs most often in childhood, often appearing after an acute infection and resolving spontaneously after a few weeks. In adults, chronic ITP is more common, affecting women more often than men. Onset is usually insidious, and fewer than 10% of cases resolve spontaneously. Occasionally, an autoimmune hemolytic anemia is associated (**Evan's syndrome**). ITP can be associated with several underlying diseases, such as SLE, lymphoproliferative diseases, or AIDS, and can appear before other manifestations of those diseases. Pregnant women with ITP deliver thrombocytopenic infants, since the antibody (usually an IgG_1 or IgG_3) can cross the placenta.

Diagnostic decisions. The diagnosis of ITP is based on the low platelet count, often with large platelets seen in the circulation, increased megakaryocytes in the marrow, absence of splenomegaly, and the absence of a history of drug ingestion or other cause of thrombocytopenia. Platelets that are present function normally when tested. Tests of platelet survival with ^{51}Cr-labeled autologous platelets show marked shortening of survival but are too expensive for routine use.

Therapeutic decisions. Treatment of ITP involves stopping any drugs that are suspected and avoiding aspirin or NSAIDs (acetaminophen is safe). If thrombocytopenia is severe, corticosteroids are given (80 to 120 mg of prednisone per day). In acute ITP of childhood, the steroids can be tapered slowly and no other therapy is usually needed. In chronic ITP, 2 to 3 months of steroid therapy can be tried. If a normal platelet count is achieved, the dose can be tapered slowly. Therapy is successful in about 70% of cases. If steroids are unsuccessful or relapse occurs, splenectomy can be considered. In some cases, steroids need to be continued after splenectomy. Immunosuppressive drugs such as vincristine may be tried, and IV gamma-globulin preparations are receiving increasing use, especially before surgery.

Other platelet abnormalities

Benign, transient thrombocytopenia is an acute but transient thrombocytopenia that can occur a few days after a transfusion in patients who have developed sensitization to a common platelet antigen (PL^AI) lacking in some people as a result of previous transfusion or pregnancy.

Consumptive coagulopathy is a syndrome in which thrombocytopenia occurs. It occurs in **thrombotic thrombocytopenic purpura (TTP)** and the **hemolytic uremic syndrome**. Both thrombosis and hemorrhage may occur. It can occur with vascular malformations such as cavernous hemangioma (the Kasabach-Merritt syndrome), which can remove platelets from the circulation. A Coombs'-negative microangiopathic hemolytic anemia is usually present in these syndromes, with shistocytes, helmet cells, and other abnormal RBC forms seen on smear. Increased reticulocytes, neurological findings, and often renal failure may develop. Corticosteroids and plasmapheresis are being tried as therapy. (See "Disseminated intravascular coagulation," below.)

Aspirin and platelet function. Aspirin and other NSAIDs inhibit the cyclooxygenase that synthesizes prostaglandins from arachidonic acid. Thromboxane A_2, the main product of this enzyme in platelets, mediates the normal platelet release reaction initiated by ADP, epinephrine, or collagen. Impaired platelet aggregation results, and the bleeding time is moderately prolonged. This effect of aspirin lasts for the life of the platelet, since the inhibition is caused by permanent acetylation of the enzyme; platelets do not possess a nucleus and therefore cannot synthesize protein and replace the enzyme. The effect of other NSAIDs is reversible, and platelet function is restored as soon as the drug is cleared from the blood. Thrombin-induced platelet activation is not affected by these agents, and thus the hemorrhagic tendency is minimized; but when a second defect exists, such as hemophilia, thrombocytopenia, or anticoagulant therapy, serious bleeding can develop following ingestion of aspirin. Gastric erosions are frequently caused by aspirin, and they often bleed profusely. In contrast, acetaminophen and nonaspirin salicylates do not inhibit platelet function and do not cause gastric erosions.

Hemophilia A

Although a positive family history with only males affected is usual, the gene for Factor VIII production has a high rate of spontaneous mutation and about 30% of cases have no family history. Carrier mothers of patients have one normal X chromosome and have about 50% of normal levels of Factor VIII; the carrier state can thus be identified, and prenatal diagnosis of affected fetuses is now possible.

Symptoms usually appear in infancy, with traumatic and spontaneous bleeding. With increasing age and physical activity, hemorrhages into joints become common and repeated hemarthroses can lead to joint deformities. Life-threatening internal hemorrhages can occur with internal trauma. Milder abnormalities occur (with about 5% of normal levels of Factor VIII), and hemorrhage appears only with severe trauma or with surgery in such cases.

Diagnostic decisions. Evaluation of patients with hemophilia A shows a normal bleeding time and PT but a markedly prolonged APTT, which is corrected by adding normal plasma. Assay of Factor VIII specifically reveals markedly decreased activity, but immunologic assay can be normal since in some families the genetic abnormality causes the synthesis of a dysfunctional but antigenically normal molecule.

Therapeutic decisions. Therapy consists of replacement of Factor VIII with concentrates. A program of regular IV injections at home at intervals determined by the frequency and severity of bleeding episodes can be designed, but the risk of hepatitis and AIDS has made use of replacement therapy more judicious. It should definitely be given for life-threatening bleeding or severe recurrent joint bleeding. When Factor VIII produced by recombinant DNA becomes available, use can again become more liberal. Since Factor VIII has a half-life of only 8 to 12 hours, frequent replacement may be needed during a severe bleeding episode; some patients develop inhibitors. Cryoprecipitate is adequate for milder episodes of bleeding, and epsilon-aminocaproic acid (EACA) decreases the rate of fibrinolysis, increasing the effectiveness of any clot formation that occurs. Joint bleeding should be treated with immobilization and ice packs. Aspirin should be avoided, but acetaminophen and narcotics, especially codeine, are safe and useful.

Von Willebrand's disease

A relatively common inherited coagulation disorder, von Willebrand's disease (VWD) affects both sexes and can be inherited as a codominant recessive trait. Platelet function becomes abnormal in this disease because of the absence of von Willebrand factor (VWF) or low factor VIII activity, since the complex of Factor VIII:VWF is necessary to obtain the action lacking in this disease. In VWD, the VWF is missing or not functional or Factor VIII activity can be mildly or markedly depressed. As a result, the APTT is prolonged, and the bleeding time is also long since platelet function is abnormal. Assays of VWF and Factor VIII show varying degrees and types of abnormalities.

The clinical manifestations of VWD vary considerably, in different affected families as well as at different times in an individual patient. The most common manifestations are ecchymoses and mucosal bleeding, such as epistaxis, GI bleeding, and menorrhagia. Hemarthoses occur in severely affected patients. Treatment of severe bleeding requires plasma or cryoprecipitate. In milder cases, infusion of desmopressin, a form of vasopressin, can raise VWF activity sufficiently to stop bleeding; this agent can be used before dental surgery. VWD usually improves during pregnancy, as the fetus replaces missing factors. Aspirin should be avoided by these patients.

Other inherited coagulation disorders

Hageman factor (XII) deficiency is usually asymptomatic, but in vitro clotting is abnormal; clotting time and APTT are prolonged. **Hemophilia B (Christmas disease)** is due to deficiency of Factor IX and produces severe bleeding problems; both boys and girls are affected. The PT is normal; APTT is prolonged and corrected by normal plasma but not barium-absorbed plasma ($BaSO_4$ absorbs vitamin K-dependent factors from the plasma, since they bind to calcium and the barium substitutes but form insoluble complexes). Fresh-frozen plasma contains the missing factor and corrects the abnormality in vitro as well as therapeutically.

Vitamin K deficiency

The most important acquired clotting disorder is vitamin K deficiency, which causes decreases in the synthesis of the factors in the prothrombin complex (Factors VII, IX, X, and proteins C and S). All have calcium-binding sites, and vitamin K is required for posttranslational gamma-carboxylation of the glutamyl residues at the amino terminal regions of the precursors of these clotting factors. Ca^{2+} is required for binding of these factors to the serine proteases on the surface of platelets. The factor with the shortest half-life, VII, is the first to decrease in vitamin K deficiency or following therapeutic administration of vitamin K antagonists such as coumarin; the next factors to decrease are Factors IX, X, and prothrombin.

Vitamin K is fat soluble but is not stored in significant quantities in the body. It is found in leafy green vegetables; deficiency occurs in clinical states with malabsorption of fat (biliary tract disease, sprue syndromes, regional enteritis), after prolonged use of oral antibiotics that alter the gut flora (which are a source of a significant amount of the vitamin K needed), as well as in newborn infants. Coumarin anticoagulants competitively inhibit the effects of vitamin K on gamma-decarboxylation of the factors in the prothrombin complex. As a result, there is prolongation of the PT. The goal of this type of anticoagulant therapy is a PT 1.5 to 2 times normal. Excessive effect can be reversed within hours by fresh-frozen plasma or prothrombin concentrates or within minutes by Factor IX concentrates.

Liver disease causes decreased synthesis of Factors V, XII, XI, fibrinogen, and plasminogen. Since most of the bleeding problems result from the low level of vitamin K-dependent factors, administration of that vitamin parenterally can correct the problem in many patients. If necessary, fresh-frozen plasma can be used.

Uremia is associated with a hemorrhagic diathesis manifested mainly as mucosal and skin bleeding. The causes include thrombocytopenia as a result of depressed bone marrow function or use of immunosuppressant drugs, platelet dysfunction, and loss of plasma proteins in the urine in patients with nephrotic syndrome (Factor IX deficiency is the main problem). Use of heparin during hemodialysis can add to the bleeding tendency.

Disseminated intravascular coagulation

DIC results from consumption of coagulation factors as a result of the activation of the clotting process in circulating plasma. It is associated with sepsis, shock, toxins, and malignancies, as well as **TTP** and the **hemolytic uremic sydrome**. Both thrombosis and hemorrhage may occur. Thrombocytopenia is usual. It develops from the release of procoagulant factors into the general circulation, such as occurs with crush injuries, hemolytic transfusion reactions, malignancies, burns, snakebite, amniotic fluid emboli, abruptio placentae, etc. Microthrombi develop in the circulation, activating fibrinolysis; the circulating plasmin depletes the levels of Factors V and VII as well as fibrinogen. The degradation products of fibrinogen and fibrin are circulating anticoagulants, delaying fibrin polymerization and impairing platelet function and leading to the tendency to hemorrhage.

Diagnostic decisions. Diagnosis is based on finding low levels of platelets and coagulation factors (fibrinogen, Factors V and VIII) and the presence of split products derived from fibrin in the plasma. The PT and APTT may be normal. A Coombs'-negative microangiopathic hemolytic anemia is usually present in these syndromes, with schistocytes, helmet cells, and other abnormal RBC forms. Reticulocyte levels are increased. Localized DIC can occur in the liver in advanced cirrhosis or in the kidney, with malignant hypertension.

Therapeutic decisions. Therapy is directed at correcting the underlying disease, replacing clotting factors with fresh-frozen plasma, cryoprecipitate, fibrinogen, and platelets if necessary. Heparin can be useful if there are problems of thromboses (but no CNS bleeding). In some cases, such as with TTP, corticosteroids and plasmapheresis are being tried as therapy.

ENDOCRINOLOGIC AND METABOLIC DISEASES

DISEASES OF THE HYPOTHALAMUS AND PITUITARY

The posterior lobe of the pituitary is actually neural tissue, and its hormones are analogous to neurotransmitters; stimulation comes directly from the hypothalamus via neural pathways. The anterior lobe is regulated by peptide and monoamine products of the hypothalamus conveyed by the hypothalamic-hypophyseal portal venous system directly to the pituitary. Hypothalamic hormones include peptides that vary from 3 to 40 amino acids in length, such as releasing factors for growth hormone (GRF), corticotrophin (CRF), gonadotrophin (GnRF), and thyrotropin (TRF), as well as an inhibitory factor for growth hormone (GH) secretion, somatostatin. Several of these neurohypophyseal hormones are found in the gut and have other functions. The hypothalamus also secretes the biogenic amines dopamine and serotonin.

Anterior pituitary hormones can be divided into three classes:

1. Corticotropin and related peptides. These hormones are secreted as a single 39-amino-acid peptide known as proopiomelanocortin, which includes adrenocorticotropic hormone (ACTH), beta-endorphin, beta-lipotropin, and melanocyte-stimulating hormone. (The last mentioned explains the pigmentation seen in Addison's disease due to adrenal destruction in which there is increased secretion of ACTH and its related hormones by the pituitary.)
2. Glycoprotein hormones, including thyroid-stimulating hormone (TSH), follicle-stimulating hormone (FSH), and luteinizing hormone (LH), which have a common alpha subunit but differing beta subunits.
3. Somatomammotropins, including GH and prolactin; they are not tropic hormones that affect function of other endocrine glands like the other anterior pituitary hormones. They affect peripheral target organs directly, as do the hormones secreted by other endocrine glands.

Diagnostic decisions. There are radioimmunoassays for these peptide hormones and stimulatory procedures to induce their secretion. Failure of such stimulation gives more convincing evidence of deficiency than basal levels, which are often quite low. For example, (1) hypoglycemia induced by insulin stimulates ACTH release; dexamethasone suppresses it in normals. (2) The TSH response to TRH stimulation and the FSH and LH response to GnRF stimulation are useful tests. (3) Prolactin secretory reserve can be evaluated by administration of dopamine antagonists such as metoclopramide or inhibitors of dopaminergic transmission, such as chlorpromazine. (4) GH secretion responds to induced hypoglycemia, or to dopamine orally, or an IV infusion of arginine.

Hypopituitarism

Hypopituitarism results from tumors such as craniopharyngiomas or pituitary tumors, postpartum necrosis (Sheehan's syndrome), hemorrhagic infarction, head irradiation or trauma, or destruction by other diseases such as histiocytosis X or tuberculosis. In children, the result is short stature and delayed puberty. Hypoadrenalism (Addison's disease) can occur, but hyperpigmentation does not occur in these cases and sodium depletion is rare (since aldosterone secretion is maintained, in contrast to destructive disease of the adrenal glands, which causes loss of all adrenal hormones). Hyponatremia can occur, since cortisol deficiency impairs water excretion. Hypothyroidism also results, but true myxedema is rare; hypothermia, hypotension, and hypoglycemia may occur.

Diagnostic decisions. The diagnosis requires ruling out multiple glandular deficiencies due to autoimmune destruction (Schmidt's syndrome), which would give the same glandular deficiencies but would be associated with *increased* levels of pituitary hormones. The finding of increased levels of prolactin, which normally is under tonic inhibition by the hypothalamus, would point to the lesion being in the hypothalamus or pituitary stalk.

Therapeutic decisions. Therapy involves replacement of deficient hormones, but it is important to begin with glucocorticoid hormone replacement and then gradually replace thyroxin, since the thyroid hormone increases turnover of glucocorticoids and acute adrenal insufficiency would result.

Pituitary adenomas

Hypersecretion of prolactin, GH, and ACTH are the most common results of hyperfunction of the pituitary. The syndromes that result are **amenorrhea-galactorrhea, acromegaly,** and **Cushing's disease.** Pituitary tumors are slow growing. Endocrine manifestations may be preceded by neurological dysfunction, especially headache with bitemporal hemianopia (usually beginning as upper quadrants of the visual fields), which results from growth of the tumor out of the sella turcica and invading the overlying optic chiasm. Extension into a nearby cavernous sinus can cause extraocular nerve palsies. A large sella is usually seen on x-ray, but such enlargement can occur without a tumor. In such instances, the empty sella syndrome, the pituitary gland is displaced because of a defect in the meningeal diaphragm lying above it, allowing CSF to enter, but endocrine function is normal.

Galactorrhea and amenorrhea

Hyperprolactinemia results from a loss of inhibitory control of the hypothalamus. Dopamine is probably the main neurotransmitter of this inhibitory mechanism. Drugs that block dopaminergic transmission, such as phenothiazines, can cause increased prolactin secretion. Other drugs known to have this effect are alpha-methyldopa, reserpine, opiates, and metoclopramide. Damage or interruption of the pituitary stalk, as occurs with tumors such as craniopharyngomas, can also result in excessive prolactin secretion. In women, hyperprolactinemia results in persistent lactation and amenorrhea. Men may also develop galactorrhea, but impotence and loss of libido are more common. When drug effect can be ruled out, a pituitary tumor (prolactinoma) is usually present; these tumors used to be called chromophobe adenomas.

Diagnostic decisions. Diagnosis is based on demonstrating markedly elevated levels of prolactin (> 150 ng/100 ml; normal < 20), but sometimes it may be necessary to test multiple samples because of secretion of the hormone in intermittent bursts. Treatment is primarily surgical, although pituitary irradiation can be helpful; bromocriptine, a dopamine agonist, can control symptoms.

Gigantism and acromegaly

Excessive secretion of GH before puberty results in **gigantism**; after epiphyseal closure it results in **acromegaly.** Findings of acromegaly include overgrowth of distal (acral) areas, including thickening of the skin; enlargement of facial features, which become coarse; frontal bossing; thickening of the tongue; and development of a deep, resonant voice because of remodeling of the nasopharynx. These patients all look similar. Fatigue, hypertension, cardiomegaly, and enlargement of other organs are also common. Headache is very frequent, and an enlarged sella turcica can usually be seen on x-ray. The tumor may extend into the optic chiasm above the sella, causing visual field defects. Impaired glucose tolerance, amenorrhea or impotence, and hyperinsulinemia are also found frequently. Frank diabetes may develop if the pancreas is unable to respond to the increased insulin need caused by the effects of GH on carbohydrate metabolism. Renal effects include increased GFR and increased tubular reabsorption of phosphate, resulting in hyperphosphatemia, which is a characteristic finding.

Diagnostic decisions. The diagnosis is established by finding elevated plasma GH levels (normal up to 5 ng/ml) that cannot be suppressed by administration of glucose. Paradoxically, administration of dopamine, which normally stimulates GH release, suppresses it in these patients.

Therapy is primarily surgical, although pituitary irradiation may be useful.

Diabetes insipidus

Axons that originate in the supraoptic and paraventricular nuclei of the hypothalamus and extend into the posterior lobe of the pituitary synthesize and secrete two peptide hormones, vasopressin and oxytocin and their carrier proteins, neurophysins. Oxytocin plays a role in release of breast milk and uterine contraction during labor. Arginine vasopressin (antidiuretic hormone [ADH]) release occurs primarily in response to increases in body osmolality. The normal plasma osmolality is about 285 mOsm/kg of body water; an increase of 1% (3 mOsm/kg), which will occur after 10 to 12 hours of water deprivation, stimulates release of ADH. Extracellular fluid volume, perceived by high-pressure baroreceptors in the aorta and low-pressure volume receptors in the left atrium, also control ADH release. Thus hypotension or decreased vascular volume will stimulate secretion of ADH and will predominate if there is a diversion of the two stimuli (i.e., hypovolemia will stimulate ADH release even in the presence of hypo-osmolality.) ADH increases the permeability of the collecting ducts and tubules in the kidney to water and urea, working via the cyclic AMP system. (This process is modulated by a number of other factors, including calcium, prostaglandins, corticosteroids, and adrenergic agents.)

Diabetes insipidus can result from head trauma, surgical hypophysectomy, granulomatous or neoplastic disease affecting the posterior pituitary, anoxic brain damage, or meningoencephalitis. Often no cause is evident. An inherited defect in renal tubular response to ADH (nephrogenic diabetes insipidus) affects males predominantly, but acquired disorders of renal function can cause a similar disorder, including lithium therapy, hypokalemia, and hypercalcemia. Diabetes insipidus causes polydipsia and polyuria, with urine volumes exceeding 3 L/day and water intake exceeding 5 L/day. Urine specific gravity is fixed at 1.010 and osmolality at under 300 mOsm/kg.

Diagnostic decisions. The diagnosis requires ruling out psychogenic polydipsia. Demonstration of serum hyperosmolality (>285) rules out a psychogenic cause, but a water deprivation test may be necessary. Table 1-10 summarizes the diagnosis of the cause of diabetes insipidus by evaluating plasma and urine osmolality after dehydration and the effect of an injection of ADH.

Treatment with chlorpropamide, which increases the renal effect of ADH, can be successful with partial deficiency states, but pitressin tannate in oil IM or a synthetic analogue by nasal insufflation every 12 to 24 hours may be necessary. Hypoglycemia with chlorpropamide may be a problem. Therapy is less effective for nephrogenic diabetes insipidus, but salt restriction to reduce the solute load and use of thiazide diuretics can help.

DISEASES OF THE THYROID

Pathophysiology of the thyroid and the basis of thyroid function tests

The thyroid gland synthesizes two hormones, thyroxine (T_4) and triiodothyronine (T_3). Peripherally, T_3 is converted to T_4. The activity of the thyroid gland can be estimated by measuring the uptake of iodine, which is done by measuring the level of **radioactive iodine (RAI)** found by counting over the gland after plateau levels are achieved (usually 24 hours after administration). Normal levels are generally 5 to 30% of the administered RAI, but this level can be lower if there has been excessive intake of iodine, resulting in a pool of iodide in the gland above the normal 10,000 μg, thus diluting the tracer and giving misleadingly low values. An elevated level is a useful indication of hyperfunction of the thyroid gland, but the low limit of normal makes the test of little value in diagnosing hypothyroidism. A low level in the face of a hypermetabolic state would be an indicator of factitious hyperthyroidism, such as occurs following ingestion of large amounts of iodine or thyroid hormone. Low levels also occur during the recovery phase of acute thyroiditis. When the RAI uptake test is done, the **scan over the thyroid** can be useful to determine if there is homogeneous uptake, increased uptake over a hot nodule, or the irregular uptake characteristic of Hashimoto's thyroiditis. **Ultrasonographic** scanning of the thyroid is useful to delineate the size and distribution of nodules and their consistency (i.e., whether or not a nodule is cystic). **Fine-needle aspiration biopsy** is a low-risk procedure done routinely to evaluate a thyroid nodule.

The thyroid suppression test, performed by administration of exogenous thyroid hormone followed by RAI, normally shows a decrease in uptake to less than half control values. Failure to suppress occurs in patients with hyperthyroidism or

with autonomous secretion of TSH. A normal suppression test is incompatible with the presence of hypothyroidism.

Most of the T_4 and T_3 in the plasma is bound to thyronine-binding blogulin (TBG), but the metabolically active fraction is the free hormone. Certain clinical states can give rise to an increase in TBG, and thus of total T_4, but do not affect free T_4 and thus do not cause a hypermetabolic state. Estrogen increases the TBG, and thus it may be elevated in patients on oral contraceptives or during pregnancy. Acute hepatitis, acute intermittent porphyria, and certain drugs (including clofibrate, 5-fluorouracil, heroin, and methadone) also raise the TBG. On the other hand, TBG levels can be low and total T_4 low (but no hypothyroidism exist) in patients with any severe illness, with advanced liver diseases (especially cirrhosis), with protein loss (e.g., nephrotic syndrome), or in patients taking anabolic steroids (e.g., androgens) or corticosteroids (e.g., prednisone).

Thyroxine is made only in the thyroid, whereas T_3 is made in the thyroid and also is formed by degradation of T_4 in peripheral tissues. The pathway of deiodination can be disturbed by acute illness of any type, resulting in misleadingly high levels of T_4 and low levels of T_3 in the blood. Thyroid function should not be evaluated until after recovery from an acute illness. The increased T_4 level in acute illnesses, including psychiatric illness, must be differentiated from true hyperfunction of the thyroid gland.

Diagnostic decisions. Measurement of serum total T_4 (normal 5 to 11 μg/100 ml) and free T_4 (1.5 to 3.5 μg/100 ml) is the best way of screening for thyroid dysfunction. Indirect methods of determining free T_4 give a "free T_4 index," which is normally 0.5 to 1.5. A parallel increase or decrease in T_4 can support a diagnosis of hyper- or hypothyroidism in the absence of an acute illness. Resin T_3 uptake (RT_3U), an older test done to estimate available TBG, is another means of estimating free T_4 and thus gives similar findings. If thyrotoxicosis is suspected but total and free T_4 are normal, total and free T_3 levels should be determined since in 5 to 10% of cases "T_3 toxicosis" can be the mechanism of the hyperthyroidism.

An elevated serum level of thyrotropin (TSH) is a useful indicator of hypofunction of the thyroid gland, since feedback inhibition of the pituitary gland is not occurring; the normal level is below 5 mU/ml. Subnormal pituitary function can be detected by the thyrotropin releasing hormone (TRH) test. After TRH injection, TSH levels rise to a peak in about 20 to 45 minutes. An increased response occurs in patients with hypothyroidism of thyroid origin, whereas in the presence of thyrotoxicosis a decreased response would be expected.

Radioimmunoassay of the thyroid-stimulating immunoglobulin (TSI, formerly called long-acting thyroid stimulator, or LATS) is very useful in diagnosing Grave's disease, since it is almost always elevated in this form of hyperthyroidism. Low values can occur in thyroiditis with hyperthyroidism.

Hyperthyroidism

The most common form of hyperthyroidism is **Graves' disease.** The usual symptoms are manifestations of the hypermetabolic state, such as heat intolerance, sweating, weight loss despite increased appetite, plus nervousness and signs of increased sympathetic tone, such as a fine tremor, tachycardia, and palpitations. Mental changes are frequent, including anxiety, irritability, restlessness, emotional lability, forgetful-

Table 1-10. Diagnosis of Diabetes Insipidus (DI)

	Urine osmolality	
	Maximum	Effect of ADH
Psychogenic DI	= plasma	Increases
True DI	> plasma	Increases
Nephrogenic DI	< plasma	No change

ness, and insomnia. On examination, an enlarged thyroid gland can usually be felt, and a bruit may be heard over it. The enhanced sympathetic tone causes a stare (widening of the palpebral fissure) and failure of the upper lid to follow the globe during downward eye movement (lid lag). Exophthalmos (proptosis) is common, and skin changes are frequent, including warmth, sweatiness, pigment changes, and sometimes a brawny edema over the shins (pretibial myxedema). Skeletal muscle weakness can occur and even dominate the picture, as can myocardiopathy with CHF.

In the elderly, classic features of hyperthyroidism may be lacking; an apathetic appearance can be the dominant feature, often accompanied by atrial fibrillation and frequently by heart failure. It is wise to screen elderly patients with new onset of CHF for hyperthyroidism if a clear etiology is not apparent, and especially if atrial fibrillation is present.

Therapeutic decisions.   Therapy of hyperthyroidism usually begins with antithyroid drugs, such as **propylthiouracil** (PTU); in pregnancy and childhood, these should be the only agents used. Permanent remission can be produced in about 30% of patients; occasionally hypothyroidism results. **RAI**, usually the definitive therapy in adults, is given after the hyperthyroidism is controlled with antithyroid agents such as PTU. Symptoms of sympathetic overactivity can be controlled with beta-blockers. **Surgery** is reserved for children whose disease cannot be controlled with antithyroid drugs and young adults with extremely large glands. Complications of surgery include recurrent laryngeal nerve injury with vocal cord paralysis and hypoparathyroidism. Hypothyroidism eventually develops in a majority of patients treated for hyperthyroidism (70% over 10 years), regardless of the method of treatment, and patients should be monitored for its development since it is usually insidious and can be missed for long periods.

In some untreated patients, **thyrotoxic crisis** can develop with high fever, disproportionate tachycardia, mental confusion, jaundice, shock, and coma. A cooling blanket (not aspirin), treatment of hypotension with fluid plus pressor agents, nutritional support, glucocorticoids, propranolol, and PTU are usually needed. Iodide is also helpful and can be given after thyroid metabolism is blocked with PTU.

Hypothyroidism

Hypothyroidism is usually due to a defect in hormone production by the thyroid gland, but pituitary or hypothalamic disease can cause secondary hypothyroidism. Autoimmune disease, such as Hashimoto's thyroiditis, is a common cause, as is treatment of preexisting hyperthyroidism. Congenital abnormalities in iodine metabolism can cause hypothyroidism in utero or in early childhood (cretinism), with failure of normal physical and mental development. Hypothyroidism appearing in later childhood can cause growth retardation and delayed puberty. In adults, hypothyroidism is less obvious and often is undetected for years.

Clinical picture.   The most common manifestations of hypothyroidism are lethargy, fatigue, cold intolerance, dry and scaly skin, hair loss, facial puffiness, deep and hoarse voice, and an enlarged tongue. Deep tendon reflexes show a characteristic delayed relaxation phase (hang-up sign). Cardiac changes, including a small pericardial effusion, myocardial changes

leading to arrhythmias, and CHF are common if the hypothyroidism is untreated. Mental changes occur and can progress from mild confusion and slow thinking and speech to severe dementia and myxedema coma. Myxedema is one of the causes of reversible psychopathology occasionally found in patients languishing in mental hospitals.

Myxedema is characterized by thickening of the skin and other tissues because of increased connective tissue proteoglycan concentration; there is increased water binding by these compounds. Excess carotene concentration in the blood gives the skin a yellowish tinge.

Diagnostic decisions.   Characteristic laboratory findings include a low total serum T_4 and free T_4. TSH is usually very high unless the hypothyroidism is due to pituitary or hypothalamic disease. If the TSH level is borderline, an exaggerated TSH response to TRH can be a useful indicator of the existence of hypothyroidism. Other laboratory abnormalities include a low serum sodium, resulting from relative excess of ADH, anemia, bradycardia, and low-voltage and conduction abnormalities on ECG. Chronic hypoventilation because of muscle weakness can result in hypoxemia and hypercapnia.

Therapeutic decisions.   Hypothyroidism should be treated with synthetic preparations of thyroxine. A full replacement dose in adults usually ranges between 100 and 150 μg/day, but it is wise to start with much lower doses, such as 25 μg/day, increasing by 25μg/day every 2 weeks, especially in elderly patients, for fear of precipitating adrenal insufficiency. However, myxedema coma is a medical emergency, and 300 to 500 μg of thyroxine should be given IV followed by 100 μg/day for 5 days. Treatment of any underlying infection, ventilatory support, and adrenal hormone replacement therapy are usually necessary. Mental function should begin to improve in 1 to 2 days if the diagnosis is correct.

Goiter

Goiter is an enlargement of the thyroid gland; the most common cause is iodine deficiency (endemic goiter), now virtually eliminated in the United States by the addition of iodine to commercial table salt. In afflicted persons, enlargement of the gland results from excess TSH stimulation in an attempt to increase the production of thyroid hormone; most patients with goiter remain euthyroid, but hypo- and hyperfunction can occur.

Congenital defects in iodine metabolism can lead to enlargement of the gland (sporadic goiter), as can various goitrogens in food, such as cabbage or turnips, which can interfere with iodine metabolism. Goiters can be smooth and uniform in consistency or multinodular. Large goiters can compress neighboring structures and cause symptoms. Dysphagia results from compression of the esophagus, hoarseness from compression of the recurrent laryngeal nerve, or dyspnea from compression of the trachea. An infiltrating malignant tumor of the thyroid can cause similar symptoms.

Therapy with T_4 can decrease a goiter by suppressing TSH secretion, but if the gland is functioning autonomously, hyperthyroidism can result. Careful monitoring of serum T_4 is therefore important. Surgery may be necessary for cosmetic reasons, for goiters that fail to suppress, or for those that cause pressure symptoms.

Solitary nodules of the thyroid are usually benign, although carcinoma is frequent among patients who have had prior irradiation of the neck, especially if during childhood. Scanning with RAI can reveal whether a nodule is functioning. A nodule that takes up more iodine than the rest of the gland is a "warm" or "hot" nodule; such nodules are usually benign. Most nodules are "cold," however, and a biopsy with a fine needle is advisable since about 5% are malignant. A growing nodule should definitely be biopsied. Malignant tumors usually are solid by ultrasonographic scanning. If no spread to lymph nodes or distant metastases are present, carcinomas of the thyroid usually can be resected, and ablative therapy with ^{131}I is often helpful. **Medullary carcinoma** of the thyroid is often familial and is a component of the multiple endocrine neoplasia syndrome. It arises from the parafollicular cells ("C cells"), which produce calcitonin.

Nodular goiters can exist for long periods and eventually cause thyrotoxicosis. Elderly patients with nodular goiters should be screened for hyperthyroidism whenever any unexplained illness develops.

Acute thyroiditis

Acute thyroiditis (de Quervain's thyroiditis) can cause fever and painful, tender enlargement of the gland. During the active phase, serum T_4 levels are usually elevated and RAI uptake depressed. Antithyroid antibodies are rarely detectable. Hyperthyroidism is usually transient and can be treated adequately with beta-blockers; hypothyroidism can result and require replacement therapy. Chronic lymphocytic thyroiditis (**Hashimoto's thyroiditis**) is much more common and is autoimmune; antithyroid antibodies are usually detectable. It commonly evolves into hypothyroidism.

Thyroiditis can give rise to transient hyperthyroidism, which can be controlled with antithyroid drugs and beta-blockers. ^{131}I is not indicated.

DISEASES OF THE ADRENAL GLAND

The adrenals are each actually two endocrine glands—the cortex, which synthesizes several hormones, and the medulla, which secretes catecholamines. In the cortex, the outer zone, the zona glomerulosa, secretes potent mineralocorticoid hormones and the inner zones, the fasciculata and reticularis, secrete glucocorticoids and small quantities of the sex steroids estrogens and androgens. The adrenals are not the primary source of catecholamines, which are neurotransmitters and are also secreted by neural tissue.

The secretion of hormones by the cortex is primarily under the control of the hypothalamicopituitary axis, which is under feedback influence from the circulating level of adrenocorticosteroid hormones, but control of aldosterone secretion is primarily in response to stimuli that originate in the kidney (the renin-angiotensin system). Reduced renal perfusion pressure or effective circulating blood volume causes renin to be released from the juxtaglomerular cells in the kidney. Renin is an enzyme that degrades its circulating substrate, an alpha$_2$-globulin that arises in the liver, liberating the decapeptide angiotensin I. Another enzyme, ACE, which is normally present in the plasma, converts angiotensin I to angiotensin II,

which stimulates the zona glomerulosa cells of the adrenal to release aldosterone. Aldosterone affects the function of renal tubular epithelial cells, increasing the transepithelial transport of sodium from lumen to plasma, increasing extracellular sodium and water and reducing the stimulus to renin secretion. Other stimuli to aldosterone secretion exist. An increase in plasma potassium stimulates secretion, and hypokalemia suppresses it. There is also evidence for a stimulatory effect of ACTH on aldosterone secretion.

Adrenocortical hypofunction

Destruction of the adrenal gland in the past was usually due to tuberculosis; metastatic carcinoma (particularly from the lung), other granulomatous diseases such as fungus infections, and adrenal hemorrhage in patients receiving anticoagulants also can cause adrenal destruction, but the most common cause in the United States today is autoimmune injury. Although infections and tumors usually destroy the entire adrenal gland, cortex and medulla, autoimmune processes usually affect only the cortex but often affect other endocrine organs simultaneously, such as the thyroid, gonads, and pancreatic islet cells, causing multiple endocrine deficiency states.

The clinical manifestations of adrenocortical deficiency (**Addison's disease**) are primarily due to cortisol deficiency, manifest primarily as weakness and fatigue, anorexia and weight loss, and general inability to withstand stress, resulting in hypotension. A medical emergency can arise, requiring immediate therapy while diagnostic laboratory tests are pending. Failure to suppress hypothalamic secretion of proopiomelanocortin results in hyperpigmentation and elevated levels of plasma ACTH. Other diagnostic laboratory tests include decreased basal plasma levels of cortisol and failure of cortisol levels to rise after stimulation with exogenous ACTH, placing the lesion in the adrenal rather than in the pituitary. Renin levels are also increased, and aldosterone levels do not rise after appropriate stimulation.

Therapeutic decisions. Therapy for adrenal insufficiency can be initiated in an emergency situation with dexamethasone, which does not affect total plasma cortisol levels sufficiently to confuse diagnostic tests. Other IV corticosteroid preparations are satisfactory when interference with diagnostic testing is not a consideration and should be given in large doses (equivalent to 200 to 300 mg/day of hydrocortisone). Parenteral salt and water are often needed as well to restore plasma volume because of the mineralocorticoid deficiency. Subsequently, lifelong replacement therapy is necessary; the usual regimen is 20 to 30 mg/day of hydrocortisone, divided into two doses (two-thirds given on arising, one-third in the evening), with increased doses given immediately at times of physiological stress. Some patients can be maintained on high salt intake without steroid hormones in the absence of stress. Another very satisfactory mineralocorticoid is fludrocortisone; usually only 200 to 300 μg/day is required. Since renin levels respond to the effective circulating plasma volume, they are usually elevated in untreated Addison's disease and can be diagnostically useful as well as valuable in evaluating the adequacy of therapy.

Secondary adrenal insufficiency, due to hypothalamic-pituitary disorders or prolonged administration of exogenous corticosteroids, usually does not need therapy in the absence of acute illness or other stress. Hyperpigmentation does not occur in these syndromes, since there is no increased hypothalamic secretion of proopiomelanocortin. Mineralocorticoid levels are usually normal, and thus there is no hyperkalemia or metabolic acidosis, but hyponatremia can develop because glucocorticoid deficiency impairs water excretion. Recovery of normal adrenal function after discontinuation of glucocorticoid therapy may take a year or longer, and extra hormonal therapy should be administered in a stressful situation, such as surgery, marked diarrhea with dehydration, or a severe infection.

Aldosterone deficiency

Aldosterone deficiency without glucocorticoid deficiency results from lack of renin secretion by the kidney rather than adrenal disease; the resulting syndrome is called **hyporeninemic hypoaldosteronism.** Lack of aldosterone due to adrenal disease is associated with elevated levels of plasma renin and can result from autoimmune processes.

Aldosterone increases renal excretion H^+ and K^+ and reabsorption of Na^+ and water. Therefore, hypoaldosteronism results in hyperkalemia, acidosis with increased plasma Cl^-, and hypovolemia.

Administration of ACE inhibitors, which block the synthesis of angiotensin II, can result in significant hyperkalemia, particularly if there is underlying renal insufficiency. Such an occurrence does not indicate underlying adrenal hypofunction.

Mineralocorticoid deficiency results from disorders that impair renal secretion of renin, such as diabetes mellitus or chronic tubulointerstitial disease of the kidney. Impaired sympathetic nervous system stimulation of the kidney in diabetics can impair renal secretion of renin, and impaired conversion of prorenin to active renin by diseased renal tubular cells is the mechanism in some other patients. Blockers of beta-adrenergic receptors and ACE inhibitors can have the same result. The administration of NSAIDs that block prostaglandin formation in the kidney also can decrease renin secretion, which is controlled by renal prostaglandin formation.

Hyperkalemia and hyperchloremic metabolic acidosis are usually present, but sodium depletion is variable. In some patients, measurements show increased total body sodium and ECF, suggesting that impaired renal excretion of salt and water is the primary process causing the decreased renin secretion.

Therapeutic decisions. Although afflicted persons are usually asymptomatic, treatment of hyporeninemic hypoaldosteronism is necessary because the hyperkalemia can cause life-threatening arrhythmias. Fludrocortisone, 100 to 300 μg/day, usually restores renal potassium and H^+ excretion but can result in so much sodium and water retention that it aggravates any underlying hypertension, causing problems especially in those patients with underlying renal disease. Furosemide, 40 to 120 mg/day, increases potassium excretion and can ameliorate the hyperkalemia and reverse the metabolic acidosis. The accompanying increased sodium and chloride excretion prevents the hypervolemia and aggravation of hypertension. Furosemide alone can be adequate therapy in some of these patients without fludrocortisone, but in others the combination of the two agents is needed.

Primary hyperaldosteronism

Primary hyperaldosteronism results from autonomous hypersecretion of aldosterone by the adrenal cortex; 75 to 85% of cases are due to a benign adenoma, and most of the remainder to diffuse bilateral hyperplasia. Less than 1% of cases are due carcinoma. It results in increased distal tubular reabsorption of sodium, expanding the ECF volume. As a result, proximal tubular reabsorption of sodium is reduced, and the increased delivery of sodium to the proximal tubule overwhelms its capacity for reabsorption. A new steady state results, with net retention of about 1.5 to 2.5 L of excess fluid, but increased secretion of potassium and hydrogen ion by the collecting duct continues. Hypernatremia, hypokalemia, and metabolic alkalosis are characteristically found, and symptoms depend on the degree of hypokalemia. Muscle weakness, polyuria, polydipsia, and paresthesias are common, but intermittent paralysis of arms and legs can occur, as can tetany. Hypertension develops, and there is suppression of renin secretion by the kidney. With severe hypokalemia, there can be autonomic dysfunction with postural hypotension.

Diagnosis of primary hyperaldosteronism is important because it causes a curable form of hypertension. The finding of elevated plasma levels of aldosterone can be misleading because of normal diurnal variation. Demonstrating increased daily urinary excretion of the hormone (or its 18-glucuronide metabolite) in the presence of decreased and nonstimulatable plasma renin activity is more useful. Autonomy of adrenal secretion of aldosterone can be demonstrated by failure to suppress hormone levels or excretion with fludrocortisone or deoxycorticosterone or IV saline, which build plasma volume and turn off the entire renin-angiotensin-aldosterone system. CT scan, iodocholesterol scan, and aldosterone levels can help localize an adenoma. Surgical removal is the treatment of choice.

Cushing's syndrome

Adrenocortical hyperfunction, Cushing's syndrome, can result from adrenocortical hyperplasia secondary to excess production of ACTH by a pituitary adenoma or ectopic sources. Pituitary tumors causing this syndrome are usually very small; when the adrenocortical hyperfunction is due to a pituitary tumor, it is called Cushing's disease. Primary adrenal adenomas and carcinomas also cause the syndrome. Cushing's syndrome is five times more common in women than in men.

Ectopic ACTH production can give ACTH levels several times higher than in Cushing's disease, yet manifestations are usually milder, perhaps because the syndrome develops more rapidly; this syndrome occurs much more often in men; small cell carcinoma of the lung, bronchial carcinoid, and medullary carcinoma of the thyroid are the most common tumors that secrete ACTH. Such patients often have markedly increased levels of deoxycorticosterone, which is a potent mineralocorticoid, and they can develop severe hypertension and hypokalemic metabolic alkalosis. Secretion of androgens or estrogens by the adrenal can cause virilization in women or feminization in men (gynecomastia is a common clinical finding in such cases).

Clinical manifestations. Cushing's syndrome causes obesity, which is more marked centrally, with a "buffalo hump" and relatively thin arms and legs. Muscle wasting and weakness are very common. Severe acne appears, and the skin is very thin, bruising and even tearing very easily. Abdominal stretch marks (striae) are usually present. Mild hypertension and mental functional changes also occur frequently. Hirsutism and amenorrhea are common in women. Impaired carbohydrate tolerance or frank diabetes mellitus develops, and osteoporosis can be marked, with collapse of multiple vertebrae.

Diagnostic decisions. The diagnosis can be made by establishing elevated levels of plasma cortisol, but secretion of this hormone may be pulsatile. It is usually necessary to demonstrate the absence of the usual diurnal variation and increased 24-hour urinary excretion of cortisol or a metabolite such as 17-OH-corticoids. The response of adrenal secretion suppression by dexamethasone is a useful diagnostic test; 1 mg is given PO around midnight, followed by determination of 8:00 A.M. plasma cortisol level. A level below 5 μg/100 ml rules out Cushing's syndrome. False-positive results (i.e., failure to suppress) can occur with phenytoin or estrogen therapy.

Measurement of plasma ACTH levels is useful in distinguishing among the causes of Cushing's syndrome. Levels are usually markedly elevated in patients with ectopic ACTH production, modestly elevated or normal in patients with pituitary tumors, and usually undetectable in patients with adrenal tumors. CT scans of the pituitary and adrenal can localize a tumor, but the pituitary lesions may be so small that no abnormality is seen in the area of the sella turcica. A high-dose dexamethasone suppression test (2 mg q 6 hours for 2 days) followed by measurement of plasma cortisol or 24-hour urinary free cortisol or 17-OH-corticoids on the second day usually reveals 50% or more suppression in cases of Cushing's disease, since the excessive pituitary function is not entirely autonomous. Adrenal neoplasms and tumors causing ectopic ACTH secretion usually do not suppress, but there are rare exceptions.

Treatment of Cushing's syndrome usually requires surgery in the case of pituitary tumors, as well as adrenal tumors and neoplasms causing ectopic ACTH production. Medical inhibition of adrenal cortisol secretion with mitotane, aminoglutethimide, or metyrapone can be of some help in inoperable cases.

Pheochromocytoma

Of the catecholamines, norepinephrine and dopamine are neurotransmitters in the CNS and postganglionic sympathetic neurons, but epinephrine originates almost exclusively in the adrenal gland. Epinephrine acts primarily on beta-adrenergic receptors, resulting in positive inotropic and chronotropic effects on the heart and vasodilatation in most vascular beds. It also increases plasma glucose by stimulating glycogenolysis in the liver and inhibiting insulin secretion by the pancreas. A variety of stimuli induce release of epinephrine from the adrenal medulla, including hypoglycemia. Norepinephrine, on the other hand, acts primarily on the alpha-adrenergic receptors, causing vasoconstriction. It has little metabolic effect. Since norepinephrine is secreted primarily by nervous tissue, adrenal medullary hypofunction causes little physiological abnormality, but hypersecretion of catecholamines causes

major pathophysiological consequences, as encountered in pheochromocytoma.

Chromaffin cells can give rise to pheochromocytoma in any sympathetic ganglion, but 90% occur in the adrenal medulla and most of the remainder occur in ganglia in the mediastinum or abdomen. Bilateral or multiple tumors occur in 5 to 10% of the cases, often in association with medullary carcinoma of the thyroid and the syndrome of multiple endocrine neoplasia type II (Sipple's syndrome). Norepinephrine is the sole product of tumors arising in extra-adrenal chromaffin tissue and may be the major secretory product of adrenal tumors. The enzyme that converts norepinephrine to epinephrine exists primarily in the adrenal medulla, and it can be the major excretory product of a pheochromocytoma of that organ.

Clinical manifestations. The main manifestation of pheochromocytoma is hypertension, usually paroxysmal, although it may be sustained with paroxysmal exacerbations. Typical spells include palpitations, sweating, flushing, and anxiety. Symptoms may be induced by ingestion of tyramine-containing foods such as cheese, particularly in patients who are taking a monamine oxidase inhibitor. Occasionally the attacks are characterized by hypotensive episodes, especially when the tumor secretes epinephrine or dopamine.

Diagnostic decisions. The diagnosis of pheochromocytoma is based on the finding of increased levels of catecholamines in the plasma or their metabolites (metanephrines and vanillyl-mandelic acid [VMA]) in 24-hour urine collections. Clonidine suppresses catecholamine levels in normals but not in patients with pheochromocytoma, and this may become the basis of a diagnostic test. CT scans can help localize tumors, which should be treated surgically; blockade of alpha receptors with phenoxybenzamine, dibenzyline, or prazosin is useful and may be necessary preoperatively. Beta-adrenergic blockade may be needed in patients who develop tachycardia.

DIABETES MELLITUS

Type I, insulin-dependent diabetes mellitus (IDDM), is characterized by little or no insulin secretion and occurs primarily in younger people (usually before age 30, with a peak age of onset between 11 and 13 years) who are not obese. There is a genetic basis, suggested by the statistical association with HLA types DR3 and DR4 and the fact that identical twins have a 50% incidence of concordance. The diabetes often begins after a viral infection, and it is thought that damage to the beta cells of the pancreas elicits an autoimmune mechanism that destroys the islets, leading to insulin deficiency, and that this process occurs in genetically susceptible individuals.

The metabolic disturbance usually begins abruptly, with symptoms of glycosuria (polyuria, polydipsia, polyphagia, and weight loss), rapid development of severe ketoacidosis, and a fatal outcome without treatment. After recovery from the initial episode, a "honeymoon phase" may appear, with restored insulin secretion, but after a few months the disease returns and lifelong insulin treatment is required. In the early years after onset, autoantibodies against pancreatic islet cells can be demonstrated, and sometimes other autoimmune diseases are associated.

Type II, non-insulin-dependent diabetes mellitus

(NIDDM), is much more common and usually begins after age 40. More than 50% of the patients are overweight. The disease may be asymptomatic, discovered by routine lab tests. It may cause symptoms that result from glycosuria, or the first manifestations may be one of the complications of long-standing diabetes, such as neuropathy or arterial insufficiency. Ketoacidosis rarely develops in type II diabetics but may appear following a stressful intercurrent illness such as a severe infection or a myocardial infarction. Type II diabetics make insulin, but in reduced amounts; occasionally basal levels are in the normal range, but there is an inadequate response to a glucose challenge. These patients are also resistant to the action of exogenous insulin because of abnormalities at the cellular level, decreased insulin binding, and decreased postreceptor effects of insulin action. Although there is no pattern of association with HLA types, an important genetic factor is present as shown by the frequent strong family history and almost 100% concordance among identical twins. Rarely, patients progress from type II to type I diabetes.

Secondary diabetes occurs following destruction of the pancreas as a result of pancreatitis or in some endocrine disorders in which hormonal action counteracts the effects of insulin, such as in Cushing's syndrome, pheochromocytoma, and glucagonoma. Many drugs can cause aggravation of underlying diabetes, including corticosteroids, phenytoin, diuretics, propranolol, and adrenergic agents.

Familial patterns. There is a low incidence of diabetes among children of diabetic parents. In IDDM, it is 2 to 5%, and in NIDDM 10 to 15%. For both types, the chances of a nonidentical sibling having diabetes is about 10%, but this figure is much higher in cases of IDDM in which the siblings have identical HLA phenotypes.

Metabolic abnormalities. Abnormal glucose tolerance, the key manifestation of diabetes, is defined as a fasting blood glucose about 140 mg/100 ml or a 2-hour blood glucose above 200 mg/100 ml after a carbohydrate-rich meal (or a standard glucose tolerance test, in which 75 g of glucose is given PO after 3 days of high carbohydrate intake and 10 hours of fasting). Many patients found to have moderate glucose elevations by these criteria never become symptomatic or need treatment. When the blood glucose exceeds the renal threshold (around 180 mg/100 ml), glycosuria results and the osmotic diuretic effect causes the polyuria and polydipsia. The caloric loss resulting from the glycosuria causes weight loss and polyphagia. Other early symptoms that can occur include fatigue, transient blurring of vision from swelling of the lens due to high blood glucose, or recurrent *Candida* vaginitis, thrush, or balanitis, despite prophylactic antifungal therapy.

Therapeutic decisions. The goals of treatment are (1) the avoidance of symptoms resulting from hyperglycemia, (2) prevention of the complications of uncontrolled diabetes, and (3) the avoidance of damaging episodes of hypoglycemia. "Tight" control seems to minimize the development of complications, but overcontrol resulting in hypoglycemia can cause life-threatening phenomena. The metabolic objective of control is fasting glucose levels between 100 and 140 and 2-hour postprandial glucoses between 100 and 200 mg/100 ml. It is best not to attempt tight control of patients who are very uncooperative (such as alcoholics or those with psychiatric

disturbances), patients who are especially susceptible to hypoglycemia (such as those with advanced liver or kidney disease, adrenal or pituitary hypofunction), or patients whose autonomic responses are blunted and cannot compensate for hypoglycemia (such as patients receiving beta-blockers or who have spontaneous abnormalities in autonomic function). In addition, patients with severe coronary artery or cerebrovascular disease could have serious damage from hypoglycemia, and it is often unwise to attempt to achieve tight control.

Type I diabetes. The most important aspect of diet is its consistency in timing and calorie content so that good control is possible. Low fat intake is important because of the frequency of vascular disease. The recommended diet is therefore 25 to 30% lipid (polyunsaturated to saturated fat ratio of 1:1 and cholesterol under 350 mg/day), 10 to 20% protein, and 50 to 60% carbohydrate. High fiber content is recommended. Insulin needs usually range between 20 and 60 units/day. A requirement over 200 units/day indicates insulin resistance, often due to circulating antibodies that bind insulin, and a change in the source species of the insulin may help (e.g., to synthetic human insulin). Allergic reactions or the development of lipodystrophy at the sites of injection are also indications for a change in the source of insulin. Table 1-11 lists different types of insulin and their duration of action.

A standard approach to insulin dosage is to give a single morning dose of an intermediate-acting insulin (e.g., NPH or lente) of 20 to 25 units, following the glucose levels at 7 A.M., 11 A.M., 4 P.M., and 9 P.M. If glucose levels during the day are high, increase the morning dose about 5 units every other day. Commonly, extra doses of regular, short-acting insulin are required with certain meals, and adjustments must be made on an individual basis. An increase in physical activity may reduce the insulin need; an intercurrent illness or stress usually raises the need. In very labile cases, an insulin pump has been used to deliver a constant basal level of insulin plus a bolus with each meal, mimicking the normal function of the pancreas more closely.

Hypoglycemia can result in rebound hyperglycemia (the

Table 1-11. Types of Insulin Available

Insulin type	Peak action (hours)	Duration of effect (hours)
Rapid acting		
Regular	2–4	6–8
Semilente	2–6	10–12
Intermediate acting		
NPH	6–12	18–24
Lente	6–12	18–24
Long acting		
Protamine zinc	14–24	36
Ultralente	18–24	36

Somogyi effect). Clinically this phenomenon occurs particularly when long-acting insulin causes nocturnal hypoglycemia, impairing glucose tolerance for breakfast. The resulting morning hyperglycemia may lead to the decision to increase the insulin dose, worsening the nocturnal hypoglycemia. The appropriate therapy is to decrease the dose of long-acting insulin.

Type II diabetes.   Treatment primarily involves diet, sometimes oral hypoglycemic agents, and in rare instances insulin. Since most of these patients are obese, calorie restriction is the most important element of therapy, and weight loss, if achieved, can improve carbohydrate tolerance. Fat and cholesterol intake should be especially restricted. In thin type II diabetics, calorie restriction is not advisable. The sulfonylureas, which lower blood glucose by increasing the secretion of insulin by the beta cells and by increasing the sensitivity of peripheral cells to the effects of insulin, are indicated when diet alone fails to control blood glucose adequately. The major complication of their use is hypoglycemia, which occurs most frequently in elderly patients, alcoholics, and patients with hepatic or renal disease. It is more common with long-acting agents, such as chlorpropramide.

Control of diabetes should be followed by home blood glucose monitoring, since urine glucose measurements are insensitive because of variations in renal threshold for glucose. Glycosylated hemoglobin, normally about 5 to 8%, can be followed as a measure of overall control status for several months. In poorly controlled diabetics, it can reach about 20%. Measurement of 24-hour urine glucose excretion is very inaccurate as a result of incomplete collections. The objective should be excretion of less than 10 g/day.

Complications of diabetes

Diabetic ketoacidosis.   Diabetic ketoacidosis occurs most often among type I diabetics, especially in childhood and adolescence, but can occur at any age. Often it is precipitated by an infection, trauma, emotional stress, omission of insulin, or an intercurrent illness. Although no precipitating factor can be identified in every case, a careful search is important since treatment of the underlying event is essential. The ketosis may present with a few days of polyuria and polydipsia, nausea, vomiting, and abdominal pain. The syndrome can mimic an intra-abdominal infection or other problem, and the differential diagnosis can be difficult. Leukocytosis and left shift occur with ketosis alone, further confounding the differential diagnosis.

Pathophysiology of ketoacidosis.   With relative hypoinsulinemia there is hyperglycemia, resulting from increased hepatic glucose production and decreased peripheral utilization. An osmotic diuresis develops, causing hypovolemia and electrolyte depletion. Plasma ketones rise because increased secretion of catecholamines causes increased release of fatty acids from peripheral adipose tissues. In the liver, fatty acids are either re-esterified or processed into ketones by the mitochondria. With hypoinsulinemic and hyperglucagonemic states, increased amounts of fatty acids enter mitochondria, resulting in accumulation of the keto acids alpha-hydroxybutyrate and acetoacetate. Acidosis develops, with decreased serum bicarbonate and an anion gap. Patients typically have tachypnea, dehydration,

and a fruity odor to the breath due to the acetonemia. They may develop confusion, somnolence, or coma. The hyperventilation resulting from acidosis is usually described as Kussmaul's respirations.

Laboratory confirmation of the diagnosis of ketoacidosis includes demonstration of elevated blood glucose and ketone bodies in the blood and urine. The usual methods of measuring ketones (the nitroprusside reaction) detect acetoacetate but do not pick up beta-hydroxybutyrate. The levels of the latter usually are higher, and in patients with lactic acidosis the alpha-hydroxybutyrate levels are considerable higher than acetoacetate levels and determination of ketones grossly underestimates the degree of acidosis. Further, treatment of diabetic ketoacidosis causes conversion of alpha-hydroxybutyrate to acetoacetate, and repeated determination of ketones can result in the misleading impression that the ketosis is getting worse.

Therapeutic decisions.   Treatment of ketoacidosis requires administration of insulin, usually 5 to 10 units/hour, preferably IV since dehydration and hypotension can restrict absorption from SC or IM routes. Because of the severe dehydration, usually resulting in a deficit of about 6 L, IV fluids should be given, initially as normal saline about 1 L/hour unless there is cardiovascular or renal disease requiring more cautious fluid administration. Although the serum potassium level may be elevated initially, these patients have depleted total potassium stores, and increased glucose utilization resulting from insulin administration will rapidly decrease plasma potassium levels; KCl (about 20 to 40 mEq/L) should be added to the IV fluids as soon as urine flow is well established and total renal function is adequate. Phosphate depletion also occurs, but replacement does not seem to be essential. Bicarbonate should be given only if the patient is severely acidotic.

As soon as the plasma glucose level decreases to about 250 mg/100 ml, glucose should be added to the IV fluids to avoid the development of hypoglycemia. Insulin administration should be tapered as soon as the ketosis is well controlled, but it must be continued to avoid a return of the ketoacidosis. Another complication of the treatment of ketoacidosis, cerebral edema, is usually seen in children and apparently results from too rapid correction of the metabolic abnormalities. Care should be taken to avoid it.

Nonketotic hyperosmolar coma.   Another complication of diabetes is the result of extremely high glucose levels, which can reach 1,000 to 2,000 mg/100 ml without concomitant ketoacidosis. This syndrome results from poor control of diabetes, with dehydration and hypovolemia. Impaired renal function and decreased renal glucose excretion may also contribute to the very high glucose levels. Often the syndrome is precipitated by a stroke, myocardial infarction, or other intercurrent illness. The high serum osmolality affects cerebral function, but it may be difficult to decide whether an underlying CNS disease has precipitated the exacerbation of the diabetes, requiring a lumbar puncture to rule out meningitis, for example. Calculation of the serum osmolality can be useful, pending actual laboratory determination of the level. A level greater than 340 mOsm/L can account for stupor or coma. The calculation is based on the following formula:

$$\text{Effective serum osmolality} = 2(\text{Na} + \text{K}) + (\text{glucose}/18)$$

Therapy for the hyperosmolar state is similar to that for ketoacidosis: Insulin, hypotonic fluids, and potassium are the main agents needed. Any underlying precipitating problem must be detected and treated. Early treatment is essential because permanent brain damage can result.

Complications of long-standing diabetes

Microangiopathy is a common result of long-standing diabetes, manifest as a **retinopathy.** Microaneurysms along with waxy and cotton-wool exudates as well as hemorrhages can be seen on funduscopic examination. The incidence of retinopathy is proportional to the duration of the diabetes. By 10 years about 50% and by 20 years about 90% of diabetics have these lesions. In a smaller proportion of the cases, a proliferative retinopathy develops characterized by formation of new vessels (neovascularization), vitreous hemorrhages, and retinal displacement. Vision loss can be severe. Laser coagulation can be helpful. Cataracts and glaucoma also occur with increased frequency among diabetics.

Diabetic renal disease is also a common development, occurring in about 50% of type I diabetics after 20 years. Proteinuria is usually the first manifestation, and it can progress to classic nephrotic syndrome; hypertension is usually associated, and progression to renal failure occurs. In general, azotemia appears 3 years after the development of significant proteinuria, and end-stage renal failure is present 3 years after the development of significant azotemia. Renal biopsy is rarely necessary in these patients, unless an active urine sediment, low serum complement, or other atypical findings such as absence of concomitant retinopathy suggest a different diagnosis. The development of renal failure requires institution of hemodialysis, peritoneal dialysis, or renal transplantation, but the outlook for these patients is not as good for other patients with chronic renal failure.

Arteriosclerotic vascular disease is increased in frequency and severity among patients with diabetes. Good control of the diabetes seems to be helpful in these patients, and other risk factors (hypertension, smoking, lipids, etc.) should be vigorously treated. **Neuropathy** is another common complication. It may occur as a symmetrical, distal polyneuropathy, with "glove and stocking" peripheral sensory loss and Charcot joints. Various dyesthesias also occur; pain is usually worse at night and can be disabling. Treatment with phenytoin, carbamazepine, or amitriptyline is reportedly helpful. Mononeuropathies also occur, including cranial neuropathy, frequently affecting the third nerve; spontaneous recovery can occur. **Autonomic neuropathy** also occurs, usually associated with distal polyneuropathy. It can cause impotence, neurogenic bladder, orthostatic hypotension, or abnormalities in GI motility. Abnormal sweating can also occur. The GI tract dysfunction can cause gastroparesis, diarrhea (often nocturnal), or constipation and anal incontinence. The abnormal GI motility can result in erratic food absorption and make the control of the diabetes more difficult.

Foot ulcers commonly develop in diabetics as a result of underlying arteriosclerosis as well as the microangiopathy and neuropathy. Progression of the ulcers to gangrene often requires amputation. Special foot care is necessary to prevent these lesions, including removal of calluses, properly fitting shoes, attention to cleanliness, and early treatment of any blisters or infection.

Hypoglycemia is usually an overdiagnosed condition, which requires a fasting blood glucose level below 50 mg/100 ml, symptoms consistent with hypoglycemia (usually those resulting from mobilization of catecholamines), and relief of symptoms by an increase in plasma glucose levels. Alcohol inhibits gluconeogenesis, and thus hypoglycemia occurs more often in alcoholics. Even moderate alcohol intake by a person who has missed a few meals can result in hypoglycemia. Because of the brain damage that can result from severe hypoglycemia, any confused or comatose patient arriving in the emergency room should immediately receive 50 ml IV of 50% glucose. An **insulinoma** can cause hypoglycemia; the diagnosis is established by demonstration of a low plasma glucose level in the presence of an inappropriately high plasma insulin level. Surreptitious self-administration of insulin can be differentiated since plasma C-peptide levels will be low and C-peptide levels reflect secretion of insulin. With an insulinoma, there are parallel increases in C peptide and insulin. Surreptitious use of oral hypoglycemia agents causes increased levels of both C peptide and insulin. Differentiation must be based on assay of blood and urine for these agents.

HYPERLIPIDEMIAS

There are several disorders of lipid metabolism that are important because of their frequency and the fact that they cause an increased incidence of atherosclerosis and its complications. The main classification of the serum lipids is based on their chemical composition (content of triglycerides and cholesterol), electrophoretic mobility, and their buoyancy in plasma when centrifuged. The most buoyant, the very low-density lipoproteins (VLDL), have the highest fat content and are most clearly associated with premature atherosclerosis. Low-density lipoproteins (LDL) are less of a risk factor, whereas high-density lipoproteins (HDL) contain less fat and are somewhat protective. The ratio between HDL and LDL is a measure of the risk of atherosclerosis.

The main lipid components of the serum and the designation of the disease with which they are associated are listed in Table 1-12.

Familial hypercholesterolemia

Familial hypercholesterolemia is an autosomal dominant disorder in which there is an increased concentration of LDL. About 1 in 500 adults in the United States are heterozygotes for this disorder and have cholesterol levels elevated to about 2 to 3 times normal. The levels in homozygotes are 6 to 8 times normal. Triglyceride levels are not abnormal. Physical examination reveals multiple tendon xanthomas, most frequently found in the gastrocnemius tendon and extensor tendons of the hands, and there are xanthelasmas about the eyes. Atherosclerosis develops at a relatively early age, causing myocardial infarction and peripheral vascular disease.

Diagnostic decisions. The diagnosis is based on the presence of xanthomas, xanthelasma, and the finding of elevated serum cholesterol with normal triglycerides.

Therapeutic decisions. Therapy with dietary restriction of saturated fats and cholesterol helps but is not adequate.

Table 1-12. Serum Lipid Components and Associated Types of Hyperlipidemia

Type based on ultracentifugation	Major lipid components	Type of hyperlipidemia
Chylomicrons	Dietary triglycerides	Alone: Type I With increased VLDL: Type V
VLDL	Hepatic triglycerides	Alone: Type IV With chylomicrons: Type V
(Remnants)	Cholesterol esters, triglycerides	Type III
LDL	Cholesterol esters	Alone: IIa With VLDL: Type IIb
HDL	Cholesterol esters	Protective effect

Cholestyramine helps by binding bile acids and, combined with nicotinic acid, can lower lipoprotein levels. With treatment, xanthelasmas slowly disappear. The effect of therapy on the progression of atheromatous disease is not yet certain.

Other inherited hyperlipoproteinemias

Familial dysbetalipoproteinemia is a rare, autosomal recessive disorder in which large "tuberous" xanthomas occur in palmar creases and over pressure points such as the elbows, knees, and buttocks. There is an increased incidence of premature atheromatous disease. Laboratory studies reveal an abnormal broad band, which migrates as a beta-globulin on electrophoresis. It contains products derived from partial catabolism of VLDL and chylomicrons. Hyperlipidemia and clinical manifestations usually do not develop until a person's 20s or 30s. This disorder is usually classified as type III (or broad beta disease). Treatment consists of reduction in dietary intake of simple sugars and cholesterol and weight reduction if there is obesity. Addition of clofibrate (500 mg 2 to 4 times daily) can result in lowering of triglyceride and cholesterol levels.

Other inherited hyperlipoproteinemias include **familial endogenous and mixed hypertriglyceridemias** and **lipoprotein lipase deficiency**, both autosomal recessive disorders characterized by eruptive xanthomas that appear over the skin surface, hepatosplenomegaly, and recurrent pancreatitis. The plasma is grossly lipemic and contains markedly elevated plasma triglycerides.

Familial multiple lipoprotein-type hyperlipidemia is a relatively common disorder characterized by elevated plasma cholesterol and triglycerides and a strong family history of myocardial infarction at relatively early ages—about 10% of people with myocardial infarction before age 60 have this disease. VLDL, HDL, or both may be elevated. The patterns are variable, but usually the same abnormality is found in all members of a given family. Treatment usually requires dietary restriction and clofibrate. If hypercholesterolemia is present, cholestyramine or nicotinic acid can be helpful.

Secondary forms of hyperlipidemias

Secondary hyperlipoproteinemia occurs in a variety of diseases. Hypercholesterolemia is seen with hypothyroidism and nephrotic syndrome, and to a lesser extent in Cushing's syndrome, anorexia nervosa, and other disease states. Sustained hypercholesterolemia can lead to premature atherosclerosis. Therapy includes correction of the underlying disorder and cholestyramine or nicotinic acid if the hypercholesterolemia is severe and persistent.

Secondary hypertriglyceridemia occurs in patients with diabetes mellitus, chronic alcoholism, chronic renal failure, acute hepatitis, and with use of oral contraceptives. Less severe changes are seen in a variety of diseases. Treatment is directed at the underlying disorder, weight reduction in obese patients, and dietary restriction of saturated fats, simple sugars, and alcohol.

LIPID STORAGE DISEASES

A group of diseases result from inherited defects in enzymes involved in the catabolism of lipids. The resulting accumulation of lipid, especially in the CNS, results in a variety of syndromes, varying from severe mental retardation with seizures and death by age two (Tay-Sachs disease), to severe neurological disease and hepatosplenomegaly affecting adults, but normal life span (Gaucher's disease). Fabry's disease can cause renal failure in males, usually by the late 30s, and Niemann-Pick disease causes extensive neurological abnormalities with cherry-red spots in the maculae. Table 1-13 summarizes the main features of these diseases.

Table 1-13. Lipid Storage Diseases

Disease	Enzyme deficiency	Stored lipid	Characteristic lesions
Tay-Sachs	Hexosaminidase A	Ganglioside	Cherry-red spots in maculae
Niemann-Pick	Sphingomyelinase	Sphingomylein	Cherry-red spots in maculae
Gaucher's	Beta-glucocerebrosidase	Glucosylceramide	Hepatosplenomegaly
Fabry's	Alpha-galactosidase	Trihexosylceramide	Neuropathy, renal failure

These diseases are all inherited as autosomal recessives, except Fabry's disease, which is a sex-linked autosomal disease. (In Fabry's, heterozygous females usually show corneal cluding but few or no other manifestations).

Diagnostic decisions.   The diagnosis can be confirmed in some instances by demonstrating decreased enzyme activity in a biopsy specimen. The source of the tissue for the enzyme assay can be WBCs in Gaucher's disease, renal or small bowel biopsy in Fabry's. The accumulation of lipid can be demonstrated histochemically in bone marrow or lymph node cells in Niemann-Pick, and in a renal biopsy in Tay-Sachs disease.

METABOLIC DISORDERS LEADING TO CRYSTAL SYNOVITIS

There are several forms of arthritis related to deposition of crystalline compounds in joints. Phagocytosis of such crystals activates neutrophils to produce mediators of chemotaxis and inflammation, including peptides (e.g., kinins) and prostaglandins. A severe form of synovitis usually results. The most common crystal synovitis is gout, which results from abnormalities in purine metabolism. A variety of syndromes can result from deposition of calcium pyrophosphate cyrstals, a process often called **pseudogout**. Apatite crystal deposition is rare but causes extensive erosion of joint and periarticular tissues.

Gout

Urate gout results from any disorder of purine metabolism that causes hyperuricemia. Most cases of gout result from incomplete renal excretion of the urate synthesized from dietary and endogenous purines. Hyperuricemia secondary to other diseases, such as myeloproliferative disorders, lymphoma, renal failure, or drug effects on renal tubular secretion of urate, can also cause gouty arthritis.

Gout can be divided into four distinct clinical syndromes:

1. Asymptomatic hyperuricemia.   Patients have elevated serum urate levels but no symptoms. The normal levels of serum urate vary with the method used. In men, 5 to 7.5 mg/100 ml is the usual range expected with the uricase method. In premenopausal women, the level is about 1 mg/100 ml lower but goes up after menopause.

Therapeutic decisions.   Since elevated serum urate levels are common without harmful sequelae in patients taking diuretics as well as some other drugs, it is rarely necessary to treat such asymptomatic patients with hyperuricemia. These patients should be warned that an attack of gout may occur. Rapid treatment can be instituted at that time. A strong family history of gout or an excessively high urate level (> 10 or 11 mg/100 ml) can warrant prophylactic treatment.

2. Acute gouty arthritis.   Attacks of gout are much more frequent in men. They are usually monarticular but can affect two or three joints at a time. About 60% of first attacks occur in the metatarsophalangeal joint of a big toe. Attacks may occur in other joints, especially the feet and legs, much less often affecting the upper extremities or spine. Subsequent attacks affect a wider distribution of joints. Characteristically, marked inflammation with severe pain, redness, warmth, and swelling typically develops within a few hours, but occasionally attacks are mild. Fever, leukocytosis, an elevated ESR are commonly present, and coupled with the severe inflammation, the syndrome often suggests infection. Untreated attacks usually subside in 1 to 3 weeks, and the patient is again clinically well.

Two carbon metabolites of ethanol, ketone bodies, and other organic acids inhibit renal tubular secretion of urate, raising serum levels. Therefore, attacks of gout can be precipitated by alcohol ingestion, ketosis following starvation (such as occurs after major surgery or a severe medical illness during which a patient does not eat), or lactic acidosis after exercise or anoxia. Attacks can result from use of drugs that raise serum urate, as do most diuretics, especially the thiazides. Uricosuric therapy or xanthine oxidase inhibitors (e.g., allopurinol) lower serum levels abruptly and can precipitate or aggravate an acute attack.

3. Intercritical gout.   After an attack has occurred, the patient may be entirely well but no longer has "asymptomatic hyperuricemia." Recurrent attacks of gout can be expected, although the interval is unpredictable, sometimes extending to several years. Once recurrent attacks begin, they tend to occur with increasing frequency. Recurrent attacks soon after the first one are more likely in younger patients, those with a stronger family history of gout, and those with a higher serum urate level. After one recurrence, subsequent attacks tend to occur with increasing frequency and may occur with intervals of a few weeks to a few months.

4. Chronic tophaceous gout.   Those patients who are producing more urate from dietary and endogenous purines than they are excreting (i.e., are in a positive urate balance) develop accumulations of urate in solid tissues, especially sites of relative acidity such as cartilage. A foreign body reaction develops, and the resulting granulomatous nodules or lumps are called **tophi**. Clinically, tophaceous masses appear most frequently in the ear lobes, in periarticular synovial tissue such as the olecranon bursae, and around joints. Tophi can ulcerate through the skin, discharging gritty, chalky material that can be demonstrated to contain urate microscopically and chemically.

Diagnostic decisions.   Gout should be considered in a patient with a sudden onset of arthritis, especially in a man, and when the arthritis affects a single joint in the lower extremity or is limited to a few joints, especially in the presence of a precipitating factor such as alcohol ingestion, ketosis, etc. A history of prior attacks with asymptomatic intervals is strongly suggestive, as is a family history suggestive of gout. Evaluation should include examination for tophi or chronic synovial thickening and aspiration of any joint to check for crystals.

Urate crystals are needle shaped and negatively birefringent with polarized light, whereas calcium pyrophosphate crystals are blunter and positively birefringent. (Memory clue: urate deposits and urate calculi are not seen on x-ray—they are radiolucent, hence think of negativity; calcium deposits and stones are visible on x-ray since they are radiopaque—think of positivity). Since differentiation from infection is the usual problem, smear and culture of joint fluid should be performed. A marked leukocytosis consisting almost entirely of neutrophils is characteristic of both gout and infection.

Workup should include a serum urate level, but this finding can be misleading. The serum urate level should not be relied on to help in the diagnosis, since it can be elevated in other forms of arthritis and can be normal in patients with gout, usually as a result of drug influences or changes in other factors that influence the renal handling of urate. (Aspirin in small doses is uricoretentive and raises the serum level, whereas high doses are uricosuric, lowering the serum level. Most people take some amount of aspirin before they consult a physician.)

Tophaceous deposits can cause destruction of joint structures, and a chronic deforming and disabling arthritis can result, resembling rheumatoid arthritis (RA). An erroneous diagnosis of coexistent RA and gout is sometimes made, but the two disease very rarely coexist in the same patient. In patients with acute attacks of gout, the rheumatoid-like manifestations are almost always due to chronic tophaceous gout, and the patient does not have RA.

Therapeutic decisions. Therapy for an acute attack can consist of colchicine and NSAIDs (other than aspirin, which is ineffective against acute gout). IV colchicine decreases the incidence of diarrhea, the most troubling side effect. After subsidence of the acute attack, prophylactic colchicine or an NSAID can prevent recurrences.

A 24-hour urine collection for urate excretion should be obtained. If it is elevated (> 600 mg/day on a diet low in organ meats for a week beforehand) or if attacks recur despite therapy, a uricosuric (e.g., probenecid) or a xanthine oxidase inhibitor (e.g., allopurinol) should be instituted. If there is a history of urinary urate calculi or intrinsic renal disease, which might impair the response to uricosurics, allopurinol is preferable. Lowering the urate level too rapidly can precipate acute attacks of gout, and initial dosage should be low.

In rare instances, prior GI side effects or disease preclude use of NSAIDs or colchicine for an acute attack. IV corticosteroids can then be used.

The incidence of renal failure in patients with gout is low, but urate deposits can develop in the kidney paraenchyma. Urate calculi occur in about 20% of patients with gout. The incidence is proportional to the 24-hour urate excretion. Chemotherapy for malignancy can cause extensive cell lysis and excessive purine catabolism, resulting in very high serum urate levels. Allopurinol therapy can prevent these complications.

METABOLIC BONE DISEASE

Osteoporosis

There is a progressive loss of bone mass with increasing age in adulthood. Loss of the effect of gonadal hormones on bone metabolism accelerates this loss, a phenomenon most marked in women after menopause. Trabecular bone, which is more metabolically active than cortical bone, shows the effects of causes of osteoporosis most markedly; sites of trabecular bone, such as vertebral bodies and the neck of the femur, are most likely to undergo pathological fractures as a result of osteoporosis.

Over the normal life span, women lose about half their bone mass and men lose about a quarter. The clinical significance of this loss depends in part on the starting level in each individual. Bone production is increased by physical stress, and bone mass is generally greater in people who have had greater physical activity. Physical inactivity, especially immobilization, aggravates bone loss. Dietary calcium depri-

vation or malabsorption also contributes to the development or severity of osteoporosis, probably by causing an increase in parathyroid hormone secretion. Administration of corticosteroids is a major factor in patients treated with such agents. Other endocrinopathies can contribute, including acromegaly or thyroid or adrenocortical hyperfunction. Similarly, chronic alcoholism, heparin administration, and some connective tissue diseases cause osteoporosis.

Osteoporosis is manifest clinically by a tendency to fractures, especially compression fractures of the vertebral bodies (especially midthoracic) and fractures of the upper femur (subcapital, neck, or intertrochanteric). Vertebral collapse causes back pain and muscle spasm, which gradually subside. Loss of height and dorsal kyphosis may become detectable. Fractured hips require surgical pinning in order to avoid prolonged immobilization and its complications, particularly thromboembolic phenomena. Despite surgery, there is a high mortality rate from a fractured hip (about 15%) and a high frequency of permanentt disability among survivors.

Radiological evidence of osteoporosis includes loss of horizontal trabeculae in vertebral bodies early, thinning of the cortex of long bones, and in advanced cases compression fractures with loss of anterior height (wedging) of thoracic vertebrae.

Prevention and therapy of osteoporosis include estrogen replacement, especially the first 5 years after menopause and in women with early onset of menopause, with progestin cycling to prevent endometrial hyperplasia which might become carcinomatous. The diet is supplemented with calcium (1 to 1.5 g/day) along with supplemental vitamin D (a minimum of 400 to 500 units/day). A program of exercises is also useful. In extreme cases, sodium fluoride is added to the regimen.

Osteomalacia

Osteomalacia is a metabolic bone disease resulting from inadequate mineralization of bone matrix (osteoid). When it develops in children, it is called **rickets**. Osteomalacia results from inadequate absorption of calcium, which results from hypovitaminosis D and lack of the hydroxylated derivatives of vitamin D, which affect calcium absorption in the intestine, especially 1,25-dihydroxyvitamin D. The disease may be caused by a dietary deficiency of vitamin D in people not exposed to sunlight and by failure of absorption of vitamin D in various intestinal malabsorption syndromes. It can also occur as a result of phosphate deficiency such as occurs with excess use of antacids or phosphate wasting with renal tubular disease.

Clinically, there may be bone aches and muscle weakness. Deformities appear in children, including bowlegs and enlargement of the cartilaginous areas of bone growth such as at the epiphyses. Similar enlargement occurs at the junction of the ribs and costal cartilages (**rachitic rosary**). The pull of the diaphragm on softened bones causes indentation of the lower ribs (**Harrison's groove**). Osteomalacia increases the incidence of fractures.

Radiological changes are similar to those of osteoporosis, but in addition pseudofractures (lucent streaks in the cortex of long bones, also known as **Looser's zones**) may be seen.

Diagnostic decisions. A relatively low serum calcium value with low serum phosphorus (due to secondary hyperaparathyroidism) is diagnostic. For the same reason, the serum alkaline phosphatase is elevated. Definitive studies are done by bone biopsy, especially with use of tetracycline labeling (administration of tetracycline at 2-week intervals), labeling the osteoid with fluorescent material that can be visualized as decalcified bone (the spaces between the fluorescent bands represent the amount of osteoid formed in the interval). Osteoid formation is depressed or low normal in osteomalacia.

CONNECTIVE TISSUE DISEASES

RHEUMATOID ARTHRITIS (RA)

RA is a chronic inflammatory disease that can affect multiple organ systems. It affects joints and periarticular tissues primarily, but the basic process is mainly a vasculitis. Therefore, in many patients the disease also affects the organs particularly susceptible to vasculitic manifestations, such as the skin, subcutaneous tissue, eyes, lungs, pleura, pericardium, spleen, and nervous system.

Pathologically, the primary lesion is inflammation of small arteries or arterioles, probably resulting from deposition of immune complexes. Local production of antibodies occurs in the lesions, especially an IgM antibody to altered gamma globulin that is called **rheumatoid factor**. Collections of immunocompetent cells appear in the lesions. As a result of local production of arachidonic acid derivatives by affected synovial cells and infiltrating inflammatory cells, there is activation of complement and the kinin system and production of toxic oxygen radicals, which lead to tissue damage, vasodilation, manifestations of inflammation, and chemotactic attraction of other leukocytes. RA is characterized by proliferation and thickening of the synovial lining of joints, causing the appearance of masses of soft tissue around joints and increased production of synovial fluid, leading to large effusions in joints.

The proliferation of synovial tissues can extend over the joint surfaces, forming a pannus or carpet of abnormal tissue that can lead to erosion and thinning of the joint cartilage and even destruction of the bone adjacent to joints. Occasionally, extensive joint erosion occurs, leading to severe deformities. Most of the deformity of affected joints is due to heaped up, thickened synovial tissue, but other deformities are caused by changes in tendons, altering their alignment and resulting in distortion of forces about the joints or shortening of muscles due to spasm, leading to contractures.

Another pathological process characteristic of RA is the appearance of granulomatous lesions in the form of nodules. They begin as areas of vasculitis and are characterized by central areas of fibrinoid deposition surrounded by macrophages (called histiocytes or epithelioid cells) and an outer zone of lymphocytes and plasma cells. These nodules appear at sites of pressure, such as around the elbows, as well as in the synovial membrane of affected joints. Occasionally such granulomatous nodules appear in other organs such as the lungs (where a solitary nodule can be confused with a tumorous coin lesion), the pleura, the heart or pericardium, and the cranial cavity (where they can be confused with brain tumors such as meningiomas). Although only about 80% of patients with RA have positive tests for rheumatoid factor (the rest are considered to have seronegative RA), all patients with nodules are seropos-

itive. A negative test is therefore useful in differential diagnosis when the nodule can be confused with another type of lesion, since it virtually rules out RA.

Clinical manifestations.   RA is more common in women and can begin at any age from early infancy to old age, but most frequently it begins in early adulthood. The onset is usually gradual, progressively affecting many joints, especially small joints of the hands and feet usually symmetrically. The disease can begin as involvement of one or a few joints but usually progresses quickly to affect several joints. Rarely the onset is explosive, with severe inflammation of most peripheral joints appearing abruptly. The patient will complain of pain, swelling, and loss of motion of affected joints, and there will be objective signs of inflammation. Usually the pain and joint stiffness are most severe on arising in the morning.

Once the disease begins, it may remain mild for many years, may be persistent and inexorably progressive, or may undergo periods of remission. It may be characterized by severe pain, effusions, and inflammation, or destructive joint changes may quickly develop.

Muscle symptoms are common, including myalgias, weakness, and atrophy. Destruction of tendinous tissue by pannus in the synovium of a tendon sheath can lead to tendon rupture with sudden loss of function (such as inability to flex a finger). An enlarged popliteal bursa (Baker's cyst) can extend down into the calf and mimic the findings of thrombophlebitis. On rare occasions, involvement of the cervical spine can lead to atlanto-occipital dislocation, with danger of cord compression. Involvement of the synovial joint between the cricoid and arytenoid cartilages can cause immobilization of the vocal cords in abduction, the resulting stridor requiring a tracheostomy.

Systemic symptoms are frequent, including ease of fatigue and weight loss; occasionally high spiking fevers are encountered, most commonly in children (the term **Still's disease** is often used for these cases). When high fever occurs in older people with RA, the term **adult Still's disease** is applied. The fever can be present before the joint symptoms and cause diagnostic difficulty. Such patients are often considered to have fever of unknown origin for long periods.

Other organs that can be involved include the eyes (episcleritis), lungs (pleural effusions, interstitial fibrosis, or solitary nodules resembling coin lesions) and heart (pericarditis). Splenomegaly with neutropenia (**Felty's syndrome**) can develop. A chronic anemia (normocytic or microcytic) is common.

The usual laboratory findings include the anemia, hypoalbuminemia, elevated ESR, and other acute-phase reactants and positive serological tests. The most useful serological test is for rheumatoid factor, which is antibody against the Fc fragment of IgG. Rheumatoid factors are usually IgM but can be IgG or IgA. Rheumatoid factors are found in about 80% of patients with RA (the seropositive cases); the others are considered seronegative and generally have milder disease. Some have one of the other syndromes described below, such as Reiter's syndrome. Rheumatoid factors are also found in some apparently normal people, and in 15 to 20% or more of patients with SLE, liver disease, and a variety of chronic infections, especially SBE. In patients with RA, rheumatoid factors can activate complement, make immune complexes insoluble, enhance chemotaxis and phagocytosis, and cause generation of inflammatory peptides including the kinins.

Therapeutic decisions.   The basic therapy for RA is the use of anti-inflammatory agents, starting with aspirin or the newer (less toxic) NSAIDs. Adjunctive physical therapy including heat, modalities including ultrasound, and exercises to preserve range of motion of joints are also helpful and should be instituted early. Locally severe inflammation or a single joint which is the main problem can be treated with intra-articular corticosteroids. Persistence of inflammatory disease despite these measures or evidence of progressive destruction or erosion of joint surfaces is an indication for use of disease-modifying agents, such as gold or penicillamine; antimalarial therapy (hydroxychloroquine) is also disease modifying but less frequently effective. If the disease remains progressive and destructive despite these agents, immunosuppressants are used.

Complications such as tendon rupture or a Baker's cyst dissecting into the calf are urgent indications for surgery. Deformities such as ulnar deviation of the fingers, which severely compromise function, also should be treated surgically early. Surgical synovectomy for thickened, inflamed synovial tissue is only of transient benefit. Extensive joint destruction can require prosthetic joint replacements, which are quite successful.

Complications such as systemic vasculitis may require systemic corticosteroid therapy, but otherwise corticosteroids such as prednisone should rarely be used and when used should be given in very small doses (< 10 mg/day).

OTHER COMMON RHEUMATIC DISORDERS

Sjögren's syndrome

Sjögren's syndrome is a connective disease characterized by dryness of the mucous membranes, especially the mouth and eyes (**sicca syndrome**). It results from inflammatory infiltration and destruction of salivary, lacrimal, and other exocrine glands. Dry, irritated eyes require therapy with artificial tears; corneal damage can occur as a result of the dryness of the eyes. The dryness of other mucous membranes also can cause considerable discomfort; a dry mouth often requires frequent water ingestion, otitis media can result from eustachian tube obstruction, dysphagia from esophageal dryness, and dyspareunia from vaginal dryness.

Associated problems include renal tubular acidosis, neuropathy, and interstitial lung disease. Biliary cirrhosis has also been observed with Sjögren's disease. Systemic lymphadenopathy is common, and localized lesions are confused with lymphomas (pseudolymphoma); true lymphomas occur with increased frequency in these patients.

A genetic basis is suggested by an association with HLA antigens B8, DR3, and DRw52. IgM rheumatoid factor is frequently found, and antinuclear antibodies to SS-A and SS-B are commonly found (see page 94).

Sjögren's syndrome occurs as a primary disease without an associated connective tissue disease and also a secondary form in association with RA, SLE, scleroderma, or polymyositis. Association with nonrheumatic systemic disease also occurs.

Diagnosis is made by establishing lack of tear formation using Schirmer's test, demonstrating lack of wetting of filter paper inserted into a corner of the eye after 5 minutes. There is a high incidence of corneal damage seen by slit-lamp examination. A definitive diagnosis can be made by biopsy of labial salivary glands, demonstrating atrophy and infiltration with lymphocytes.

Psoriatic arthritis

Psoriatic arthritis occurs in about 5% of patients with psoriasis. The clinical manifestations are similar to those of RA, with a few extra features. Involvement of the distal interphalangeal joint is common. When this occurs, the overlying nail is usually thickened and hyperkeratotic. Spondylitis is common, resembling the clinical and radiological findings in the spine seen in Reiter's syndrome and ankylosing spondylitis (AS). The course can be limited to disease of the distal interphalengeal joints, or there can be severe inflammation and extensive erosion of joint surfaces (arthritis mutilans).

When the spine is affected, back pain and stiffness usually occur, with radiological evidence of scaroiliitis.

The arthritis frequently flares simultaneously with flareups of the skin lesions, but occasional cases occur with minimal skin involvement, sometimes limited to seborrheic dermatitis of the scalp. There is an association with HLA-B27 antigen; it is found in 60% of patients with psoriatic spondylarthropathy (but only 8% of the white population in general). B17, Bw38, Bw39, and DRw4 are increased in patients with peripheral psioratic arthritis.

Treatment of psoriatic arthritis is similar to that for RA; gold compounds and other immunosuppressants are often needed.

Reiter's syndrome

Reiter's syndrome is characterized by mucocutaneous and joint lesions leading to the triad of urethritis, conjunctivitis, and arthritis. Diarrhea and skin lesions also are frequently associated. The disease is recognized much more commonly in men. A venereal etiology is suspected in a high proportion of the cases, but the offending organism is in doubt (a similar syndrome occurs in association with gonorrhea, but the term *Reiter's syndrome* is not usually applied to these cases). Dysentery due to *Salmonella, Shigella,* or *Yersinia* can lead to the same syndrome. Some cases are familial, and a spondyloarthropathy often occurs. There is a high association of the B27 antigen (75% in white, 37% in blacks with Reiter's).

Joint lesions are usually inflammatory, with large effusions. Multiple joints, including the spine, are involved, but often the process is not symmetrical, in contrast to RA. Many cases are transient, but a chronic arthritis can develop. Extensive joint erosions rarely occur.

Ankylosing spondylitis

The syndrome of AS occurs as an idiopathic disease (formerly known as rheumatoid spondylitis). It also occurs in association with Reiter's syndrome, psoriatic arthritis, ulcerative colitis, regional enteritis, and Whipple's disease. These syndromes are characterized by an **enthesiopathy**, which is involvement of the insertion of ligaments into bones. The new periosteal bone formation that results at these sites can be painful, particularly when developing. There are characteristic radiological findings. Sacroiliitis, spondylitis, inflammatory disorders of the uveal tract of the eye, and an asymmetric peripheral arthritis that is rarely erosive also occur. There is a high frequency of HLA-B27 antigen in all of these syndromes, highest in idiopathic AS. The rheumatoid factor is negative, hence these diseases are known as seronegative spondyloarthropathies.

Idiopathic AS is more common in whites and is especially common in American Indians. It is much more common in men (at least 3:1), but isolated sacroiliitis is about equally common in men and women. Family history is often positive for the same disease.

Symptoms usually start in the late teens or 20s, with soreness and pain in the lower spine, along with stiffness. The pain often radiates into the buttocks and down the posterior aspect of the legs ("sciatic" pain). Enthesiopathic pain occurs in a variety of places where tendons or ligament insert into bones; examples include Achilles tendinitis, iliac crest pain, pain in the buttocks due to inflammation of the ischial tuberosities, plantar fasciitis, and rib cage pain. Peripheral arthritis occurs, especially in the shoulders and hips, occasionally in the knees and other joints. The peripheral arthritis is rarely erosive. Extensive involvement of the spine can occur, extending from the sacroiliac area to the neck.

Eye involvement, which is usually an iridocyclitis, causes pain, photophobia, and redness. Involvement of the aortic root occurs and can lead to aortic valvular insufficiency and to left ventricular failure.

On physical examination, there is usually spasm of the paravertebral muscles with decreased mobility of the spine. The lumbar lordosis is decreased. Involvement of the costovertebral joints can limit chest cage motion on inspiration. When severe, impaired drainage of secretions from the lungs leads to pulmonary infections and COPD. Progression of the disease can lead to fixed forward flexion of the spine and a stooped posture. Flexion of the neck can impair the ability to see ahead, but severe disability is uncommon. The pain eventually subsides as the inflammation recedes, but increasing stiffness and loss of motion of the spine frequently develop.

Radiologically, early there is evidence of widening of the sacroiliac joint space with fuzziness of the joint surfaces, progressing to narrowing and fusion of these joints. Vertebral bodies becomes squared as the periosteal bone production resulting from the enthesiopathy fills in the normal anterior concavity of the vertebral bodies. Erosions of the superior and inferior margins of the bodies occur, followed by fibrosis and calcification of the ligaments that surround the vertebral bodies. New bone formation can occur, bridging the intervertebral spaces. Ultimately the appearance is that of a "bamboo spine," with calcific density surrounding the entire length of the involved spine. Other laboratory tests are normal except for the ESR and the B27 antigen, which is present in 90% of whites with the disease and 50% of blacks, but only 8% of the unaffected white population and 4% of blacks. The diagnosis can be made without testing for this antigen, and the majority of people with a positive test for the antigen do not have AS. It is therefore rarely indicated to order this test.

Treatment of AS consists primarily of NSAIDs and exercise therapy to maintain the spine as straight as possible.

Ankylosing spondylitis in other syndromes

AS occurs in association with **ulcerative colitis** and **regional enteritis.** In both, there is a lower ratio of men to women than in true AS and a high frequency of B27 antigen, although not as high as in true AS. Spondylitis occurs in roughly 5% of people with ulcerative colitis and about 7% of people with regional enteritis. Isolated sacroiliitis occurs with a higher frequency in both conditions. Peripheral arthritis also occurs in both types of inflammatory bowel disease, as can iridocyclitis and erythema nodosum.

The peripheral arthritis is rarely erosive and usually subsides when the bowel disease goes into remission. The spondylitis is similar to that of idiopathic, true AS both clinically and radiologically. It does not improve as often as the peripheral arthritis when the bowel disease subsides.

OSTEOARTHRITIS

Osteoarthritis (OA) primarily affects older people since it is essentially a wear and tear process that causes slow destruction of articular cartilage. Erosions of articular cartilage are the fundamental lesions in the disease, with secondary proliferation of bone, both at the joint margins (forming outgrowths called osteophytes) and of the underlying articular cortical bone because of the extra stresses to which it is subjected. This thickening of the articular cotrical bone is called eburnation, because the resulting dense bone is like ivory. Increased osteoclast as well as osteoblast activity occurs, leading to areas of erosion of the subchondral bone in some instances.

Flaking of cartilage from the surface where erosions are occurring causes a secondary synovitis, partly because of phagocytosis of these fragments. Synovitis, however, is a relatively minor feature of this disease, in contrast to RA, which is primarily an inflammatory process.

OA is classified as primary when no other form of musculoskeletal disease is playing a causative role. Often some postural abnormality such as knock-knees, bowlegs, or scoliosis is identifiable, putting extra physical stress on focal areas of specific joints and leading to the osteoarthritic breakdown. Secondary OA often develops in patients who had epiphysitis or congenital subluxation of a hip, altering the contour of the joint and leading to increased stresses. Chondromalacia of the patella (breakdown of the cartilage on the posterior surface of the patella) is very common.

OA is a focal process, affecting some joints or even parts of a joint but sparing other areas (in contrast to RA, which is a generalized process affecting multiple joints in each patient.)

The most common joints affected by OA are the intervertebral and facet joints of the spine, the hips, the knees and the distal interphalangeal joints of the fingers. The disease is characterized by pain that is aggravated by joint use, morning stiffness, muscle atrophy, and gradual loss of motion. On examination, bony enlargement may be evident and tenderness is common over parts of affected joints. Small effusions may be present.

Laboratory examination usually shows no significant abnormalities unless other diseases are present. In contrast to RA, the ESR is usually normal in OA, since inflammation is such a minor aspect of this disease. X-rays of affected joints demonstrate narrowing of joint spaces (due to destruction of the cartilage that occupies the space seen on x-ray), osteophyte formation, and increased density of underlying bone, as well as erosions. The clinical manifestations do not correlate well with the extent of the x-ray findings.

Therapeutic decisions. Therapy should consist of analgesics, usually in the form of NSAIDs such as aspirin. Acetaminophen is quite useful even though it is not anti-inflammatory, since it is analgesic and has much less gastric toxicity than other agents. Steroids are not useful systemically, although intra-articular injections can give temporary benefit, especially when a flare-up has occurred, probably representing a traumatic synovitis. Frequent injection, however, can lead to progression of the disease. Physical therapy is quite useful, including heat and various modalities to relieve pain. Exercises to strengthen the muscles that protect and move specific involved joints are an essential component of therapy. When joint destruction is extensive and pain is severe, replacement joint surgery is very effective, especially for hip disease.

PAINFUL NECK AND SHOULDER SYNDROMES

Pain arising from the cervical spine is often due to disk disease; it is usually felt in the neck and the back of the head and is aggravated by movements of the neck. Limitation of motion of the neck is frequently detectable, especially lateral bending and rotation (turning of the head). The pain may radiate to the shoulder and arm. If a nerve root is affected, such as C6 or C7, pain and sensory and motor abnormalities in the shoulder and arm are usually present (see page 107).

Pain arising at the thoracic outlet, such as that caused by a cervical rib, is usually felt over or between the shoulders posteriorly. It is induced by movements of the arm or neck, and usually there is tenderness over the supraclavicular space. A palpable lesion may be found in that fossa, such as an aneurysm of the subclavian artery, a cervical rib, or a tumor originating in the lung. The pulse may be obliterated when the patient takes a deep breath with the head turned or the neck extended (Adson's test), and there may be unilateral Raynaud's phenomenon and trophic changes including interosseus muscle atrophy, as well as sensory loss over the ulnar side of the hand. X-rays may show the lesion, and electromyographic studies can point to disease affecting the brachial plexus.

Disease of the tendinous cuff of the shoulder causes pain localized to the shoulder, often worse at night, with local, even point tenderness. The symptoms are usually aggravated by abduction, internal rotation, and extension, and there is usually limitation of these motions. The site of the pathology may be the supraspinatus tendon, the infraspinatus, or inflammation of the subjacent subdeltoid bursa. Rupture of the rotator cuff causes marked weakness of abduction and forward flexion and sometimes a palpable gap in the tendinous cuff.

Inflammation of the tendinous structures of the shoulder can result in **adhesive capsulitis** with marked limitation of motion (**frozen shoulder**). Findings of nerve root compression are absent in these syndromes.

Diagnostic decisions. Calcification, which often appears in sites of necrosis in the tendinous cuff, can be visualized on x-ray. An arthrogram is useful to confirm a rupture of the cuff.

No other laboratory tests are needed unless extensive destruction has occurred, in which case electron-microscope examination of aspirated joint fluid can reveal apatite crystals, indicating the presence of Milwaukee shoulder.

Therapeutic decisions. Therapy for inflammatory lesions of the structures around the shoulder, especially those with focal tenderness on examination, usually respond to local injection of corticosteroids. NSAIDs are also useful, as are physical measures such as ultrasound and heat. Exercises are important to preserve joint motion.

SYSTEMIC LUPUS ERYTHEMATOSUS

SLE is a disease of unknown etiology that is mediated primarily by immune mechanisms. It affects women about eight times more often than men, and black women about three times more often than white. Small blood vessels are the primary site affected, and manifestations can appear in almost any organ but are most frequent in skin, joints, kidneys, serosal surfaces, and the CNS.

Immunoglobulins, complement components, and immune complexes can be demonstrated in lesions in most organs, including in the skin at the dermal-epidermal junction even at apparently unaffected sites in patients with the disease (the **lupus band test**), as well as in affected glomeruli. The inflammation affecting capillaries and small arteries and venules can cause skin lesions that on biopsy are described as leukocytoclastic vasculitis, a type of pathology encountered in a variety of connective tissue diseases. The vessels show areas of necrosis, deposition of fibrinoid, interruption of the vessel wall, endothelial cell hypertrophy, local hemorrhage, and cellular infiltrate around the vessel, which is usually leukocytic but can be lymphocytic.

Clinically, SLE is very variable, and affected patients often have remissions and exacerbations over many years. The disease usually starts in early adulthood, and the primary group affected are women during childbearing years. There are 11 manifestations that are on the list of official criteria developed to assist in the diagnosis of SLE. A patient is considered to have enough criteria to warrant a diagnosis of SLE if four are present. The official criteria include the following (in each instance, other causes of these phenomena must be ruled out):

1. A **skin rash**, commonly red macules, most often over the malar areas of the face, giving a butterfly distribution, but occasionally more generalized and even petechial or hemorrhagic.

2. A more destructive local skin change, with scaliness and pigmentary changes, as well as atrophy of skin appendages, which is called a **discoid rash**. It has a characteristic pathology.

3. **Photosensitivity**, which occurs in many patients, resulting in a flare-up of systemic manifestations of the disease following exposure to sunlight (or ultraviolet light of other origin).

4. **Mucosal ulcers**, especially in the mouth or nasopharynx. These are usually superficial and painless and frequently become secondarily infected with *Candida* and thus appear as white patches.

5. **Joint pains**, often with minor objective signs of inflam-

mation. The most frequent manifestations of SLE, these arthralgias usually affect multiple small joints of the hands as well as large joints. (Rheumatoid factor can be found in about 20% of patients with SLE, and the distinction from RA may be difficult, especially since RA can cause serositis and other systemic manifestations. However, RA does not cause kidney disease, and nodules like those seen in RA are rare in SLE, as are joint erosions, contractures, and deformities.)

6. **Serositis** is common, manifested as pleurisy (pain and friction rub, with or without effusions) or pericarditis. Echocardiograms usually reveal the presence of an effusion.

7. **Renal disease.** The kidney involvement can give a picture of acute glomerulonephritis with an active sediment (RBC and WBC casts) plus some proteinuria, or a nephrotic syndrome with severe proteinuria and edema. Hypertension and renal failure can develop, requiring maintenance dialysis (see below).

8. **CNS involvement.** Not rare, it can consist of convulsive seizures, a frank psychosis, a sterile meningitis, and vasculitic lesions of the spinal cord. Peripheral neuropathy is not as common as in cases of periarteritis nodosa, which affects larger arteries.

9. **Hematologic abnormalities.** A leukopenia (<1,500/ mm^3) occurs during flare-ups of the disease, and a neutropenia can also occur. A mild, normochromic normocytic anemia is common, but a frank acquired hemolytic anemia also occurs and can be severe. Thrombocytopenia is not rare, and many cases that begin as ITP develop other lesions characteristic of SLE. A circulating anticoagulant can develop in patients with SLE, paradoxically leading to problems of thromboembolic disease, including peripheral phlebitis, pulmonary emboli, and strokes.

10. **Antinuclear antibody** (see discussion below).

11. **Immunologic findings.** In addition to ANA and LE cells, low complement levels are frequently observed during active SLE, and antibodies to a variety of antigens can be found in these patients. The term **immunologic epilepsy** was used to describe this syndrome. These antibodies can become a special problem when they cause transfusion reactions, and finding compatible blood when cross-matching patients with SLE can occasionally be extremely difficult. Biologic false-positive tests for syphilis are common in SLE.

Other manifestations of SLE occur but are not included in the basic criteria for the diagnosis because of rarity or lack of specificity. These include the following:

Raynaud's phenomenon occurs frequently, sometimes with mild skin thickening over the fingers distally, which can resemble the changes seen in early scleroderma.

Abdominal pain is probably due to vasculitic lesions in the abdomen. Acute pancreatitis can develop as a result of the vasculitis in that organ. Splenomegaly and generalized adenopathy are occasionally noted. Hepatomegaly is infrequent, and hepatitis is rare. A syndrome called **lupoid hepatitis**, once thought to result from SLE, is probably unrelated to true SLE. It is a chronic active viral hepatitis with a positive ANA.

Myalgias and frank myositis can occur, with proximal muscles affected more severely than distal muscles, resembling the findings seen in polymyositis.

Secondary infections are frequent in patients with SLE.

Urinary tract infections are most common, but pneumonia is a frequent problem and can become life threatening. Therapy requires appropriate antibiotics plus concomitant corticosteroids to suppress the basic disease.

Pregnancy can cause an exacerbation of SLE, but in most cases no change or a remission occurs. After delivery, the patient usually returns to the previous level of disease activity. The fetus is usually not affected, but there has been a rather high frequency of failure to thrive after delivery, with death in infancy. Cord blood contains ANA, but this apparently does no significant harm to the fetus, except for antibodies to ribonucleoprotein (anti-RNP), which have been associated with a high frequency of congenital heart block. Pacemakers are required by such infants.

Drug-induced SLE can result from a variety of agents that induce a positive ANA and many of the manifestations of SLE. This syndrome develops in both men and women. Arthritis, rashes, fever, pleurisy, pericarditis, plus leukopenia and occasionally other hematologic changes are the most common manifestations of drug-induced SLE. Hypergammaglobulinemia, positive ANA, and occasionally a positive VDRL occur, but renal and CNS disease do *not* develop in these patients and the entire syndrome disappears within a few months of stopping the drug. No anti-dsDNA or anti-Sm antibodies (see below, under "Immunologic findings") appear in drug-induced SLE. Procainamide is the most frequent cause of drug-induced SLE, occurring in up to 30% of patients receiving it for long periods, but hydralazine, isoniazid, phenytoin, pencillamine, quinidine, and other drugs have been implicated.

Therapeutic decisions. Therapy of SLE consists first of NSAIDs for treatment of mild symptoms, including mild fever and arthralgias. More serious manifestations such as high fever and systemic manifestations require corticosteroids, which can be lifesaving and may be necessary in high doses. Steroid toxicity can be a serious problem, including moon face, acne, muscle weakness, striae, thin skin, and ecchymoses. Truncal obesity, impaired carbohydrate tolerance, and susceptibility to infections also occur. Since the drugs are often needed for long periods, osteoporosis can become a major problem.

When the renal disease is severe, renal biopsy is usually performed to determine the type of kidney involvement, and a decision is then made whether to switch to immunosuppressant therapy. In the presence of diffuse proliferative glomerulonephritis or severe systemic disease unresponsive to steroids, cyclophosphamide is usually used to induce a remission, followed by azathioprine for maintenance.

Immunologic findings in SLE and other systemic connective tissue diseases

ANA is characteristic of SLE, and the diagnosis is rarely made in its absence. It is usually demonstrated by immunofluorescence, based on the binding of the antibody in patient's serum to a source of nuclei, such as sections of rat liver, followed by addition of a labeled antibody against human IgG. many of these antibodies are directed against DNA. Similar antibodies exist against other nuclear components and some against cytoplasmic antigens.

Antibody against native, double-stranded DNA (dsDNA) is most specific for SLE and correlates with the presence of active renal disease; in general the titer of anti-dsDNA reflects the degree of activity of the disease process and is a useful parameter to follow. The overall titer of ANA does not correlate well with disease activity.

Antibody to single-stranded DNA is not as specific for SLE.

Antibodies to histones (the protein component of many nucleoproteins) occur in 30 to 60% of SLE sufferers but are present in almost all cases of drug-induced lupus and about 20% of patients with RA.

Anti-Sm (so called for a patient named Smith) antibodies are directed against another nuclear component that is not degraded by ribonuclease but is not a histone. It is quite specific for SLE but is present in only about 40% of cases.

Anti-RNP antibody is directed against a nuclear antigen that is degraded by ribonuclease and protease. It is particularly common in **overlap syndrome**, in which there are features of SLE, polymyositis, and scleroderma concomitantly. It also occurs occasionally in other rheumatic syndromes.

Antibodies to SS-A (also called anti-Ro) and SS-B (anti-La), which usually cause a speckled pattern on immunofluorescent assay, are another ANA. Anti-SS-A is transmitted across the placenta and is found in infants with neonatal lupus, especially those with heart block. It is also seen in Sjögren's syndrome (about 60%) and SLE (about 30%). Anti-SS-B is less frequent.

In patients with scleroderma, anti-Scl-70 and anti-centromere antibodies are seen as well; the latter seems to correlate with CREST syndrome (calcinosis, **R**aynaud's syndrome, esophageal dysmotility, sclerodactyly [i.e., sclerodermatous changes of the distal parts of the fingers], and telangiectasia). It occurs in about 80% of patients with this form of scleroderma.

ANAs seen in polymyositis or dermatomyositis include PM-1, which occurs in about 50% (and in over 80% of patients with overlap syndrome). LO-1 antibody occurs in about a third of patients with polymyositis but only about 5% of patients with dermatomyositis. Another antibody, Mi-2, occurs in about a third of patients with dermatomyositis.

LE cells were the first manifestations of ANA to be detected, but the test for them is rarely indicated today, since it requires a great deal of technician time. The test can be performed on an emergency basis, however, and may be ordered when the diagnosis is in doubt and an immediate answer is needed, whereas the ANA is usually available only on a routine basis.

Complement consists of series of enzymes and cofactors that generate products that promote chemotaxis and phagocytosis and can cause lysis of cell membranes. The classic pathway begins when antigen-antibody complexes bind to Clq, activating other components of Cl (C1r, C1s). C4 and C2 are subsequently activated, followed by C3, which is cleaved, generating two fragments, C3a and C3b.

The alternative (properdin) pathway can be activated by IgA, bacterial polysaccharides, endotoxins, and probably also IgE. The factors in this pathway include factor B, factor D, and properdin (P). They also generate the active components derived from cleavage of C3.

The terminal sequence of complement is activated by products of C3 generated by either the classic or alternative pathway and is called the attack sequence. It includes components C5, C6, C7, C8, and C9. The C5–9 complex binds to target cells, lysing the cell wall (e.g., RBC or bacterial cells).

The components of the complement sequence are consumed faster than they can be replaced during some immunologic reactions, including the binding of some autoantibodies to antigens, decreasing levels in the plasma. Measurement of complement levels can be useful in following the activity of some autoimmune diseases, especially SLE. Assays are reported as CH_{50} (50% hemolytic activity) or as assay of individual components, especially C3 or C4. A decrease in one or more of these levels indicates increased activity of the disease. Therapy can result in return of levels toward normal. Congenital complement deficiencies exist and can be misleading.

OTHER SYSTEMIC CONNECTIVE TISSUE DISEASES

Polymyalgia rheumatica and giant cell arteritis

Muscle aches, primarily in the shoulder and pelvic girdle, occur in older people (generally over 50) in association with a high ESR. This syndrome, called polymyalgia rheumatica (PMR) is of unknown etiology. Low-grade fever, generalized achiness and stiffness, fatigue, headache, anorexia, and weight loss are common symptoms. There are no specific physical findings, and other laboratory tests are normal, including muscle enzymes (CPK, aldolase, SGOT), electromyography, and immunologic tests such as ANA and rheumatoid factor. The ESR is over 35 mm/hour, and sometimes over 100. It must be performed using a long tube (the Westergren method). Laboratories that use a short tube (the Wintrobe method) for performing ESR cannot detect ESRs over about 50, and the important clue to the existence of this disease can be missed.

Treatment of PMR usually requires steroids, but small doses are adequate (e.g., prednisone, 10 mg t.i.d. at first until the symptoms and ESR are controlled, tapering to under 10 mg/day fairly quickly).

Some cases of PMR are associated with clinical evidence of a giant cell arteritis, which primarily affects medium-sized arteries in the upper part of the body, especially temporal arteries, vessels in the scalp, and muscles of mastication. Hence there is often pain on chewing (jaw claudication) or a tender nodule on a temporal or scalp artery. Occlusions of these arteries can develop. Involvement of the ophthalmic artery is common, and unilateral blindness can develop suddenly. Lesions of other arteries also occur, including coronary vessels, and myocardial infarction can develop on this basis.

Diagnostic decisions. Biopsy of a temporal artery can establish the diagnosis of giant cell arteritis. A large segment of artery (about 5 cm) must be obtained and the entire specimen examined, since the lesions can be focal. Granulomas in the vessel wall are found, with abundant macrophages and giant cells, some with phagolysosomes containing fragments of elastin. The lesions develop only in arteries with an elastic layer, and fragmentation of the elastin can be seen. Since the retinal artery has no elastic layer, it is not affected. Patients with vision symptoms including blindness do not show changes in the fundus. The ophthalmic artery, which contains elastin, is the site of the lesions that are behind the eye.

Therapeutic decisions. Treatment of giant cell arteritis requires higher doses of prednisone. Usually 20 mg t.i.d. (60 mg/day) is given at first, and the dose slowly tapered as long as the ESR stays under control. Treatment should be started as soon as the diagnosis is considered because of the possibility of sudden onset of blindness or some other vascular catastrophe. A biopsy taken within the first few days of steroid therapy will still show the lesions.

Other forms of vasculitis

The classification of vasculitis is unsatisfactory; there is a form called **hypersensitivity vasculitis**, as well as **allergic granulomatosis** and Wegener's syndrome, all of which are characterized by granulomatous lesions and a generalized vasculitis of small arteries. Pulmonary involvement is common, and asthma, rhinitis, and hypereosinophilia occur. In Wegener's there are large granulomas in the respiratory tract, either in the sinuses, the nasal passages, or the lungs. Renal involvement is common but usually not severe. Skin lesions occur, including areas of infarction or hemorrhage, and palpable purpura occurs, especially in the lower extremities. Abdominal pain is common as a result of vasculitic lesions of the intestine. Henoch-Schönlein purpura is a similar vasculitis affecting skin with hemorrhagic lesions in the intestine with abdominal pain, as well as causing a nephritis due to the vasculitis.

Periarteritis nodosa is a form of vasculitis affecting larger, more muscular arteries. It causes widespread lesions, including renal involvement and hypertension, but pulmonary lesions are absent unless there has been antecedent hypertension of the pulmonary circulation. In the past, some cases were due to antecedent systemic hypertension.

Diagnostic decisions. Laboratory tests in general are non-specific, but biopsy of lesions can reveal the vasculitis and granulomatous lesions. Renal biopsy can be helpful. Rheumatoid factor and ANA may be present. Cryoglobulins are often present. Many cases of these syndromes have been reported as a result of infection with hepatitis B, and antibodies to that virus can be detected in the serum. In periarteritis nodosa, angiograms are more helpful in diagnosis than in syndromes affecting smaller vessels. Aneurysmal lesions can be visualized, especially in the renal vascular bed.

Therapeutic decisions. Therapy of these syndromes is generally unsatisfactory. Steroids are usually tried first. Immunosuppressants, especially cyclophosphamide, are particularly successful in the therapy of Wegener's syndrome.

POLYMYOSITIS AND DERMATOMYOSITIS (PM/DM)

PM/DM is characterized by muscle weakness, affecting proximal muscles more severely then distal, as is characteristic of inflammatory and metabolic disorders in contrast to neuropathic muscle diseases. The disease is apparently of autoimmune origin, but specific autoantibodies have not been demonstrated. A rash is common during at least part of the course, and hence the two terms refer to the same disease process. The weakness can be severe and cause respiratory muscle failure requiring ventilator support at least for a period. In general it is more common in women, possibly even with a ratio of 9:1.

Many cases of PM or DM have an underlying malignancy, but the association is controversial. Exacerbations of the muscle disease occur with recurrences of malignancy, such as the appearance of metastases, but the general association is not frequent enough to warrant a special workup of patients with PM for an underlying malignancy beyond a careful history and physical examination. Any findings suggestive of a malignancy should be followed up, however. For example, an iron deficiency anemia, a lung lesion, or a breast mass should be carefully investigated, as they should in anyone else.

Diagnostic decisions. PM/DM causes elevations of muscle enzymes, including the CPK and aldolase. The 24-hour excretion of creatine in the urine may be increased and that of creatinine decreased when there is sufficient loss of functioning muscle to fail to remove all the creatinine made each day by the liver. In the muscle it is converted to creatinine, which is excreted in an amount proportional to the functioning muscle mass. Electromyographic findings are useful, showing polyphasic potentials, fibrillations, and bizarre discharges. ANA and rheumatoid factor tests are often positive. Muscle biopsy shows infiltration with inflammatory cells, degeneration of muscle fibers resulting in variations in the width of the remaining fibrils, and proliferation of sarcolemmal nuclei.

Therapeutic decisions. Corticosteroids are effective in managing the skin lesions and the acute inflammatory muscle lesions. Large doses are often needed for the muscle pathology. Immunosuppressants are also helpful, especially for their steroid-sparing effects. Methotrexate and azathioprine are used most frequently.

PROGRESSIVE SYSTEMIC SCLEROSIS (SCLERODERMA)

Scleroderma is associated with interstitial fibrosis in many organs, hence the term *progressive systemic sclerosis*. Skin lesions are diagnostic, with an early phase characterized by edema that pits very slowly, synovitis affecting peripheral joints primarily, followed by thickening and tightening of the skin beginning in the distal parts of the fingers and the face but often extending over wide areas. Raynaud's phenomenon is usually present and can be severe. The primary lesion may be in the intima of small arteries, and the deposition of collagen secondary. Muscle involvement, with weakness and tenderness, is also common. The tightness of the skin results in loss of motion, contractures, and considerable functional disability.

In addition to the skin and muscle, the next most commonly affected organ is the gut, especially the esophagus. Dysphagia, reflux esophagitis, and abnormal motility are found commonly on investigation. More extensive lesions of the gut can occur, affecting the small bowel and leading to malabsorption and malnutrition. Pulmonary lesions are common, with an interstitial fibrosis. Loss of pulmonary function can dominate the clinical picture. Cardiovascular lesions are also frequent, and heart failure can develop due to myocardial fibrosis, although valvular lesions, pericardial fibrosis, or arrhythmias can develop. Involvement of the vessels in the kidneys can lead to sudden onset of malignant hypertension that if left untreated can lead to rapidly progressive renal failure, heart failure, or a cerebral hemorrhage.

Diagnostic decisions. Laboratory findings are generally non-specific. ANA is often positive. Skin biopsies are usually unsatisfactory, since criteria for thickening are vague. A biopsy from an area of marked involvement will heal poorly and should not be performed. Biopsies of equivocally involved areas yield equivocal results. The physical and radiological findings are usually sufficient for diagnosis. Therapy of scleroderma in general is unsatisfactory. Vasodilators are helpful for the Raynaud's phenomenon and essential for the hypertension.

Variants of scleroderma include the **CREST syndrome** (see above), which is often mild, and the **overlap syndrome**, in which manifestations of SLE or PM may dominate the picture. Both of these syndromes are usually more benign than the usual form of the disease; therapy is similar to that for similar problems in each of the basic diseases described.

DISEASES OF THE NERVOUS SYSTEM

WORKUP OF THE PATIENT WITH NEUROLOGICAL DISEASE

The approach to diagnosis of neurological disease is easier if, after analysis of the problem, an attempt is made to decide the most likely etiologic category. The nine categories of neurological disease, in alphabetical order, are as follows: degenerative, developmental (or genetic), environmental (or toxic), immunologic, infectious, metabolic/nutritional, neoplastic, traumatic, and vascular.

Points to check especially carefully in the physical examination are as follows:

Level of arousal: alert, drowsy, lethargic, stuporous (responds only to external, relatively strong stimuli), comatose (not responsive even to strong stimuli).

Mental state: orientation (person, place, time); short-term memory, which is the most vulnerable (e.g., repeat three unrelated words 5 minutes later), ability to abstract (recognize similarities, e.g., child/dwarf).

Stance and walk: If patient can walk on toes and heels, turn quickly, do deep knee bend, motor strength and coordination are fine.

Cranial nerve exam, including fundi.

Motor strength of arms and legs.

Sensation including recognition of objects placed in hand, position and vibration sense in hands and feet.

Diagnostic procedures

Lumbar puncture indications include suspicion of infection and as a check for hemorrhage before instituting anticoagulant therapy for cerebrovascular disease. A relative indication is suspected, undiagnosed CNS disease. Contradictions include infection at the site the needle would penetrate, increased intracranial pressure, and bleeding tendency (e.g., thrombocytopenia, anticoagulation) because of danger of spinal epidural hematoma.

Muscle biopsy is done primarily to distinguish neuropathic from myopathic weakness. Select an affected muscle, but one not too atrophic to show diagnostic changes. Biochemical and electron microscope examination are often helpful in addition to ordinary microscopic examination. Neuropathy leads to grouped areas of atrophy; myopathy produces random changes and variation in fiber size within individual groups, usually with migration of nuclei from central to peripheral location in fibers; infiltration with inflammation cells may be observed.

Peripheral nerve biopsy is rarely needed. It is done to check for amyoid, vasculitis, or leprosy. It is usually done on the sural nerve near the ankle, separating fibers and taking only half to minimize anesthesia of the foot.

Brain biopsy is performed open or by needle. It is done to identify the nature of an inflammatory lesion; brain biopsy used to be required to diagnose HSV encephalitis, but currently a trial of antiviral agents is given first. Biopsy may be useful for diagnosis of Alzheimer's disease or slow virus diseases such as Creutzfeldt-Jakob disease, but it is rarely indicated in view of lack of effect of the biopsy information in determining therapy.

CT scan is often done with injection of contrast material to identify increased permeability of the blood-brain barrier (contrast enhancement). The main indication is identification of anatomic changes in the brain or spine. The size of ventricles and any shift can be seen; edema formation, mass lesions, hemorrhage and infarcts identified; and subdural hematomas or brain atrophy visualized. It can miss early infarcts and other "isodense" lesions.

MR imaging gives better resolution than CT, is unaffected by bone, can visualize structures in any plane (CT is limited to coronal and horizontal planes), and can visualize areas of demyelination. It is especially useful to identify bony lesions or protruding intervertebral disks impinging on spinal cord or nerve roots. MR is contraindicated in patients with pacemakers and in those with metal clips on intracerebral aneurysms, because of the high magnetic field generated. Newer instruments are becoming much faster, and the problem of keeping patients immobile for 30 to 45 minutes will be solved.

Myelograms used to be valuable for identifying mass lesions (such as tumors or herniated disks) narrowing the spinal canal. This test has largely been replaced by the new imaging procedures.

Angiography has been improved by computerized digital subtraction techniques and is the best test for visualizing vascular lesions such as aneurysms and arteriovenous anomalies; it is indicated whenever surgical correction is possible.

Electroencephalography is useful whenever seizure activity is suspected. **Sensory evoked potentials** test the integrity of various nerve pathways. For example, visual evoked potentials can detect early, asymptomatic lesions of the optic nerve and thus help in the diagnosis of multiple sclerosis.

Nerve conduction studies distinguish between muscle disease and neuropathy as a cause of weakness. This technique helps to differentiate demyelinating neuropathy from axonal neuropathy, since demyelinating neuropathies affect mainly large fibers and thus slow conduction velocity, whereas when axons are also damaged, the decreased number of active units decreases the size of the action potential. These studies also can distinguish radiculopathy from peripheral neuropathy.

Electromyography (EMG) can reveal fibrillation potentials, indicating disease of the muscle membrane. Visible fasciculations may be seen. Damage to nerve axons results in a decreased number of active muscle units and their voluntary action potentials but an increase in the size of the action potentials. Degeneration of muscle fibers causes a decrease in size of the action potentials. The distribution of muscle or nerve abnormalities can be determined. Repeated electrical stimulation of the neuromuscular junction can reveal diminution in responses typical of myasthenia gravis or abnormal facilitation seen in the Eaton-Lambert pseudomyasthenic syndrome accompanying malignancies.

CNS INFECTIONS

The most common CNS infections—meningitis and encephalitis—are discussed in the section on infectious diseases, as are syphilis, tuberculosis, and fungal infections of the nervous system.

Epidural and subdural abscesses usually arise by direct extension from adjacent sites of infection, such as mastoiditis, paranasal sinusitis, or intervertebral disk infection. The main clinical manifestations are those of the original site of infection, but if untreated, extension may occur to produce meningitis or brain abscess. CT scan is generally the most helpful diagnostic test, and the organism can usually be identified from cultures of the original site of infection. Treatment with antibiotics is usually successful, but surgical drainage is sometimes necessary, especially with subdural abscess (empyema). Lumbar puncture should *not* be performed in patients suspected of having a subdural abscess, since organisms are not usually recovered and the CSF is usually under considerably increased pressure. The rapid changes in pressure due to the tap can induce cerebral herniation. When the abscess develops in the spine from direct extension from intervertebral disk infection or vertebral osteomyelitis, staphylococci are usually responsible. There may be local tenderness, distribution of the pain along a nerve root, fever, and leukocytosis. A high ESR is common. CT scan is usually helpful in these cases. Lumbar puncture is safe, and a pleocytosis is usually found along with elevated protein and normal glucose levels. Prolonged antibiotic therapy is necessary, since osteomyelitis of a vertebra is usually the basic, initial lesion.

Brain abscesses also arise by direct extension along venous channels from paranasal sinuses, but most develop as a result of seeding via the bloodstream following dental or urologic surgery or from septic emboli arising in acute bacterial endocarditis, a process most commonly encountered in heroin addicts. A variety of organisms cause brain abscess. Streptococci, staphylococci, *Clostridium, Actinomyces, Nocardia*, and tuberculosis are the most frequent. Symptoms resemble those of a brain tumor but progress much more rapidly, including headache and localizing signs that depend on the site of the lesion. Fever and leukocytosis are often absent. Lumbar puncture is contraindicated because of the danger of cerebral herniation. CT scan usually shows a hypodense region surrounded by a ring or halo of increased density. Differentiation from a brain tumor may be impossible before surgical exploration, and surgical aspiration may be necessary to determine the nature of the infecting organism. Most patients with brain abscess respond to appropriate antibiotics. Anticonvulsants may be needed until the lesion resolves.

Malignant external otitis, an infection primarily afflicting diabetic patients, is due to *Pseudomonas aeruginosa*. There is ear pain from the outset, but the infection spreads from the ear to the neighboring soft tissue, including the parotid gland, temporomandibular joint, and masseter muscle, and often involves the cranial nerves VI through XII. Purulent drainage is usually absent. Treatment with carbenicillin and gentamicin is required. Infection with Phycomycetes (mucormycosis) also occurs in diabetics. It usually begins in the nose or palate and spreads to the orbit. Cavernous sinus occlusion can occur. Proptosis of the affected eye and extraocular muscle paralyses

develop, along with high fever, headache, and toxicity. A black necrotic patch can usually be seen in the nose or on the palate, and scraping reveals the presence of the organism. Although antifungal agents are helpful, a fatal outcome is usual. Treatment is based on the clinical findings while awaiting the cultures.

Coccidioidomycosis and **cryptococcosis** occur in both immunocompromised and nonimmunocompromised hosts. Diagnosis is based on finding the organisms or antigens in the CSF. The most important parasitic infection is **cysticercosis**, which is due to *Taenia solium* tapeworm acquired by eating inadequately cooked pork. Brain lesions occur in about 60% of infected people, with single or multiple cysts detectable on CT or MR scans. There is increased intracranial pressure, and seizures are common. Eosinophilia and positive serological tests (primarily hemagglutination) are usually present. Therapy with the anthelmintic antibiotic praziquantel is useful. If intraventricular cysts cause obstruction to flow of CSF, a shunt may be necessary.

Reye's syndrome is a type of encephalopathy that occurs in relation to infection with influenza A or B or varicella virus, usually beginning as the viral infection clears. The syndrome is characterized by loss of liver and brain function, apparently due to abnormalities in mitochondria, which are evident by altered morphology as well as function. Metabolic derangements that develop include hyperammonemia, lactic acidosis, and elevation of free fatty acids. Hyperbilirubinemia and hypoglycemia also develop, especially in children. The syndrome usually begins with severe headache and intractable vomiting, lethargy, stupor, and coma. CSF shows high pressure but otherwise is normal. When coma develops, the mortality is high. Mortality is lower in adults. Management includes measures to decrease the intracranial pressure and correct the metabolic derangements including the acidosis and hypoglycemia. In children, the administration of aspirin has been associated with occurrence of Reye's syndrome, and it is important to avoid using this agent in any suspected infection with influenza or varicella. Acetaminophen should be used instead as an antipyretic and analgesic.

CNS TRAUMA

Brain injury occurs at the site of trauma and on the side directly opposite due to the acceleration-deceleration of the brain in the skull. **Concussion** is a brief loss of consciousness without any immediate or delayed residual effects. During the period of unconsciousness, the pupils can be fixed and dilated and there can be apnea and bradycardia. A greater degree of **diffuse injury** can produce unconsciousness lasting an hour, and recovery of orientation and behavior are slower. Pathologically, and by MR scan, no lesions may be seen, but scattered small ecchymoses and contusions may be evident. There may be some permanent behavioral change or loss of intellectual function, especially in older people. **Severe diffuse injury** is defined as trauma resulting in more delayed complications such as brain edema, ischemic infarcts, or hemorrhages, which may be extradural, subdural, or intracerebral. These are the patients who "talk and then die." With severe brain trauma there is immediate unconsciousness, and decorticate or decerebrate posturing may occur with noxious stimuli. Bilateral pupillary fixation or loss of oculovestibular responses (doll's eyes) indicates brain-stem damage and a very poor prognosis (fewer than 15% recovering reasonably satisfactorily.)

Treatment of head injury first requires putting the patient supine and flat, avoiding twisting or flexing the neck or spine in case there is a fracture. Opiates must be avoided to prevent interference with interpretation of findings. Unresponsive patients should be intubated as soon as possible. Oxygen and mechanical ventilation may be needed. Hemorrhage or fluid loss should be treated. Dehydration is not an advantage in these patients, but monitoring of serum sodium and glucose is necessary to prevent hyponatremia and hyperglycemia. Any seizure activity should be treated with diazepam and phenytoin IV. Level of consciousness and vital functions should be monitored every 30 to 60 minutes. Corticosteroids are not indicated. Aspiration pneumonia is a serious danger, and antibiotics should be started as soon as there is any indication of pulmonary or other infection. Fluid balance should be controlled and, in the absence of renal pathology, urine output about 1,500 ml/day maintained. If massive cerebral edema has developed, passive hyperventilation to reduce cerebral blood flow and 20% mannitol IV are indicated. As patients regain consciousness, codeine may be needed for pain, diazepam for mild agitation, or halperidol for severe agitation. Benzodiazepines should be given for early signs of tremulousness to prevent seizures.

Progressive deterioration at a time when improvement is expected usually means **intracranial bleeding**. CT and MR scanning are essential to detect areas of edema or hemorrhage, which can be extradural, subdural, or intracranial. If neither CT nor MR is available, arteriorgraphy should be performed, seeking evidence of shifts of intracranial structures. Skull x-rays are of some value in the absence of scanning procedures. Fracture across the middle meningeal artery groove in the temporal bone can lead to tears of the artery, with extradural bleeding. If untreated, such hemorrhages can lead to uncal or tentorial herniation. Basal skull fractures can open channels from the paranasal sinuses to the subarachnoid space, leading to CSF rhinorrhea and meningitis, which can be recurrent. Depressed skull fractures carry a high risk of posttraumatic epilepsy if not corrected.

After head injury producing unconsciousness, patients may note giddiness and irritability along with difficulty concentrating. Complete recovery is rare in adults who are comatose for a week or more. About 5% develop late epilepsy. Prophylactic phenytoin is often given for about 2 years following severe head injury.

Chronic subdural hematoma can follow apparently trivial or severe head injury by weeks to months. Alcoholism, anticoagulation, and advanced age increase the likelihood of a subdural hematoma. Sustained headache, somnolence, confusion, impaired mentation, and occasionally hemiparesis can appear. Symptoms often fluctuate in severity, perhaps because of impaired autoregulation of cerebral arteries. CT scan or MR shows the hematoma directly or indirectly through shift of the brain or, in the case of bilateral hematomas, abnormally small ventricles. After a few weeks the hematoma may become isodense and not be visualized by CT scan, but this problem does not occur with MR imaging.

Spinal cord injury if severe can cause spinal shock, with flaccidity and hypoactive deep tendon relfexes. If complete transection has occurred, bowel and bladder function is lost, as well as all sensation and motor function below the site of the injury. A Babinski's sign usually appears after a few days. Partial spinal cord injury can give a variety of syndromes. More severe local paralysis and loss of sensation can occur. **Cervical hyperextension** injury, such as occurs with a whiplash, produces primarily painful paresthesias in the arms and loss of position and vibratory sense below the lesion. **Hyperflexion** injury can damage the anterior spinal artery, causing an infarct of the cord with quadriplegia. Combinations of these injuries can occur. The **Brown-Sequard syndrome** of unilateral cord injury is rare. Treatment of spinal cord injury includes placing the patient on a flat surface and avoiding twisting or flexion, ventilatory assistance if necessary, immobilization of the neck, and treatment of any fracture-dislocation. Surgical decompression can be helpful. Rehabilitation of spinal cord injuries is slow and tedious, requiring transfer to a specialized center.

APPROACH TO THE PATIENT WITH ALTERED CONSCIOUSNESS

Coma can result from diffuse cortical damage or lesions of the tegmental reticular activating system, which is located from the most rostral position of the pons to the paramedian posterior hypothalamus.

Various levels of reduced arousal. These include coma, stupor, obtundation (drowsiness, reduced alertness), confusion, delirium, a vegetative state, a locked-in state, and brain death. The **locked-in state** occurs when efferent neural pathways are inoperative—even a very severe motor polyneuropathy can cause it—and the patient is fully aware and conscious but cannot communicate in any manner except, sometimes, by vertical eye movements. A similar state occurs when a patient is intubated and passively ventilated with blockage of motor pathways (e.g., by succinylcholine). It is important for the medical staff to be aware that such patients are totally conscious and very frightened.

Causes of stupor and coma. Supratentorial causes include lesions of the posterior ventromedial diencephalon, such as infarcts or neoplasms, or compression-herniation of the diencephalon against the midbrain, such as occurs with large intracerebral or subdural hemorrhages or tumors. These cases usually show intact pupillary and eye movements or have abnormal conjugate eye movements (doll's eyes). Compression of the brain stem can produce third nerve dysfunction. Subtentorial causes of coma include pontine or cerebellar hemorrhage, infarction, or tumor. Diffuse metabolic causes include anoxia, hypoglycemia, electrolyte abnormalities, liver or kidney failure, hypothryoidism, poisonings, and infections, including meningitis or encephalitis, concussion, and postictal states.

Subtentorial causes of coma often show accompanying brain-stem dysfunction, indicated by abnormal pupils, which may be pinpoint (pons), fixed (midbrain), irregular or unequal (both pons and midbrain). Apneustic breathing (sustained inspiratory pauses), paralysis of cranial nerve V or VII, unilateral cerebellar signs, and bilateral motor signs (flaccid or decerebrate) also can be present.

Clues to seek in the diagnosis of coma. **Fever** would suggest infection but can occur with atropine or scopolamine poisoning. **Hypothermia** suggests myxedema, hypoglycemia, or brain-stem infarction. **Stiff neck** suggests meningitis or an extensive subarachnoid hemorrhage. **Signs of trauma** would suggest concussion, cerebral contusion, or subarachnoid hemorrhage. **Hypertension** points to severe hypertensive encephalopathy or a major hemorrhage, whereas **hypotension** points to a cause of shock, low cardiac output, or depressant drugs. **Cardiac arrhythmia** suggests myocardial infarction or a tricyclic drug overdose. **Hyperventilation** points to a cause of acidosis (e.g., diabetic ketosis, uremia, salicylate poisoning), whereas **hypo-ventilation** suggests anoxia due to depressant drugs (e.g., opiate overdose), low brain-stem infarct, or hemorrhage. The presence of **petechiae** would point to thrombocytopenia with hemorrhage, meningococcemia, or bacterial endocarditis with embolic infarct or abscess. **Cherry-red lips** or pink skin suggests carbon monoxide poisoning.

Drug overdoses usually leave intact pupillary light reflexes except when due to strong anticholinergic drugs (e.g., atropine), street drugs (especially narcotics, which cause marked pupillary constriction), or deliberate use of mydriatics.

After necessary life-support measures are instituted, workup should proceed, including measurement of blood electrolytes, BUN and creatinine, glucose, and ketone bodies, ABGs, skull films, and a CT scan. If no major space-occupying lesion or hemorrhage is seen on CT scan, lumbar puncture is indicated. EEG is of little help early in the workup. If no obvious cause is found, self-induced drug overdose is likely, and tests for a variety of street drugs and pharmaceutical findings are included on workup.

Transient loss of consciousness. Syncope can be due to a vasodepressor reflex or any cause of decreased cardiac output (arrhythmia, bleeding, severe heart failure, cardiac tamponade, or any transient cause of decreased right heart filling, including coughing). Fainting due to emotional cause is common, often familial. Alcohol and hunger increase susceptibility to attacks of syncope, and hypoglycemia can cause attacks. The position the patient was in during an attack is an important clue. True syncope does not occur with a patient supine. Incontinence is unusual. Cerebral causes are rare, and extensive neurological workup is rarely necessary.

DRUG ABUSE

The problems with drug abuse, including alcohol, narcotic and other street drugs, include **psychological dependence**, craving and desire for the effects on mood and sensation; **tolerance**, requiring increased doses to achieve the desired effects; and **physical dependence**, the development of withdrawal symptoms. The psychological effects of all these drugs vary with the individual, especially when tolerance has developed. The physical effects lead to many medical problems.

Marijuana, used primarily by inhalation for the effects of delta-9-tetrahydrocannabis, causes autonomic changes, including conjunctival congestion, tachycardia, flushing, orthostatic hypotension, dry mouth, and at times vomiting. It also causes irritation of the respiratory tract and decreased sperm formation. Chronic use leads to apathy, depression, paranoia, and frank toxic psychosis.

Depressant drugs such as the benzodiazepines (e.g., Valium), barbiturates, methaqualone (Quaalude), and others are used mainly to combat anxiety, but overuse can lead to withdrawal symptoms such as increased depression, anxiety, insomnia, and some mild autonomic changes.

Cocaine, used primarily by inhalation, causes local anesthesia, fever, tachycardia, hypertension, pupillary dilatation, peripheral vasoconstriction, tachypnea, and anorexia. It produces a particularly strong craving, with a severe "crash" on withdrawal. It is therefore very addictive and socially destructive. A cerebral angiitis has been reported with cocaine and with **amphetamine** abuse.

Opiate overdose, most frequently with heroin or morphine, causes pupillary constriction, irregular breathing with hypoventilation, fall in blood pressure and body temperature, and sometimes seizures and acute pulmonary edema. Naloxone, repeated frequently, is useful in therapy. Chronic opiate abusers develop restlessness, anxiety, yawning, and rhinorrhea after receiving naloxone, effects that may be relieved by clonidine. Intravenous users often develop local infections and sepsis, including acute staphylococcal endocarditis and brain abscess. Viral hepatitis is very common, as is the development of AIDS, because of sharing of contaminated equipment.

Phenylcyclidine (PCP), recently the most frequently used hallucinogen, can cause ataxia, confusion, prolonged psychotic states characterized by aggressive behavior, convulsions, and coma. Urinary acidification with NH_4Cl and continuous gastric suction can hasten excretion of the drug and shorten a "bad trip."

The most frequently abused agent is **ethanol**. This drug is cleared by the liver and the lungs at a rate of about 8 ml/hour, which clears about 15 mg/100 ml/hour from the blood. Chronic drinkers develop tolerance to high blood levels, but legal intoxication begins at 100 g/100 ml. Lethargy usually begins at 200 mg/100 ml, and stupor at 300 to 350. After recovery from acute intoxication, withdrawal symptoms are usual, varying from a hangover (headache, difficulty concentrating, nausea, tremulousness) to severe tremors and delirium tremens (DTs). Convulsions ("rum fits") can occur. Diazepam may be necessary, sometimes in large doses, to control the seizure activity. An EEG is usually nonspecific, but if seizures are focal, a CT scan should be obtained to check for a local lesion such as a subdural hematoma. DTs, which usually follow withdrawal by 3 to 5 days, include severe tremulousness, hallucinations, and beta-adrenergic autonomic hyperactivity (sweating, tachycardia, and hypertension). Huge amounts of diazepam may be needed. Thiamine should also be given in large quantities, since alcohol overuse often is associated with malnutrition. Thiamine deficiency is particularly common, since the metabolism of alcohol uses cocarboxylase, a thiamine metabolite. Peripheral neuropathies are frequent and sometimes very painful. The full syndrome of **beriberi** can develop, including a high-output form of heart failure with massive edema. **Wernicke's syndrome** can result from axonal demyelination and other pathological changes in the nervous system. Ophthalmoplegia is common, but any cranial nerve can be affected, and diffuse anesthesia can be noted. Tachycardia, hypotension, and hypothermia can develop, and the syndrome can be fatal if not treated promptly with thiamine. Glucose given before the thiamine can aggravate the syndrome since it uses cocarboxylase in its metabolism. **Korsakoff's syndrome** also is related to alcohol abuse. It often follows Wernicke's syndrome and is characterized by a defect in recent memory accompanied by confabulation (wrong answers to questions requiring memory, convincingly given but completely different when the question is repeated).

Other syndromes produced by alcohol overuse include gastritis and hepatitis, which can cause severe liver failure and can progress to cirrhosis (see the section on GI disease), a cardiomyopathy, optic atrophy due to an optic neuritis, cerebral atrophy, and a peripheral myopathy. Peripheral myopathy can be acute, with muscle pain, cramps, weakness, and elevated CPK, and can include myoglobinemia and secondary acute renal failure. The myopathy can be chronic with diffuse, primarily proximal muscle atrophy. A localized form of cerebellar degeneration can occur with ataxia but no nystagmus or loss of coordination in the arms. A demyelination in the brain stem, **central pontine myelinosis**, can occur, with dilirium and quadriparesis. It is not directly related to alcohol but can occur in other malnourished people with hyponatremia that is corrected too rapidly. The lesions can be visualized by CT scan after a week and are slowly reversible.

HEADACHE

Most headaches are not due to structural disease and do not require expensive workup. Headaches of recent origin, especially beginning after age 30 if focal or following trauma, require a CT scan. Lumbar puncture is indicated for an unusual headache that is acute or very severe and is accompanied by fever, but if possible a CT scan should be obtained first.

Vascular headaches including **migraine** may be precipitated by certain foods, red wine, menstrual periods, certain environmental stimuli such as bright sun, or emotional stress. Classic migraine usually has an "aura" of up to half an hour, with vision changes (e.g., hallucinations of flashing lights, or vision field defects). Persons with basilar artery migraine can have vertigo, ataxia, and diplopia, sometimes with hemiparesis or sensory changes. Migraine headaches tend to be familial, can awaken patients from sleep, and are relieved by ergotamine preparations. Other therapy that can be useful, especially as prevention, includes beta-blockers such as propranolol. The diagnosis of migraine can be made on the basis of the history without investigation. If severe neurological disability occurs, CT scan or angiography may be indicated to rule out a structural or vascular lesion.

Cluster headaches occur in attacks of severe, usually unilateral head pain, lasting 1/2 to 2 hours, often recurring several times a day for several weeks (i.e., in clusters) and then disappearing for months or years before recurring. Clusters tend to recur in spring and fall. During an attack, there is often pain in a nostril or behind the eye, spreading to the frontal area and accompanied by rhinorrhea from the affected nostril and often tearing of the ipsilateral eye. A Horner's syndrome may develop. Alcohol often induces an attack, and oxygen can give relief. The serotonin inhibitor methysergide sometimes gives relief.

Tension headaches are due to muscle spasm, are of long duration (days to months), and are often accompanied by tenderness of cervical, temporalis, or masseter muscles. Pro-

longed work in unusual postural attitudes is often responsible.

Trigeminal neuralgia, pain in the distribution of one of the branches of the fifth cranial nerve, can be triggered by stimuli to the lips or mouth and is often very severe but usually brief, even lightning-like, occurring in clusters of attacks. Carbamazepine is often effective in giving relief. Phenytoin or baclofen can also be useful. **Glossopharyngeal neuralgia** is a similar syndrome occurring in the distribution of the glossopharyngeal or vagus nerves. The trigger is often in the tonsillar area, pain is felt in the angle of the jaw and ear, and bradycardia and syncope can occur. The same drugs can be useful, but nerve section may be needed for either of these syndromes.

CEREBROVASCULAR DISEASE

Cerebrovascular accidents (CVAs) or stroke occurs in older people. The incidence is increased by several risk factors, including untreated hypertension, smoking, diabetes mellitus, alcoholism, familial hypercholesterolemia, and underlying heart disease. Hematocrits above 55% increase viscosity and also predispose to strokes. The use of combined progesterone-estrogen oral contraceptives increases the incidence about threefold.

Heart disease is the most frequent underlying factor in patients with CVAs. Arrhythmias (especially atrial fibrillation), mitral valve prolapse, anterior wall myocardial infarcts, bacterial endocarditis, prosthetic heart valves, calcific mitral or aortic valve disease, and chronic CHF all are associated with an increased incidence.

Examination of patients with cerebrovascular disease may reveal bruits over one or both carotid arteries, representing areas of stenosis. In general, the harsher the bruit the more severe the stenosis, especially if accompanied by a thrill. Such bruits can be distinguished from murmurs originating in the aortic valve area or elsewhere by the fact that they diminish in intensity toward the clavicle.

TIAs are periods of focal loss of nervous system function lasting minutes to a few hours and followed by complete recovery. They are due to vascular insufficiency. Many TIAs are caused by emboli that cause spasm and then move peripherally to a silent area or dissolve, or they may be due to temporary changes in cardiac output or cerebral blood flow without actual occlusion. Such emboli may arise in the internal carotid artery, the aorta, or the heart. The term **reversible ischemic neurological defects (RINDs)** is used for deficits in CNS function that persist for 24 to 36 hours but resolve completely, as opposed to **completed stroke**, which refers to permanent necrosis or infarction of nervous tisue. The syndrome of a TIA depends on the area of the brain affected by the ischemic episode. A typical syndrome of a TIA is **amaurosis fugax**, unilateral blurring or loss of vision lasting seconds to minutes. Retinal examination during an attack may reveal marked vascular narrowing both arterial and venous, and even segmentation of blood within vessels. TIAs resulting from obstruction of vessels in the area supplied by the middle cerebral artery can cause temporary loss of motor function of an arm or hand, or even a transient hemiparesis. Sometimes there is accompanying sensory loss. Transient aphasia or loss of consciousness can occur, but seizures are rare. TIAs precede major strokes in at least 20% of cases. TIAs rarely affect the anterior cerebral artery.

Major vascular occlusions are the main cause of strokes. The manifestations usually develop rapidly, with the neurological defect dependent on the vessel that becomes occluded. Headache is a common symptom at onset. Generalized seizures are infrequent. The results of internal carotid artery occlusion depend on the rate at which occlusion occurs and the extent of anastomotic compensation. In about half the occlusive lesions of the internal carotid artery found by arteriography, the patient is not aware of having had symptoms. Middle cerebral artery occlusions are more often symptomatic. Typically the patient awakens with aphasia (if the dominant hemisphere is affected) or a major motor deficit, such as a hemiplegia affecting the contralateral side. Major strokes involving the nondominant hemisphere can produce confusion and varying degrees of spatial and emotional abnormalities.

TIAs resulting from changes in the vertebrobasilar artery system are common and are quite varied in clinical manifestations. They can cause transient global aphasia, diplopia, paroxysmal drowsiness, ataxia, dysarthria, or even transient hemiparesis or tetraparesis. Lesions affecting the circumferential branches of the basilar artery system can cause vertigo, paresthesias on one side of the face or body, visual scintillations, or episodic hemianopia. Occlusion of major vessels in this part of the intracerebral circulation can cause loss of consciousness with varying pupillary and eye muscle functional changes. Decorticate or decerebrate motor posturing and extensive paralysis or sensory impairment can occur. Dysconjugate eye movements, unequal pupils, and upper motor neuron hemiparesis occur if the lesions are in the caudal part of the distribution of the basilar artery circulation. Complete basilar artery occlusion can produce ischemic functional transection of the brain stem, with deep coma, tetraplegia, pinpoint or irregular unequal pupils, bilateral paralysis of conjugate gaze, and ophthalmoplegia. Such strokes are usually fatal within a few days. Vertebral artery or posterior cerebellar artery occlusion can be asymptomatic but can produce ipsilateral lower motor neuron paralysis of the ninth, tenth, and twelfth cranial nerves, coupled with loss of pain and temperature sense ipsilaterally on the face and contralaterally on the body.

Acute cerebellar infarction can follow occlusion of one of the main vessels to the cerebellum, with headache (usually predominantly ipsilateral and occipital), vomiting, cranial nerve defects, and loss of cerebellar function. Progression causes bilateral headache, stupor, and bilateral upper motor neuron signs in the extremities. CT scans often show evidence of obstruction of the fourth ventricle, with internal hydrocephalus requiring immediate surgical drainage to prevent further damage.

SEIZURE DISORDERS

In children under age 2, seizures are generally due to metabolic disorders, congenital malformations, or perinatal injury. In older children and adolescents, hereditary factors are more frequent. After age 20, the onset of seizures suggests a space-occupying lesion, trauma, drug or alcohol withdrawal, or cerebrovascular disease. Encephalitis or meningitis can initiate seizures at any age.

Classic epileptic seizures consist of an aura, an attack that can last from a few seconds to a few minutes, and a postictal period of drowsiness or confusion that can last from a few hours to several days. Partial seizures (simple, affecting only one type of neurological function without loss of awareness, or complex, which progress to affect more than one function), also occur. The nature of the symptoms often correlates with the portion of the brain that is abnormal. **Partial complex seizures of temporal lobe limbic origin** are the most frequent form of chronic epilepsy, representing about 40% of the cases. Usually beginning before age 25, there frequently are anatomic abnormalities in that area. This type of epilepsy frequently follows febrile convulsions in childhood, trauma, or, in older patients, cerebral ischemia or focal atrophy.

Absence seizures (petit mal epilepsy) are episodes of 1 to 2 seconds duration characterized by a blank stare, often with movements of eyelids. There may be no awareness of these attacks. More obvious, prolonged attacks can occur, lasting up to a minute. The onset of petit mal epilepsy most commonly occurs in childhood, and the attacks usually stop by age 20, but about half develop generalized epilepsy. EEG findings are characteristic, and there is a high incidence (40%) of EEG abnormalities in family members.

Myoclonus, brief uncontrollable muscle jerks during presleep drowsiness, have no relation to epilepsy and are benign.

Generalized (grand mal) epilepsy can begin at any age. Attacks are usually preceded by an aura lasting a few minutes and sometimes by prodromal symptoms, such as mood changes, lasting several hours. There is usually a cry, myotonic contractions beginning with hyperextension, then repetitive clonic muscle jerks and finally relaxation. Pupils may be fixed and dilated during an attack. Hyperactive reflexes and extensor plantar responses can last several minutes after an attack. Patients often bite their tongue or empty their bowels or bladder during a seizure. Drowning in a bathtub or suffocation under bedclothes during an attack are dangers about which patients should be warned. After a seizure, confusion or somnolence can last several hours (the postictal phase). EEG changes show characteristic spiking discharges during an attack and between attacks usually show diagnostic mixtures of spike waves and slow activity.

Diagnosis of epilepsy is based on history, EEG, and negative CT scan. Lumbar puncture should be done in the absence of a contraindication such as papilledema or CT findings that suggest a tumor. The CSF is usually normal, but repetitive major seizures can cause the appearance of up to 100 cells/mm^3 and raise the protein level.

Reflex epilepsy, generalized seizures that can be precipitated by repetitive light patterns (strobe lights, sunlight passing through a row of trees, etc.), can consist of absence attacks or grand mal seizures. Therapy of reflex epilepsy with valproate is usually effective. Lightning pains, severe painful flashes seen in luetic tabes dorsalis or diabetic neuropathy as well as trigeminal neuralgia, can also be treated successfully with anticonvulsants.

Management of epilepsy. The most important drugs for grand mal seizures include phenytoin and phenobarbital, carbamazepine, and primidone. For absence attacks, ethosuximide, valproate, trimethadione, and clonazepam are used.

Seizures can be completely controlled with anticonvulsants in 60% and partially controlled in about 20%. Single attacks that do not recur need no therapy, but if there is a positive family history, a history suggestive of a traumatic focus or other finding making repeat attacks a likelihood, preventive therapy is appropriate. Single febrile convulsions in a child need no therapy, but care should be taken to give antipyretics early during future febrile illnesses. If single drugs do not control attacks, combinations can be given. Monitoring of blood levels is useful, especially if therapy is not fully effective or to improve compliance. Consideration can be given to discontinuing medication if there have been no seizures for 3 to 5 years, but EEG monitoring is advisable. Most adults with a history of several seizures should not stop medication. Care should be taken if medication is discontinued to do so gradually, to avoid precipitating status epilepticus.

Status epilepticus, a state in which repeated seizures occur, new ones beginning before the manifestations of a previous episode have cleared, requires intensive therapy. Maintenance of airway together with IV fluids with glucose and diazepam should be started immediately. Phenytoin and then phenobarbital are given in addition if necessary. If control is not obtained, general anesthesia with halothane and neuromuscular blockade are the next steps. If anesthesia is not available, IV lidocaine can be tried.

Febrile convulsions lead to generalized epilepsy in about 10% of affected children, mostly when onset is before age 1, when attacks come in clusters or last over 15 minutes, or if there is a family history of epilepsy. Counseling of parents with epilepsy is important. Figures show that 4 to 10% of adults with generalized epilepsy have children who are affected. Figures for inheritance of other types of epilepsy are less clear.

CNS TUMORS

The terms *benign* and *malignant* are confusing when applied to CNS tumors. Many tumors are of multifocal origin, distant metastases are rare, and histologically benign focal lesions can recur after removal and can cause death. In this passage, the term *benign* therefore is used to mean relatively benign.

The most common CNS tumors in adults are of glial origin. Benign **astrocytomas** are usually multifocal, and **gliobastoma multiforme** is very malignant. The most common mesothelial tumors are **meningiomas**, which are usually benign but can recur after removal. The most frequent sites of menigiomas are along the dorsal surface of the brain, often affecting the motor cortex, the frontal areas, the base of the skull, the falx, the sphenoid ridge, and the lateral ventricles.

Many manifestations of tumor growth depend on alterations in the blood-brain barrier, which occur for several reasons, including new vessels forming in the tumor and compression of surrounding tissue altering the vessels. As a result, edema formation is common, adding to the mass effect of the enlarging tumor. The brain has no lymphatic system, and removal of edema fluid is slow. Tumors also can affect function of specific neural pathways.

Brain tumors usually present with headaches, diffuse or in the area of the tumor. Since benign headaches are very common, appearance of headaches in a patient not previously prone to them or changes in the headache pattern are important clues. Papilledema is common in children but rare in adults. Vomiting without preceding nausea, especially on arising in the morning, is also common, especially with posterior fossa tumors. Altered consciousness is common. Other manifestations depend on the site of the tumor and often are localizing. For example, compression of the underlying motor cortex by a meningioma can cause epileptiform seizures.

In workup of suspected brain tumors, a CT scan is the first test, with and without injected contrast material. Skull films and radionuclide scans add little. If there is no evidence for increased intracranial pressure, a lumbar puncture can be performed. The CSF usually has elevated protein, low glucose, and increased cells. Malignant cells may be seen. MR scan, arteriography, and myelography are sometimes indicated. Treatment is primarily surgical; radiation can be helpful with some lesions.

Neurofibromatosis is an inherited, autosomal dominant trait that is characterized by pigmented skin lesions (café au lait spots) and multiple neurofibromas of peripheral nerves. Often there are associated intracranial meningiomas, fibrous dysplasia of bone, pheochromocytomas, and other endocrine tumors.

Malignant tumors outside the nervous system can produce neurological manifestations (**paraneoplastic syndromes**) that can be confused with a variety of CNS diseases. Such syndromes include the following: **Subacute cerebellar degeneration** produces a progressive syndrome characterized by ataxia, dysarthria, and vertigo. **Subacute sensory neuronopathy** is a rare entity that causes loss of sensation with preservation of motor power. CSF protein is usually elevated. A **myasthenic syndrome** resembling myasthenia gravis is especially common in men over 40 with intrathoracic tumors. It is called the **Eaton-Lambert syndrome**. In contrast to true myasthenia, strength usually increases with repetitive contractions. The defect is apparently due to deficient release of acetylcholine at the myoneural junctions. Electromyography is diagnostically useful. Cholinesterase inhibitors are not useful in therapy, but guanidine hydrochloride is helpful. Polymyositis (PM/DM), another syndrome sometimes associated with underlying malignancy, is described in the section on rheumatology.

Pseudotumor cerebri is usually of unknown etiology, but some cases probably result from venous occlusion since it often follows head trauma, middle ear disease, oral contraceptive use, pregnancy, or polycythemia vera. Some cases follow withdrawal of corticosteroids or use of other medications, including vitamin A and tetracycline. It occurs most often in young females and consists of headache, papilledema, and sometimes vision disturbances. Workup including CT scan is negative; CSF pressure is elevated (usually >300 mm H_2O) but is otherwise normal. Digital venous angiography may be necessary if venous obstruction is suspected. Usually only symptomatic therapy is necessary, although corticosteroids are sometimes given.

Hydrocephalus, enlargement of the ventricular system, usually results from stenosis or obstruction of the flow of CSF. It can appear acutely (e.g., following meningitis) and be rapidly progressive and fatal if not corrected. Headache, vomiting, lethargy, dementia, and coma can result. CT scan is usually diagnostic, and lumbar puncture confirmatory. Ventricular shunting may be needed. Hydrocephalus ex vacuo results from atrophy of the cerebral cortex. CSF pressure is normal and therapy is of no value.

DISEASES OF THE SPECIAL SENSES

Systemic diseases affecting vision. Vision field defects fall into patterns depending on the location of the lesion in the pathways conducting vision (Table 1-14). **Optic neuritis** of any cause can cause unilateral focal scotomata or complete blindness. Demyelinating processes such as multiple sclerosis are a common cause. Papillitis of the optic nerve head can be seen on fundus examination. Transient or permanent unilateral blindness of acute onset can occur with giant cell arteritis or small emboli to a retinal artery. Bilateral blindness can occur acutely as a result of increased intracranial pressure, often due to a tumor, but the most common systemic cause of gradual, chronic blindness is diabetes. Hereditary degenerative conditions such as retinitis pigmentosa are also relatively common. **Glaucoma** causes vision loss that can be rapid and associated with pain if sudden, narrow-angle closure has occurred. In these cases, inflammation of the eye can be present. A deeply cupped optic disk may be seen, and tonometry reveals increased pressure.

Pupillary changes. Causes of **small pupils** are as follows: Effect of opiates or pilocarpine, Argyll Robertson pupils (due to autonomic neuropathy, usually resulting from syphilis or diabetes), pontine hemorrhage, Horner's syndrome (partial ptosis of the upper lid, anhidrosis, and small pupil due to loss of sympathetic innervation). Small pupils also can result from old age. Causes of **large pupils** include mydriatic drops, atropine, glutethimide or amphetamine overdose, anxiety, posttraumatic iridoplegia, Holmes-Adie's pupil (an autonomic neuropathy affecting parasympathetics in which the pupil reacts very poorly to light but slowly to accommodation), and cerebral death. Large pupils also occur physiologically in childhood.

Extraocular palsies. The sixth nerve innervates the external rectus, which if weak results in loss of abduction. The fourth nerve innervates the superior oblique muscle (remember ER_6SO_4), which moves the eye down and in. All other muscles are innervated by the third nerve. These nerves are closest in the cavernous sinus, and lesions that compress or occlude that sinus cause multiple unilateral ocular palsies. Brain-stem lesions (usually vascular, tumors or demyelination) affect individual nerves and cause associated neurological abnormalities. Vascular lesions of the third nerve (e.g., diabetes) often spare the pupil, whereas compressive lesions (e.g., tumors or aneurysms) usually affect the pupil. Conjugate gaze to the opposite side is often paralyzed with unilateral lesions of a hemisphere, such as tumors, hemorrhage, or infarct. The eyes are often deviated toward the affected side. Lesions of the brain stem, on the other hand, cause paralysis of conjugate movement to the affected side, with slight eye deviation away from that side.

Deafness. Deafness can be conductive if due to disease in the ear itself (external, middle, or inner). Bone conduction exceeds air conduction, and the Weber test lateralizes to the deaf side. Loss of nerve function affects high-frequency sounds early; air conduction exceeds bone conduction, and the Weber's test lateralizes to the normal side. **Otosclerosis** results from thickening and calcification of the annular ligament attaching the stapes to the oval window. Surgery can be helpful. Drugs cause deafness by affecting the cochlear hair cells. Aminoglycosides cause a permanent effect that is proportional to the blood level. Salicylates, furosemide, and ethacrynic acid cause tinnitus and reversible deafness.

Vertigo. A false sensation of movement, vertigo results from abnormal vestibular fucntion. It should be distinguished from dizziness or light-headedness, which is often due to cerebral anoxia (such as can occur with postural hypotension) and can be accompanied by actual loss of consciousness (fainting). The clinical sign of vestibular disease is nystagmus. The "dizzy" patient should be evaluated with special attention to the cardiac status and blood pressure, evidence of hyperventilation (which can lower the PCO_2), cerebellar or other neurological disease that can cause ataxia, and the presence of nystagmus. Vascular disease of the brain stem can cause vertigo associated with nausea and vomiting, and vertigo can be a sole symptom of TIAs. Neuropathy of the eighth nerve can produce vertigo. The most common cause is herpes zoster, which can produce the **Ramsay Hunt syndrome** (vertigo, deafness, sometimes with facial paralysis, associated with herpetic lesions of the external ear and sometimes the palate). Vertigo is treated with drugs that sedate the vestibular apparatus, such as scopolamine, meclizine, and diazepam.

Anosmia. Permanent anosmia can result from basal skull fractures that disrupt the olfactory nerves, brain tumors in the frontal fossa, and occasionally herpes zoster, vitamin B_{12} deficiency, and multiple sclerosis.

MUSCLE WEAKNESS

Upper motor neuron weakness affects mostly skilled movements. Weakness is more marked in distal than in proximal muscles and is combined with some degree of spasticity. Deep tendon reflexes are increased, and abnormal reflexes develop, including the Babinski reflex. The face is seldom paralyzed.

Basal ganglia lesions cause weakness, but usually it is mild and the main difficulty occurs with starting a movement. There is rigidity rather than spasticity of the extremities. Reflexes may be normal and the Babinski's is absent.

Lower motor neuron disease causes weakness in the area of the affected nerve cells, resistance to passive motion is

Table 1-14. Defects in the Field of Vision

Pattern of defect	Location of lesion
Unilateral blindness	Optic nerve
Bitemporal hemianopia	In optic chiasm, centrally
Homonymous hemianopia	Behind optic chiasm (e.g., in optic tract)
Quadrantic anopsia	Temporal lobe damage if superior Parietal lobe damage if inferior
Focal scotomata	Occipital optic cortex (also encountered with intraocular lesions)

decreased, deep tendon reflexes are diminished or absent, Babinski reflex is absent, fasciculations appear, and muscle atrophy develops. EMG findings are typical of denervation.

Myopathy, disease of the muscle itself, usually causes progressive weakness, the pattern of findings varying with the disease process. Proximal muscles are usually affected to a greater extent than distal muscles. Muscle enzymes typically are elevated.

Myotonia results from postsynaptic muscle membrane abnormality, which causes repetitive depolarization after a stimulus, resulting in sustained shortening of the muscle fibers.

Diseases of the neuromuscular junction, such as **myasthenia gravis**, are described below.

Workup of patients with muscle weakness. Determine which specific muscle functions are affected, to help to decide if there is generalized asthenia or focal muscle weakness. Proximal weakness affects putting objects onto high shelves, getting out of chairs, crossing the legs, or, if severe, turning over in bed. Ability to grip objects firmly and to walk on the toes and heels may be preserved. Such proximal weakness suggests disease of the muscle rather than the nervous system. Diplopia, ptosis, and other eye muscle abnormalities suggest myasthenia gravis. Difficulty puckering the lips or whistling suggests muscular dystrophy (fascioscapulohumeral type). The pattern of progression is helpful diagnostically. Slow development over many months suggests dystrophy or a metabolic myopathy. Rapid onset is more typical of PM/DM or peripheral neuropathy. Periodicity suggests a form of periodic paralysis. Unusual contractions can be due to fasciculation, suggesting denervation or myotonia.

Laboratory exam should include serum muscle enzymes (CPK, aldolase), which if high suggest an inflammatory myopathy or dystrophy; thyroid function tests; evaluation for diabetes; acetylcholine receptor antibodies, which are diagnostic of myasthenia gravis; EMG and nerve conduction tests to distinguish myopathy from neuropathy; and biopsy of an affected muscle, planning on histochemical enzyme studies as well as morphology to help define a metabolic myopathy or a lipid or glycogen storage disease.

SPECIFIC DISEASES AFFECTING MUSCLE FUNCTION

The **muscular dystrophies** are inherited and cause progressive painless muscle weakness, usually beginning in childhood. **Duchenne's dystrophy** is X linked and therefore affects boys almost exclusively. Weakness is maximal in the pelvic girdle, less in shoulder muscles, and least distally. Pseudohypertrophy may develop, especially in calf muscles. Motions are awkward, especially when running, and **Gower's sign** is typical: The hands are used to get up from the floor by "walking" them up the legs. The CPK is elevated. Progression usually requires a wheelchair by adolescence, and death is frequently due to aspiration pneumonia.

Limb-girdle dystrophy is an autosomal recessive with a high rate of new mutations, affecting muscles of both shoulder and pelvic girdles. It occurs with equal frequency in boys and girls. **Fascioscapulohumeral dystrophy** affects predominantly the perioral and ocular muscles, as well as the latissimus dorsi, causing winging of the scapulae. Shoulder and pelvic girdle muscles become affected, and scoliosis frequently develops.

Progression is usually very slow. Therapy is supportive; there is no effective treatment for any of the inherited dystrophies.

PM and DM are one disease, differing only in the presence of a generalized, erythematous, macular skin rash, often with heliotrope discoloration around the eyes (see the section on rheumatic diseases). An underlying malignancy is occasionally found in adult cases, but extensive workup is not indicated. Specific leads (such as occult blood in the stool) should be pursued. A similar syndrome can accompany other forms of connective tissue disease, including SLE or scleroderma. Corticosteroid therapy is usually effective, but immunosuppressants may be needed.

Another connective tissue disease, **PMR**, causes pain and stiffness but no weakness predominantly of the muscles of the neck, shoulder, and upper back. The ESR is typically very high (}50, sometimes }100 mm/hour); this syndrome is often associated with giant cell arteritis (see the section on rheumatic diseases). Both syndromes respond well to corticosteroid therapy, but smaller doses are needed for PMR alone.

The most common endocrine forms of myopathy occur in hyperthyroidism and hypothyroidism. Muscle weakness, twitching, even fasciculations may occur, and the syndrome can resemble a limb-girdle form of dystrophy or myasthenia gravis. A peculiar form of percussion myopathy is sometimes encountered in myxedema, in which a local band of contraction occurs where the muscle is rubbed firmly. Thyroid function tests are vital to diagnosis.

Drug-induced myopathies are noted with penicillamine, clofibrate, guanethidine, emetine, ipecac, vincristine, and epsilon-aminocaproic acid (EACA). Hypokalemia resulting from diuretics can also cause weakness and, if severe, muscle necrosis and elevated CPK.

Myopathy also occurs with the glycogen and lipid storage diseases. **McArdle's disease**, the most common form of glycogen storage disease, results from the absence of muscle phosphorylase. Patients are unable to degrade muscle glycogen during exercise, and painful muscle cramps develop. Myoglobinemia, myoglobinuria, and renal failure may occur. Similarly, myoglobinemia can result from extensive crush injuries to muscle, with similar functional damage due to plugging of the renal tubules.

Periodic paralysis occurs with very high or low serum potassium levels. It causes attacks of flaccid paralysis that usually begin in childhood and that last minutes to days.

Myasthenia gravis is an autoimmune process that results in the formation of antibodies that affect the acetylcholine receptors at the myoneural junctions. Typically it begins in early adulthood with weakness of eye muscles. Ptosis and diplopia occur early, followed by difficulty chewing and swallowing. Nasal regurgitation or aspiration is common. Generalized weakness then develops, and respiratory muscle function can be severely impaired. Repetitive contraction of muscles aggravates the weakness and can cause ptosis to worsen. EMG confirms the decline in action potential with repetitive stimulation, and the Tensilon (edrophonium HCl) test is helpful in diagnosis, since this rapidly acting anticholinesterase causes marked but transient improvement. Antibodies to the acetylcholine receptor can be found in the serum. **Therapy** is primarily the use of anticholinesterase drugs, such as neostigmine or pyridostigmine. Thymectomy is sometimes helpful. The **Eaton-Lambert syndrome** is a similar patho-physiological process that occurs in the presence of malignant tumors. It also affects neuromuscular junctions, but distal muscles are more affected than proximal, and muscle function improves with repeated contractions. Neither disease causes muscle atrophy, spasticity, or abnormal reflexes.

Botulism is caused by an exotoxin of the organism **C. botulinum**, present in contaminated, improperly canned food. It interferes with release of acetylcholine at the neuromuscular junction. GI symptoms usually develop first, with nausea, vomiting, and diarrhea. Muscle weakness usually appears within a few days, rapidly progressing to paralysis of the arms, legs, and cranial and respiratory muscles, requiring ventilatory assistance. Autonomic nerve transmission is also affected, and loss of visual accommodation occurs early. CSF findings are normal.

Tick paralysis is a severe form of weakness developing 4 to 5 days after a tick becomes embedded in the skin, typically near the hairline and often unnoticed. The disease therefore develops more often in girls. Paresthesias and a flaccid paralysis of the extremity and respiratory muscles develop as a reult of a neurotoxin that blocks transmission at the neuromuscular junction, similar to the toxin of botulism. CSF protein is normal. The paralysis improves very rapidly after the tick is removed.

Aminoglycoside antibiotics can affect neuromuscular transmission, causing severe respiratory paralysis. Typically this syndrome appears acutely postoperatively, especially in patients who have renal failure and who develop high blood levels.

DEMYELINATING DISORDERS OF THE NERVOUS SYSTEM

The demyelinating disorders probably result from immune processes and are characterized by an increase in CSF IgG compared with plasma IgG. The oligodendroglial cells, the cells that produce and maintain the myelin, are primarily affected. In demyelinated areas, the axons themselves may become damaged.

A demyelinating disorder of apparently immune origin, **multiple sclerosis** (MS) usually begins between the ages of 20 and 40. It is characterized by exacerbations and remissions, with flare-ups occurring at varying rates, averaging about one every 2 years, lesions appearing in different sites in the nervous system over the years. In mild cases, only a few attacks may occur over a lifetime, with no permanent functional loss, but continuously progressive disease occurs in other patients. The lesions are characterized by loss of myelin in the white matter of the CNS, brain, brain stem, or spinal cord. After a few weeks, the myelin is restored and function returns, but repeated flare-ups usually lead to progressive permanent loss of function. After 10 years, about 60% of patients remain fully functional, but after 30 years only 25 to 30% are still functional. Although disability may occur, life expectancy is not decreased, but infections, especially of the urinary tract, can become life threatening. The disease is more common in temperate zones, among people with haplotype DRW2 (65% versus 15% of controls) and is rare among Orientals and blacks.

The oligodendroglial cells that are responsible for the production and maintenance of myelin are probably the primary targets of the disease process. Inflammatory infiltrates, primarily lymphocytic, appear at the site of subsequent demyelination, and there is evidence of production of immunoglobulin in the nervous system, with an elevated CSF-to-serum ratio of IgG. When disease is severe, other structures are damaged, including astrocytic cells and nerve axons.

The typical manifestations of MS include muscle weakness, spasticity and ataxia, transient partial vision field loss or blindness in one eye, ophthalmoplegias, diplopia, vertigo, dysarthria, intention tremor, and electric shock-like pains initiated by neck flexion and radiating to the extremities (Lhermitte's sign). Mental changes, dysphagia, and convulsions can occur. On examination, spasticity or hyperreflexia, Babinski's sign, absent abdominal reflexes, intention tremor, and nystagmus are the most frequent findings. Facial nerve paralyses, loss of position and vibration sense, regional loss of pain sensation, and other sensory changes can occur. Neurological manifestations become worse, and new findings may appear with fever.

The characteristic diagnostic aspect of the examination is the finding of evidence for more than one lesion in the CNS, such as optic nerve abnormality (vision loss) plus loss of extraocular muscle functions or a spinal cord lesion with loss of vibratory and position sense. Visual-evoked responses may help to establish that there are multiple sites of lesions.

The pattern of onset and progression of clinical manifestations is a strong feature suggesting the diagnosis, especially when there are exacerbations after fever and evidence for more than one focal lesion in the nervous system. Supporting lab data include elevated IgG in the CSF, with separate oligoclonal bands on electrophoresis, the finding of myelin basic protein by radioimmunoassay, CT evidence of hypodense areas, and MR images of similar abnormalities, most frequently seen near the lateral ventricles with both techniques. Visual-evoked potentials are usually abnormal because of the high frequency of optic nerve lesions.

Treatment is not satisfactory. Corticosteroids are apparently helpful during exacerbations, and some clinicians use them as maintenance therapy as well. Immunosuppressives may be of value in rapidly progressive cases.

Acute disseminated encephalomyelitis produces a similar demyelinating disorder. It usually begins abruptly 7 to 10 days after an acute viral infection or after vaccination. Headache, fever, and multifocal neurological signs develop. The CSF shows 20 to 200 lymphocytes and increased IgG; glucose is normal. Myelin basic protein is demonstrable in the CSF. EEG is usually abnormal but does not show the characteristic focal and sharp-wave activity seen in HSV encephalitis. Severe cases progress to stupor and coma; seizures are common. Therapy is ineffective.

NEUROPATHIES

Neuropathy can effect cell bodies, axons, or myelin sheaths. Distal areas are affected predominantly because longer nerves are more metabolically active. Demyelinating neuropathies are usually due to immunologic or infectious damage and tend to spare the thinner pain and temperature fibers, whereas axonal neuropathy tends to affect those modalities disproportionately.

Demyelinating neuropathies can affect cranial nerves. CSF protein concentration may be elevated since the spinal roots can be affected. Recovery from demyelinating neuropathies is relatively fast, from axonal degeneration slower. Nerve cell damage is usually permanent.

Focal neuropathies are common and are usually due to trauma or compression producing ischemia and then demyelination. For example, "Saturday night paralysis" results from compression of the radial nerve on the humerus over the back of a chair during a stuporous sleep. The **carpal tunnel syndrome** is very common. It produces tingling, numbness, or pain over the median or ulnar nerve distribution in the hand. Sometimes pain is felt above the wrist as well. Weakness and atrophy of thenar muscles may develop. Pain may be reproduced by percussion over the wrist (Tinel's sign). The pain typically is most severe at night because flexion of the wrist during sleep adds to the pressure on the nerves. Treatment begins with wrist splints worn at night. Local corticosteroid injection in the flexor retinaculum area of the wrist helps, but surgical decompression may be necessary. **Lateral femoral cutaneous neuralgia** (meralgia paresthetica) is pain in the lateral thigh as a result of compression of that nerve in the inguinal ligament.

Guillian-Barré syndrome is a severe polyneuropathy, usually developing following a viral respiratory tract infection. One outbreak followed use of influenza vaccine. It often begins with tingling paresthesias in the hands and feet and progresses to ascending paralysis of voluntary muscles, including those supplied by cranial nerves. Deep tendon reflexes are lost. Respiratory paralysis can occur. Autonomic dysfunction and pain can also develop. The paralysis usually begins in the legs and ascends to the face (**Landry's ascending paralysis**). CSF protein rises after the first few days, usually to levels above 100 mg/100 ml, without an increase in cells (albuminocytological dissociation). After progressing a few weeks, the weakness usually stabilizes and recovery gradually occurs. There are reports that recovery is hastened by plasmapheresis. Other immune neuropathies, causing both sensory and motor changes, include a syndrome associated with multiple myeloma and one with benign monoclonal gammopathy.

Diabetic neuropathy is common, affecting about 40% of those with diabetes of 25 years duration. It causes a variety of syndromes, primarily with sensory abnormalities. A process affecting large nerve fibers is most common, causing paresthesias and decreased sensation in the feet, with diminished ankle jerks. Another variety affects primarily small nerve fibers, causing dull or burning pain in the feet, especially at night, with diminished touch and pain perception but without loss of ankle jerks or position sense. Autonomic neuropathy causes impaired gastric emptying and intestinal motility, with constipation and often nocturnal diarrhea as well. Orthostatic hypotension, impotence, and loss of bladder control can also occur. A syndrome resembling tabes dorsalis occurs, and Charcot joints can develop, especially in the feet and ankles. More limited mononeuropathy also occurs, usually with pain. The third nerve is often affected, with headache and weakness of eye muscles.

A variety of drugs can cause **toxic neuropathy**. Most produce typical peripheral neuropathy with mixed sensory and motor abnormalities (e.g., gold, glutethimide, hydralazine,

lithium, vincristine), but isoniazid produces a sensory neuropathy whereas nitrofurantoin produces primarily a motor neuropathy. Lead, organophosphates, and a variety of other environmental toxins also produce neuropathies.

A **herniated intervertebral disk** produces pain by compression of sensory nerves to the dura and often nerve roots as well. Back pain, often aggravated by minor trauma, is worst when sitting and least when lying flat. Pain may be felt in the distribution of the specific nerve root compressed. Typical findings include paravertebral muscle spasm, loss of normal spinal curvature, and pain on straight leg raising. Radicular pain, along the distribution of spinal root, may be sharp or dull and is usually aggravated by phenomena that raise CSF pressure such as a sneeze, cough, or strain, with radiation of the pain from proximal to distal areas. At times pain is made worse by walking, probably because of compression of the vascular supply by the disk. Pain along the sciatic nerve is common. Segmental sensory changes, such as paresthesias, impairment of pain and touch receptors, and motor symptoms (spasm, cramp, twitching, atrophy, fascicular twitching, loss of deep tendon reflexes) are relatively common. Functional changes of the sphincter usually appear late.

Workup includes CT scan or MR imaging. Myelography is still being done, at least preoperatively. Treatment consists of rest while lying flat, with analgesics. Lumbar support is helpful during exacerbations. Conservative management is usually successful, but long-term management and prevention of recurrences require strengthening of abdominal muscles. Surgery is indicated for incapacitating, intractable pain, cauda equina compression producing bladder dysfunction, or definite nerve root compression with functional motor loss. Injection of the disk with chymopapain to cause dissolution is still being evaluated.

A **herniated cervical intervertebral disk** usually results from trauma, especially sudden hyperextension such as occurs with a whiplash injury, although many cases develop without definite antecedent trauma. The main symptoms are pain and limitation of motion of the neck. If the disk has herniated laterally, unilateral nerve root compression can result. A lesion at C5-C6 affects the sixth cervical root. Typically it causes pain over the trapezius, in the shoulder and upper arm anteriorly, sometimes radiating down the radial side of the forearm to the thumb and index finger. The same areas may show paresthesias and hypersensitivity. There may be motor weakness of the biceps and flexors of the forearm as well as supinators, with diminution of deep tendon reflexes in those areas. If the disk is between C6 and C7, it affects the seventh cervical root and causes pain in the region of the scapula, axilla, posterolateral upper arm, elbow and middle of the forearm, third and forth fingers or all fingers. Tenderness is usually most severe over the medial aspect of the scapula at the level of T3 and T4. Sensory loss is most severe over the third and forth fingers. Weakness is present in the extensors of the forearm and wrist, including the triceps. Grip strength is weakened, and triceps reflex is diminished. Biceps and supinator strength and reflexes are normal. Increasing the pressure on a compressed nerve root by coughing, sneezing, or downward compression of the neck by pressure on the head can increase the pain, whereas traction can relieve it. Incomplete syndromes are common.

Spinal stenosis is due to osteophyte formation compressing the spinal cord. It typically produces increasing weakness without pain. Atrophy and fasciculation occur, and the process can be confused with spinal cord disease. Surgery is often successful. Cervical stenosis, osteophyte formation resulting from cervical disk disease, can cause narrowing of the intervertebral canal or lateral compression of nerve roots. Mild neck pain with flare-ups and limitation of motion (especially lateral bending and rotation) are common, but severe flare-ups can occur. Nerve root impingement can give severe pain radiating down an arm, numbness of one side of the hand or two or three fingers, and hyporeflexia of the affected area.

Spinal cord compression can result from posterior osteophyte formation and thickening of ossification of the ligamentum flavum, especially if there is a developmentally narrow spinal canal. Symptoms usually begin subtly and progress slowly over several years. Spastic weakness of one or both legs and posterior column signs (loss of position and vibratory senses and ataxia). Minimal or indefinite sensory changes are often present in one or both arms and hands, with or without mild motor abnormalities. Narrowing of the spinal canal can be visualized by lateral x-rays, myelography, and CT or MR scan. Localized severe narrowing by a lesion at C4-C5 can produce an increase in all tendon reflexes in the arms. Narrowing at C5-C6 can cause loss of the biceps reflex, leaving the triceps and finger reflexes intact. If there is a lesion at C6-C7, the triceps reflex is diminished. Herniated intervertebral disk, diabetic neuropathy, pernicious anemia with myelopathy, and amyotrophic lateral sclerosis (ALS) are the main differential diagnostic problems. Analgesics, rest, cervical traction, support of the neck with an orthopedic collar, and a proper pillow at night can give relief in milder cases, but laminectomy and decompression of the cord or affected nerve roots may be necessary.

In **lower spine stenosis**, lesions of the conus medullaris (i.e., lower sacral segments of the spinal cord) cause early disturbances of the bladder and bowel, back pain, hypesthesia and anesthesia over sacral dermatomes, a lax anal sphincter and loss of anal and bulbocavernosus reflexes, and sometimes weakness of the gluteus and hamstring muscles.

A Babinski's sign means that there is a lesion above the third lumbar segment of the spinal cord.

AMYOTROPHIC LATERAL SCLEROSIS

ALS affects both upper and lower motor neurons, afflicting all four extremities. It increases in incidence with advancing age, occasionally with a familial pattern that tends to affect younger individuals. It often begins with bulbar involvement, and such cases progress rapidly. A milder form, called progressive muscle atrophy, affects primarily lower motor neurons and progresses more slowly. ALS typically begins with asymmetric weakness affecting distal muscles, especially in the hands. Muscle fasciculations and atrophy appear early. There may be cramps but no other sensory symptoms. Upper motor neuron abnormalities appear, including spasticity, hyperreflexia, and extensor plantar responses. The disease spreads to involve all muscle groups, but the eye muscles are usually spared. CSF is normal, as are muscle enzyme levels. Nerve conduction velocities are normal, differentiating ALS from neuropathies. EMG shows evidence of muscle denervation. Therapy is limited to supportive measures.

DISEASES AFFECTING BASAL GANGLIA

The basal ganglia affect control over planned and skilled motor functions and have distinct neurotransmitter physiology. Afferents from the cortex and thalamus secrete glutamine. Within the substantia nigra and striatum, dopamine is the main transmitter, but cholinergic neurons oppose the dopaminergic input. The major transmitter of the output from the basal ganglia is gamma-aminobutryic acid. Therapeutically, drugs that enhance dopamine effect and anticholinergic agents are currently in use.

Parkinsonism, the most important disease of the basal ganglia, results from idiopathic or postencephalitic degeneration of dopamine-secreting neurons that connect the substantia nigra to the striatum. Drugs that block dopamine receptors in the striatum cause a similar syndrome. The idiopathic form of the disease is most common in men over 40. It progresses gradually, beginning with weakness or tremor, stiffness, and ease of fatigue. It may affect a single extremity or be bilateral. A typical, slow resting tremor occurs in most but not all patients. Those with marked rigidity may not show it. Patients with parkinsonism typically walk stiffly, stooped forward, with little movement of the arms and a mask-like facies. Hands show a pill-rolling tremor (flexing at the metacarpophalangeal joints). Failure of blinking, spontaneous as well as after stimulation of the brow (Myerson's sign) is common. Deep tendon reflexes may be normal or abnormal, and Babinski's signs may appear late in the course. There is a steady resistance to passive movement of the extremities, combined with a tremor, resulting in cogwheel rigidity. Depression is usual and dementia may develop.

Treatment of Parkinson's disease usually begins with amantadine, which helps many patients and is low in toxicity. Levodopa, usually combined with a peripheral dopa-decarboxylase inhibitor, is the main form of therapy for advanced cases. Anticholinergic drugs are also useful, alone or in combination. They are of particular benefit for the tremor, whereas dopamine helps mainly with the rigidity. Antidepressants are also useful.

Drug-induced parkinsonism can follow use of several antipsychotic drugs, especially the phenothiazines and butyrophenones, which block dopaminergic receptors. Patients may have acute dystonic motor abnormalities, including oculomotor dystonia (oculogyric crises), which respond to anticholinergic, antihistamine, or diazepam therapy. The symptoms of parkinsonism usually do not respond to therapy with dopamine. Another form of toxic drug reaction, tardive dyskinesia, is more serious. It consists of involuntary movements of the mouth, trunk, or extremities and typically appears following withdrawal of antidopaminergic antipsychotic agents, especially the phenothiazines. It can appear after short periods of use of such agents. Reserpine may be of benefit, but the condition is usually irreversible.

Wilson's disease, another basal ganglia syndrome, is described under metabolic disorders.

Disorders of cerebellar function result in generalized weakness (asthenia), an ataxic gait, inability to control movements of the arms, particularly inability to synchronize movements that involve several joints. Tremor and dysarthria are frequent, as is nystagmus, with the fast component toward the side of the lesion. Cerebellar diseases may be inherited degenerative process (e.g., Friedreich's ataxia), inherited metabolic abnormalites (e.g., Refsum's disease), or acquired (e.g., alcoholic/nutritional cerebellar degeneration). Vascular insufficiency and toxins (alcohol, sedatives, phenytoin, others) can also cause cerebellar dysfunction. A variety of rare nervous system disorders also can affect the cerebellum.

BIBLIOGRAPHY

Adams RD, Victor M: Principles of Neurology, 3rd ed. McGraw-Hill, New York, 1985.

Andreoli IE, et al: Cecil Essentials of Medicine. WB Saunders, Philadelphia, 1986.

Braunwald E (ed): Heart Disease, 2nd ed. WB Saunders, Philadelphia, 1984.

Braunwald E, et al (eds): Harrison's Principles of Internal Medicine, 11th ed. McGraw-Hill, New York, 1987.

Brenner BM, Rector FC (eds): The Kidney, 3rd ed. WB Saunders, Philadelphia, 1986.

Cupps TR, Fauci AS: The Vasculitides. WB Saunders, Philadelphia, 1981.

DeGroot LG, et al (eds): Endocrinology. Grune and Stratton, Orlando, 1987.

Fishman AP (ed): Pulmonary Diseases and Disorders, 2nd ed. McGraw-Hill, New York, 1987.

Fitzpatrick TB, et al (eds): Dermatology in General Medicine. McGraw-Hill, New York, 1983.

Kelley W, et al (eds): Textbook of Rheumatology, 2nd ed. WB Saunders, Philadelphia, 1985.

Mandell GL, et al (eds): Principles and Practice of Infectious Diseases, 2nd ed. John Wiley & Sons, New York, 1985.

Rodnan GP, Schumacher HR (eds): Primer on the Rheumatic Diseases, 8th ed. Arthritis Foundation, Atlanta, 1983.

Schlesinger J, Fortran JS (eds): Gastrointestinal Disease, 3rd ed. WB Saunders, Philadelphia, 1983.

Sherlock S: Diseases of the Liver and Biliary System, 7th ed. FA Davis, Philadelphia, 1985.

Smith LH Jr, Thier SO (eds): Pathophysiology—The Biologic Principles of Disease. WB Saunders, Philadelphia, 1985.

Snider GL: Clinical Pulmonary Medicine. Little, Brown & Co., Boston, 1981.

Stanbury JB, et al (eds): The Metabolic Basis of Inherited Disease. McGraw-Hill, New York, 1983.

Williams WJ, et al (eds): Hematology. McGraw-Hill, New York, 1983.

Wilson JD, Foster GW (eds): Williams' Textbook of Endocrinology. WB Saunders, Philadelphia, 1985.

SAMPLE QUESTIONS

DIRECTIONS: Each question below contains five suggested answers. Choose the **one best** response to each question.

1. Skin lesions that are clues to the existence of bacterial sepsis are seen in all of the following infections EXCEPT

    A. *Pseudomonas aeruginosa*
    B. meningococcemia
    C. gonococcemia
    D. *Hemophilus influenzae*
    E. Gram-negative sepsis

2. All of the following are major complications of diabetes mellitus EXCEPT

    A. nephropathy with renal failure
    B. blindness due to retinopathy
    C. peripheral neuropathy with pain in the extremities
    D. autonomic neuropathy with nocturnal diarrhea
    E. Korsakoff's syndrome

3. All of the following statements are true EXCEPT that

    A. drug-induced lupus is usually benign, without renal involvement
    B. drug-induced lupus subsides after the specific drug is stopped
    C. smaller arteries are affected by lupus more often than in other forms of vasculitis, such as periarteritis nodosa
    D. low serum complement levels are inaccurate indicators of lupus activity
    E. giant-cell arteritis most frequently affects medium-sized arteries in the scalp and head

4. Sinus bradycardia occurs in all of the following EXCEPT

    A. well-trained athletes
    B. increased intracranial pressure
    C. hypothyroidism
    D. hypothermia
    E. pericardial effusion

5. The rate of elevation of the BUN in a patient with renal failure is influenced by all of the following factors EXCEPT

    A. the amount of dietary protein ingested
    B. the protein catabolic rate, which is increased by tissue necrosis
    C. muscle mass of the patient
    D. hypovolemia
    E. liver failure, decreasing synthesis of urea

6. Abnormalities in renal tubular function can result in all of the following EXCEPT

   A. glycosuria
   B. aminoaciduria
   C. hypouricemia
   D. proteinuria
   E. hypophosphatemia

DIRECTIONS: Each question below contains four suggested answers of which **one** or **more** is correct. Choose the answer:

A if 1, 2, and 3 are correct
B if 1 and 3 are correct
C if 2 and 4 are correct
D if 4 is correct
E if 1, 2, 3, and 4 are correct

---

7. Skin lesions are often associated with which of the following infections?

   1. Syphilis
   2. Lyme disease
   3. Rocky Mountain spotted fever
   4. Streptococcal infection

8. Acidosis as a result of renal tubular dysfunction can result from which of the following abnormalities?

   1. Failure of normal tubular secretion of H^+ by the proximal tubule
   2. Defect in hydrogen ion transport in the distal tubule
   3. Interstitial renal disease affecting response of collecting tubules to aldosterone
   4. Excessive secretion of bicarbonate due to deficiency of carbonic anyhydrase

9. Skin tests as a means of diagnosing infection

   1. are useful in the diagnosis of tuberculosis, since the majority of people who do not have active infection have negative skin tests
   2. should be performed as a clue to the existence of infection with *Histoplasma* or *Coccidioides immitis*
   3. are not interpretable when negative unless control antigens (e.g., mumps or *Candida*) reveal positive results
   4. are useful for diagnosing streptococcal infections

10. Infections that are acquired by exposure to animals or insects include

    1. Q fever
    2. brucellosis
    3. leptospirosis
    4. toxoplasmosis

11. Which of the following statements about pelvic inflammatory disease are true?

    1. Chlamydia is now a common cause of this syndrome
    2. Sterility is a frequent sequela
    3. Occurrence of PID is increased by intrauterine devices
    4. *Neisseria gonorrhoeae* is reponsible for over 50% of the cases

12. Which of the following statements about staphylococci are true?

    1. Staphylococci are frequent causes of urinary tract infection
    2. They are particularly common causes of infection among diabetics
    3. Positive blood cultures of any species of staphylococcus indicate serious infection
    4. They frequently colonize the nose and can be spread by picking the nose

13. Which of the following statements about anaerobes are true?

    1. Anaeroebic organisms are commensals that inhabit the skin, mucosal surfaces, and intestinal tract without producing infection
    2. Anaerobes in the mouth can cause severe gingivitis
    3. Aspiration of mouth organisms into the lung often causes serious pulmonary infection, e.g., putrid lung abscess
    4. Although most anaerobes are sensitive to penicillin, abdominal infections with these organisms usually require other antibiotics, such as metronidazole

14. Gram-negative bacteria are important causes of which of the following clinical states?

    1. Shock due to endotoxemia
    2. Cystitis and pyelonephritis
    3. Nosocomial pneumonias
    4. Endocarditis in drug abusers

15. Which of the following statements about patients with chronic obstructive pulmonary disease are true?

    1. The extra work of breathing increases caloric expenditure and contributes to weight loss
    2. They tend to have a mixed respiratory and metabolic acidosis because of CO_2 retention and metabolic acidosis from anoxia
    3. They usually require use of accessory muscles of breathing
    4. Loud breath sounds are usually found on physical examination

16. In study of the nature of pleural effusions,

  1. transudates show a pleural fluid to plasma ratio of total protein > 0.5
  2. a high eosinophil count suggests an allergic origin
  3. a low glucose level compared with serum glucose in a patient with rheumatoid arthritis suggests superimposed infection
  4. the presence of blood in the absence of trauma suggests malignancy

17. Which of the following statements about hypoventilation are true?

  1. It occurs in patients with sleep apnea syndrome
  2. It occurs in very obese patients (pickwickian syndrome)
  3. It occurs with inhibition of central centers by drugs such as narcotics
  4. It can result in polycythemia, pulmonary hypertension, and cor pulmonale

18. Which of the following statements are true?

  1. GI x-rays using barium are better than endoscopy for identification of submucosal or compressive lesions of the esophagus
  2. Endoscopy is preferable to barium studies for identification of sites of bleeding in the stomach
  3. Barium studies are contraindicated if obstruction is suspected
  4. Gallstones are better identified by oral cholecystography than by ultrasonography

19. Which of the following statements about inflammatory bowel disease are true?

  1. Development of fistulas between bowel and skin or bladder suggests granulomatous bowel disease, e.g., regional enteritis
  2. Severe hypotension with fever, leukocytosis, and abdominal distension suggests development of toxic megacolon, which usually requires immediate surgery
  3. Occult bleeding occurs in both ulcerative colitis and regional enteritis, but gross bleeding is more characteristic of ulcerative colitis
  4. Pseudopolyps developing in ulcerative colitis do not become malignant

20. Which of the following statements about inflammatory bowel disease are true?

  1. Arthritis, affecting peripheral joints or the spine, occurs in both ulcerative colitis and regional enteritis
  2. The increased incidence of gallstones in regional enteritis is attributed to decreased absorption of bile salts
  3. There is an increased incidence of kidney stones in regional enteritis
  4. Surgery is recommended early in the treatment of both types of inflammatory bowel disease to avoid complications

21. Which of the following statements about GI tract cancer are true?

  1. Stomach cancer has become infrequent among most groups of native Americans but is more common in Orientals
  2. Stomach cancer occurs in association with gastric achlorhydria
  3. Iron deficiency anemia is a common mode of presentation of carcinoma of the right colon
  4. In the absence of familial polyposis, colonic polyps rarely become malignant

22. Which of the following statements about mitral valve prolapse are true?

  1. The condition is common and occurs most frequently in women
  2. There is an increased incidence of bacterial endocarditis in these patients
  3. Ventricular arrhythmias are a common complication
  4. Atrial enlargement and pulmonary edema commonly develop in these patients

23. Which of the following statements are true?

  1. The reticulocyte count will be decreased following transfusion
  2. A low reticulocyte count is found in iron deficiency anemia
  3. An increase in reticulocyte count after administration of folic acid establishes folate deficiency as the cause of anemia
  4. Correction of the reticulocyte count compensates for decreased red cell volume diluting the number of reticulocytes made each day

24. Which of the following statements are true?

  1. Folate is present in leafy vegetables, but since it is heat labile it may be lacking in the diets that contain cooked vegetables
  2. The intestinal conjugase that aids in absorption of folate is inhibited by phenytoin
  3. Red cell folate levels are a better measure of body stores of the vitamin than plasma levels
  4. Folate is capable of reversing the hematologic and CNS abnormalities that occur as a result of vitamin B_{12} deficiency

25. Which of the following statements are true?

  1. The bone marrow is capable of increasing red cell production by up to eightfold with severe hemolysis of bleeding
  2. An autoimmune thrombocytopenia may accompany autoimmune hemolytic anemia
  3. Active hemolysis is characterized by an increased reticulocyte count
  4. Hyperbilirubinemia seen with active hemolysis consists primarily of direct-reacting bilirubin

26. Which of the following statements are true?

  1. Splenomegaly due to any cause can be accompanied by hypersplenism
  2. The pancytopenia seen in hypersplenism is accompanied by active blood cell production in the bone marrow ("empty blood, full marrow" syndrome)
  3. Autoimmune hemolytic anemia is characterized by positive test for antibody bound to red cell membranes (Coombs' test)
  4. "Innocent bystander" type of hemolysis, resulting from antibodies to drugs bound to plasma proteins, would not be expected to be severe enough to cause anemia.

27. Which of the following statements are true?

  1. Patients with sickle cell anemia often have serious infections with *Salmonella* and pneumococci.
  2. The incidence of sickle cell trait is higher in certain parts of Africa than among American blacks
  3. Patients with sickle cell anemia tolerate the anemia well, but red cell transfusions are often needed before surgery or during pregnancy
  4. Children with sickle cell anemia typically have normal renal function

28. Common complications of advanced alcoholic cirrhosis of the liver include which of the following?

  1. Portal hypertension with massive ascites
  2. Apathy, restlessness, and abnormal motions of the extremities
  3. Splenomegaly with neutropenia due to hypersplenism
  4. Development of primary hepatic carcinoma

29. Which of the following statements regarding the workup of patients with polycythemia are true?

  1. Arterial blood gas determination is useful to rule out underlying pulmonary disease
  2. Splenomegaly points to polycythemia vera
  3. Polycythemia can occur secondary to renal lesions
  4. An increased red cell mass distinguishes between polycythemia vera and secondary polycythemia

30. Which of the following statements are true?

  1. In an emergency, type O Rh+ red cells can be given uncrossmatched to a type B Rh− recipient who has not received blood previously
  2. Platelet transfusions are useful in thrombocytopenic states with bleeding
  3. Coagulation factors can be supplied with fresh-frozen plasma
  4. Transfusion for anemia should consist of whole blood

31. Appropriate precautions to take in patients with severe neutropenia (WBCs < 1,000) include

  1. reverse isolation precautions
  2. use of stool softeners
  3. rapid institution of antibiotic therapy if fever develops
  4. immediate administration of granulocyte transfusion

32. Regarding complications of multiple myeloma, which of the following statements are true?

  1. Overwhelming infections with pneumococci occur frequently and prophylactic use of pneumococcal vaccine is worthwhile
  2. Renal failure can result from deposition of light chains in the renal tubules
  3. Use of radiopaque materials for an IVP can precipitate renal shutdown
  4. Back pain and anemia in a patient over age 50 are often a diagnostic clue to the presence of multiple myeloma

33. Which of the following statements are true?

  1. Bleeding time is primarily a measure of platelet function
  2. Prothrombin time measures the activity of several coagulation factors that are made in the liver
  3. Synthesis of the coagulation factors that determine the prothrombin time is affected by vitamin K
  4. Serum calcium determinations are indicated as part of the workup of patients with a bleeding disorder

34. Which of the following questions about pituitary tumors are true?

  1. Galactorrhea, acromegaly, and Cushing's disease are syndromes that result from tumors causing hyperfunction of the pituitary gland
  2. Extension of pituitary tumors into the cavernous sinus often produces ocular muscle palsies
  3. Extension of a pituitary tumor above the sella turcica can cause bitemporal hemianopsia
  4. The empty sella syndrome is characterized by a hypopituitary state

35. Which of the following statements about thyroid disease are true?

  1. Excessive intake of iodine before a test with radioactive iodine can result in misleadingly low uptake of iodine over the thyroid gland
  2. The circulating level of triiodothyronine (T_3) can be decreased by acute illness of many types, and therefore it is usually useless to determine the serum level in an acutely ill patient
  3. Elevated levels of serum thyrotropic hormone (TSH) can provide evidence for hypothyroidism even in an acutely ill patient
  4. In elderly patients, usual features of hyperthyroidism may be lacking and congestive heart failure may be the presenting manifestation

36. Which of the following questions about adrenal insufficiency are true?

1. Emergency therapy can be instituted with dexamethasone without interfering with diagnostic assay of plasma hormone levels
2. Thyroid hormone replacement should be begun early in the therapy of adrenal insufficiency due to hypopituitarism
3. Emergency therapy should include large amounts of salt and water, preferably parenterally
4. Hyperpigmentation occurs in adrenal insufficiency whether it is due to primary adrenal disease or to pituitary failure

37. Which of the following questions about Cushing's syndrome are true?

1. The syndrome can result from production of ACTH in tumor tissue in a variety of organs, such as lung tumors
2. Severe hypertension and diabetes are often part of this syndrome
3. Redness appearing in old scars and development of abdominal stretch marks is a characteristic findings in this syndrome
4. When the syndrome is due to a pituitary tumor, the tumor is usually large and easily detected radiologically

38. Which of the following questions about diabetes mellitus are true?

1. The likelihood of children developing diabetes is higher if the diabetic parent has noninsulin-dependent diabetes than if the parent has the insulin-dependent form of the disease
2. In diabetic ketoacidosis, there is usually marked hypovolemia due to the antecedent severe diuresis
3. Coma can result from hyperglycemia without ketoacidosis
4. In childhood diabetes, the likelihood of a nonidentical sibling developing the disease is the same as for an identical twin

39. Which of the following statements are true?

1. Vitamin D is made in the skin through the effect of ultraviolet light on a precursor and therefore it is not a necessary component of the diet
2. Vertebral fractures in patients with osteoporosis are the usual cause of sudden onset of back pain
3. Hip fractures in patients with osteoporosis can be successfully corrected surgically, but there is still a high frequency of death or permanent disability
4. The value of postmenopausal estrogen in prevention of osteoporosis does not outweigh the risk of uterine cancer in women who are put on replacement therapy

40. Which of the following statements about the treatment of hypertension are true?

1. An initial step in therapy should be weight reduction if the patient is obese
2. Reduction in alcohol consumption is an important aspect of therapy
3. Sodium restriction is useful
4. Institution of diuretics is usually the first step in pharmacologic therapy

41. Which of the following statements about sarcoidosis are true?

1. There can be blunted T-cell function resulting in negative skin tests to tuberculin, mumps, *Candida*, etc.
2. There can be blunted T-cell function resulting in frequent pulmonary infections with organisms such as *Pneumocytis carinii*
3. The finding of an increased serum level of angiotensin-converting enzyme is a useful diagnostic test
4. Hypercalcemia often occurs as a result of excessive ingestion of vitamin D

42. Which of the following statements are true?

1. Increased myocardial wall tension increases oxygen consumption and can aggravate anoxia due to coronary artery arteriosclerotic disease
2. Vasodilators can decrease both cardiac preload and afterload, resulting in improvement in cardiac function
3. Oliguria occurs as a manifestation of shock
4. Angina may occur at rest as a result of coronary artery spasm

43. Unstable angina is correctly described as

1. the new onset of anginal pain after exertion that previously led to no symptoms
2. an increase in the severity of preexisting angina
3. angina appearing with a degree of exertion that was previously well-tolerated
4. the first appearance of angina at rest or while asleep

44. Laboratory evidence for myocardial infarction includes

1. elevation of CPK
2. elevation of the sedimentation rate
3. leukocytosis
4. fever

45. Which of the following statements about pericarditis are true?

1. The presence of a friction rub means that there has been myocardial damage
2. A pulsus paradoxus is defined as an inspiratory rise in systolic blood pressure
3. The development of a large effusion makes tuberculosis the most likely cause
4. Constrictive pericarditis can follow any type of acute pericarditis

46. Which of the following statements about valvular heart disease are true?

1. Arterial emboli occur as a complication of rheumatic mitral valvular disease
2. The diastolic murmur of mitral stenosis usually loses its presystolic accentuation when atrial fibrillation develops
3. Oral penicillin should be administered prophylactically before dental surgery in patients with mitral valve disease
4. Mitral regurgitation is most frequently due to rheumatic valvular deformity

47. Which of the following statements about chronic renal failure are true?

1. Patients on chronic dialysis can need increased frequency of dialysis if they develop an acute illness
2. The bone disease associated with renal failure is in part related to increased parathyroid function
3. Acute inflammation of the soft tissues or joints can occur as a result of calcium pyrophosphate crystal deposition
4. Neuropathies including disturbances in GI motility and blood pressure control occur

48. The frequency of ventricular premature contractions can be increased by

1. ingestion of alcohol
2. smoking
3. hyperthyroidism
4. fever

49. Raynaud's syndrome may be initiated or aggravated by

1. frostbite
2. scleroderma
3. use of beta-blockers
4. emotional stress

50. Which of the following statements about accelerated hypertension are true?

1. Necrosis of arterial walls develops, with deposition of fibrinoid
2. Papilledema develops
3. Renal failure can develop rapidly
4. Development of left ventricular failure would not be an expected complication

51. Which of the following statements about Reye's syndrome are true?

1. It usually follows a viral respiratory tract infection such as influenza
2. In children, the use of aspirin has been associated with the occurrence of the syndrome; therefore, aspirin should not be given to children with respiratory tract infections
3. Abnormalities in liver and brain function are associated with morphological abnormalities in mitochondria in these organs
4. Mortality due to Reye's syndrome is just as high in adults as in children

52. Which of the following statements about head trauma are true?

1. Basal skull fractures can open tracts from paranasal sinuses, leading to cerebrospinal fluid rhinorrhea and recurrent meningitis
2. A concussion causes a reversible loss of consciousness without any residual loss of function
3. If cerebral function deteriorates after trauma, when recovery of function is expected, investigation for active intracranial bleeding is warranted
4. Bilateral pupillary fixation and loss of oculovestibular reflexes (doll's eyes) indicate brain stem damage

53. Which of the following statements about the relationships of renal function and drug effects are true?

1. Drugs that produce marked lowering of blood pressure can result in accumulation of other drugs that are mainly excreted by the kidney
2. Short-acting drugs in general are excreted by the kidney, and the dosage should be adjusted in the presence of renal failure
3. Blood level determinations are the best way of adjusting drug dosage in patients with chronic renal failure
4. Inhibitors of the synthesis of prostaglandins (e.g., nonsteroidal anti-inflammatory drugs) can cause an irreversible azotemia due to changes in renal perfusion

54. Which of the following statements about subdural hematomas are true?

1. Chronic subdural hematomas can follow apparently trivial head injury
2. Symptoms often fluctuate in severity
3. Factors that increase the likelihood of subdural hematoma include advanced age, alcoholism, and the use of anticoagulants
4. Older subdurals can become isodense and may not be visualized by CT scan

55. Which of the following statements about the locked-in state are true?

1. In the locked-in state, patients are fully aware and conscious but cannot respond and can appear to be comatose
2. This state can result from severe polyneuropathy
3. Care must be taken regarding communication to such patients since they are awake
4. This state results from irreversible brain-stem injury and is always fatal

56. During recovery from a bout of alcoholism, a patient has a focal seizure. You would take which of the following steps?

1. Treat with diazepam to control seizure activity
2. Obtain a CT scan to check for a subdural hematoma
3. Treat with large doses of thiamin
4. Avoid all habit-forming sedative drugs

57. Which of the following statements about transient ischemic attacks (TIAs) are true?

1. Unilateral blurring or loss of vision for a few minutes is typical of a TIA
2. Temporary loss of motor function (e.g., paralysis or severe weakness) of an arm or leg can occur
3. Since a major stroke may follow a TIA, hospitalization is often indicated
4. Transient sensory loss does not occur as part of a TIA

58. Neuromuscular syndromes that can be associated with underlying malignant tumors outside the nervous system include

1. a myasthenia gravis-like picture
2. polymyositis
3. subacute cerebellar degeneration
4. pseudotumor cerebri

59. Neuropathy due to long-standing diabetes mellitus typically results in

1. pain or numbness in the feet
2. rapidly progressive destruction of a joint such as an ankle
3. constipation and nocturnal diarrhea
4. impotence

60. Severe muscle weakness typically occurs in

1. excessive blood levels of aminoglycoside antibiotics
2. food poisoning with *Clostridium botulinum* toxin
3. the continued presence of a toxin-producing tick
4. food poisoning with a toxin produced by *Staphylococcus aureus*

61. Which of the following statements about carpal tunnel syndrome are true?

1. It is very common without any specific underlying disease
2. Pain is especially severe at night
3. Percussion over the wrist may reproduce the pain
4. A similar syndrome can occur in the feet due to tarsal tunnel nerve entrapment

DIRECTIONS: The groups of questions below consist of lettered choices followed by several numbered items. For each numbered item, select the one lettered choice with which it is most closely associated. Each lettered choice may be used once, more than once, or not at all.

Questions 62–65. For each of the types of blood cells listed below, select its life span.

A. 6 hours
B. 1 day
C. 7 to 10 days
D. 1 to 2 weeks
E. 120 days

62. Red blood cells

63. Neutrophils

64. Platelets

65. Reticulocytes

Questions 66–70. For each of the types of infections listed below, choose the usual causative agent.

A. *Campylobacter* sp.
B. *Hemophilus influenzae*
C. *Staphylococcus aureus*
D. Pneumococcus
E. *Bacteroides fragilis*

66. Skin infections

67. Paranasal sinus infection

68. Otitis and mastoiditis

69. Peritonitis

70. Gastroenteritis

ANSWERS

1. D	19. A (1, 2, 3)	37. A (1, 2, 3)	54. E (all)
2. E	20. A (1, 2, 3)	38. A (1, 2, 3)	55. A (1, 2, 3)
3. D	21. A (1, 2, 3)	39. A (1, 2, 3)	56. A (1, 2, 3)
4. E	22. A (1, 2, 3)	40. E (all)	57. A (1, 2, 3)
5. C	23. C (2, 4)	41. B (1, 3)	58. A (1, 2, 3)
6. D	24. A (1, 2, 3)	42. E (all)	59. E (all)
7. E (all)	25. A (1, 2, 3)	43. E (all)	60. A (1, 2, 3)
8. A (1, 2, 3)	26. A (1, 2, 3)	44. E (all)	61. E (all)
9. B (1, 3)	27. A (1, 2, 3)	45. D (4)	62. E
10. E (all)	28. E (all)	46. A (1, 2, 3)	63. A
11. E (all)	29. A (1, 2, 3)	47. A (1, 2, 3)	64. C
12. C (2, 4)	30. A (1, 2, 3)	48. E (all)	65. B
13. E (all)	31. A (1, 2, 3)	49. E (all)	66. C
14. E (all)	32. E (all)	50. A (1, 2, 3)	67. D
15. A (1, 2, 3)	33. E (all)	51. E (all)	68. D
16. D (4)	34. A (1, 2, 3)	52. A (1, 2, 3)	69. E
17. E (all)	35. E (all)	53. A (1, 2, 3)	70. A
18. A (1, 2, 3)	36. B (1, 3)		

2

SURGERY

Richard M. Stillman

HEAD AND NECK MASSES

Clinical features

A variety of systemic neoplastic or infectious disorders may present as a neck mass or oral cavity lesion. The vast majority of malignancies of the upper aerodigestive tract are squamous cell cancers arising from the mucosal lining. These tend to spread to cervical lymph nodes. Half of neck masses are located in the midline area and are thyroidal in nature. Half of lateral neck masses in adults are metastatic lymphadenopathy. Most arise from the upper aerodigestive tract or skin; a minority arise from primary tumors of the lung, GI tract, or kidney.

Diagnosis

The head and neck are inspected and palpated in a systematic fashion, noting characteristics of any abnormalities. Anterior rhinoscopy is indicated for epistasis or if an intranasal or paranasal sinus tumor is suspected. Posterior rhinoscopy is indicated for any thorough head and neck examination and is especially useful for the evaluation of cervical lymphadenopathy, nasopharyngeal lesions, posterior epistaxis, and cranial nerve deficit. Sonography is useful for thyroidal masses to determine whether they are cystic or solid. Radioactive iodine thyroid scanning is useful to determine function, because nonfunctional (cold) nodules are more likely to be malignant than functioning (hot) thyroidal nodules. For all head and neck masses, biopsy will be necessary to establish the diagnosis. If carcinoma is confirmed, a search for metastatic tumor is undertaken.

1. **Anterior oral cavity cancers** appear initially as either a fleshy exophytic lesion or persistent heaped-up ulceration. They then infiltrate adjacent structures causing referred pain, loosening of teeth, and impairment of speech.
2. **Tumors of the tonsillar fossa or posterior gingiva** (retromolar trigone) that infiltrate the lateral pterygoid muscle may produce trismus.
3. **Early tumors of the true vocal cords** (glottis) are associated with hoarseness.
4. **Neoplasms arising from the extrinsic larynx or hypopharynx** progress insidiously until dysphagia or pain and cervical metastases develop.
5. **Nasopharyngeal tumors** cause a variety of nasal, aural,

and neuro-ophthalmic symptoms such as nasal obstruction, ear symptoms, and optical motor nerve palsy.
6. **Maxillary sinus neoplasms** cause cheek swelling, palatal bulging, or invasion of the orbital floor.
7. **Thyroidal masses** move with deglutition and are found in the lower anterior neck.

Therapeutic decisions

Treatment of head and neck cancers must provide adequate local control of disease, preferably avoiding disfiguring resections and circumventing resection of vital structures. Sometimes this limits surgical therapy and requires a combination of surgical, radiation, and chemotherapy.

ARTERIAL DISEASE

Clinical features

Atherosclerosis is characterized by invasion of a damaged arterial intima by plaque consisting of lipid, necrotic cells, cholesterol crystals, and connective tissue. Although these atherosclerotic plaques are initially asymptomatic, discovered only by diminished pulses or the presence of a bruit on physical examination, progression of disease results in ischemia of the anatomic sites supplied by the atherosclerotic arteries.

Diagnosis

Symptoms. **Intermittent claudication** implies pain or fatigue occurring in the muscles of the calf, hip, or buttock on walking a reproducible distance ranging from several steps to several blocks. The symptom subsides with a few minutes rest.

If the pain occurs at rest or in bed at night (**ischemic rest pain**), is aggravated with elevation, or is relieved by dependency of the foot, it is considered rest pain and suggests advanced ischemia.

If severe pain occurs suddenly and is accompanied by paresthesias and progressive paralysis of the involved extremity, **acute arterial occlusion is suspected** (and urgent treatment is indicated). In this case, it is vital to obtain a history concerning cardiac disease or arrhythmia (suggests a possible embolic source), preexisting chronic arterial disease (suggests acute thrombosis of a chronically atherosclerotic vessel), abdominal aortic disease, or aneurysm (possible source of atheroembolism).

Physical examination. Physical exam is vital in determining the location and severity of peripheral arterial occlusive disease.

A **pulsatile midabdominal mass**, especially one that appears to extend to the left of the midline, suggests abdominal aortic aneurysm. A bruit may be audible over the midepigastrium or flank. If the pulsatile mass is also tender, if there is ecchymosis or hematoma of the flank or perimubilical area, or bulging of the flank (especially the left flank), or ecchymosis of the scrotum, rupture or impending rupture of an aortic aneurysm is likely and urgent treatment is vital.

The **foot** is examined for evidence of arterial ischemic changes including atrophy of the muscle, skin, or nails; loss of hair; coolness to touch; slow capillary refilling; cyanotic rubor; pallor; or necrosis.

Claudication that is vascular in origin is associated with absent or diminished distal **pulses** and/or the presence of bruits.

Noninvasive peripheral vascular studies. **Doppler pressures** are obtained by listening to the posterior tibial or dorsalis pedis artery while inflating a blood pressure cuff around the calf. **Plethysmography** provides tracings of overall segmental limb flow.

Routine blood tests. Routine blood tests include blood glucose (diabetes mellitus is associated with a high incidence of infrapopliteal occlusive disease), cholesterol and triglycerides (hyperlipoproteinemia will require dietary management), hematocrit (polycythemia is associated with high blood viscosity that interferes with arterial perfusion), and BUN and creatinine (assessment of renal status is vital prior to angiography).

Angiography. Angiography is the definitive test for determining arterial anatomy but is indicated only if operative intervention is planned.

Aortic ultrasonography. Aortic ultrasonography is diagnostic for aneurysm.

The diagnosis and treatment of arterial occlusive disease are summarized in Figure 2-1.

Therapeutic decisions

Intermittent claudication. The risk of limb loss in patients with intermittent claudication alone without evidence of impending tissue ischemia is 1% per year. Hence, medical management is indicated. This includes control of underlying risk factors (cigarette smoking, diabetes, hypertension, obesity, hyperlipidemia), exercise, and pentoxifylline. Acute arterial occlusion requires anticoagulation with heparin and urgent operative thrombectomy or embolectomy. If disabling claudication continues despite the above, if there is ischemic rest pain, or if the feet show signs of ischemia, surgery is considered. Possible options include percutaneous transluminal angioplasty (for short-segment high-grade stenotic lesions, especially of the iliac artery), bypass using autogenous saphenous vein or prosthetic graft, and endarterectomy (removal of plaque and diseased underlying intima, appropriate for short-segment accessible lesion).

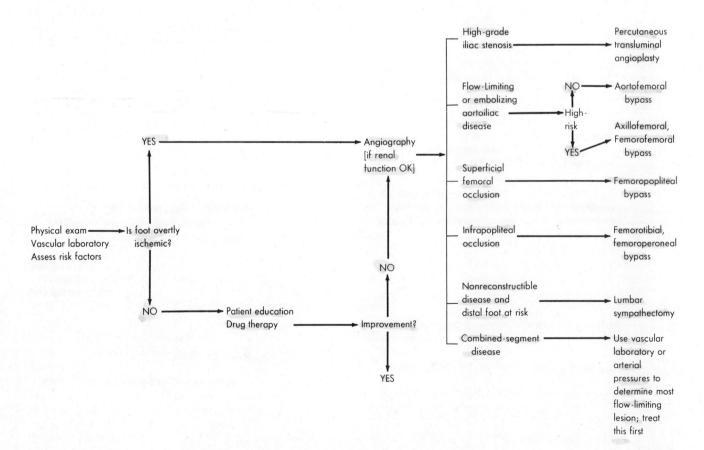

Figure 2-1. Peripheral arterial occlusive disease: Diagnosis and treatment.

Aneurysm. Abdominal aortic aneurysm requires elective operative resection (risk of rupture is 50% within 2 years, 80 to 90% within 5 years).

Postoperative complications

Possible postoperative complications include hemorrhage, graft thrombosis, embolization of plaque ("trash foot"), infection, erosion into adjacent structures (aortoduodenal fistula), renal failure (especially after ruptured aortic aneurysm), intestinal ischemia (especially after interruption of flow to the inferior mesenteric artery during aortic surgery), ureteral injury, spinal cord ischemia (may occur with interruption of flow in the great radicular artery of Adamkiewicz during aortic surgery), impotence (with interruption of hypogastric arterial flow), and lymphedema (common following femoropopliteal bypass procedures).

THORACIC SURGERY

HEMOPTYSIS

Clinical features

The most common causes of hemoptysis are bronchitis, tuberculosis, foreign bodies, pneumonia, pulmonary embolus, bronchiectasis, aspergillosis, carcinoma, sarcoma, cystic fibrosis, arteriovenous malformation, mitral stenosis, tracheo-innominate artery fistula, and pulmonary artery erosion from thermistor-tipped, flow-directed pulmonary artery catheter. The diagnosis will not be made in 10%, even after an extensive workup.

Diagnosis

Smoking history suggests an inflammatory or neoplastic etiology. Fever, chills, night sweats, and productive cough all suggest an inflammatory etiology. Malaise and weight loss may suggest malignancy. The presence of a diminished gag reflex may lead to foreign body aspiration. The presence of deep vein thrombosis suggests the possibility of pulmonary embolism. End-stage mitral stenosis may lead to hemoptysis; associated features will include dyspnea on exertion, orthopnea, paroxysmal noctural dyspnea, pulmonary edema, chronic cough, atrial fibrillation, hepatomegaly, ascites, and a history of repeated respiratory infections. Exsanguinating hemoptysis will occur from tracheoinnominate fistula, a complication of long-term tracheal intubation. Asymptomatic hemoptysis may be due to carcinoma, sarcoma, or arteriovenous malformations. Chest x-ray may help differentiate infiltrative inflammatory processes, lung abscesses, neoplasms, and foreign bodies. Apical scarring suggests tuberculosis. Air-fluid levels suggest an abscess cavity. Bronchography is useful if bronchiectasis is suspected. Bronchoscopy may reveal tracheitis, bronchitis, endobronchial lesions, and foreign bodies.

Therapeutic decisions

Immediate treatment is indicated for gross hemoptysis. It includes intravenous fluids, NPO, 45-degree angulation of the bed, antimicrobial agents, mild sedation, and cough suppression. Sputum is collected for examination and culture. If there is dyspnea or tachypnea, oxygen is provided by mask or nasal cannula. Emergent control may require bronchoscopic locali-

zation of the responsible lung and insertion of a special endotracheal tube to allow selective ventilation of the normal side. Definitive treatment of the underlying lesion may include operative exploration for lobectomy or pneumonectomy and angiographic embolization of arteriovenous fistulas.

DYSPHAGIA

Clinical features

Dysphagia may result from congenital or acquired problems. Congenital problems include esophageal atresia or duplications, short esophagus, vascular anomalies, or esophageal webs. Acquired causes include achalasia, reflux esophagitis, esophageal malignancy, esophageal diverticula, lye stricture, or extrinsic compression (by aortic aneurysm, goiter, exostoses of cervical vertebrae, mediastinal neoplasm, lymphadenopathy, left atrial enlargement, or vascular anomalies). Some systemic problems may give rise to dysphagia. These include scleroderma, pellagra, and myasthenia gravis.

Diagnosis

The duration of the symptom and presence of weight loss may suggest the etiology. Ask where the patient believes the food lodges— this may well accurately localize the lesion. Ask about associated nausea, vomiting, hematemesis, melena, fever, pain, weakness, malaise, weight loss, halitosis, and regurgitation of undigested food particles. A barium swallow will define the location and often the nature of the lesion. Esophagoscopy will allow biopsy and confirm the diagnosis by pathological examination of the specimen. In some cases, cytological examination of a nasogastric aspirate will demonstrate malignant cells.

Therapeutic decisions

Therapy is directed toward the underlying disease process.
1. **Achalasia.** Pneumatic or hydrostatic dilatation or modified Heller's myotomy (sectioning the hypertrophied muscular layers).
2. **Diverticula.** Surgical correction.
3. **Lye stricture.** Early dilatation; esophagectomy and cervical esophagogastrostomy for chronic stricture.
4. **Leiomyomas.** Enucleate (they are submucosal).
5. **Carcinoma.** After metastatic disease is ruled out, resection is indicated.
6. **Strictures resulting from long-standing reflux esophagitis.** Dilatation, correction of the cause of reflux (hiatal hernia repair).
7. **Upper esophageal webs.** Correct the underlying metabolic or nutritional deficiency; periodic dilatation may be necessary.
8. **Foreign bodies.** Airway obstruction may require the Heimlich maneuver or cricothyrotomy; otherwise, endoscopic removal may be necessary.

BREAST MASS

Clinical features

Breast cancer is the second most common malignancy (skin cancer is first) in females, affecting 1 of every 14 women. However, only one in four breast masses will prove to be malignant. Benign breast masses in patients younger than 30 years are usually fibroadenoma, papillomatosis, breast abscess, cystosarcoma phylloides, or mesothelial neoplasms. After the age of 30, breast cysts, fibrocystic disease, breast cancer, breast abscess, fat necrosis, and cystosarcoma phylloides are common. Breast pain may be due to premenstrual mastodynia, fibrocystic mastopathy, breast abscess, or traumatic fat necrosis. Bilateral nipple discharge is usually due to pregnancy or lactation but may rarely persist for years. Unilateral nipple discharge suggests a local problem within the ductal system of the breast, usually an intraductal papilloma.

Diagnosis

History. *Determine the presence of risk factors for breast cancer.* The incidence of breast cancer increases with age. Countries with high daily fat intake have the highest incidence of breast cancer. Long menstrual life (i.e., early menarche and late menopause) is associated with an increased risk of developing breast cancer. Multiple pregnancies decrease the length of the menstrual life and thus have a protective effect. Papillomatosis and gross cystic disease are associated with a higher incidence of later development of breast cancer. Family history of breast cancer— especially in the patient's mother, maternal aunt, sister, or grandmother— is associated with an increased risk of breast cancer. A history of prior breast cancer is associated with a higher incidence of subsequent development of another breast cancer.

Physical examination. Focus on the size, consistency, fixation, nipple involvement, and axillary node involvement associated with the mass.

Biopsy and needle aspiration. Biopsy is the definitive procedure for any patient with a breast mass. However, if the mass appears cystic, needle aspiration may be attempted. If this results in resolution of the mass, then surgical excision is avoided. If the mass persists or recurs, surgical biopsy under local anesthesia is required. If the mass appears solid or suspicious, surgical biopsy is of course mandatory. The surgical specimen is brought to the pathologist without preservative. This allows immediate diagnosis (by frozen section examination); if malignancy is discovered, hormonal receptor assays are performed on the fresh tissue.

Routine screening examinations

1. Women 20 years of age and older should perform breast self-examination every month.
2. Women 20 to 40 years of age should have a physical examination of the breasts every 3 years.
3. Women over 40 should have a physical examination of the breasts every year.
4. If there is a strong family history or positive risk factors, breast examinations should start at age 35.
5. Women between the ages of 35 and 40 should have a baseline mammogram.
6. Women over 50 years old should have a mammogram every year when feasible.
7. Women with the presence of any risk factors defined above should undergo mammography every other year from ages 40 to 50.
8. Any suspicious mass found on examination or on mammography must not be ignored.
9. If the mass is not palpable, mammographic injection of methylene blue or needle localization will help guide surgical excision.
10. Mammography is also indicated for follow-up of some benign lesions (e.g., fibrocystic mastopathy), nipple discharge without a palpable lesion, breast pain without a clinical explanation, and in some patients with severe cancerphobia.

Therapeutic decisions

Therapeutic decision is based on the staging of the tumor (Table 2-1). The possibility of metastatic disease is investigated with chest x-ray, bilateral mammography, complete blood

Table 2-1. Tumor-Node-Metastasis (TNM) Staging of Breast Cancer

T (Tumor)

Tis	Carcinoma in situ and Paget's disease of the nipple with nonpalpable tumor.
T0	Metastases present in the axillary nodes or elsewhere in the body in the patient with a nonpalpable tumor of the breast and nothing suggesting malignancy on mammography.
T1	Tumor measures less than 2 cm.
T2	Tumor measures 2 to 5 cm.
T3	Tumor measures greater than 5 cm.

T1, T2, and T3 may be subclassified as

a	Not attached to pectoral fascia or muscle.
b	Attached to pectoral fascia or muscle. Nipple retraction or skin tethering does not affect the T classification.
T4	Tumor is massive, has ulcerated through the skin, is associated with peau d'orange, or is fixed to the chest wall.

N (Nodes)

N0	The nodes are not clinically palpable.
N1a	Nodes are palpable and are thought to be hyperplastic.
N1b	Nodes are thought to contain metastases.
N2	The metastases in the nodes have extended beyond the capsule as manifested by fixation of the nodes to one another, to the skin, or to the deep tissues.
N3	Ipsilateral apical or supraclavicular nodes are thought to contain metastases.

M (Metastases)

M0	Distant metastases are not found clinically or on preoperative investigations.
M1	Distant metastases have been found.

count, liver function tests, and serum calcium determination. In the absence of documented metastatic disease or grave local signs, the treatment options include modified radical mastectomy or lumpectomy (i.e., wide local excision of the lesion and axillary lymph node removal, followed by radiation therapy). Advanced cancer requires systemic therapy. Hormonal manipulation is indicated for premenopausal women, especially when the tumor has estrogen or progesterone receptors in high concentration. Radiotherapy is effective for control of pain due to bony metastases. Systemic chemotherapy is indicated when hormone receptor assays are negative.

THYROID LESIONS

Clinical features

Toxic (hyperthyroid) disorders may be diffuse (Graves' disease), multinodular, or solitary (toxic adenoma). Nontoxic (euthyroid) disorders may be multinodular or solitary. Single nontoxic nodules may be colloid or congenital cysts or benign or malignant tumors. Thyroglossal duct cysts and dermoid cysts are developmental abnormalities that present as midline neck masses.

Diagnosis

Thyroid function tests (T_3, T_4, TSH) determine whether the patient is hyperthyroid, euthyroid, or hypothyroid. (For more detail, see Chapter 1, Internal Medicine.) Grave's disease is a diffuse, symmetrically enlarged gland usually with an audible bruit. Toxic multinodular goiter is irregular, firm, and asymmetric. Toxic adenoma is a hyperfunctioning, solitary, firm nodule that suppresses function of the remainder of the gland. The radionuclide thyroid scan is useful to determine the extent and function of diseased thyroid gland. Nontoxic multinodular colloid goiter is characterized by multiple, usually bilateral, nodules with varying degrees of functional activity. Functioning (hot) thyroid nodules are far less likely to be malignant than nonfunctioning (cold) nodules. Ultrasonographic examination of the thyroid gland will distinguish cystic (usually benign) from solid masses. Needle biopsy is useful in equivocal or nonsuspicious thyroid masses, whereas surgical exploration and lobectomy are required for suspicious masses.

Therapeutic decisions

Graves' disease is treated with antithyroid drugs (prophylthiouracil or methimazole), radioactive iodine therapy (^{131}I), or surgery (subtotal thyroidectomy). Each modality has its benefits and risks. Surgical therapy is required for thyroid cancer or nodules suspected to be malignant. The appropriate surgical procedure for cancer includes total lobectomy, isthmusectomy, and ipsilateral paratracheal lymph node removal. High-grade malignancies or those with suspected lymph node metastases will require more radical surgery, including total thyroidectomy or radical neck dissection.

ABDOMINAL PAIN

Clinical features

Prompt diagnosis and treatment of abdominal pain are essential because delay significantly increases mortality. In many cases, the exact pathology may remain elusive until laparotomy. Nevertheless, history and physical examination provide clues to the etiology and determine whether urgent operation is indicated.

Diagnosis

The nature, duration, and location of the pain relate directly to the offending problem (Table 2-2).

Characteristics of the pain. **Sudden onset of excruciating pain** suggests a ruptured hollow viscus, sudden obstruction of the cystic duct or ureter, or ruptured aneurysm. **Sudden onset of severe, constant pain** suggests strangulation obstruction of the small bowel, acute pancreatitis, or ruptured ectopic

Table 2-2. Etiology of Abdominal Pain

Usual nature of pain	Usual location of pain	Typical causes
Abrupt and excruciating	Right upper quadrant	Biliary colic
	Generalized or epigastric	Perforated peptic ulcer
	Midabdominal with possible radiation to back	Ruptured aortic aneurysm
	Flank or lower quadrant, possible radiation to groin	Ureteral colic
	Midsternal or epigastric	Myocardial infarction
Severe and constant with rapid onset	Epigastric with possible radiation to back	Pancreatitis
	Midabdominal	Mesenteric ischemia
	Hypogastric	Ruptured ectopic pregnancy
Intermittent and colicky with pain-free intervals	Midabdominal	Small bowel obstruction
	Hypogastric	Inflammatory bowel disease
Gradual and steady	Right upper quadrant	Acute cholecystitis, acute cholangitis, or acute hepatitis
	Periumbilical shifting to right lower quadrant	Acute appendicitis or acute salpingitis
	Left lower quadrant	Diverticulitis

pregnancy. **Intermittent colicky pain with pain-free intervals** suggests small bowel obstruction or inflammatory bowel disease. **Gradual onset of steady pain** suggests peritonitis secondary to diverticulitis, appendicitis, cholecystitis, cholangitis, hepatitis, or salpingitis.

Visceral versus somatic pain. **Visceral pain** results from distension of a hollow viscus and is referred to the midline area, corresponding to the embryologic origin of the involved viscus. **Epigastric pain** will result from distension of the stomach, duodenum, gallbladder, and pancreatic ducts—all outgrowths of the foregut. The initial pain of acute pancreatitis, perforated duodenal ulcer, and cholecystitis is typically epigastric. **Periumbilical pain** results from distension of the small bowel from the ligament of Treitz to the midtransverse colon, those organs of the midgut supplied by the superior mesenteric artery. The initial pain of acute appendicitis and of small bowel obstruction is typically periumbilical. **Hypogastric pain** is characteristic of distension of the hindgut, the colon from the midtransverse region to the rectum, supplied by the inferior mesenteric vessels. The initial pain of sigmoid diverticulitis is typically hypogastric.

Somatic pain results from mechanical or chemical irritation of the parietal peritoneum and is noticed in the area actually involved. Pain in this area is increased by maneuvers that stretch or place tension on the involved area, such as a bumpy ride to the hospital.

Associated symptoms

Anorexia. The presence of anorexia in association with abdominal pain is variable but is often an early sign of an acute abdominal problem, particularly appendicitis. If, however, an inflamed appendix is surrounded by intact omentum, peritonitis may not occur and anorexia may be absent. Hence, the presence of anorexia should arouse suspicions of peritonitis, although the absence of anorexia does not rule out acute abdominal pathology.

Nausea and vomiting. Distension of a hollow viscus induces reflex vomiting often not associated with nausea. If the pain is not relieved by vomiting, it suggests a closed-loop obstruction of the small bowel or a biliary or GU tract obstruction. Vomiting secondary to simple mechanical small bowel obstruction will temporarily relieve the colicky pain.

Change in bowel habits. **Obstipation** suggests intestinal obstruction. **Diarrhea** suggests viral gastroenteritis but may also occur with pelvic peritonitis, especially appendiceal abscess. **Bloody diarrhea** suggests ulcerative colitis, colonic regional enteritis, dysentery, or colonic ischemia.

Fever. **High spiking fever** suggests pylephlebitis, pelvic inflammatory disease, abscess, or infection of the CNS, lung, or urinary tract. **Intermittent chills and fever** suggest acute cholangitis or acute pyelitis. **Moderately high fever** occurs with perforation of a hollow viscus or ischemic bowel. Appendicitis is usually associated with **low-grade fever**. Conversely, however, a **normal temperature** does not rule out any abdominal pathology.

Signs

Inspection. The presence of surgical scars in the patient with intestinal obstruction suggests obstruction due to **adhe**sions. **Dilated abdominal wall veins** suggest portal hypertension or may be present in severe abdominal distension due to other causes or to inferior vena cava obstruction. A generalized abdominal **skin rash** suggests systemic toxemia, viral infection, or septicemia. **Distention of the small bowel due to paralytic ileus or intestinal obstruction** is the most common cause of abdominal distension in the patient with acute abdominal pain. **Ascites** is suggested by abdominal distension with bulging flanks. There is anterior tympany, a fluid wave, and shifting dullness. The presence of **shifting dullness** is determined by percussing the level of dullness in the flanks with the patient supine and then turned to one side. Considerable shift in this level suggests the presence of free intraperitoneal fluid.

Advanced pregnancy may be diagnosed by the presence of abdominal distension and engorged breasts, softening of the uterine cervix, palpation of the fetus, and auscultation of the fetal heartbeat. A massively **enlarged liver** or spleen may also fill much of the abdominal cavity and can be distinguished from other causes of abdominal distension by percussion or palpation.

A suprapubic bulge suggests a distended bladder or pregnancy. Incisional **hernia**, epigastric hernia, and umbilical hernia are obvious on examination. Large inguinal hernias are obvious, but small ones may be subtle, requiring digital examination through the inguinal canal to detect the defect, bulge, or impulse. Approximately 3 cm medial to the pulsating femoral artery, a bulging mass suggests **femoral hernia**.

Pulsation of the midportion of the abdomen suggests a transmitted pulse from the aorta through a retroperitoneal or intra-abdominal mass or the presence of an aortic aneurysm. However, in the very thin patient with a scaphoid abdomen, this finding may be normal.

Percussion. A shrunken **liver** is compatible with advanced cirrhosis, whereas an **enlarged liver** is compatible with hepatitis, early cirrhosis, or metastatic tumor.

Auscultation. **Loud, prolonged high-pitched hyperactive** sounds occur in intestinal obstruction. **Absent bowel sounds** (silent abdomen) suggest advanced peritonitis.

Palpation. Palpation is the portion of the physical examination most likely to reveal those dramatic findings suggesting peritonitis; nevertheless, it is discussed last to emphasize the fact that history, inspection, auscultation, and percussion all have their place in the physical diagnosis of abdominal pain.

Tenderness noted during quick withdrawal of the palpating fingers is termed **rebound tenderness**. This is characteristic of irritation of the parietal peritoneum. **Tenderness at McBurney's point** is characteristic of appendicitis. This point is located just below the midpoint of a line between the umbilicus and the anterior superior iliac spine. It represents the usual location of the base of the appendix. Much attention should be paid to the presence of muscle **guarding** during the examination of the patient with abdominal pain. **Involuntary guarding** is highly suggestive of peritonitis, with rare exceptions (uncommon neurological disorders and renal colic). Voluntary guarding is muscle spasm resulting from pain caused by the examination.

Other signs may also accompany abdominal disease. In the **psoas sign**, hyperextension of the thigh stretches the psoas major muscle and causes pain if a retrocecal appendix overlying this muscle is inflamed. In the **obturator sign**, internal

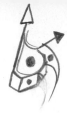

rotation of the patient's thigh will stretch the obturator muscle and cause pain if an inflamed retrocecal appendix overlies this area. In **Murphy's sign**, deep right subcostal palpation during deep inspiration will allow the examiner's fingers to compress a distended gallbladder and cause pain if there is acute cholecystitis. On **rectal and pelvic examination**, tenderness on cervical motion suggests adnexal inflammation. A retrocecal appendix or a pelvic abscess will be palpable when tender on rectal examination.

Specific diagnostic techniques

Laboratory studies may be necessary to prepare the patient for a safe operation. When operation is not indicated, laboratory tests may help confirm a nonsurgical diagnosis or follow the progress of the underlying pathology. These laboratory tests include serum electrolytes, hematocrit, white cell count, amylase, and urinalysis.

Obtunded patients with suspected abdominal pathology may be subjected to careful **abdominal paracentesis and lavage** to determine the presence or absence of pus, blood, or amylase.

Abdominal flat plate and upright films and chest x-ray should routinely be done. Subphrenic free air (suggesting perforated viscus) is best seen on an upright chest film in which the diaphragm is adequately visualized. **Abdominal films** will demonstrate obscured borders of liver, spleen, kidneys, or psoas muscle; differential air-fluid levels in the small bowel, suggesting obstruction; absence of gas or feces in the colon, suggesting colonic obstruction; and abnormal calcifications, suggesting fecalith in the appendix, stones in the gallbladder, chronic calcific pancreatitis, abnormal lymph nodes, or a calcified aortic aneurysm. The unusual finding of differential air-fluid levels with calcific density along the small bowel and air in the biliary tract is highly suggestive of gallstone ileus.

Sonography (real-time or B-mode ultrasonography) is useful in defining the nature of abdominal masses (solid or cystic), confirming the presence or absence of aortic aneurysm, and localizing intra-abdominal abscess. Ultrasonography is very accurate in the evaluation of the pancreaticobiliary tract (dilated pancreatic or common bile duct suggesting distal obstruction, edematous pancreas suggesting acute pancreatitis, pancreatic pseudocyst, cholelithiasis, edema of gallbladder wall suggesting acute cholecystitis) and of the urinary tract (renal mass lesions and hydronephrosis). Sonography may occasionally be helpful in directing percutaneous aspiration or drainage of certain selective intra-abdominal lesions. It is a noninvasive and inexpensive procedure that can even be performed at the bedside.

CT scan provides information similar to but more accurate than that provided by sonography but requires more time and is considerably more costly. It is indicated when sonography is nondiagnostic, when sonography is inaccurate (e.g., in obese patients), and when the increased diagnostic sensitivity and specificity are vital, as in localization of small intra-abdominal abscesses or metastatic disease.

Contrast studies of the GI tract are usually avoided in acute abdominal pain but in rare cases may be useful. Such a case is the alcoholic whose history, physical examination, and laboratory plain x-ray studies cannot distinguish between acute pancreatitis and perforated peptic ulcer. In this case, a water-soluble contrast material administered through a nasogastric tube may help determine the need for exploratory laparotomy.

Angiography is rarely indicated in the workup of abdominal pain, although it is invaluable in the diagnosis and treatment of massive GI hemorrhage. If chronic mesenteric ischemia is suspected, selective visceral angiography is indicated to assess the site and degree of disease.

Pipida scanning is useful in the diagnosis of suspected acute biliary tract obstruction.

Findings suggesting nonsurgical causes of abdominal pain

1. **Myocardial infarction.** Abnormal ECG and elevated creatinine phosphokinase (CPK).
2. **Acute hepatitis.** Liver tenderness; elevated prothrombin time, bilirubin, and serum glutamic-oxaloacetic transaminase (SGOT).
3. **Acute porphyria.** Porphobilinogen in the urine (Watson-Schwartz test).
4. **Acute epidemic pleurodynia.** Tenderness over lower thoracic wall.
5. **Pneumothorax.** Visualized on chest x-ray.
6. **Pneumonia.** Visible on chest x-ray.
7. **Vasculitis** (i.e., systemic lupus erythematosus or polyarteritis nodosa). Differential diagnosis may be impossible because, although vasculitis may cause nonsurgical abdominal pain, it may also be associated with visceral ischemia that does require laparotomy.

Therapeutic decisions

Analgesics should be withheld until a diagnosis is made or until the need for laparotomy is ascertained. If peritonitis is suspected, broad-spectrum antibiotics are administered. Insertion of an intravenous line for hydration with the appropriate solution is performed on admission to the emergency room. If generalized peritonitis, intestinal obstruction, or paralytic ileus is present, a nasogastric tube is passed immediately. Otherwise, this may be performed with the patient under anesthesia at the time of laparotomy. The need for laparotomy is usually determined by the diagnosis made on the basis of the history and physical examination. After laboratory and radiological examination, if the need for laparotomy is still uncertain, the patient is admitted to the hospital and observed. Laparotomy is undertaken if there is increasing or severe local tenderness, involuntary guarding or rigidity, suspected mesenteric ischemia (unexplained acidosis), or clinical deterioration during nonoperative therapy. In addition, radiological or laboratory findings documenting perforation, abscess, intractable bleeding, or obstruction warrant operative intervention.

INTESTINAL OBSTRUCTION

Clinical features

If the patient has previously had an abdominal operation, the chances are nine to one that small bowel obstruction is the result of **adhesions**. If the patient has not had a previous operation, a **visible external hernia** is the most frequent cause of the obstruction. Other less likely causes of small bowel obstruction include small bowel neoplasms, intussusception, and inflammatory lesions, particularly due to untreated appendicitis or Crohn's disease. The most common cause of mechanical large bowel obstruction is cancer, usually located in the rectosigmoid. Other less common causes include sigmoid or cecal volvulus, diverticulitis, fecal impaction, and Ogilvie's syndrome (idiopathic adynamic ileus). Mortality in patients with intestinal obstruction is related to two problems: (1) inadequate correction of fluid and electrolyte deficits and (2) inordinate delay before operative intervention, allowing progressive ischemia, acidosis, and sepsis.

Diagnosis

Evaluation of the patient with constipation or obstipation, abdominal pain, distension, nausea, or vomiting is directed toward (1) assessing correctable secondary problems such as dehydration and electrolyte imbalance and (2) determining the location (i.e., small bowel or large bowel) and cause (i.e., mechanical, ischemic, or paralytic) of obstruction to determine the need for and appropriate timing of operative intervention. Once a diagnosis of mechanical or ischemic obstruction is suspected, endoscopic or radiological workup may occasionally delineate the cause of the problem, but nothing short of exploratory laparotomy will determine the viability of the bowel so involved.

Obstipation and intermittent cramping abdominal pain occur early. Proximal lesions cause early bilious vomiting and little distension. Distal obstructions cause more pronounced abdominal distension and late feculent vomiting. With simple mechanical small bowel obstruction, episodes of vomiting will at least temporarily relieve the pain. If the pain is not relieved by vomiting, closed-loop obstruction or ischemic bowel is suspected. Temperature will be normal to slightly elevated. Small bowel obstruction is accompanied by hyperactive and high-pitched bowel sounds, abdominal distension, and possibly diffuse minimal abdominal tenderness. Peritoneal signs such as rebound or guarding suggest either bowel ischemia or an inflammatory process.

Rectal examination usually reveals an empty rectal vault but may disclose occult blood (suggesting an intraluminal lesion or ischemic bowel) or tenderness (suggesting a pelvic abscess or retrocecal appendicitis). Elevated hematocrit and hemoglobin suggest hemoconcentration and dehydration. White blood cell count may be somewhat elevated, but major elevations (over 14,000 cells/mm^3) suggest strangulation, obstruction, or peritonitis. Serum electrolytes typically reveal loss of sodium, potassium, chloride, and acid secondary to vomiting of gastric contents. Abdominal x-ray will reveal distended intestine proximal to the obstruction and collapsed intestine with absent gas distally. With mechanical obstruction, air-fluid levels will be **differential** (J-loops) because of the effect of peristalsis attempting to move air and fluid toward the obstruction. For large bowel obstruction, proctosigmoidoscopy may reveal a neoplasm or inflammatory lesion but will be nondiagnostic if the lesion is above the reach of the proctoscope (25 to 30 cm from the anus).

If the plain film reveals a classic massive sigmoid dilatation and crow's beak appearance of sigmoid volvulus, proctosigmoidoscopy with insertion of a rectal tube beyond the kink will allow explosive decompression and immediate temporary relief. If there is intermittent, questionable, or early large bowel obstruction, a contrast enema may be performed after rectal examination and proctosigmoidoscopy. For colonic obstruction with a palpable abdominal mass suggesting a diverticular abscess, ultrasonography of the abdomen is indicated.

Therapeutic decisions

Intestinal obstruction requires operative relief after correction of fluid, electrolyte, and acid-base abnormalities. Operative correction depends on the cause.

1. **Single adhesive band.** Lysis.
2. **Multiple adhesions.** Lyse all of them; the offending adhesion is the one occurring at the transition between the proximal distended and distal collapsed intestine.
3. **Intrinsic lesions or ischemia.** Resect.
4. **Massively distended bowel.** Decompress by long tube passed orally or nasally.
5. **Recurrent adhesive obstruction.** Intestinal plication or stenting.
6. **Obstruction due to hernia.** Repair hernia and correct any resultant small bowel problem as above.
7. **Distension of the cecum** over 12 cm. Urgent operative decompression, because the cecum is the earliest portion of the large bowel to undergo necrosis and perforation.
8. **Left colonic obstruction.** Decompressive colostomy or cecostomy if bowel is unprepared; resection later after bowel preparation.
9. **Colon obstruction with perforation.** Resection, proximal colostomy, drainage of abscess.
10. **Sigmoid volvulus.** Proctoscopic decompression; elective resection to prevent recurrence (common).
11. **Transverse or right colon obstruction.** Primary resection and anastomosis may be considered even with unprepared bowel because of the lower bacterial concentration on the right side of the colon.
12. **Cecal volvulus.** Cecopexy.

GASTROINTESTINAL BLEEDING

Clinical features

Upper GI bleeding may result from duodenal ulcer, gastric erosion (stress, burns, drug-induced), gastric ulcer, esophageal or gastric varices, Mallory-Weiss tears, hiatal hernia, neoplasm, vascular lesions, trauma (hemobilia), or aneurysmal or vascular graft erosion into the GI tract.

Lower GI bleeding may arise from diverticulosis, neoplasm, ulcerative colitis, vascular malformations, ischemic bowel disease, and aortoenteric fistula.

Diagnosis

Ascertain if there is a prior history of bleeding, peptic ulcer disease, alcoholism, or ingestion of steroids, salicylates, or anticoagulants. Obtain a nasogastric aspirate. "Coffee grounds" material suggests slow or stopped bleeding with retention of blood in the stomach until it is converted to acid hematin. Red blood suggest rapid bleeding. GI endoscopy is over 90% accurate

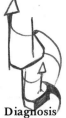

in upper GI bleeding. Because of the inability to properly cleanse the colon, it is often not useful for lower GI bleeding. Arteriography is indicated for upper GI bleeding if endoscopy fails to visualize the site of the bleeding or for treatment of continuing or recurrent bleeding. Arteriography is the diagnostic, and often therapeutic, procedure of choice for rapid lower GI bleeding. Bleeding rates as low as 1/2 ml/minute may be visualized. Note that actual bleeding from the esophagus is rarely visualized by arteriography, but it may demonstrate the presence of portal hypertension (i.e., retrograde portal vein flow), hepatic collaterals, varices, or tortuosity of intrahepatic arteries. Barium contrast study is not useful for acute bleeding and obscures the view on subsequent arteriogram. Barium study is appropriate for elective workup of intermittent or slow bleeding. A trial of balloon tamponade may be useful in patients with suspected portal hypertension and massive upper GI bleeding; control of massive bleeding by the Sengstaken-Blakemore tube suggests a variceal cause.

Therapeutic decisions

Intravenous fluid replacement and blood transfusion are instituted. Nasogastric suction and intermittent gastric lavage are begun. Antacids may be administered via nasogastric tube. Histamine H_2 blockers are titrated to maintain gastric aspirate pH above 5. Endoscopic sclerotherapy is useful for variceal bleeding. Angiography with Gelfoam or autogenous clot embolization or vasopressin (Pitressin) infusion may also be therapeutic. Colonic bleeding is far more likely to cease spontaneously than is upper GI bleeding. Operative treatment is indicated for rapid bleeding beyond the ability to replace losses, for recurrent bleeding, for loss of more than 2,000 ml total or 1,000 ml rapidly, for bleeding vessel seen on endoscopy, and when transfusion is impossible (e.g., refusal of blood or rare blood type). The operative procedure depends on the bleeding site.

1. **Duodenal ulcer.** Oversewing of bleeder and vagotomy and pyloroplasty.
2. **High gastric ulcer.** Oversewing and biopsy of ulcer; vagotomy and pyloroplasty.
3. **Low gastric ulcer.** Antrectomy.
4. **Coexisting gastric and duodenal ulcers.** Antrectomy and vagotomy.
5. **Stress ulcers, erosive gastritis.** Oversewing, possible vagotomy and pyloroplasty, possible near-total gastrectomy.
6. **Mallory-Weiss tears.** Oversewing of bleeders.
7. **Variceal bleeding.** Portal decompression by shunt, variceal ligation, or portoazygous disconnection.
8. **Colonic hemorrhage.** Colon resection.

JAUNDICE

Clinical features

Jaundice may result from hemolysis, hepatic disease, or extrahepatic biliary obstruction. Clinical examination and laboratory examination will differentiate the causes. The presence of biliary tract obstruction requires determination of the lesion, preoperative stabilization of nutritional, hematologic, and renal status, and operative correction.

Diagnosis

History. Anorexia, fatigue, malaise, or nausea suggests viral hepatitis. Gradual weight loss and anorexia suggest malignancy. Colicky upper abdominal pain perhaps radiating to the subscapular area, intolerance of fatty foods, and intermittent jaundice suggest biliary tract disease. Gnawing midabdominal pain, often with radiation to the back, suggests pancreatic disease. Fever and chills are associated with cholangitis. Recent transfusion may be associated with hemolytic jaundice. A variety of drugs may cause a hemolytic reaction or hepatotoxicity.

Physical examination. On physical examination, icterus is best seen in the sclera and oral mucous membranes. Vascular spiders, palmar erythema, cutaneous xanthomata, and dilated periumbilical veins suggest cirrhosis. A firm nodular liver edge suggests postnecrotic cirrhosis or metastatic liver neoplasia. An enlarged, palpable, nontender gallbladder (Courvoisier's sign) suggests malignant obstruction of the common bile duct.

Blood testing. Comparison of the direct and indirect fractions of bilirubin will help differentiate obstructive from hemolytic causes. A disproportionate increase in the indirect fraction suggests hemolysis or impaired hepatic uptake. A high direct fraction suggests obstructive jaundice. Large increases in serum alkaline phosphatase occur with obstructive jaundice. Elevated SGOT and serum glutamic-pyruvic transaminase (SGPT) occur in hepatocellular disease. Prolongation of the prothrombin time suggests vitamin K deficiency or hepatic disease. Advanced hepatic disease leads to decreased serum albumin. Renal function should be evaluated preoperatively, because patients with jaundice are prone to develop postoperative renal insufficiency.

Sonography. Ultrasonic imaging of the liver, biliary tract, and pancreas will delineate masses, calculi, inflammation, and ductal dilatation.

CT scanning. CT scan is a somewhat more sensitive and specific though more expensive test that provides information similar to that obtained by ultrasonography.

Endoscopic retrograde cholangiopancreatography. ERCP is useful in outlining the biliary tract with contrast and may allow biopsy of suspicious periampullary masses, or even section of the sphincter of Oddi to allow passage of retained common duct stones. It may be complicated by cholangitis or pancreatitis.

Percutaneous transhepatic cholangiography. PTC is useful when there are dilated intrahepatic ducts (usually demonstrated beforehand by ultrasonography or CT scan) and provides an excellent radiographic image of the biliary system. PTC may also allow preoperative drainage of the obstructed biliary system, though the value of this preoperative drainage is debated. It may be complicated by hemorrhage.

Therapeutic decisions

Preoperative preparation. The preoperative preparation of the patient with obstructive jaundice depends on the chronicity and urgency of correction of the underlying problem. If time allows, parenteral nutritional supplementation and correction of vitamin K deficiency and coagulation abnormalities are performed. Antibiotic therapy is directed toward gram-negative organisms. Renal function is protected with adequate hydration and avoidance of nephrotoxins.

Surgical procedures. The choice of surgical procedure depends on the underlying pathology. For **choledocholithiasis,** after cholecystectomy is performed, the common bile duct is opened and the stones removed. A T-tube is inserted to allow intraoperative cholangiography and postoperative drainage. If there are multiple common duct stones, sphincteroplasty or choledochoduodenostomy is performed to prevent subsequent obstruction of the duct by residual stones.

Pancreatic or periampullary **carcinoma** is treated by pancreaticoduodenectomy (Whipple procedure). Unresectable pancreatic malignancy is palliated by gastrojejunostomy and/or cholecystojejunostomy. A variety of procedures are available for the resection or palliation of cholangiocarcinoma, including hepaticojejunostomy, placement of a U-tube, and retrograde and intrahepatic cholangiojejunostomy (Longmire procedure).

Cholangitis requires emergent surgery. Possible postoperative complications include subhepatic abscess, bleeding, bile peritonitis, biliary or duodenal fistula, mechanical problems with the T-tube, retained stones, pancreatitis, cholangitis, stricture formation, and renal insufficiency.

HERNIA

UMBILICAL HERNIA AND OMPHALOCELE

Clinical features

In the infantile type of **umbilical hernia**, there is faulty closure of the umbilicus during obliteration of the umbilical vessels that is possibly familial. The incidence is 1 to 10% in white children and up to 80% in black children. There is usually spontaneous closure before age 3 years. **Omphalocele** is a sac consisting of peritoneum internally and amniotic membrane externally, with lack of covering by skin. Omphalocele represents a congenital failure of complete return of eviscerated organs to the abdominal cavity during early fetal development, often accompanied by insufficient enlargement of the abdomen for acceptance of the viscera. Adult umbilical hernia usually contains omentum adherent to sac.

Diagnosis

Infantile umbilical hernia is usually asymptomatic during the first year of life. In older children with a large hernia, there may possibly be pain in the affected area, together with digestive disturbances. There is a soft swelling covered by skin that protrudes while crying or straining. A translucent hernial sac at the base of umbilical cord is an omphalocele. In adult umbilical hernia, the transverse colon is pulled by omentum, causing pain or intestinal obstruction. This may be exacerbated by factors that increase intra-abdominal pressure, such as chronic cough, ascites, pregnancy, and possibly obesity.

Therapeutic decisions

Because of the possibility of incarceration, surgical repair is indicated for adults and for children with persistent umbilical hernia after age 3 years. Omphalocele requires immediate surgical treatment to avoid rupture, necrosis of the intestine, and peritonitis.

INGUINAL HERNIA

Clinical features

Indirect inguinal hernia results from a persistently patent processus vaginalis; it is therefore familial. The hernia begins at the internal inguinal ring and passes through the inguinal canal, emerging at the external inguinal ring. In the complete form, the contents of the hernia extend into the tunica vaginalis of the testis into the scrotum. When there is a large abdominal ring, the visceral contents in the scrotal sac may be huge. In the incomplete form, there is obliteration of the lower portion of the processus vaginalis, preventing communication of the tunica vaginalis with the hernia sac. The most common groin hernia is the indirect inguinal hernia, accounting for 60%. The highest incidence is in the first year of life and is often present at birth. Indirect inguinal hernia is 10 times more common in males.

Direct inguinal hernia is a defect in the posterior inguinal wall inferior to the Hesselbach's triangle. It results from a weak posterior inguinal wall, inborn weakness of connective tissue, or a sudden increase in intra-abdominal pressure. Direct inguinal hernia comprises 20% of groin hernias. It is rare in females.

Sliding inguinal hernia is a direct or indirect inguinal hernia in which there is incorporation of a hollow viscus into the sac wall. It is more common in elderly males and occurs more frequently on the left, often containing the sigmoid colon. It may also contain the cecum or bladder.

Femoral hernia results from a defective femoral ring associated with increased abdominal pressure, as in pregnancy or obesity. The main sac extends into the femoral canal, although subsidiary loculi into the scrotum or labia majora may occur (Cooper's hernia). Femoral hernia is three to four times more common in females than males, accounting for 7% of groin hernias and 3 to 4% of parietal abdominal hernias.

Diagnosis

Inguinal hernia. Inguinal hernia presents as an inguinal lump that is possibly painful and is relieved by recumbency. It is often accompanied by a dragging sensation. Direct inguinal hernia usually presents as a painless inguinal swelling and a feeling of heaviness that is noticed more when standing or straining. There is a visible, palpable mass protruding through the posterior inguinal wall, medial to the inferior epigastric vessels in the area bounded by the Hesselbach's triangle. The mass often disappears with recumbency.

Femoral hernia. With femoral hernia, there may be a painless inguinal swelling or a palpable mass below the inguinal ligament lateral to the pubic spine. Femoral hernia usually persists with recumbency and is therefore usually nonreducible. There may be associated dysuria, urinary frequency, or hematuria, possibly preceding palpable evidence of the femoral hernia. This results from a portion of the bladder being caught in the hernia.

Incarceration. Incarceration (irreducibility, trapping) is suggested by increased pain in the region of the hernia without reduction on reclining. Anorexia, nausea, vomiting, constipation, abdominal distension, and passage of blood-stained mucus suggest intestinal obstruction. Abdominal x-ray may reveal the location and type of obstruction.

Strangulation. Strangulation implies loss of blood supply to the incarcerated viscus. Although strangulation may be recognized by the onset of fever, leukocytosis, and peritonitis, the presence of necrotic bowel is often determined only during emergent repair of an incarcerated hernia. This implies that the absence of signs of strangulation does not rule out this possibility.

Richter's hernia. An incarcerated hernia with only part of the circumference of the bowel trapped in the hernial ring is called a Richter's hernia.

Therapeutic decisions

Surgical repair of a hernia is required to prevent incarceration of bowel with resultant intestinal obstruction, strangulation (loss of blood supply) of bowel, necrosis, and perforation. Urgent repair of incarcerated hernia is essential.

INCISIONAL HERNIA AND EPIGASTRIC HERNIA

Clinical features

Incisional hernia results from postoperative failure of healing of musculoaponeurotic and fascial layers of the wound. It is most common with vertical surgical incisions. This failure of normal healing may be precipitated by infection, drains through the abdominal wall favoring infection, incomplete closure of the wound, inadequate hemostasis, unduly tight sutures, avascular necrosis, or preoperative influences such as obesity, malnutrition, hypoproteinemia, vitamin C deficiency, tissue edema, postoperative cough, and abdominal distension.

Epigastric hernia is a combination of a congenital aponeurotic defect with increased intra-abdominal pressure and muscular effort. Epigastric hernia usually occurs at the linea alba between the xiphoid and the umbilicus and may be multiple. There first is protrusion of fat; later, there is protrusion of attached peritoneum. It is most common in males 20 to 50 years old.

Diagnosis

A large incisional hernial defect may cause severe discomfort, but even small incarcerated hernias may be very painful. The incisional defect will be noticeable and palpable as a protruding abdominal mass, possibly multiple defects, or separate hernial rings incarcerated within the hernial sac. Epigastric hernia is associated with pain in the upper abdomen after eating, relieved by reclining, possibly mimicking the pain of peptic ulcer, cholecystitis, or pancreatitis.

Therapeutic decisions

Treatment is usually by surgical repair. The repair of very large incisional hernias may require the use of a prosthetic mesh.

RARE TYPES OF HERNIAS

Sciatic hernia is a congenital defect exiting through the greater or lesser sacrosciatic foramen; the sac is adjacent to the gluteal vessels or sciatic nerve, emerging beneath the gluteus maximus. There may be localized or radiating pain, often simulating an attack of sciatica. Rarely, it can present as a posterior protrusion below the fold of the buttock.

Lumbar hernia may result from a congenital absence of layers of the internal oblique muscle, deficient muscular floor in the inferior lumbar triangle, constant vascular lacuna, failure of union of muscle following incisions for nephrectomy, and trauma. The hernia occurs through the inferior lumbar Petit's triangle or through the superior lumbar Grynfelt's triangle. The sac usually contains retroperitoneal fat. Findings include backache, dragging sensation, disturbances of the GI tract, and bulging with exertion or during coughing.

Obturator hernia results from a congenitally large obturator canal. The sac emerges caudad and medial to the obturator vessels, passing through the obturator foramen beneath the pectineus muscle. Obturator hernia is most common in elderly women. Findings include intermittent thigh pain radiating to the knee (Howship-Romberg sign). Strangulation is signaled by generalized abdominal pain and rigidity. The mass is palpable on rectal examination.

Retroperitoneal hernia may be congenital or acquired, possibly due to defective suturing of the mesentery. Retroperitoneal hernia may be paraduodenal, paracecal, or intersigmoid. Findings are those of intestinal obstruction, including severe cramping abdominal pain, nausea, vomiting, obstipation, abdominal distension, and hyperactive high-pitched bowel sounds. Untreated, this will progress to peritonitis, shock, and death.

Spigelian hernia is a ventral hernia protruding through the linea semilunaris (Spigelius's line), usually at the junction of the semilunar line and the semicircular line of Douglas. A congenital defect in the aponeurosis of the transversus abdominis muscle and internal oblique muscle is thought to be responsible. This hernia may result from violent muscle strain, as in pregnancy, and is aggravated by obesity. Spigelian hernia is usually asymptomatic, though there may be lower abdominal pain. It may be mistaken for a neoplasm or pelvic disease, especially an ovarian lesion. Because there may be local tenderness near the location of the appendix, it can be confused with appendicitis. The depth and location of the hernial sac may make diagnosis difficult because of overlying fat or rigidity of the overlying external oblique aponeurosis.

FLUID, ELECTROLYTE, AND ACID-BASE DERANGEMENTS

Clinical features

Water requirements are the sum of minimal urinary output and insensible losses (water lost from evaporation from the skin and respiratory tract) minus the endogenous water produced by metabolism. The normal kidney can reduce renal sodium excretion to a minimal quantity with slight volume depletion. Thus, total curtailment of sodium intake for days will not result in significant volume depletion. In contrast, the kidney cannot conserve potassium as effectively until there is substantial potassium depletion. There is also an obligatory fecal loss of potassium of about 10 mEq/day. Overall, adequate parenteral maintenance therapy can then be provided as 500 ml 10%

dextrose + 20 mEq potassium chloride (KCl) over 12 hours and 1,000 ml 5% dextrose in 0.45 or 0.9% saline + 20 mEq KCl over the next 12 hours. In addition to maintaining these baseline requirements, the body must replenish losses of water and electrolytes. These losses include insensible losses from the skin and lungs, GI losses, urinary losses, and internal sequestration of fluid. Body weight, urine output, temperature, measurement of actual losses, and measurement of blood values help to delineate the magnitude of abnormal fluid and electrolyte loss and therefore guide adequate replacement therapy.

Diagnosis and therapeutic decisions

Hyponatremia.   Hyponatremia is the most common electrolyte abnormality observed in clinical practice. This is because antidiuretic hormone (ADH, or vasopressin) secretion is frequently increased in the immediate postoperative period for various reasons such as surgical stress, pain, and the use of analgesics. Hyponatremia produces symptoms because it leads to hypoosmolality of the body fluids and, hence, intracellular accumulation of water. Most cases of true hyponatremia are due to an impaired ability of the kidneys to excrete dilute urine (water). Clinical manifestations of hyponatremia are the result of brain edema and range from minimal disturbances of mentation to seizures and coma. Therapeutic options include correction of arterial volume disturbances or the use of hypertonic saline.

Hypernatremia.   The maintenance of hypernatremia is possible if (1) the thirst mechanism is lost, (2) the patient is unable to drink water because of confusion, coma, restraints, or esophageal obstruction, or (3) there is no access to water. The clinical manifestations of hypernatremia are primarily neurological and result from brain dehydration. They range from minimal disturbances of mentation to seizures and death. The acute therapy of hypernatremia is administration of intravenous 5% dextrose in water.

Hypokalemia.   Hypokalemia is usually but not always accompanied by a reduction in total body potassium content. When hypokalemia occurs as a result of intracellular shift of potassium, body potassium content is not reduced. Hypokalemia may result from low potassium intake or an intracellular potassium shift due to alkalosis, glucose and insulin administration, an anabolic state, familial hypokalemic paralysis, epinephrine release (beta-stimulatory effect), or excessive potassium loss (extrarenal or renal). The clinical manifestations of hypokalemia include muscle weakness and paralysis, rhabdomyolysis, cardiac arrhythmias, impairment of insulin release, nephrogenic diabetes insipidus, and paralytic ileus. Treatment includes administration of potassium to correct the deficit and correction of the underlying disorder.

Hyperkalemia.   **True hyperkalemia** implies increased extracellular potassium concentration. This must be differentiated from **pseudohyperkalemia,** which implies increased serum potassium only in the local blood vessel or in the test tube. Pseudohyperkalemia may result from a high platelet count, severe leukocytosis, or hemolysis in the blood collection tube. True hyperkalemia may result from excessive potassium intake, extracellular potassium shift (due to acute acidosis, rhabdomyolysis from crush injury or gangrene, hemolysis,

increased catabolism, barium intoxication, or hyperkalemic periodic paralysis), or reduced renal excretion of potassium. The latter may result from aldosterone deficiency (Addison's disease, heparin therapy, congenital enzymatic defect, hyporeninemic hypoaldosteronism), tubular unresponsiveness to aldosterone, use of potassium-sparing diuretics, or renal failure. Hyperkalemia can result in cardiac arrhythmias, often ventricular tachyarrhythmias. Severe hyperkalemia causes neuromuscular weakness or paralysis. Treatment options for hyperkalemia include (1) reduction in total body potassium using an ion exchange resin to increase fecal potassium excretion, (2) dialysis, (3) induction of an intracellular potassium shift by administration of glucose and insulin or sodium bicarbonate, and (4) antagonism of the effects of potassium on the cardiac cell.

Metabolic acidosis.   Metabolic acidosis usually results from endogenous production of acid, such as ketoacidosis (uncontrolled diabetes) or lactic acidosis (inadequate tissue perfusion), although a number of other causes are also possible. Clinical manifestations of metabolic acidosis include arteriolar dilatation and impaired cardiac contractility in acute cases and osteomalacia in chronic cases. Acute treatment is administration of sodium bicarbonate and correction of the underlying condition.

Metabolic alkalosis.   Metabolic alkalosis is an increase in extracellular pH secondary to an increase in bicarbonate concentration. This may result from endogenous production of bicarbonate (nasogastric suction or vomiting) or administration of exogenous alkali (bicarbonate). Metabolic alkalosis is compensated by renal excretion and hypoventilation. Renal compensation is less effective in the face of hypokalemia, because the kidneys will tend to excrete acid in order to preserve potassium, thus exacerbating the alkalosis. Clinical manifestations include tetany and increased neuromuscular irritability, followed by confusion, stupor, and coma. Treatment includes administration of intravenous fluids containing potassium. Emergent treatment rarely requires administration of dilute acidic solutions or the use of acetazolamide, a carbonic anhydrase inhibitor.

Respiratory alkalosis.   Respiratory alkalosis results from hyperventilation leading to carbon dioxide loss. Hyperventilation may be caused by hypoxia, drugs or toxins (salicylate) that stimulate the respiratory center, CNS disorders (meningitis or cerebrovascular accident), or psychogenic factors. There will be compensation by tissue buffering and a reduced renal threshold for bicarbonate, with generation of lactic acid. Chronic respiratory alkalosis is usually asymptomatic because of the efficacy of compensatory mechanisms. Dizziness, nervousness, paresthesias, altered level of consciousness, and tetany will occur as the process progresses. Treatment is by correction of the underlying disorder, use of a rebreathing bag, or sedation if psychogenic hyperventilation is the problem.

Respiratory acidosis.   Respiratory acidosis is the result of inadequate ventilation leading to carbon dioxide retention. Causes may include pharmacologic suppression of the CNS (residual anesthetic agents, narcotics, or barbiturates), neuromuscular dysfunction (splinting secondary to fractured ribs, thoracic or upper abdominal incision), airway obstruction, pulmonary disease, and primary alveolar hypoventilation. Compensation is by tissue buffering and then renal generation and retention of bicarbonate. Chronic respiratory acidosis may be asymptomatic because compensatory mechanisms will maintain normal blood pH. When symptoms are present, they are usually a manifestation of hypoxemia. Acute elevation of PCO_2 produces asterixis, headache with papilledema, obtundation, and coma. Treatment is by correction of the underlying disorder.

Hypocalcemia.   Hypocalcemia may result from hypoparathyroidism (postsurgical damage to the parathyroid glands), pseudohyperparathyroidism (hypocalcemia, hyperphosphatemia, multiple somatic abnormalities, and high levels of parathyroid hormone), vitamin D deficiency, or hyperphosphatemia. Serum calcium levels are intimately related to serum phosphate and pH. Clinical manifestations of hypocalcemia include neuromuscular irritability and tetany (Chvostek's and Trousseau's signs), prolonged Q-T interval on ECG, and chronic cataracts. Treatment is by correction of the underlying disorder. Acute therapy includes infusion of elemental calcium. Chronically, oral calcium and vitamin D may be required.

Hypercalcemia.   Hypercalcemia is often the result of osseous invasion by tumor but may also result from primary hyperparathyroidism, vitamin D toxicity, immobilization, milk-alkali syndrome, sarcoidosis, tuberculosis, thiazide diuretics, hyperthyroidism, adrenal insufficiency, vitamin A intoxication, or familial hypocalciuric hypercalcemia. Most cases of hypercalcemia are asymptomatic, but severe hypercalcemia may result in disturbances of consciousness, ECG abnormalities, polyuria, nephrocalcinosis, renal failure, anorexia, nausea, vomiting, constipation, and extraskeletal calcification. Treatment is by intravenous volume expansion, furosemide to increase urinary calcium excretion, inorganic phosphate to induce calcium precipitation into bone (contraindicated in the face of renal insufficiency or hyperphosphatemia), and mithramycin to inhibit bone resorption. In severe cases, dialysis may be required to lower serum calcium rapidly.

Hypophosphatemia.   Hypophosphatemia results from inadequate phosphate intake (total parenteral nutrition), reduced intestinal absorption, increased renal excretion, and intracellular shift (acute pH increase). Clinical manifestations include metabolic encephalopathy, rhabdomyolysis, hemolysis, myocardial dysfunction, and muscle weakness (resulting in pulmonary hypoventilation). Treatment is with oral phosphate supplementation.

Hyperphosphatemia.   Hyperphosphatemia may result from renal failure, increased renal threshold (hypoparathyroidism and pseudohypoparathyroidism), or increased phosphate load (acute acidosis or rhabdomyolysis). Acute hyperphosphatemia causes hypocalcemia (tetany and metastatic calcification). Treatment is by administration of intestinal phosphate binders (aluminum hydroxide or aluminum carbonate).

Hypomagnesemia.   Hypomagnesemia may result from poor intake, GI disorders interfering with absorption, or excessive renal loss. Clinical manifestations include paresthesias, tetany, carpopedal spasm, hyperreflexia, seizures, a prolonged Q-T interval, and arrhythmias. Treatment is with parenteral magnesium sulfate.

Hypermagnesemia.   Hypermagnesemia may occur in renal failure, or it may be induced by exogenous magnesium sulfate administration (in the treatment of eclampsia). Clinical manifestations include diminished deep tendon reflexes, respiratory depression, and cardiac conduction defects. Treatment is by intravenous administration of calcium to antagonize the cardiac effects of hypermagnesemia.

CONDITIONS REQUIRING NUTRITIONAL SUPPORT

Clinical features

An average adult patient resting in bed requires 25 kcal/kg of body weight per day (about 1,800 kcal/day). The stress of illness and surgery substantially increases this baseline requirement to 40 to 60 kcal/kg/day. Carbohydrate administration is important to avoid protein catabolism and therefore permit efficient incorporation of protein into healing tissue. Healthy adult females require 44 g of protein daily. Healthy adult males require 56 g of protein daily. Protein cannot be replaced by any other food and cannot be stored. Very ill or severely injured patients should be given 100 g of protein daily, except for patients with hepatic or renal insufficiency, for whom oral protein intake must be limited to avoid hyperammonemia. Some tissues, such as the brain, heart, and skeletal muscle, can adapt to the use of ketones instead of carbohydrates to fulfill their energy needs. Although this fat may arise from mobilization of adipose tissue reserves, administration of exogenous fat is beneficial. Water-soluble vitamins are required daily. Recommended daily doses are as follows: vitamin B_1 (thiamine), 5 to 10 mg; vitamin B_2 (riboflavin), 5 to 10 mg; niacinamide, 100 mg; pantothenic acid, 20 mg; vitamin B_6 (pyridoxine) 2 mg; folic acid, 1 mg; vitamin B_{12}, 4 μg; and vitamin C, 30 mg. Because vitamin C losses increase in severe trauma or illness, 500 mg daily should be provided. The required fat-soluble vitamins include vitamin A, 4,000 to 5,000 IU/day; and vitamin E, 8 to 10 IU/day. Vitamin K is synthesized by intestinal bacteria, and vitamin D is produced by the human body.

Diagnosis

Nutritional support is required when oral intake is inadequate to meet nutritional demands. This may result from GI failure, starvation, or dysmetabolism. GI failure may result from enterocutaneous fistula, prolonged ileus, chronic intestinal obstruction, severe inflammatory bowel disease, or acute ulcerative colitis. Starvation implies that oral intake is inadequate to meet nutritional needs. Initially there is a period of adaptation when the body first uses its glycogen stores, then fatty stores, while preserving structural and muscle protein. However, eventually even proteins are metabolized for energy. Dysmetabolism implies the presence of abnormal hormones and mediators that interfere with mobilization of fatty stores and impair energy production from glycolysis. Dysmetabolism is usually a consequence of malignancy.

Therapeutic decisions

The choice between enteral and parenteral nutrition is based on the clinical circumstances, GI tract function, and a consideration of the potential complications of each of these alternatives. Enteral nutritional support has many advantages over parenteral support, including lower cost, physiological utilization of the bowel, portal presentation of substrates for hepatic metabolism, and relative ease of access. However, because enteral nutrition requires GI function and motility, parenteral nutrition is often required in postoperative or posttrauma patients. Enteral support may employ oral feeding, flexible nasogastric tube feeding, or feeding via gastrostomy or jejunostomy. Complications of enteral feeding include gastric retention leading to regurgitation and aspiration, osmotic diarrhea, abdominal cramps, nausea and vomiting, and exacerabation of active pancreatitis. Total parenteral nutrition (TPN, or intravenous hyperalimentation) is given by central venous catheter. Complications of total parenteral nutrition are many and diverse. They include catheter-related problems such as pneumothorax, catheter breakage and embolization or thrombosis of the catheter, septic complications, and metabolic derangements of glucose, electrolyte, magnesium, calcium, phosphate, ammonia, and acid-base balance. Vitamin, mineral, and fatty acid deficiency may also occur during prolonged parenteral nutrition.

SHOCK

Clinical features

Inadequacy of at least one of the following circulatory components launches the patient's descent into the shock state: (1) Pump (heart), (2) Peripheral resistance (vessels), or (3) Perfusate (blood volume). The physiological response to failure of one of these P's is compensation by the other two P's. The only factor common to all forms of shock is inadequate tissue perfusion. The immediate hormonal response to inadequate tissue perfusion includes secretion of vasopressin (ADH), adrenocorticotropic hormone (ACTH), aldosterone, and catecholamines. The kidneys are thus prompted to preserve sodium chloride and water at the expense of potassium and urine volume. Oliguria occurs early. Lactic acidosis occurs because of anaerobic metabolism in oxygen-deficient tissue. Hyperglycemia results from glucagon secretion, breakdown of glycogen, and deficiency of insulin secretion. Terminally, sluggish blood flow results in capillary thrombosis and cell death.

Shock progresses through three clinical stages termed **preshock, shock, and irreversible shock.** At first, the patient is asymptomatic because of the efficacy of the compensatory mechanisms. For example, with hemorrhage of up to 10 to 20% of blood volume, blood pressure may be maintained at normal levels by intense peripheral vasoconstriction. An unexplained tachycardia may be the only hint that there is any problem. This has been termed preshock, though it is indeed an integral part of the spectrum of shock. As the initial physiological insult persists, compensatory mechanisms begin to rob vital organs of needed perfusion and the patient enters the shock state. During this second stage, blood pressure drops and cerebral and renal perfusion decrease. Restlessness, hypotension, tachycardia, and oliguria occur. In a patient with underlying coronary artery disease, angina or myocardial infarction may occur. In a patient with underlying renovascular disease, irreversible renal failure may occur. As irreversible shock approaches, organ hypoperfusion increases and vital organs cease to function. Compensatory mechanisms eventually attempt to maintain blood pressure by such severe restrictions of blood flow that tissue hypoperfusion leads to stagnation of blood flow, acidosis, and cell death. It is in this third stage when the process may become irreversible.

Diagnosis

Typically, the patient in shock is described as having cold, clammy, pale skin; hypotension; rapid and thready pulse; and diminished central venous pressure, urine output, mental status, and venous PO_2. However, there is much variability in clinical presentation, depending on the underlying cause. In preshock, there is increasing thirst and muscle weakness. Urine output decreases. After initial signs of agitation, consciousness diminishes. Skin and mucous membranes become pale (or cyanotic), cold, and clammy when vasoconstriction is a predominant compensatory mechanism. When vasoconstriction is blocked by bacterial toxins, the skin may be deceptively warm and dry. Skin capillary filling as assessed by response to pressure blanching is slow. Later on, blood pressure decreases and the pulse becomes rapid and thready.

Therapeutic decisions

Immediate therapy is directed toward restoring normal hemodynamics, often without regard to the underlying cause. Coronary and cerebral perfusion are improved by placing the patient in the head-down (Trendelenberg's) position. The airway and oxygenation are assured, maintaining the arterial PO_2 around 70 mm Hg. Urine output and vital signs are monitored. Bleeding is controlled and blood volume is replaced. Pain relief may be necessary, but analgesics must be used with caution to avoid further respiratory or circulatory depression. The treatment of shock is adequate when urine output, central venous pressure, and mentation return to normal. The Swan-Ganz pulmonary artery catheter is useful in monitoring intravascular volume status (wedge pressure reflects right atrial pressure), cardiac output (measured by thermodilution technique), and peripheral vascular resistance.

Hypovolemic shock may be secondary to trauma, hemorrhage, third space loss (unmeasurable losses into the bowel, peritoneal cavity, or as edema), severe vomiting, diarrhea, or burns. Hypovolemic preshock is characterized by cold, clammy extremities and tachycardia, whereas hypotension suggests frank hypovolemic shock. Improvement in the patient's hemodynamic parameters and clinical appearance after fluid volume challenge is characteristic of hypovolemic shock. Continued correction of ongoing volume losses and control of the source of hypovolemia are then undertaken.

Cardiogenic shock may occur with cardiac arrhythmias, myocardial infarction, pericardial tamponade, acute valvular or papillary muscle disruption, or congestive heart failure. There may have been preexisting salt and water retention in the patient with chronic cardiac insufficiency. Treatment of cardiogenic shock requires optimizaiton of volume status judged by progress of the pulmonary capillary wedge pressure and serial estimation of cardiac output. Cardiac output may be improved by pharmacologic manipulation.

Neurogenic shock may occur with spinal anesthesia or quadriplegia. Loss of sympathetic control of resistance vessels causes a sudden decrease in peripheral resistance with pooling of blood in dilated capacitance vessels. The compensatory mechanism is tachycardia. Immediate treatment requires placing the patient in the Trendelenburg's position and rapid volume loading with intravenous fluids (saline) to relieve life-threatening hypotension. Definitive treatment may require the use of a vasopressor such as ephedrine. When the occurrence of neurogenic preshock can be anticipated, such as with spinal anesthesia, volume loading may be preventive.

Septic shock is the most complex variety of shock; it tends to include components of hypovolemia, cardiogenic, and neurogenic shock. Septic shock results from infection, most often from the urinary tract, the respiratory system, the peritoneum, or from septic abortion. The organism is usually gram negative. Initially, when compensatory mechanisms are functional, there is vasodilatation and tchycardia; the patient's extremities are warm (hyperdynamic septic shock). As the toxemia progresses, compensatory mechanisms are blocked, cardiac output decreases, vasoconstriction occurs, and hypodynamic septic shock ensues. Bacterial endotoxins cause an increase in capillary permeability. This results in pooling of blood in the microcirculation. This and associated fluid loss cause severe hypovolemia. Therefore, although treatment is eventually directed to the underlying cause, initial therapy must maintain adequate tissue perfusion. This includes volume replacement, antibiotics, and vasopressor therapy (used with caution because vasopressors raise blood pressure at the expense of tissue perfusion). If peripheral perfusion is threatened by severe vasoconstriction or if there is associated myocardial ischemia, vasodilators are useful; however, the best vasodilator in the hypovolemic patient is intravenous fluid. The use of corticosteroids in the treatment of sepsis is controversial; recent data suggest that the use of steroids may cause a higher mortality rate in patients with elevated serum creatinine levels or in those who develop a secondary infection after steroid therapy is begun.

Postresuscitative care

Postresuscitation hypertension is due to rapid mobilization of sequestered third space fluid causing hypervolemia after volume loading. It can lead to respiratory failure, hematuria, or encephalopathy. Continued monitoring of pulmonary capillary wedge pressure or central venous pressure and careful fluid management will help avoid or treat this complication. Pulmonary insufficiency (adult respiratory distress syndrome, ARDS) usually first manifests as hypoxemia unresponsive to increasing inspired oxygen. Low compliance causes a "stiff lung" with a fall in functional residual capacity. Chest x-ray shows a pattern of diffuse interstitial edema. Treatment is ventilatory support and careful monitoring. Fraction of inspired oxygen (FiO_2) may have to be increased but will be deleterious above levels of about 40%. Therefore, positive end-expiratory pressure (PEEP) is instituted to help overcome low compliance. Alterations in oxygen transport occur for several reasons. As oxygen tension rises, hemoglobin oxygen saturation rises in a sigmoid-shaped curve. The P_{50} value is that tension at which saturation is 50%. This normally is about 27 mm Hg. Factors that shift the curve to the right (increase P_{50}) are advantageous because an equivalent amount of oxygen can be released at a lower PO_2. Decreased diphosphoglycerate (DPG) and alkalosis

shift the curve to the left and should therefore be avoided during resuscitation of the patient in shock.

TRAUMA

NECK TRAUMA
Clinical features

Even serious neck injuries may be asymptomatic. Airway injuries give rise to stridor, hoarseness, dyspnea due to hematoma or aspiration, and subcutaneous emphysema. Esophageal injuries may cause chest pain, dysphagia, and eventually mediastinitis. Esophageal injuries are often associated with other injuries, such as those of the spinal cord. Spinal cord injuries are associated with paralysis, cervical pain or tenderness, and diminished consciousness. Vascular injury gives rise to hemorrhage or hematoma. A bruit suggests arteriovenous fistula. Air embolism may occur with venous injury. Neurological injury is associated with specific findings:

1. Hypoglossal. The tongue points to the side of injury.
2. Bilateral vagus. Hoarseness and dysphagia.
3. Phrenic. Elevated hemidiaphragm.
4. Spinal accessory. Paralysis of the sternomastoid and deltoid.
5. Brachial plexus. Sensory or motor deficits of an upper extremity.

Diagnosis

Rule out associated injuries, then perform a neurological examination. Obtain chest x-ray, looking for widened mediastinum. Obtain a lateral x-ray of the neck; this may show anterior displacement of the phayrnx by air. Endoscopy is indicated for suspected injury of the larynx, pharynx, or esophagus. Gastrografin swallow is warranted for suspected esophageal injury. Arteriography is usually not required.

Therapeutic decisions

In the emergency room, ensure a patent airway. This may require intubation, cricothyrotomy, or tracheostomy. Control external hemorrhage by digital compression. Administer intravenous fluids. Immobilize the cervical spine if spinal injury is suspected. Whenever the platysma is penetrated, operation is considered. Prepare for cervicothoracic incision if the wound is near the base of the neck. Obtain proximal and distal vascular control prior to exploring any hematoma surrounding a major vessel. To prevent air embolism, maintain the patient in head-down position until venous bleeding is controlled.

1. Trachea or larynx. Tracheostomy, suture, or stent.
2. Esophagus. Suture and drain; pass a nasogastric tube to locate the problem.
3. Cervical spine or cord. Immobilization; laminectomy.
4. Carotid artery. Repair, unless neurological deficit has already occurred (in that case, ligate).
5. Vertebral artery. Repair or ligate.
6. Venous injury. Keep head down until bleeding is controlled by ligation.
7. Air embolism. Place the patient left side down. This keeps air out of the right ventricular outflow tract.

Trendelenburg's position increases pulmonary perfusion and prevents further air embolism. Maintain circulation by cardiac compression. Aspirate air after advancing the central venous pressure line into the heart. Stop nitrous oxide, which enters the air bubble rapidly.

8. Lymphatic injury. Ligate.
9. Nerve injury. Neurorrhaphy.

CHEST TRAUMA

Clinical features

Chest trauma may range from rib contusion or fracture to major injuries giving rise to a flail chest, inadequate oxygenation, or cardiac penetration.

Diagnosis

Treatment depends on stability of vital signs, physical examination of the chest, and sometimes results of chest x-ray studies.

Therapeutic decisions

1. **Rib fracture.** Rib fractures are treated with observation, analgesia, and rib strapping if they are severely painful.
2. **Flail chest.** If a portion of the chest wall is isolated by major rib fractures and moves paradoxically with respiration, ventilation will be compromised. This is termed a flail chest. Flail chest may require use of a ventilator for 2 to 3 weeks until healing occurs.
3. **Hemothorax and pneumothorax.** Hemothorax and pneumothorax are treated by use of a tube thoracostomy (chest tube) connected to underwater drainage.
4. **Sucking wounds.** Sucking wounds require application of an occlusive dressing.
5. **Ruptured bronchus.** A ruptured bronchus is suggested by the presence of a persistent air leak or pneumomediastinum. Treatment is bronchial repair or resection.
6. **Aortic injury.** An aortic tear is usually located just distal to left subclavian at the ligamentum arteriosum. Urgent aortography and operative repair are required, though few patients with an aortic laceration survive the trip to the hospital.
7. **Cardiac injury.** Cardiac injuries are treated by pericardiocentesis for immediate relief of tamponade, then operative repair.
8. **Diaphragmatic injury.** Diaphragmatic injuries (which are usually located on the left hemidiaphragm) are repaired operatively. If unrecognized at the time of injury, diaphragmatic trauma may present years later with herniation.
9. **Pulmonary injury.** Pulmonary contusion presents with blood-tinged secretions, dyspnea, cyanosis, and lung "white-out" on x-ray. Treatment is fluid restriction, Swan-Ganz catheter, and respiratory care.
10. **Adult respiratory distress syndrome.** (ARDS, shock lung) typically occurs within 1 week of multiple trauma or is associated with sepsis. Treatment is fluid restriction and PEEP ventilation.
11. **Continued bleeding.** Thoracotomy is indicated for rapid bleeding or continuous bleeding. Usually, an intercostal vessel is the source of bleeding.
12. **Associated abdominal injury.** Thoracoabdominal injury (especially penetrating wounds) is associated with a very high mortality rate if unrecognized. In order to avoid overlooking abdominal injury in patients with chest trauma, abdominal paracentesis and lavage are useful.
13. **Esophageal injury.** Esophageal injuries present with pain, fever, subcutaneous emphysema, and mediastinal crunch (Hamman's sign). Esophageal injury is confirmed by a chest x-ray revealing widening of the mediastinum and a left pleural effusion. Although Gastrografin swallow is useful to demonstrate the location of the injury, false-negatives are common. Treatment is nasogastric suction, then operative closure and drainage.

ABDOMINAL TRAUMA

Clinical features

Abdominal trauma is perhaps the most difficult traumatic problem because of the diversity of possible organs that can be injured and the multitude of types of injury.

Diagnosis

The fully conscious patient who presents with peritoneal signs (tenderness, rebound tenderness, guarding, diminished bowel sounds) will require little further diagnostic testing before laparotomy. The fully conscious patient who presents with a normal abdominal examination and stable vital signs may require little more than hematocrit, urinalysis, chest x-ray, and abdominal x-ray prior to hospital admission and close observation.

X-ray studies. X-ray studies may help locate a bullet that may be in an apparent location or may have entered a blood vessel and embolized to an unsuspected location. X-rays will also reveal free air or fluid, ileus pattern, or loss of anatomic borders, suggesting injury to adjacent organs.

Evaluating the unconscious patient. The unconscious patient (unconsciousness due to associated head trauma or drug or alcohol intoxication) presents a diagnostic problem. Because even life-threatening abdominal injuries may be present in the face of a normal abdominal x-ray, there are two better techniques for evaluating the extent of intra-abdominal injury when physical examination is unreliable. These techniques include the classic abdominal paracentesis and lavage and the CT scan.

The **paracentesis and lavage** rely on the fact that even localized injury to an abdominal viscus will lead to release of blood or amylase into the peritoneum. The lavage fluid will be tinged pink from even the smallest amount of free intraperitoneal blood.

CT scanning appears to be highly sensitive and specific for delineating the anatomic location and extent of intra-abdominal injury. It can define small hematomas or free intraperitoneal blood.

Suspected retroperitoneal injury. Abdominal tap and lavage often do not detect the presence of an isolated injury to retroperitoneal structures. Hence, if retroperitoneal injury is suspected because of the nature of the injury, the path of a bullet, or clinical findings, obtain serum amylase, Gastrografin series, sonography, an x-ray of the lumbar spine, an intravenous pyelogram, and angiography.

Hematuria. If there is hematuria, an intravenous pyelogram, cystogram, or contrast-enhanced CT scan is indicated.

Unstable vital signs. Despite the additional information that may be obtained using sophisticated diagnostic tests, any patient with unstable vital signs and obvious substantial abdominal trauma requires exploratory laparotomy as the **first and only** diagnostic procedure.

Therapeutic decisions

Begin with assuring an adequate airway, breathing, and circulation. Administer intravenous fluid resuscitation. Send blood for type and crossmatching. Insert a nasogastric tube and urethral catheter. Locate all exit and entry wounds. Immobilize fractures (beware of cervical spine fracture). Insert a chest tube if indicated.

The choice of operative procedure depends on the exact nature and extent of the injury. Common organ-specific **therapeutic options** are listed here:

1. Kidney. Resection or nephrectomy, but try to conserve as much tissue as possible.
2. Ureter. Transverse suture, resection and anastomosis, ureteroneocystostomy, ureteroureterostomy, or autotransplantation of the kidney to the pelvis.
3. Bladder. Suture, suprapubic cystostomy, drainage.
4. Urethra. Indwelling catheter.
5. Spleen. Splenorrhaphy or splenectomy (beware of the possibility of overwhelming postsplenectomy sepsis that may occur after splenectomy, especially in children, usually due to gram-positive cocci).
6. Gallbladder. Cholecystectomy.
7. Common bile duct. Insert T-tube, anastomose over T-tube, Roux-en-Y choledochojejunostomy.
8. Pancreas. Drainage, distal pancreatectomy (for injury to tail of pancreas), debride and drain (for contusion with capsular tear), pancreatectomy or pancreaticoduodenectomy (for injury to head of pancreas).
9. Stomach. Debride and suture.
10. Duodenum. Transverse suture, pyloric exclusion and gastrojejunostomy, rarely pancreaticoduodenectomy.
11. Small bowel. Transverse suture, resection and anastomosis.
12. Colon. Primary closure, or resection with diverting colostomy.
13. Rectum. Debridement and irrigation, perineal drainage, diverting colostomy.

THERMAL INJURIES

Clinical features

The skin is the largest organ of the body; it has a surface area of 19 square feet (1.8 m^2). Thermal injuries result in loss of water barriers, thermoregulation, and protection against bacterial invasion. Therefore, the management of the burn victim requires major supportive care aimed at fluid and electrolyte balance and prevention of infection, pending skin grafting or spontaneous healing.

Diagnosis

History and circumstances of injury. Inhalational injury is suspected if the burn occurred in a closed space or if the fire resulted in deaths. **Associated internal or musculoskeletal injuries** are suspected if the burn occurred as the result of an explosion. Scalding usually results in a partial-thickness injury. **Flame burns** are potentiated by involvement of the patient's clothing and therefore result in deep involvement. **Flash burns** are usually partial thickness. **Chemical burns** may result in coagulation necrosis (acid) or liquefaction necrosis (alkali). **Radiation burns** vary from the superficial involvement of mild sunburn (ultraviolet) to the deep involvement of nuclear radiation. **Electrical injuries** often result in considerable deep-tissue damage, which may not be apparent from the extent of the visible burn.

Physical examination. Physical examination of the burn victim concentrates on determining the location, depth, and surface area of the burn.

A **first-degree** burn is erythematous and dry, with only slight swelling, associated only with discomfort. These burns heal completely with no scarring. **Superficial second-degree burns** are hyperemic with a pink base and often bright red spots. Blister formation (separation of the epidermis from the dermis due to accumulation of exudate) occurs within 24 hours. The burns appear moist as a result of constant exudation of fluid, and there is usually associated swelling. In the absence of infection, healing occurs spontaneously within 10 to 14 days by regeneration and coalescence of dermal appendages. **Deep second-degree burns** appear pale but may leave scarlet red spots of varying intensity. These burns are also moist and may form small blisters. Healing requires separation of the necrotic eschar to allow regeneration of the epithelium from adjacent deeper layers of the epidermis, and hyperplasia of the dermis. The result is often poor-quality generated skin that is prone to infection, scarring, and breakdown. **Third-degree burns** present as pale brown or black lesions. They may be dark pink in the elderly or the young. The skin is dry, hard, and devoid of the usual elasticity, and thrombosed superficial vessels may be visible. At least initially, the patient experiences little or no pain because of damage of the nerve endings. In third-degree burns, separation of the eschar occurs after 3 to 5 weeks. Small areas may heal by contraction, whereas larger areas will require skin grafting. It may require several days to distinguish between deep second-degree burns and third-degree burns, and infection may convert a deep second-degree burn to a third-degree burn.

The **surface area** of burn is the principal factor by which fluid and electrolyte therapy is determined. This is best estimated from an age-specific chart (Lund-Browder chart) but may be estimated by the **rule of nines**, in which the body surface regions are divided into areas that are multiples of 9%: head, entire upper extremity, one-half of one lower extremity, one-half of the anterior trunk surface, or one-half of the posterior trunk surface. The perineum represents the remaining 1%.

Laboratory tests. Baseline laboratory tests include urinalysis

Laboratory tests. Baseline laboratory tests include urinalysis to check for myoglobinuria or hemoglobinuria, electrolyte determinations, and hematocrit (hemolysis is common).

Therapeutic decisions

The airway is assured and vascular access is obtained. All clothes are removed to assess the extent of the injury. Associated injuries are treated. Chemical burns require copious irrigation. Vital signs and urine output are monitored. A nasogastric tube is indicated if the surface area exceeds 25% because of the likelihood of a profound paralytic ileus and gastric distension. Analgesia is often necessary, but respiratory depression must be avoided. Tetanus immunization must be assured. Stress ulcer prophylaxis with histamine H_2 blockage is indicated. **Isotonic crystalloid** is the standard resuscitative fluid used during the initial 24 hours. The required sodium replacement may be given in a smaller volume of fluid by using a hypertonic saline solution. This solution, however, may cause hypernatremia and cellular dehydration. **Protein colloid solutions** such as Plasmanate or salt-poor albumin may help to counteract capillary protein leak. Hetastarch (Hespan) or low-molecular-weight dextran may also help replete intravascular volume. The exact volume of resuscitative fluid required is calculated by either the Brook formula (Baxter formula) or Parkland formula. Wound management includes obtaining a culture to identify bacterial or fungal colonization early, escharotomy for deep restrictive eschar that interferes with respiration or extremity perfusion, splinting of affected joints in the position of function, range of motion exercises to avoid contractures, topical antimicrobial agents, and biologic dressings (porcine xenografts or split-thickness meshed skin grafts).

WOUND HEALING AND INFECTION

Clinical features

When there is loss of skin, migration of cells adjacent to the wound results in **epithelial regeneration**. This process ceases when the contact between adjacent epithelial cells is reestablished. If there is a deep wound, **contraction** occurs simultaneously. This involves migration of the full thicknesses of skin and subcutaneous tissues, slowly pulling the wound edges closer together. Myofibroblasts provide the special force necessary for this form of repair. The **formation of connective tissue** is the most vital and prolonged phase of wound healing and results in the lasting strength of the healed wound. When a wound is closed primarily with sutures or tape, it heals by a combination of epithelial regeneration and connective tissue formation. This is called **healing by first intention**. When a wound is left open and allowed to heal spontaneously, it heals by a combination of all three mechanisms. This is known as **healing by second intention** (granulation). Because contaminated subcutaneous tissue is more susceptible to infection when the skin is closed, in severely contaminated wounds the subcutaneous tissues and skin are left open. After about 5 days, when there is some protective granulation tissue, the skin is closed. This is called **healing by third intention**, or healing by delayed primary closure. Multiple factors influence the ability of wounds to heal normally. Acute problems with wound healing include wound infection and dehiscence. Chronic wound healing problems include hernia formation and excessive fibrosis. Factors that adversely affect wound healing can be remembered by the mnemonic **DIDN'T HEAL**: Drugs, Infection, Diabetes, Nutrition inadequate, Tissue necrosis, Hypoxia, Excessive tension on wound edges, Another wound (competition for substrates), and Low temperature.

Definitions

The incidence of wound complications, especially infection, is directly related to the preoperative status of the wound. A **clean wound** is a surgically created wound in a sterilely prepared field for a procedure that does not enter a contaminated viscus. A **clean-contaminated wound** occurs when a potentially contaminated viscus is entered without spillage. A **contaminated wound** is one in which there is gross spillage from a contaminated viscus, a preexisting infection, or a gross break in operative technique. A **dirty wound** is one in which there is continued contamination of the wound itself.

Diagnosis and therapeutic decisions

A **seroma** is a serous fluid collection occurring in a surgical wound. Seroma presents as a fluctuant swelling deep in the skin wound closure or deep to a flap and is diagnosed and treated by needle aspiration under strict aseptic conditions.

Wound dehiscence implies a disruption of the fascial closure of a surgical wound. The skin remains intact. Wound dehiscence is heralded by serous or serosanguineous wound drainage, often preceded by a popping or tearing sensation experienced by the patient. Treatment is operative closure.

Evisceration occurs when dehiscence is accompanied by disruption of the skin as well, resulting in extrusion of abdominal contents. Treatment is immediate operative repair.

Hematoma implies bleeding into the wound and results from inadequate operative hemostasis, especially in patients with a coagulation abnormality. Small hematomas may be observed, but large or expanding hematomas, those near prosthetic material, or those that compromise respiration require operative evacuation.

Cellulitis is an invasive, nonsuppurative connective tissue infection that starts as erythematous and edematous skin. It is often accompanied by high fever and chills. It advances particularly rapidly in ischemic extremities and in persons with severe venous stasis disease, diabetes, and alcoholism. The treatment is penicillin or erythromycin because the usual organism is *Streptococcus*.

Clostridial infections are a spectrum of soft-tissue infections with a variety of manifestations ranging from those of superficial lesions to lethal gas gangrene. A Gram stain of the exudate showing large gram-positive rods is diagnostic of a clostridial infection. Treatment includes surgical debridement, administration of appropriate antibiotics, blood volume replacement, and sometimes hyperbaric oxygen therapy.

1. **Simple contamination** of an open wound with clostridia may result in a brown seropurulent exudate. If surrounding tissue is well vascularized, invasive gangrene will not occur.
2. **Gas abscess** occurs about 1 week after contamination. The brown exudate develops a foul odor, and gas may be present. Fever and tachycardia may occur.

3. **Crepitant clostridial cellulitis** occurs when the surrounding tissue becomes ischemic, leading to rapid spread to the subcutaneous fascia with resultant crepitation and surrounding edema.

4. **Localized clostridial myositis** implies involvement of the underlying muscle. There is fever, tachycardia, wound crepitation, edema, and a foul-smelling odor.

5. **Gas gangrene** implies diffuse clostridial myositis and is heralded by a rapid increase in wound pain and edema with progressive systemic toxicity. The disease is self-perpetuating, as surrounding tissues lose blood supply and allow spread of the clostridial invasion. Fever and crepitus are not always present.

6. **Edematous clostridial gangrene** is an especially aggressive and lethal variant of clostridial gangrene in which muscle edema, not gas formation, predominates.

Necrotizing fasciitis occurs after infection of a traumatic or surgical wound. Infectious spread along the fascia causes thrombosis of skin vasculature. Skin necrosis first manifests as hemorrhagic bullae, then rapidly progressive edema, erythema, tenderness, and sometimes crepitation. Progressive necrotizing fasciitis is accompanied by fever, leukocytosis, tachycardia, systemic toxicity, and finally cardiovascular collapse. The patient is often remarkably alert until the terminal stages. Gram-stained smears of the exudate will reveal a mixed flora. Treatment includes surgical debridement, antibiotics, and blood volume replacement.

BIBLIOGRAPHY

Davis JH, et al (eds): Clinical Surgery. CV Mosby, St. Louis, 1987. 3,000 pages of clearly illustrated, well-written information about clinical surgery. Highly recommended for those who aspire to careers in surgery and its specialties.

Schwartz S: Principles of Surgery, 4th ed. McGraw-Hill, New York, 1984. A 3,000-page compendium of surgery. Appropriate as a major source of pathophysiological, diagnostic, and therapeutic information for those with a major interest in surgery and its specialty areas.

Stillman RM: General Surgery: Review and Assessment, 3rd ed. Appleton & Lange, E. Norwalk, 1988. A basic review of general surgery in outline format, peppered with mnemonics, and including board-type multiple-choice questions.

Way LW: Current Surgical Diagnosis and Treatment, 8th ed. Appleton & Lange, E. Norwalk, 1987. A 1,300-page well-organized and complete text of surgery. Highly recommended as an introduction to surgery. Most appropriate for senior medical students interested in surgery and for surgical residents during their first year.

SAMPLE QUESTIONS

DIRECTIONS: Each question below contains five suggested answers. Choose the **one best** response to each question.

1. A 21-year old patient has sustained severe trauma. Ligation of which of the following vessels is most likely to result in loss of the extremity or infarction of the organ supplied by that vessel?

    A. Inferior mesenteric artery
    B. Brachial artery
    C. Left renal vein
    D. Popliteal artery
    E. Internal iliac artery

2. The major determinant of operability in patients who have a ventricular septal defect is the

    A. size of the defect
    B. age of the patient
    C. pulmonary artery pressure
    D. location of the defect
    E. pulmonary vascular resistance

3. The sole communication between the pulmonary circulation and the bronchial arteries is

    A. small muscular pulmonic arteries
    B. arteriovenous fistulae
    C. interlobar and segmental pulmonary veins
    D. pre- and postarteriolar capillary plexus
    E. patent ductus arteriosus

4. Thirty minutes after an uneventful cholecystectomy, a 30-year-old woman is noted to be restless and cyanotic. Blood pressure is 120/70, pulse is 110, and respiration is 12/minute and shallow. The most appropriate procedure at this point is to

    A. start heparin therapy
    B. ventilate
    C. obtain a lung scan
    D. start antibiotic therapy
    E. sedate

5. Bright red blood streaking of stool associated with excruciating pain on defecation suggests

    A. rectal cancer
    B. condylomata acuminata
    C. internal hemorrhoids
    D. anal fistula
    E. anal fissure

6. A 72-year-old man is admitted to the hospital because of severe abdominal pain after meals and constipation alternating with flatulence. He has lost 40 pounds in 3 months. Physical examination reveals an abdominal bruit. The suspected diagnosis is

    A. peptic ulcer disease
    B. GI arteriovenous malformation
    C. an occult carcinoma
    D. abdominal angina (mesenteric ischemia)
    E. a malabsorption syndrome

7. After major intra-abdominal surgery, a 60-year-old woman is noted to have diffuse bleeding. Platelet count is 20,000/mm³, Factor V <20% of normal, prothrombin time is 22 seconds, partial thromboplastin time is 85 seconds, and fibrinogen 50 mg/100 ml. The most likely diagnosis is

    A. acidosis
    B. hemophilia A
    C. hemophilia B
    D. von Willebrand's disease
    E. disseminated intravascular coagulopathy

8. Which of the following is NOT associated with peptic ulcer or gastric hypersecretion?

    A. chronic liver disease
    B. chronic respiratory insufficiency
    C. hypoparathyroidism
    D. chronic renal failure
    E. massive intestinal resection

9. A 50-year-old man presents with abdominal pain and on gastroscopy is found to have an ulcer of the lesser curvature of his stomach. Four biopsies are taken and are benign. He is treated with antacids and diet for 1 month, at which time he is free of symptoms. Appropriate management is

    A. angiography
    B. further workup only if symptoms recur
    C. serum gastrin levels and analysis of blood type
    D. repeat gastroscopy and biopsy
    E. gastrectomy

10. The initial treatment of a lung abscess includes systemic antibiotics and

    A. lobectomy
    B. tube drainage of the abscess
    C. pneumonectomy
    D. bronchoscopy
    E. segmental resection

11. The right middle lobe syndrome most commonly results from

    A. mucoviscidosis
    B. bronchiectasis
    C. hilar lymphadenopathy
    D. bronchial stenosis
    E. foreign body aspiration

12. A 30-year-old male is admitted with a gunshot wound of the left chest in the midaxillary line. Blood pressure is 90/60 mm Hg, pulse is 120, and respirations are 30/minute. After 2 L of normal saline intravenously, central venous pressure rises to 30 cm. The most likely diagnosis is

    A. tension pneumothorax
    B. flail chest
    C. cardiac tamponade
    D. ruptured pulmonary artery
    E. myocardial infarction

13. Following drainage of a subphrenic abscess, a patient who weighs 70 kg is placed on a volume ventilator with the following settings: tidal volume, 500 ml; respiratory rate, 12/minute; inspiration:expiration ratio, 1:2; inspired oxygen concentration, 0.40. Arterial blood gas determinations reveal PO_2=100, pH=7.35, and PCO_2=52. Appropriate management is to

    A. increase the FiO_2 to 1.0
    B. add 10 cm H_2O positive end-expiratory pressure
    C. increase the tidal volume to 1,000 ml
    D. increase the respiratory rate to 20/minute
    E. change the inspiration:expiration ratio to 1:3

14. In a patient with reversal of flow in a vertebral artery, the obstruction is most commonly found in the

    A. internal carotid artery
    B. distal subclavian artery
    C. proximal subclavian artery
    D. common carotid artery
    E. external carotid artery

15. The sum of tidal volume, inspiratory reserve volume, and expiratory reserve volume is called the

    A. vital capacity
    B. forced expiratory volume
    C. maximal voluntary ventilation
    D. tidal volume
    E. residual volume

16. Methods of decompressing the portal system may make use of any of the following EXCEPT the

    A. hepatic vein
    B. portal vein
    C. superior mesenteric vein
    D. inferior vena cava
    E. left renal vein

17. Of the following, the type of thyroid cancer most likely to be familial is

    A. follicular
    B. anaplastic
    C. medullary
    D. papillary
    E. associated with Hashimoto's thyroiditis

18. Prevention of postoperative pseudomembranous enterocolitis requires

    A. avoidance of unnecessary antibiotics
    B. avoidance of nonabsorable colonic sutures
    C. adequate resection margins
    D. antibiotic bowel preparation
    E. use of preoperative stool softeners

19. Which of the following anesthetic agents is contraindicated in patients with porphyria?

 A. Thiopental sodium
 B. Ethylene
 C. Ether
 D. Nitrous oxide
 E. Cyclopropane

20. In patients with von Willebrand's disease requiring operation, preoperative preparation should include

 A. small doses of epsilon-aminocaproic acid
 B. packed cells
 C. vitamin K_1 oxide
 D. fresh-frozen plasma
 E. fibrinogen

21. A 70-year-old man presents with right upper quadrant abdominal pain. His abdominal x-ray shows multiple stepladder air-fluid levels throughout the abdomen and tubular air shadows in the right upper quadrant. The most plausible explanation is

 A. internal hernia
 B. cancer of the colon
 C. obstruction due to adhesions
 D. sigmoid diverticulitis
 E. gallstone ileus

22. The major risk of an untreated insulinoma involves damage to the

 A. central nervous system
 B. liver
 C. kidney
 D. spleen
 E. pancreas

23. The most common pathological type of lung cancer is

 A. adenocarcinoma
 B. undifferentiated large cell
 C. bronchiolar carcinoma
 D. epidermoid
 E. oat cell

24. The most appropriate initial therapy for the majority of patients with low cardiac output secondary to myocardial infarction is

 A. Isuprel administration
 B. intra-aortic balloon
 C. epinephrine administration
 D. nitroprusside administration
 E. volume replacement

25. Open reduction is indicated in all of the following fractures in an adult EXCEPT

 A. comminuted fracture of the head of the radius
 B. fracture of middle third of the clavicle with overriding
 C. fracture of the olecranon
 D. fracture of middle third of the clavicle without overriding
 E. transverse fracture of the patella

26. The need for surgical intervention in sliding hiatus hernia is best determined by

 A. size of hernia
 B. amount of sequelae of reflux
 C. duration of symptoms
 D. weight loss
 E. sphincter tone

27. Resection of a "mixed tumor" of the parotid gland might lead to paresis of which of the following cranial nerves?

 A. III
 B. V
 C. VII
 D. IX
 E. XI

28. A 40-year-old woman presents with an aortic systolic murmur detected on routine physical examination by her gynecologist. On further questioning, she admits having occasional syncopal attacks. Cardiac catheterization reveals a 75-mm Hg gradient across the aortic valve. Appropriate management includes

 A. antibiotics and observation for 1 year
 B. digitalis, diuretics, and observation for 1 year
 C. observation for 1 year without drug therapy
 D. Holter monitoring and probable insertion of transverse pacemaker
 E. aortic valve replacement

29. The most common cause of surgical wound infection is

 A. trauma due to overretraction
 B. wound dressings removed too early
 C. inadequate skin preparation
 D. contamination during the operation
 E. anergy

30. A temporary or permanent cardiac pacemaker is LEAST likely to be required for a patient who

 A. requires cholecystectomy and develops asymptomatic complete heart block
 B. has congestive heart failure with complete heart block
 C. has Stokes-Adams attacks
 D. has sinus bradycardia with angina pectoris
 E. has atrial fibrillation and a ventricular rate of 55

31. Cerebrospinal rhinorrhea secondary to an otherwise asymptomatic skull fracture is best managed with

    A. diuretics
    B. nasal packing
    C. immediate surgical closure
    D. culture and appropriate antibiotics
    E. surgical closure after brain scan ruling out intracranial lesion

32. Complications of an undescended testis include all of the following EXCEPT

    A. exposure to trauma
    B. renal failure
    C. abnormal spermatogenesis
    D. torsion
    E. malignancy

33. Which of the following is LEAST likely to be associated with an increased risk of breast cancer in the female?

    A. Nulliparity
    B. Breast-feeding
    C. Family history
    D. Early menarche
    E. Cancer of the uterine corpus

34. Anemia secondary to chronic infection results from

    A. unrecognized hereditary spherocytosis
    B. iron deficiency
    C. vitamin B_{12} deficiency
    D. hemolysis
    E. erythropoietic depression

35. Complications of postoperative hypothermia in infants include all of the following EXCEPT

    A. increased blood viscosity
    B. hypotension
    C. metabolic acidosis
    D. respiratory depression
    E. tachycardia

36. An adenocarcinoma found on rectal examination at 3 cm from the anal verge is best treated by

    A. anterior resection of the colon
    B. abdominoperineal resection
    C. radiotherapy and chemotherapy only
    D. left hemicolectomy
    E. total proctocolectomy

37. The most common presentation of breast cancer is

    A. nipple retraction
    B. focal fixation of the skin
    C. a painless lump
    D. "orange-peel" skin
    E. warm red hyperemia of the entire breast

38. Of the following, the LEAST likely manifestation of Crohn's disease is

    A. weight loss
    B. bowel obstruction
    C. diarrhea
    D. enterocutaneous fistulas
    E. bleeding

39. A 26-year-old man 2 weeks after blunt upper abdominal trauma develops jaundice, abdominal pain, and hematemesis. The diagnosis is best made by

    A. oral cholecystography
    B. sonography
    C. rose bengal scan
    D. percutaneous liver biopsy
    E. arteriography

40. Volkmann's ischemic contracture is associated with

    A. carpal navicular fracture
    B. chronic hypercalcemia
    C. greenstick fracture of the forearm
    D. fracture of the olecranon
    E. supracondylar fracture of the humerus

41. A 74-year-old male with generalized peritonitis secondary to perforated diverticulitis develops bibasilar rales and anuria several hours after exploratory laparotomy. His central venous pressure is normal. Which of the following studies would be most useful in following his state of hydration?

    A. Pulmonary wedge pressure
    B. Arterial blood gases
    C. Arterial pressure tracings
    D. Urine to serum creatinine ratio
    E. Electrocardiogram

42. Following a severe chest injury caused by hitting the steering wheel, a truck driver is found to have distended neck veins, tachycardia, a narrow pulse pressure, and a paradoxical pulse. The most likely diagnosis is

    A. mediastinal shift
    B. massive atelectasis
    C. cardiac tamponade
    D. tension pneumothorax
    E. pulmonary embolism

43. The treatment of most cases of diverticulitis is

    A. medical management
    B. Mikulicz's resection
    C. transverse colostomy
    D. primary resection and anastomosis
    E. resection, anastomosis with proximal colostomy

44. The surgical procedure most likely to be indicated in intractable ascites due to portal hypertension is

A. end-to-side portacaval shunt
B. mesocaval H-graft
C. distal splenorenal shunt
D. central splenorenal shunt
E. peritoneojugular shunt

45. Following a bite by a black widow spider, the associated abdominal pain can be best controlled by

A. aspirin
B. steroids
C. adrenalin
D. calcium gluconate
E. potassium chloride

46. A 59-year-old woman is examined in the recovery room 2 hours following a Whipple procedure. Her blood pressure is 80 by palpation, and pulse is 140. She is restless, pale, and has cool, moist skin. The first step is to

A. obtain arterial blood gases
B. check hematocrit
C. obtain a chest x-ray
D. inspect the drain sites
E. obtain an electrocardiogram

47. In an otherwise healthy patient, a deficiency of which of the following would have the LEAST effect on wound healing?

A. Vitamin A
B. Vitamin C
C. Alpha-ketoglutarate
D. Iron
E. Oxygen

48. The most important step in the treatment of both septic shock and hemorrhagic shock is

A. antibiotics
B. Swan-Ganz catheter
C. Foley catheter
D. intravenous fluids
E. vasopressors

49. D-tubocurarine can be reversed with

A. neostigmine
B. succinylcholine
C. epinephrine
D. atropine
E. isoproterenol

50. A patient with intractable heart failure, coronary occlusive disease, and angiocardiographic studies that show an area of akinesis of the left ventricular wall would be a candidate for

A. heparin therapy
B. heart transplant
C. mitral valve replacement
D. excision of akinetic ventricular wall
E. increasing ventricular rate by pacemaker stimulation

51. Early management of a severely contaminated traumatic wound includes all of the following EXCEPT

A. debridement
B. irrigation
C. tetanus prophylaxis
D. hemostasis
E. primary closure

52. A 40-year-old woman who has been receiving total parenteral nutrition through a subclavian vein for 2 weeks becomes comatose while crossmatched blood is being administered through the subclavian catheter. The most likely cause of this problem is

A. sepsis
B. hypoglycemia
C. ketoacidosis
D. transfusion reaction
E. hyperosmolar nonketotic coma

53. The treatment of hypercalcemia of malignancy includes all of the following EXCEPT

A. mithramycin
B. prednisone
C. furosemide
D. dipyridamole
E. phosphosoda

54. All of the following are true of papillary carcinoma of the thyroid EXCEPT that

A. radical neck dissection is usually indicated
B. thyroid lobectomy and isthmusectomy are usually indicated
C. psammoma bodies may be seen histologically
D. it often appears as a nonfunctioning nodule on thyroid scan
E. it has a better prognosis than anaplastic thyroid cancer

55. All of the following are true of intermittent claudication EXCEPT that

A. the drug pentoxifylline is approved as a therapeutic agent
B. superficial femoral artery occlusion may be discovered
C. Doppler pressures are a valuable diagnostic index
D. the risk of amputation is 25% during the first year after onset
E. it is usually a result of atherosclerotic disease

ANSWERS

1.	D	15.	A	29.	D	43.	A
2.	E	16.	A	30.	E	44.	E
3.	D	17.	C	31.	D	45.	D
4.	B	18.	A	32.	B	46.	D
5.	E	19.	A	33.	B	47.	A
6.	D	20.	D	34.	E	48.	D
7.	E	21.	E	35.	E	49.	A
8.	C	22.	A	36.	B	50.	D
9.	D	23.	D	37.	C	51.	E
10.	D	24.	D	38.	E	52.	B
11.	C	25.	B	39.	E	53.	D
12.	C	26.	B	40.	E	54.	A
13.	C	27.	C	41.	A	55.	D
14.	C	28.	E	42.	C		

3

OBSTETRICS AND GYNECOLOGY

Hugh R. K. Barber and David H. Fields

EMBRYOLOGY

DEVELOPMENT OF THE FEMALE PELVIC ORGANS

Functionally, the urogenital system can be divided into two entirely different components: the **urinary system**, which excretes waste products and excess water by means of an intricate tubular system in the kidney; and the **genital system**, which assures continuation of the human race by producing germ cells as well as the incubator in the passage areas where the human being passes to be born.

Embryologically and anatomically, however, both systems are interwoven. Both develop from a common ridge formed by proliferation of mesoderm along the posterior wall of the abdominal cavity, and the excretory ducts of both systems initially enter a common cavity, the cloaca.

Because the urinary and genital systems are so closely related anatomically, and more particularly embryologically, it is almost impossible to study one and ignore the other. However, just the internal and external genitalia will be presented here.

In the development of both excretory and reproductive organs, **mesoderm** plays the major part, but entoderm and ectoderm also make important contributions.

The genital organs begin to differentiate and become identifiable in the fifth week of intrauterine life, when the embryo is approximately 10 mm long. At this stage, the primitive gut is suspended from the dorsal aspect of the coelomic cavity in the midline by mesentery, and this is flanked on either side by a longitudinal ridge, covered by coelomic epithelium. This is produced by the mesonephros; the wolffian (mesonephric) duct lies on the lateral side.

Almost the entire reproductive and urinary systems of both sexes are formed from the wolffian body, a large and important bilateral structure occupying the posterior or dorsal portion of the primitive peritoneal cavity. On the lateral side of each wolffian ridge, a groove appears and later becomes converted into a tube known as the paramesonephric (ovarian) duct. The female ducts, unlike those of the male, are not part of the urinary system but develop independently and serve no purpose except that of the female genital ducts.

The **müllerian ducts** begin to develop in embryos of about 10 mm (35 to 36 days) when the mesonephros is at its greatest stage of development. Each duct begins as an ingrowth of the peritoneal epithelial covering, the mesonephros near its anterior end. This ingrowing mesothelium forms a short groove that becomes deeper and sinks beneath the surface as a tube. The anterior end is the first part to form and opens into the peritoneal cavity as the osteum abdominalis of the tube. From this beginning, the duct, by independent growth at its tip, grows caudally beneath the peritoneum and parallel to the mesonephric duct, until in the embryo of about 24 mm (8 weeks) it reaches the urogenital sinus, where it ends blindly, closely adjacent to the mesonephric ducts, in an elevation known as **Müller's tubercle.**

The two müllerian ducts are at first separate throughout their course, but about the time they reach the urogenital sinus, their caudal portions unite to form the uterovaginal canal while the cephalic portions remain separate.

In the female, the uterus and vagina develop from the uterovaginal canal, and the two uterine tubes (fallopian tubes) from the separate portion of the müllerian ducts. In this development there forms about the duct, especially the uterovaginal portion, a dense mass of mesenchyme, from which develop the muscular and fibrous parts of the organs. The epithelial lining of these organs develops from the müllerian ducts except at the lower end of the vagina (possibly its entire length), where recent studies have shown the lining to be formed of entodermal epithelium migrating from the urogenital sinus and replacing the original mesodermal lining. Nevertheless, the vagina is fundamentally derived from the müllerian ducts. The vagina for a time has a solid core of epithelium in which, at about 18 weeks, the lumen begins to form by breaking down of the central cells, the stratified squamous lining being left in place. The fimbriated ostia of the uterine tubes develop from the primary ostia of the müllerian ducts. The **hymen** makes its appearance as a fold on the wall of the vagina, with its external opening at the position of Müller's tubercle. There are rod cells present. These rod cells regress, and a solid cord of epithelial cells derived from the urogenital sinus grows upward in its place, extending as far as the cervix. The central cells of this cord break down to form the lumen of the vagina. The hymen marks the site from which this upward growth of sinus and cells begins. The surrounding mesoderm of the genital septum gives rise to the musculature of both the vagina and the uterus.

The **ovary** and upper part of the müllerian duct, which becomes the **fallopian tube**, develop in the upper part of the coelom and receive their blood supply from the corresponding segment of the aorta. During fetal life, the ovary and fallopian tubes gradually descend into the pelvis, and the blood vessels lengthen accordingly.

OVARY DEVELOPMENT

The sex of the embryo is genetically determined at the time of fertilization. The gonads do not acquire male or female morphological characteristics until the seventh week of development.

The gonads appear initially as a pair of longitudinal ridges on the posterior abdominal wall and are designated the **genital** or **gonadal ridges**. They are formed by proliferation of coelomic epithelium and a condensation of the underlying mesenchyme. The germ cells do not appear in the genital ridges until the sixth week of development. In human embryos, the primordial germ cells appear at the very early stage among the endodermal cells in the wall of the yolk sac. They migrate by an amoeboid movement along the dorsal mesentery of the hindgut and invade the genital ridge at about the sixth week of development. If they fail to reach the genital ridge, no gonad is formed, and therefore the primitive germ cell is an inductive influence on the development of the gonad into ovary or testis. At about the time that the germ cells reach the genital ridge, there is proliferation of the surface epithelium, and this penetrates the underlying mesenchyme. This gives rise to a series of irregular sex cords, which are called the **primitive sex cords**. In both male and female embryos, these cords are connected to the surface epithelium, and it is impossible to differentiate between the male and female gonad. Therefore, at this point the gonad is called the **indifferent gonad**.

In the presence of an **XX** sex chromosome complement, the primitive sex cords are broken up into regular cell clusters. These clusters contain groups of primitive germ cells and are mainly located in the medulla. These primitive germ cells disappear and are replaced by a very vascular stroma called the **medulla** of the ovary.

The surface epithelium of the female gonad, unlike that of the male, continues to proliferate. In the seventh week it gives rise to a second generation of cords called the **cortical cords**, which penetrate the underlying mesenchyme but remain close to the surface. In the fourth month, these sex cords split into isolated clusters of cells that surround one or more primitive germ cells. The germ cells subsequently develop into the **oogonia**, and the surrounding epithelium that comes from the surface gives rise to the follicular cells.

The oogonium becomes an oocyte when it enters the first of its two meiotic divisions. The first oocytes can be recognized at about 8 weeks and are most numerous at about 5 months, when they number about 4 million. At the time of birth, no oogonia remain and the oocytes have been reduced to 2 million. By the seventh postnatal year, only about 300,000 oocytes remain.

The ovary, like the testis, has a **gubernaculum**; this extends from the inferior pole of the ovary to the internal inguinal ring. In addition, it becomes incorporated into the uterine wall at the point of entry of the fallopian tube. It persists in the adult as the ovarian ligament and the round ligament of the uterus.

The mesonephros degenerates almost completely, but a few tubules may persist in the broad ligament, where they may give rise to cysts in adult life. In the male, the wolffian duct forms the vas deferens, but it degenerates in the female fetus. It can sometimes still be traced in the adult female, when it is known as **Gardner's duct**. This duct runs medially through the broad ligament and down the side of the vagina, or cysts may form in it.

EXTERNAL GENITALIA DEVELOPMENT

At an early stage, the hindgut and the various urogenital ducts open into a common cloaca. A **septum** (urorectal) grows down between the allantois and the hindgut during the fifth week. Eventually this septum fuses with the cloacal membrane, dividing the cloaca into two compartments—the rectum dorsally and the urogenital sinus ventrally. At the same time, the developing uterus grows down and makes contact with the **urogenital sinus**. The urogenital sinus—which forms the bladder, urethra, and vestibule—develops as a ventral diverticulum from the hindgut. At the end of the seventh week, the urogenital membrane breaks down so that the urogenital sinus opens onto the surface. The developing uterus and vagina push downward and cause an elongation and narrowing of the upper part of the urogenital sinus. This will form the **urethra**.

At first the urogenital sinus and the hindgut open into a common cavity, the **cloaca**, which at this stage is separated from the exterior by the cloacal membrane. Later this sinus is completely separated from the hindgut by a septum, the mesoderm, which divides the cloacal membrane into a posterior part, which temporarily closes the future anus, and an anterior part, the **urogenital membrane**.

On the surface of the embryo around the urogenital sinus, five swellings appear. At the cephalic end a midline swelling grows, the **genital tubercle**, which will become the **clitoris**. Posterior to the genital tubercle and on either side of the urogenital membrane, folds are formed—**urethra folds**. Lateral to each of these, a further swelling appears—the genital or labial swelling. These swellings approach each other at their posterior ends, fuse, and form the posterior commissure. The remaining swellings become the **labia majora**.

Certain small but clinically important glands are formed in and around the urogenital sinus. In the embryo, epithelial buds arise from the urethra and also from the epithelium of the urogenital sinus. In the male, these two sets of buds grow together and give rise to the glands of the prostate. They remain separate in the female, and the urethral buds form the urethral glands and the urogenital buds giving rise to the paraurethral **Skene's glands**. The ducts of the latter open into the vestibule on either side of the urethra.

Two other small glands arise by budding from the epithelium of the posterior part of the vestibule, one on either side of the vaginal opening. These are the greater vestibular or **Bartholin's glands**. Similar smaller glands also arise in the anterior portion of the vestibule.

In summary, in front of the urogenital membrane arises a midline tubercle, the **phallic tubercle**. On either side two ridges develop, the inner called the genital folds, and the outer the genital swellings. Eventually the phallic tubercle forms the clitoris. The inner genital folds form the **labia minora** and the frenulum and prepuce of the clitoris. The outer genital swellings give rise to the **labia majora**. Finally, the urogenital membrane disappears so that the vestibule communicates with the exterior through the **vulva**.

ANATOMY OF THE FEMALE PELVIC ORGANS

Knowledge of anatomy assists in gynecologic diagnosis and is essential for gynecologic surgery.

EXTERNAL GENITALIA

The external genitalia consist of the mons pubis, the labia majora, the labia minora, the clitoris, the vestibule, the vestibular bulbs, the Bartholin's glands (vestibular glands), and the hymen.

The **vulva** includes those portions of the female genital apparatus that are externally visible in the perineal region. The mons veneris is composed of fibrofatty tissue that covers the bodies of the pubic bones. The mons veneris, overlying the symphysis pubis, is a fatty prominence covered by crisp, curly hair. From it, two longitudinal folds of skin, the labia majora, extend in an elliptical fashion to enclose the vulvar cleft.

The **labia majora** are two folds of skin in subcutaneous fat that merge posteriorly into the perineum, where they are joined together by the fourchette. The skin covering them contains sebaceous and sweat glands and a few specialized apocrine glands. The lateral aspects of the labia majora bear hair follicles. In the deepest part of the labia majora, there is a core of fatty tissue continuous with that of the inguinal canal, and the fibers of the round ligament terminate here. During development of the diverticulum of the peritoneal cavity, their processus vaginalis accompanies the round ligament into the inguinal canal. It usually disappears but may persist as the canal of Nuck.

The **labia minora** are thin, firm, pigmented, redundant folds of skin that anteriorly split to enclose the **clitoris**; laterally, they bound the vestibule, and diminish gradually as they extend posteriorly. The skin of the small labia is devoid of hair follicles, poor in sweat glands, and rich in sebaceous glands. The labia minora are very sensitive and contain some erectile tissue.

The **clitoris**, a small cylindrical erectile organ situated at the lower border of the symphysis, is composed of two crura, a body, and a glans. The two crura diverge posteriorly to attach to the descending rami of the pubic bones. The glans is covered with modified skin containing many nerve endings. The body and the crura are composed of erectile tissue. The ischiocavernosus muscles surround the crura and, by their contraction, produce erection of the clitoris.

The **vestibule** becomes apparent on separation of the labia. It is bounded anterolaterally by the labia minora and posteriorly by the fourchette. Into the vestibule open the urethra, the ducts of Bartholin's glands, and the vagina. The external urethral meatus is situated on a slight papilla-like elevation 2 cm below the clitoris. In the posterolateral aspect of the urinary orifice, the openings of the bilateral Skene's ducts are evident. They run below and parallel to the urethra for a distance of about 1.5 cm. Bartholin's ducts are visible on each side of the vestibule, in the groove between the hymen and labia minora, at about the junction of the middle and posterior third of the lateral boundary of the vaginal orifice. The vestibular bulbs are two oblong masses of erectile tissue that lie on either side of the vaginal entrance from the vestibule.

The **Bartholin's glands** (vestibular glands) are two small, racemose glands situated on either side of the vaginal orifice, deep to the posterior ends of the labia minora. During sexual excitement, they secrete thin mucus that serves as a lubricant. A duct on each side opens in the groove between the labia minora and the hymen.

The **hymen** is a membrane composed of thin, vascularized membrane that separates the vagina from the vestibule. It is covered on both sides by a stratified squamous epithelium of the mucous membrane variety. As a rule, it shows great variation in thickness and in the size and shape of the hymenal openings (annular, septate, cribriform, and fimbriate). The hymen is partially ruptured at the first coitus and further disrupted during childbirth. Any tags remaining after rupture are known as carunculae myrtiformes.

INTERNAL REPRODUCTIVE ORGANS

The **vagina** is a muscular canal lined by stratified squamous epithelium and leading from the uterus to the vulva. Its length averages 10 cm, with the posterior being longer than the anterior part of the vagina. The vagina meets the anteverted uterus at a right angle. The cervix projects into the vaginal vault, which is described as having four fornices—anterior, posterior, and two lateral. The posterior vaginal wall is longer than the anterior wall, so that the posterior fornix is deeper than the anterior. The vaginal walls are rugose, with transverse folds.

Laterally, the vagina is supported by the strong cardinal ligaments (transverse cardinal ligaments), which form a sling extending from the side walls of the pelvis to the vaginal vault and supravaginal cervix. The vagina is also supported in its middle third by the medial edges of the levator ani muscles, from which fibers are given off to blend with the muscular coat of the vagina. Posteriorly, the lower part of the vagina is supported by the perineal body.

The **uterus** is normally anteverted and anteflexed. The superior surface is convex and directed forward. The anterior surface is flat and looks downward and forward, resting on the bladder. Its peritoneal covering is reflected at the level of the isthmus to the upper aspect of the bladder, creating the vesicouterine pouch. The posterior surface of the uterus is convex and lies in relation to the pelvic colon and rectum. The peritoneum of the posterior wall covers the body and upper cervix and then extends over the posterior fornix of the vagina to the rectum to form the rectouterine pouch or Douglas's cul-de-sac.

In adult life, the uterus weighs about 70 g and is about 7.5 cm long, with walls about 2 cm thick. It consists of two unequal parts: an upper corpus, or body, which is about 5 cm long; and a lower cervix, or neck, which is about 2.5 cm.

The **cervix** is directed downward and backward to rest against the posterior vaginal wall. Only the upper half of the posterior surface is covered by peritoneum. The external os of the cervix lies about the level of the upper border of the symphysis pubis in the plane of the ischial spine.

The cervix is cylindrical in shape and continuous above with the body of the uterus. It is described in two parts—supravaginal and vaginal. The vaginal surface of the cervix is covered with squamous epithelium, which extends to the margin of the external os.

The fallopian tube on either side extends outward from the uterine cornua to end near the ovary. At the abdominal ostium, the tube opens into the peritoneal cavity, which is therefore in communication with the exterior of the body via the uterus and vagina. The tubes or oviducts convey the ova from the graafian follicles to the uterus. Each fallopian tube is about 10 cm long.

Each tube lies between the two layers of the broad ligament, and, passing outward and backward, its outer half comes to lie in direct contact with the ovary, where it ascends over the meso-varian border and tubal pole, descends on the free border, and finally comes to rest on its medial surface. Each tube is described as consisting of four parts. A narrow portion within the wall of the uterus, called the interstitial part, is about 2.5 cm long. This leads into a straight part called the isthmus, about 2.5 cm long. This is followed by a tortuous part called the ampulla, about 5 cm long. Finally, the tube ends in a dilated trumpet-shaped portion called the infundibulum, which opens at the abdominal ostium.

The ovaries are two almond-shaped solid organs, measuring about 3.5 cm in length, 2 cm in depth, and 1 cm in thickness. In the nullipara, the ovary lies in a shallow peritoneal fossa on the lateral pelvic wall known as the Waldeyer's fossa ovarica. Its long axis lies in the vertical plane, so that it has an upper and a lower pole, an anterior and posterior border, and a medial and a lateral surface. The fossa ovarica lies immediately below the bifurcation of the common iliac artery, and one of the most important relations of the ovary is the ureter, which lies immediately behind it. The ovary is not covered with peritoneum; it is attached at its hilum to the posterior surface of the broad ligament. The most natural part of the broad ligament is called the infundibulopelvic fold, and this supports the outer pole of the ovary. The inner pole is suspended from the cornua of the uterus by the ovarian ligaments. This is continuous with the round ligament, which is also attached to the cornua below the fallopian tube.

PELVIC DIAPHRAGM

The pelvic diaphragm forms a musculotendinous, funnel-shaped partition between the pelvic cavity and the perineum. It is composed of the levator ani and coccygeus muscles, sheathed in a superior and inferior layer of fascia. The muscles of the pelvic diaphragm extend from the lateral pelvic walls downward and medially to fuse with each other and are inserted into the terminal portions of the urethra, vagina, and anus. Anteriorly, they fail to meet in the midline just behind the pubic symphysis, exposing the gap in the pelvic floor that is completed by the urogenital diaphragm. In this area, the inferior fascia of the pelvic diaphragm fuses with the superior fascia of the urogenital diaphragm.

The levator ani muscles may be subdivided into an anterior pubococcygeus and a posterior iliococcygeus portion. The medial borders of the pubococcygeus muscle pass on either side from the pubic bone to the preanal raphe. They thus embrace the vagina, and on contraction have some sphincteric action. The nerve supply is from the third and fourth sacral nerves. The muscles support the pelvic and abdominal viscera, including the bladder. The most medial part of each muscle is described as the pubococcygeus portion. The medial edge of this passes beneath the bladder and lateral to the urethra, into which some of its fibers are inserted. Together with the fibers from the opposite muscle they form a loop that maintains the angle between the posterior aspect of the urethra and the bladder base. During micturition, this loop relaxes to allow the bladder neck and upper urethra to open and to descend.

The coccygeus muscles are triangular, arise from the ischial spines, and are inserted into the lateral border of the lower sacrum and upper coccyx. They lie on the pelvic aspect of the sacrospinous ligaments.

PERINEUM

The perineum refers to the anatomic region at the inferior end of the trunk, below the pelvic floor. With the thighs abducted, it is diamond-shaped. On the surface it is bounded by the mons veneris in front, the buttocks behind, and the thighs laterally. More deeply, it is limited by the margins of the pelvic outlet—namely, the pubic symphysis and arcuate ligament, the ischiopubic rami, the ischial tuberosities, the sacro-tuberous ligaments, the sacrum, and the coccyx. A transverse line joining the ischial tuberosity divides the perineum into an anterior urogenital and a posterior anal triangle.

The perineal floor is bounded by skin and two layers of superficial fascia. The deep fascia of the perineum is not included in the floor, for it covers the muscles that bound the ischiorectal fossa.

The superficial fascia consists of a superficial fatty layer and a deeper membranous layer (the Colles' fascia). The deep portion of the superficial fascia is continued anteriorly as the Scarpa's fascia on the lower abdominal wall. It surrounds the vestibule and its contents and then winds around the transverse perineum muscles to blend with the base of the urogenital diaphragm immediately in front of the ischial tuberosities. Laterally, it is attached to the ischial pubic rami.

The urogenital diaphragm (triangular ligament) is a structure peculiar to humans. It consists of a sheath of muscles enclosed between two triangular fascial membranes. The muscular sheath is swamped by the transversus perinei profundus and the sphincter urethra membranous muscles. The urogenital diaphragm encloses the deep perineal compartment. It is a strong muscular membranous partition stretched across the anterior half of the pelvic outlet, beneath which are contained the deep perineal muscles, the sphincter of the membranous urethra, and the pudendal vessels and nerves. It is pierced by the urethra and vagina.

The anal triangle contains the termination of the anal canal and its sphincters, the anococcygeal/ischiorectal body, and the ischial rectal fossa, together with the blood vessels, nerves, and lymphatics in this region.

The muscles of the perineum include the bulvocavernosus, the ischiocavernosus, the superficial and deep transverse perineal muscles, the sphincter of the membranous urethra, and the external anal sphincter.

The **central point** of the perineum is often referred to by the obstetrician simply as the perineum. It lies at the base of the urogenital diaphragm, between the vulva and anal orifice. It consists of a fibromuscular mass, muscle fibers predominantly, for at this point seven muscles meet and fuse. This central point is in the very vulnerable position at parturition and is easily torn; its constitution, therefore, is a matter of great importance. The muscles that blend at the central point are the sphincter ani externus, the two levator ani muscles, the two transversus perinei muscles, the bulbocavernosus muscle, and the recto-urethralis muscle.

The **anococcygeal body** is a mass of fibrous and muscular tissue between the tip of the coccyx and the anal orifice. The levator ani and sphincter ani externus make up the muscular part. It serves as support for the anal canal.

OVARIAN LIGAMENT AND ROUND LIGAMENT

The ovarian ligament lies beneath the posterior layer of the broad ligament and passes from the medial pole of the ovary to the uterus just below the point of entry of the fallopian tube. The round ligament is the continuation of the same structure and runs forward under the anterior leaf of the peritoneum to enter the inguinal canal, ending in the subcutaneous tissue of the labia majora. Together, the ovarian and round ligaments are homologous with the gubernaculum testis of the male. The round ligament is seldom tense enough to prevent the uterus from becoming retroverted; it has no other supporting function.

ARTERIES SUPPLYING THE PELVIC ORGANS

Ovarian artery

The ovary develops on the posterior abdominal wall and migrates from about T10 down into the pelvis. It derives its blood supply directly from the abdominal aorta. The ovarian artery arises from the aorta just below the renal artery and runs downward on the anterior surface of the psoas muscle to the pelvic brim, where it crosses in front of the ureter, and then passes into the infundibulopelvic fold of the broad ligament. The artery divides into branches that supply the ovary and tube and then run on to reach the uterus, where they anastomose with the terminal branches of the uterine artery.

Internal iliac (hypogastric) artery

The hypogastric artery measures about 2 cm in length and begins at the bifurcation of the common iliac artery in front of the sacroiliac joint. It quickly splits into anterior and posterior divisions; the branches that supply the pelvic viscera all are from the anterior division.

The **uterine artery** provides the main blood supply to the uterus. The artery runs downward on the lateral wall of the pelvis, in the same direction as the ureter. It then turns inward and forward, lying in the base of the broad ligament. By this change of direction, the artery crosses above the ureter at a distance of about 2 cm from the uterus at the level of the internal os. On reaching the wall of the uterus, the artery turns upward to run tortuously to the upper part of the uterus, where it anastomoses with the ovarian artery. In this part of its course, it sends many branches into the substance of the uterus.

The artery supplies a branch to the ureter as it crosses it, and shortly afterward another branch is given off to supply the cervix and upper vagina.

The **vaginal artery** is another branch of the internal iliac artery, and it runs at a lower level to supply the vagina.

The **vesicle arteries** are variable in number. They supply the bladder and the terminal ureter. One occasionally runs in the roof of the ureteric canal.

The **middle hemorrhoidal artery** often arises in common with the lowest vesicle artery.

The **pudendal artery** is another branch of the internal iliac artery. It leaves the pelvic cavity through the sciatic foramen and, after winding around the ischial spine, enters the ischiorectal fossa, where it gives off the inferior hemorrhoidal artery. It terminates in branches that supply the perineal and vulvar structures, including the erectile tissue of the vestibular bulbs and clitoris.

The **superior hemorrhoidal artery** is a continuation of the inferior mesenteric artery and descends in the base of the pelvic mesacolon. It divides into two branches, which run on either side of the rectum and supply numerous branches to it.

PELVIC VEINS

The veins around the bladder, uterus, vagina, and rectum form plexuses that intercommunicate freely. Venous drainage from the uterine, vaginal, and vesicle plexus is chiefly into the internal iliac veins.

Venous drainage from the rectal plexus is via the superior hemorrhoidal veins to the inferior mesenteric veins, and the middle and inferior hemorrhoidal veins to the internal pudendal veins and so to the iliac veins.

The ovarian veins on each side begin in the pampiniform plexus, which lies between the layers of the broad ligament. There are at first two veins on each side, and these accompany the corresponding ovarian artery. Higher up, the vein becomes single; that on the right ends in the inferior vena cava, and that on the left in the left renal vein.

PELVIC LYMPHATICS

The lymphatic vessels and nodes lie in the extraperitoneal connective tissue and, since they are embedded in adipose tissue, are extremely difficult to locate or demonstrate unless they are the seat of some pathological disturbance. Lymphatics are developed from veins, and the lymphatic vessels tend to follow the course of the veins draining a particular region. The lymphatic nodes, which are filters lying along the course of the vessels, are usually aggregated into small groups lying in close contact with the larger blood vessels. The groups of lymph nodes that are concerned with draining the pelvis and perineum are the external, internal, and common iliacs, the aortic, and the inguinal groups.

The lymphatic vessels from individual parts of the genital tract drain into this system of pelvic lymph nodes in the following manner:

Vulva and perineum. Medial to the labial crural folds, these contain superficial lymphatics, which pass upward toward the mons and then curve laterally to the superficial inguinal and femoral nodes. Damage from these is through the fossa ovalis and to the deep femoral nodes. The largest of these, which lie in the upper part of the femoral canal, is known as the node of Cloquet.

Vagina.   The lymphatics of the lower third follow the vulva drainage to the superficial inguinal nodes, those from the upper two-thirds pass upward to join the lymphatic vessels of the cervix, and the middle third goes either into the channels drained by the cervix or into the lower part drained by the vulva.

Cervix.   The lymphatics pass either laterally in the base of the broad ligament or posterior wall in the uterosacral ligaments to reach the sidewall of the pelvis. Most of the vessels drain to the internal iliac, obturator, and external iliac nodes, but vessels also pass directly to the common iliac and lower para-aortic nodes, so that radical surgery for carcinoma of the cervix should include removal of all these node groups on both sides of the pelvis.

Corpus uteri.   Nearly all the lymphatic vessels join those leaving the cervix and therefore reach similar groups of nodes. A few vessels at the fundus follow the ovarian channels, and there is an inconsistent pathway around the round ligament to the inguinal nodes.

Ovary and fallopian tubes.   These structures have a plexus of vessels that drain along the infundibulopelvic fold to the para-aortic nodes on both sides of the midline. These are around the left renal pedicle, while on the right there may be only one node intervening before the lymph flows into the thoracic duct, thus accounting for the rapid early spread of metastatic carcinoma to distant sites such as the lungs.

Bladder and urethra.   The drainage is into the iliac nodes, whereas the lymphatics and lower part of the urethra follow those of the vulva.

Rectum.   The lymphatics from the lower anal canal drain to the superficial inguinal nodes, and the remainder of the rectal drainage follows pararectal channels accompanying the blood vessels to both the internal iliac nodes (middle hemorrhoidal artery) and the para-aortic nodes at the origin of the inferior mesenteric artery.

NERVES OF THE PELVIS

The **pudendal nerve** arises from the second, third, and fourth sacral nerves. As it passes along the outer wall of the ischiorectal fossa, it gives off an **inferior hemorrhoidal branch** and divides into the **perineal nerve** and the **dorsal nerve** of the clitoris. The perineal nerve gives the sensory supply to the vulva; it also innervates the anterior part of the external anal sphincter and levator ani, the superficial perineal muscles. The dorsal nerve of the clitoris is sensory.

The sensory fibers from the mons and labia also pass in the ileoinguinal and genital femoral nerves to the first lumbar root. The posterior femoral cutaneous nerve carries sensation from the perineum to the small sciatic nerve and thus to the first, second, and third sacral nerves.

The main nerve supply of the levator ani muscles comes from the third and fourth sacral nerves.

The pelvic organs are supplied by the autonomic nervous system. The vagina, uterus, bladder, rectum, and medial portions of the fallopian tubes are innervated by sympathetic nerve fibers from the pelvic plexus and by parasympathetic fibers through the nervi erigentes. The ovaries, the outer portion of the fallopian tubes, and the broad ligaments derive their nerve supply separately through the ovarian plexus of the sympathetic system. In general, the sympathetics inhibit peristalsis, contract sphincters, inhibit glandular secretion, and act as vasoconstrictors. The parasympathetics are antagonistic.

The anatomic relations of the **presacral nerve** or superior hypogastric plexus are of importance because resection of the presacral nerve is sometimes performed for the relief of intractable pelvic pain. Beneath the peritoneum, at the level of the bifurcation of the aorta, the superior hypogastric plexus will be found embedded in loose areolar tissue, overlying the middle sacral vessels in the bodies of the fourth and fifth lumbar vertebrae. Usually a broad, flattened plexus consisting of two or three incompletely fused trunks is found. In about 25%, a single nerve is present. Fine nerve strands pass from the lumbar sympathetic ganglion beneath the common iliac vessels to the presacral nerve. The right ureter is visualized as it crosses over the iliac vessel at the brim of the true pelvis. If the presacral nerve is interrupted by a presacral neurectomy, pain from the bladder and uterus can be blocked. Apart from a transient pelvic hyperemia, there is no change in the motor function of either the bladder or uterus. At an ordinary hysterectomy the ureterovaginal plexus is not disturbed, but after a more extensive Wertheim's operation there may be painless atony and distension of the bladder, which is attributed to loss of bladder sensation because the sacral connections of the uterovaginal plexus have been divided.

The myometrium contains both alpha- and beta-adrenergic receptors and also cholinergic receptors. In the nonpregnant uterus, the balance of their action is uncertain; but during pregnancy, strong stimulation of beta receptors with beta-mimetic drugs such as isoxsuprine will inhibit myometrial activity.

THE EVENTS LEADING TO CONCEPTION

The events leading to and making reproduction possible are complex and interwoven and span many years. Production of gametes, development of sex drive, and mediation of ovarian, cervical, and uterine changes to allow fertilization and successful nurturing of the newly established life are the subject of this chapter. The basis of reproduction is the ovarian cycle. From it arise the ova to be fertilized and the hormones that make the rest of the reproductive system cooperate. Although we think of this cycle as beginning with the onset of menses each month in the woman of reproductive age, it actually starts during embryonic life.

EMBRYOLOGIC DEVELOPMENT OF OVA AND OVARIES

Germ cell formation begins in the 3-week embryo in the yolk sac. These cells then migrate to the gonadal ridges, where they enter the **germinal epithelium** and proliferate. The rapidly dividing cells of the germinal epithelium give rise to the medulla and cortex of the ovary. Similarly, the germ cells increase in number by mitosis to form **oogonia**. At 2 months gestational age, the oogonia number 600,000, and by 5 months they have increased to a peak of almost 7,000,000. After the fourth month, the oogonia progressively enter the **first meiotic division**, becoming **primary oocytes**. They pass through the **leptotene, zygotene,** and **pachytene** stages of **prophase**, but are arrested in the **diplotene** stage. The ova remain in the diplotene stage of prophase of the first meiotic division until they are recruited during menstrual cycles for ovulation, up to 40 years later. Each oocyte is encased in a layer of germinal epithelial cells, **follicle cells**, and the unit is called the **primordial follicle**. Although there are approximately 7,000,000 by midgestation, their number gradually decreases so that, at birth, there are about 2,000,000 within the ovaries, and, by menarche, only about 400,000.

No further development occurs until puberty, when the primordial follicles that remain are recruited at monthly intervals, in the process creating the hormonal events of the menstrual cycle. The selection basis for follicles in any one cycle is not known, but of the many that begin maturation, only one, or occasionally two, become **graafian follicles**.

OOGENESIS

Oogonia in the fetal ovary are **diploid**, carrying the 46,XX chromosome complement. Multiplying by **mitosis**, they form primary oocytes, each genetically identical to the parent oogonia, still in the fetal ovary. Primary oocytes next begin **meiosis**, or reduction division. In the **prophase** they first enter the **leptotene** stage, during which the double-stranded chromosomes become thread-like. Next, in the **zygotene** stage, the 23 homologous pairs line up along the equator of the cell in apposition. **Synapsis** (unwinding and duplication) occurs, resulting in 46 **tetrads** or **chromatids**, each set bound by a **centromere**. The **pachytene** stage is entered when the chromatids separate and recombine to form new genetic combinations from the parent oocytes. In the **diplotene** stage, the newly formed strands separate into 46 **bivalents**. Primary oocytes remain in the diplotene stage of meiosis 1 for the rest of the fetal period and throughout life until they are recruited during a given menstrual cycle. Those oocytes will then complete meiosis 1 during the formation of the graafian follicle.

During follicular recruitment during a cycle, the primary oocyte enters the **metaphase** of meiosis 1 when the bivalents align at the cellular equator and become bound by the **spindle**. During **anaphase**, one of each of the homologous pairs migrates toward each pole. Meiosis I is then completed during the **telophase**, with the reformation of the cell membrane separating the two daugher cells, each carrying the **haploid** chromosome number of 23,X. However, the genetic complement is still twice haploid, as each of the chromatids is a pair. Although the two daughter cells are genetically equivalent (to each other but not to the parent primary oocyte), they are not equal. One of the two has received almost all the cytoplasm (**secondary oocyte**) and the other almost none (**first polar body**). The first polar body is discarded between the **vitelline membrane** and the **zona pellucida** of the secondary oocyte, which is the structure that is released during ovulation.

The second meiotic division follows only if fertilization occurs, initiated by the penetration of the zona pellucida by the sperm. The events of meiosis 2 are similar to those of meiosis 1, except for the duplication and redistribution of genetic material in the zygotene and pachytene stages. These steps are absent in meiosis 2, so that at its completion, the second polar body has been ejected and the remaining oocyte (about to be fertilized by the penetrating sperm) has 23 single-strand chromatids (23,X). When fertilization is successful, the egg is joined by a sperm of similar chromosome content (23,X or 23,Y) (having undergone two similar meiotic divisions) to reconstitute the normal diploid chromosome complement (46,XX or 46,XY) in the conceptus.

PHYSICAL EVENTS OF OVULATION

The events of ovulation begin with the awakening of several follicles in each ovary, caused by pituitary secretion of follicle-stimulating hormone (FSH). As these follicles begin to grow, secreting estradiol, one or two mature more rapidly, becoming progressively more avid gatherers of FSH. These will become dominant follicles. The formation of these graafian follicles begins with an increase in the size of the oocyte, followed by a changing of the **granulosa** (follicular) cells from flat to cuboidal. Coincident with an increase in the number of granulosa cells, **antralization** occurs—the formation of a fluid-filled space within the follicle. This begins acentrically, with the **liquor folliculi** accumulating at one pole and the bulk of the granulosa cells containing the ovum (cumulus oophorous) at the other. At about the same time, the entire structure becomes encased in a clear mucoid layer, the **zona pellucida**. Next, around the granulosa cell layer but separated from it by a membrane, the ovarian stroma gives rise to the **theca interna** and theca externa.

As the follicle develops, the oocyte within completes the first meiotic division, resulting in the formation of the **secondary oocyte** (containing most of the cytoplasm) and the atretic **first polar body**, which will be discarded. The secondary oocyte will go on to the **second meiotic division** at fertilization, extruding the **second polar body**, so that only the haploid egg remains to be fertilized.

Near midcycle, the follicle has grown so that it nears the surface of the ovary. Antralization has progressed to the point that the oocyte and its surrounding granulosa cells (**corona radiata**) float within the follicle. The thinnest area of the follicle then begins to necrose, possibly mediated by granulosa cell production of an enzyme called plasminogen activator, which causes the production of plasmin, a proteolytic enzyme within the follicular fluid. At rupture, the liquor folliculi along with the oocyte and its corona are extruded into the peritoneal cavity.

After ovulation, the theca and those granulosa cells remaining in the ovary undergo rapid change. Luteinized by the luteinizing hormone (LH) surge, the theca vacularizes the granulosa, which begins to produce large quantities of both estradiol and progesterone. The lipids produced as part of this process give the **corpus luteum** its characteristic yellow color. If pregnancy does not occur, the corpus luteum functions for 9 to 12 days and then begins to degenerate, its hormone production waning. The cells are resorbed over time, eventually only a small scar remaining. In the event of conception, feedback from the zygote maintains the corpus luteum, resulting in continued hormonal support for at least 2 to 3 months.

HORMONAL EVENTS OF THE MENSTRUAL CYCLE

While the physical events of ovulation occur within the ovary, the hormonal events involve at least three organs—the hypothalamus, pituitary, and ovary (Table 3-1).

The menstrual cycle is usually thought of in terms of a 28-day period beginning with the onset of menstrual bleeding. Since endometrial shedding is the result of estrogen and progesterone withdrawal, it follows that the hormonal cycle will be several days in advance. In fact, the hormonal cycle begins when estrogen and progesterone levels have dropped sufficiently that the hypothalamus recognizes their relative absence. It signals the pituitary by secreting gonadotropin releasing hormone (Gn-RH) into the portal system, resulting in the production by the anterior pituitary of FSH and LH. FSH is secreted into the systemic circulation, causing the recruitment of multiple follicles in the ovaries. These follicles have a varying affinity for FSH. Those with the most receptors grow most quickly, one or two eventually outstripping the others. As the follicles grow, their granulosa and theca cells produce increasing amounts of estradiol, which seems to increase their affinity for FSH, thereby enhancing their own growth.

Table 3-1. Glossary of Hormones

Follicle-stimulating hormone: A glycoprotein produced by anterior pituitary; MW 30,000; composed of alpha and beta chains; alpha chain is same for all glycoprotein hormones, beta chains are individual to each; in first half of menstrual cycle causes follicular maturation and estrogen production.

Luteinizing hormone: A glycoprotein produced by anterior pituitary; MW 30,000; released as a surge at midcycle to cause a ripe follicle to ovulate; if released tonically, causes ovary to increase androgen production.

Estrogen: Any hormone resulting in female sexual development or activity, primarily evidenced by mating behavior and maturation of the female genital tract; in humans they are 18-carbon structures based on the estratriene nucleus.

Estradiol: C18 steroid hormone; major estrogen produced by the granulosa cells of developing follicles in the ovary; most potent of the estrogens; distinguished from estrone (OH, =O) and estriol (OH, OH, OH), by the presence of two hydroxyl groups; major actions are (1) stimulation of LH receptors on graafian follicle, (2) preparation of proliferative endometrium to be acted on by postovulatory progesterone, and (3) maturation and maintenance of secondary sex organs (breasts, vagina, cervix, uterus, tubes); major metabolic products are glucuronides found in feces and urine.

Estrone: C18 steroid hormone of same nucleus as estradiol, but hydroxylated in only the C3 position; derived from extraglandular (primarily in adipose tissue) conversion of androstenedione, which is in turn produced in the ovary and adrenal gland.

Estriol: Triply hydroxylated estrogen found mostly in pregnancy and produced by the fetoplacental unit.

Progesterone: C21 steroid hormone; produced in greatest quanity by the corpus luteum and in lesser amounts in the adrenal gland; primary actions are (1) conversion of proliferative endometrium to secretory, (2) inhibition/reduction of estrogen receptors, (3) quieting of smooth muscle (especially the uterus to maintain pregnancy, but also smooth muscle of ureter, gut, and vascular system), (4) further development of estrogen-primed breast, toward lactation capability, and (5) natriuresis; major metabolic products are pregnanediol and pregnenolone found in feces and urine.

Prostaglandins: Cellular messengers derived from the fatty acid arachadonic acid, which is converted into C20 structure, prostanoic acid; major obstetrically/gynecologically active agents are PGF and PGE-locally active at sites throughout the body; among their many actions are (1) initiation of both menstruation and labor, (2) mediation of inflammatory reactions, (3) rhythmic contraction of smooth muscle, including uterine and vascular, (4) cervical ripening, and (5) maintenance of patency of ductus arteriosus before birth.

Human chorionic gonadotropin: A glycoprotein hormone; MW 37,000; composed of alpha and beta chains; alpha chain is identical in all glycoprotein hormones; beta chain is distinctive, but closely related to the beta chain of LH; produced by syncytiotrophoblast throughout pregnancy; maintains corpus luteum function for first 2 months, actions after that time unknown; is the hormone detected by pregnancy tests.

Human placental lactogen: A peptide hormone, single chain; MW 20,000; produced by syncytiotrophoblast from early pregnancy; lipolytic and anti-insulinic in mother; increases protein synthesis and glucose availability to fetus.

While this is in process, LH is being produced, but not released by the anterior pituitary. However, when serum estradiol levels have increased sufficiently, usually to at least 200 ng/ml, the pituitary releases a large amount of LH at once—the LH surge. This LH surge, usually occurring when the dominant follicle has reached 18 to 20 mm in diameter, triggers ovulation. It also causes luteinization of the postovulatory granulosa and theca cells, a result of lipid accumulation and necessary for subsequent progesterone production.

Production of estradiol and progesterone by the corpus luteum (LDL> cholesterol> pregnenolone> progesterone) increases from several hours after ovulation to peak levels from 5 to 9 days later. During the luteal phase, high levels of both estradiol and progesterone have a negative feedback effect on the hypothalamus, switching off pituitary production of both FSH and LH. After approximately the ninth postovulatory day, ovarian steroid production begins to fall unless conception has occured. By the 11th or 12th postovulatory day, corpus luteum function has effectively ceased and the cycle begins again at the beginning.

ENDOMETRIAL EVENTS OF THE MENSTRUAL CYCLE

The menstrual cycle is dated from the first day of bleeding. In reality, this means that we count from the end of one cycle to the next. For clarity, however, we think of the endometrial cycle as beginning in the **proliferative phase**, actually about the fifth or sixth day after the onset of menses.

At the start of the proliferative phase, the endometrium is very thin, with short, narrow glands. As estradiol is secreted by the developing follicles in increasing amounts, it enters the nuclei of the endometrial cells and acts as a growth hormone. It also induces the formation of progesterone receptors. Gland and stromal mitoses characterize the proliferative phase, increasing the thickness of the lining and the length and tortuosity of its glands and arteriolar vessels. The cells become taller, with nuclei at varying heights, giving the appearance of a multilayer lining (pseudostratification).

In the postovulatory **secretory** phase, progesterone from the corpus luteum causes the glands of the endometrium to undergo secretory changes and the rapid mitoses characteristic of the proliferative phase to cease. The mechanism for this is, at least in part, the reduction in endometrial estradiol receptors effected by progesterone.

These alterations, under normal circumstances, are so specifically timed that the endometrium may be "dated." The usual convention for dating is to assign ovulation to day 14. The lining differentiates into three layers: the basal, the spongy, and the compact. Most secretory changes occur in the two more superficial layers, the basal not changing much throughout the cycle. The middle spongy layer becomes filled with the tortuous glands, while in the superficial compact layer the glands are less contorted and are filled with secretion.

In the first 2 days after ovulation (days 14 through 16), secretions collect in subnuclear vacuoles. In the next two (17 and 18), the vacuoles have increased in size sufficiently to move the nuclei upward. During days 19 and 20, the vacuoles migrate past the nuclei and begin shedding their secretions into the glandular lumens. Most of the stromal edema characteristic of the middle and later secretory periods has appeared in the compact layer by days 20 to 21. The spiral arteries, resulting from extremely rapid vascular growth, also are most prominent in the compact layer at this time. By about the time a conceptus would implant (postovulatory 6 to 8 days), the endometrium is succulent and extremely well vascularized. Continued progesterone stimulation results in early **decidual** changes (increased stromal cytoplasm) in the compact layer around the spiral arteries during the 23rd and 24th days.

If pregnancy has not occurred, corpus luteum function begins to wane by the ninth postovulatory day (23). This is accompanied within a day or two by leukocytic infiltration of the endometrium and the beginnings of degeneration in the spongy and compact layers (25 through 26). Increased coiling of the spiral arteries being folded upon themselves by their loss of support is associated with decreased circulation to the endometrium and vasodilatation. Probably secondary to the action of locally produced **prostaglandins**, vasoconstriction

follows the dilatation, resulting in ischemia of the two superficial layers. Within 1 day, the structure of the endometrium disintegrates and menstrual bleeding begins, sloughing necrotic tissue. The first several days of the menses are characterized by cyclic relaxation and spasm of the spiral arteries (probably prostaglandin mediated), resulting in alternating periods of local hemorrhage and ischemia, eventually eliminating all but the basal layer. During the last few days of bleeding, estradiol production by a new crop of follicles has begun, resulting in regeneration of the spongy and compact layers and the beginning of a new cycle.

CERVICAL CYCLE

During most of the month, cervical mucus is thick and relatively impassable. As such, it is a barrier between the contaminated environment of the vagina and the sterile world of the endometrial cavity. It is necessary, however, to allow passage of sperm for conception. As the follicular development progresses and estradiol levels increase, cervical glandular cells undergo changes similar to but less pronounced than their endometrial counterparts. They become more tortuous and increase their secretory capacity. Additionally, increasing estrogen levels change the quality of the mucus. Its sodium chloride content increases (manifested by its crystallization into the so-called fern pattern upon drying), and it becomes largely acellular. As a result of these alterations, the mucus becomes permeable to sperm a variable number of days (1 to 7) prior to ovulation.

These changes are rapidly reversed within 1 to 3 days after ovulation by the action of progesterone, which lowers the salt content (loss of ferning), increases the viscosity, and results in reestablishment of the cervical barrier.

FERTILIZATION

Ovulation releases the secondary oocyte within its corona radiata into the peritubal peritoneal space. Sperm deposited in the vagina during coitus at the right time of the month (i.e., any time after maturation of the cervical mucus) migrate through the cervix into the uterine cavity, tubes, and peritoneal space, undergoing capacitation in the process. Sperm trapped in the hostile environment of the vagina (primarily pH related) die within 6 to 8 hours, but those passing through the cervical mucus may live for up to 10 days and seem to be capable of initiating fertilization for at least a significant portion of that time. The egg, however, remains fertilizable for less than 24 hours. The event of fertilization, therefore, is closely tied to the timing of ovulation, but not necessarily so closely to coitus.

As the sperm penetrates the zona pellucida, the secondary oocyte undergoes the second meiotic division, discarding the second polar body. The pronuclei of the egg and sperm (now within the vitelline membrane) fuse, resulting in the **zygote**. Whether fertilization occurs in the peritoneal space behind the uterus or in the ampulla of the tube is uncertain. In either case, the egg (or zygote) is transported by the tube through a combination of peristaltic and ciliary motions toward the uterus, where it will implant in several days if the necessary hormonal events described above have occurred.

THE ZYGOTE

After ovulation and/or fertilization, transport through the tube to the uterus continues for 3 to 4 days. During this time, the zygote has begun to divide into **blastomeres**. The pattern roughly approximates geometric progression. By the 12 to 16-cell stage, the blastomeres have formed a solid ball-like structure, the **morula** (mulberry). The morula accumulates fluid within it, becoming a **blastocyst**, which differentiates into an **inner cell mass** (embryo) at one end and an **outer cell mass** (trophoblast-to-be) at the other. The blastocyst arrives in the endometrial cavity by the third or fourth postovulatory day and remains unattached for several days, until the zona pellucida dissolves. The blastocyst then implants into the endometrium (sixth to eighth postovulatory day), becoming the **embryo**. At this time, the inner cell mass begins to differentiate into the **syncytiotrophoblast** and **cytotrophoblast**.

THE EMBRYONIC PERIOD

The developing fetus is termed an embryo from the time of implantation until completion of the formation of the major organ systems at approximately eight weeks after conception. The events of the embryonic period are described below and will be dated counting conception as day one. A concurrent series of events in the endometrium will be detailed afterward.

Shortly after implantation (day 7 to 8), the outer cell mass begins to differentiate into cytotrophoblast and syncytiotrophoblast while the inner cell mass, or future fetus, becomes **ectoderm** and **endoderm**.

By day 9 to 10, the syncytiotrophoblast begings to develop **lacunae**, while the ectoderm of the embryo assumes a dorsal orientation and the endoderm, ventral. The **amniotic cavity**, surrounded by the **amniotic membrane**, forms dorsad to the ectoderm, while the **exocoelomic cavity** (future **yolk sac**), bounded by Heuser's membrane, forms ventrad to the endoderm. The entire structure is surrounded by the just formed extraembryonic mesoderm, then the cytotrophoblast, and, finally, the syncytiotrophoblast. Concurrent with this, the syncytiotrophoblast invades the maternal vessels in the now decidualized endometrium, causing blood to fill the developing lacunae. (The syncytiotrophoblast, although it forms the invasive leading edge of the villi, is not capable of mitosis. It appears, instead, that the cytotrophoblast is the actively dividing part of the trophoblast and supplies the syncytiotrophoblast with cellular mass and nuclei.) Sprouts of trophoblast, the **primary villi**, grow into the blood-filled lacunae, at first solid but shortly invaded by the rapidly dividing mesenchyme, to become **secondary villi**. The **tertiary villi** are formed early in the third week when the villi become vascularized by fetal vessels.

During this same period, the extraembryonic mesoderm cavitates to form the **extraembryonic coelom**, which becomes lined by the **chorion**. Simultaneously, the extraembryonic mesoderm coalesces to form the precursor to the umbilical cord, the **body stalk**, which connects the embryo to the chorion for nutrition, while cells from the endoderm migrate out to line the yolk sac and cells from the ectoderm similarly

line the amniotic cavity. The **mesoderm** arises from a thickened ridge, the **primitive streak**, between the endoderm and ectoderm. The three layers from which all fetal structures are derived have now developed. The endoderm will form the entire lining of the GI tract, liver and pancreas, thyroid and parathyroids, urinary bladder, germ cells, and respiratory tree. The ectoderm will become the skin and its appendages (e.g., hair, sebacaeous and sweat glands, and teeth) the nervous system and its derivative organs (the lens and retina of the eye), the adrenal medulla, and the pituitary gland. The muscles, vascular system, urinary and genital systems (other than the bladder and gametes), adrenal cortex, and connective tissues all will arise from mesoderm.

WEEKS 3 AND 4

As above, by early in the third week after conception, the embryo has progressed to the three-layer stage, the amnion and chorion have formed, and the tertiary villi have developed. During the third week, the embryo develops **cephalic** and **caudal poles**. The primitive streak grows rapidly, giving rise to the **notochord** and segmented blocks of tissue, the **somites**, which are the forerunners of the segmented musculoskeletal system. A **neural groove** is formed in the midline of ectoderm (dorsal to the notochord), surrounded by the rapidly growing **neural folds**. The neural groove expands at its cephalic end to give rise to the brain and elongates caudally to form the spinal cord. At the end of the third week, approximately half of the embryonic mass is primitive brain and head.

Also during this week, rapid expansion of the amnion and ectoderm convert the trilaminar embryonic disk to a tubular structure by enfolding the mesoderm and endoderm within, creating the "tube within a tube" design characteristic of all animals phylogenetically beyond the flatworms. The embryo now consists of a three-layered tubular structure within the amniotic cavity, connected to the developing placenta by the body stalk, or soon-to-be umbilical cord.

Coincident with this rapid development, the entire unit has been penetrating further into the developing decidua and is completely covered over by the middle of the third week. After conception, the continued production of high levels of estrogen and progesterone have caused the secretory endometrium to become **decidualized**. The zona compacta and zona spongiosum become quite edematous and filled with the now extremely tortuous spiral arteries, which will provide maternal blood flow to the placenta. Together, they are known as the zona functionalis, as they provide the bulk of the endometrial response to pregnancy. The underlying zona basalis is less responsive and will serve mainly as a source for new endometrial growth after delivery, as it does after menstruation.

The decidua overlying the pregnancy, now separating it from the uterine cavity, is known as the **decidua capsularis**, while that below it is the **decidua basalis**. The rest of the decidua, remote from the implantation site, is termed the **decidua vera**. (As the pregnancy enlarges, the decidua capsularis will balloon into the endometrial cavity and eventually fuse with the decidua vera, obliterating the old cavity.) Inside the fetoplacental unit, the chorion apposed to the decidua capsularis will become the **chorion laeve**, in which the villi will degenerate, while that near the decidua basalis becomes the **chorion frondosum**, which forms the fetal part of the placenta. Some of the villi in the chorion frondosum grow all the way to the decidua basalis and into it, without arborizing. These form the supporting structure binding the fetal (chorion frondosum coalesced into the **chorionic plate**) and maternal (decidua basalis or **basal plate**) halves of the placenta into a unit. Between the two, the villi branch into smaller and smaller units, projecting into the **intervillous space**, which is filled with maternal blood from the eroded decidual vessels.

Meanwhile, back at the fetus, the conversion of the trilaminer disk into a tube within a tube has incorporated some of the yolk sac within the endodermal space. The rest protrudes from the midgut and will be progressively reduced in size. The resultant body stalk will become the umibilical cord. Lagging slightly behind the villous expansion in the chorion frondosum, the heart and vascular system of the fetus have begun to develop from the previously described somites. Connected to the villous system in the chorion by two umbilical arteries and one vein, the beating fetal heart has established a placental circulation by the early part of the fourth week after conception. By the end of this week, limb bud and eye formation have begun.

WEEKS 5 THROUGH 8

Over the next 4 weeks, placental anatomy is defined (see "Placental Structure and Function"). The embryo completes the early definition of all major body systems, increasing in size from a few millimeters to approximately 4 cm. The umbilical cord has been completely clothed in amnion, and the fetus floats freely in the amniotic cavity. The body cavity has been transected by the progenitors of the diaphragm. In the chest cavity, the lobar and bronchiolar structure of the lungs is evident and the heart has developed to the four-chambered stage. Correspondingly, the basis for the arterial and venous systems has been laid. The gut, liver, and pancreas all are extant. The fetal kidneys, ureter, and bladder have been defined, although sexual differentiation is not apparent. Fingers and toes are clearly defined. The brachial arches have differentiated into their cephalic counterparts, and midline fusion of the nose and palate is complete. The brain has developed its basic divisions, and the foundations of the autonomic and somatic nervous systems are in place. Eye and ear formation are far advanced.

THE FETUS

After the eighth week (tenth menstrual week), the fetus will grow and mature, but essentially all organs and systems found in the neonate have been formed. What follows is a system-by-system catalog of fetal development.

CARDIOVASCULAR SYSTEM—PLACENTA AND FETUS

All of the fetal needs, both nutritional and excretory, are met via the placenta. The placenta is anchored into the decidua basalis by villi, which grow all the way to the basal plate, and is divided into **cotyledons** by fibrous septa of maternal origin. Each cotyledon has a floor (basal plate) that is

perforated by a spiral artery. Maternal blood enters the **intervillous space** through these spiral arteries and cascades upward, fountain-like. It exits under residual pressure through randomly placed venous sinuses, also in the basal plate. From the roof of the intervillous space (chorionic plate), each cotyledon is penetrated by one stem villas and its hundreds of progressively smaller rami, the fetal circulation of the placenta. These are supplied with blood from the **umbilical arteries** and return their flow to the fetus via the **umbilical vein**.

Exchange of wastes and nutrients occurs in the intervillous space by several mechanisms. Simple **diffusion** accounts for transfer of most smaller molecules, nutrients and wastes including oxygen, carbon dioxide, glucose, sodium, potassium chloride, and urea. **Active transport** of some substances, such as iron and vitamin C, concentrates them in the fetus in amounts greater than in maternal blood. In general, highly ionized substances like heparin and more complex proteins like insulin cross the placental barrier poorly, if at all, whereas steroid hormones and other nonpolarized compounds have more access. A notable exceptable to this is IgG (especially important in consideration of Rh sensitization), which crosses the placental barrier in spite of its size and complexity.

Early in the course of pregnancy, the placenta meets fetal needs by sheer size. In the 59-cell stage, only 5 cells are destined to become fetus whereas 54 will be placenta. By term, however, the average fetus outweighs its placenta by 6 to 1. In this respect, pregnancy may be thought of as the fetus progressively outgrowing its supply line. The placenta meets these demands by becoming more efficient. As it matures, the branching of the villi increases while the amount of connective tissue separating the two vascular systems decreases. In addition, as maternal cardiac output increases into the late second trimester, maternal flow through the placenta increases accordingly. By term, the maternal supply to the placenta is more than 500 ml/minute.

The placenta and fetus are connected by the umbilical cord. As the amniotic cavity expands to encompass the fetus, layers of amnion ensheath the body stalk. The vessels within it (two arteries, one vein—the right umbilical vein is obliterated) traverse to the fetal circulation. The arteries are coiled around the vein within the cord and packed in a gelatinous material called **Wharton's jelly**, which cushions them. The umbilical arteries are branches of the **hypogastric arteries** of the fetal systemic circulation and carry blood from the fetus to the placenta, while the umbilical vein transports it back to the fetal vena cava.

The fetal circulatory system differs from the adult in several major ways. Before birth, blood flow through the lungs is minimal, since they are not expanded and resistance is high. Instead, most of the output of the right heart is passed into the "systemic system" through two temporary communications, the foramen ovale and the ductus arteriosus, which will be obliterated shortly after birth. Blood enters the right atrium from two sources: The **superior vena cava** returns venous blood from the head, and this blood is passed primarily to the right ventricle; the **inferior vena cava** brings in a mixture of lower trunk return and oxygenated blood from the placenta, and this blood is largely shunted across the **foramen ovale** into the left atrium. This more oxygenated blood is pumped by the left ventricle into the **aorta,** while the less oxygenated blood from the right ventricle enters the **pulmonary arteries.** Most of the flow through the pulmonary arteries is diverted through the **ductus arteriosus** into the aorta, decreasing its oxygen content, but only after the **coronary** and **carotid** arteries have received undiluted blood to supply the heart and brain. The descending aorta then carries approximately half this mixed blood to the trunk and viscera and half to the placenta. The portion that remains in the fetus is returned via the inferior vena cava; the placental supply passes from the hypogastrics into the umbilical arteries through the villi, where it is oxygenated, and back into the umbilical vein. The oxygenated blood of the umbilical vein is then transported to the liver, where most of it is mixed into the inferior caval return via the **ductus venosus.**

The effect of this shunting and mixing of more and less oxygenated blood is to have varying oxygen content at different places in the system. Compared with an oxygen tension of 95 mm Hg in maternal arterial blood, the fetus operates at partial pressures of oxygen (PO_2) that would be fatal after birth. The highest PO_2 in the fetal circulation (umbilical vein) is approximately 30 mm Hg, slightly less than that of the intervillous space. After dilution by the blood from the inferior cava, the PO_2 drops to approximately 20 to 25 mm Hg, which is about the best any fetal organ (brain, heart) experiences. The less critical systems supplied by the aorta below the ductus arteriosus operate at even lower levels. How does the fetus prosper in such an atmosphere?

Three factors seem to compensate. The fetal cardiac output is much higher per unit of body weight than after birth, so that even if the oxygen supply is poor per unit of blood, there is more supplied per unit of time. Secondly, fetal hemoglobin (see the next section) is a much more efficient deliverer of oxygen at low pressures. Lastly, fetal hematocrits are higher than adult, again enabling greater oxygen transport at low oxygen tensions.

HEMATOPOIETIC SYSTEM

During the course of intrauterine life, the fetus produces several different hemoglobins. All are four-chain globin molecules, but the kinds of chains in each differ. In the first 2 months, the yolk sac produces Gower I (four epsilon chains) and Gower II (two alpha and two epsilon chains) hemoglobins. Next the liver becomes the major hematopoietic organ, producing the predominant fetal hemoglobin, F (two alpha, two gamma chains). Lastly, beginning in midpregnancy, hemoglobin A, adult hemoglobin (two alpha, two beta chains), is made by the bone marrow. Importantly, however, hemoglobin F remains the major form until after birth. This is critical because Hb F has higher affinity for oxygen, binding more at lower PO_2 than Hb A, which results in a preferential transfer of oxygen to the fetus from the mother, enabling the fetus to survive at lower oxygen tensions.

Additionally, fetal red cells are nucleated and contain more hemoglobin than their adult counterparts. By term, Hb F concentrations are often greater than 17 g/100 ml and hematocrits over 60%.

Leukocyte concentrations are not markedly different from after birth, but immunoglobin production is. The fetus is not a

good producer of antibodies. IgM is made under stress, but IgG appears to be of maternal origin, transported across the placenta.

While platelet counts are the same as after birth, most coagulation factors are present in decreased amounts (fibrinogen [I], II, VII, IX, X, XI, XII, XIII).

RESPIRATORY SYSTEM

By the beginning of the second trimester, fetal breathing movements may be seen with ultrasonography. The basic structure of bronchi branching into bronchioles ending in alveoli is elaborated on over the next several months, probably at least in part because of the "breathing" of amniotic fluid in and out of the chest cavity. Aside from the mechanical growth of the respiratory tree, amniotic fluid plays an important role in lung maturation.

In order to facilitate easy expansion of the lungs after birth and to prevent atelectasis, chemicals called **surfactants** are necessary. These phospholipids, **lecithins,** are surface tension-lowering agents that appear in amniotic fluid in increasing amounts in the third trimester. Initially, two lecithins,, **phosphatidylcholine** (PC) and **phosphatidylinositol** (PI) are produced by the **type II pneumocytes** in the alveoli. Four to five weeks before term, however, PI production gives way to **phosphatidylglycerol** (PG). These chemicals are secreted by the pneumocytes and carried by the fetal breathing movements into the amniotic fluid. The likelihood of respiratory distress syndrome (RDS, hyaline membrane disease) may be estimated by measuring the concentrations of these lecithins in the amniotic fluid.

In general, these concentrations are expressed in relation to the amount of another phospholipid, **sphingomyelin,** as the **lecithin/sphingomyelin** ratio, or L/S ratio. It has been experimentally determined that the likelihood of RDS is extremely small when the L/S ratio is greater than 2 and PG is present. If the L/S ratio is between 1.5 and 2, RDS may occur in 25 to 40% of births but will rarely be fatal. The most common exceptions to this are pregnancies complicated by diabetes, where the L/S ratio may be higher than 2 but PG may still be absent, and in births complicated by asphyxia, where these measurements may be irrelevant.

GASTROINTESTINAL SYSTEM

The gut has been fully formed as a continuous tube through the fetus by the end of the embryonic period. Swallowing occurs as early as the beginning of the second trimester. As with the respiratory tree, the intake of amniotic fluid probably plays a role in the formation of the viscera. Obviously, as the fetus grows it swallows progressively greater amounts of fluid and, by late in the second trimester, is capable of processing this material into an excretory product, **meconium,** which consists of swallowed amniotic fluid, bile pigments, and GI epithelial cells.

The presence of bile in the GI tract is evidence that the fetal liver functions as a secretory organ. It does so, however, in a very limited fashion, even late in fetal life. It is capable of conjugating bilirubin in only very small amounts until almost term, and even then is far less efficient than it will be several months after birth. Although not important to the fetus, since unconjugated bilirubin crosses the placenta and is disposed of via the mother's liver, this is a major factor in the development of neonatal jaundice, when the liver is called on to conjugate the large amounts of bilirubin resulting from rapid hemolysis in the first week of postnatal life.

Like the liver, the pancreas is capable of secreting digestive enzymes from midpregnancy but, in reality, is called on to do little.

URINARY SYSTEM

The kidneys, complete with functioning nephrons, are active by the end of the first trimester. Like the digestive organs, however, they are functional in spirit only. Although urine is produced, it remains unconcentrated until after birth, as fluid balance is controlled largely by the mother. Hypotonic urine is excreted into the amniotic fluid and seems to be a major source of its volume.

ENDOCRINE SYSTEM

The endocrine systems of the fetus seem to be largely functional by the end of the first trimester. The pituitary produces growth hormone, prolactin, FSH, LH, and adrenocorticotrophic hormone (ACTH) by the tenth week. Insulin and glucagon have been detected from the pancreas by the ninth week. Thyroid and parathyroid hormones are also detectable in the first trimester. In fact, because maternal thyroxine crosses the placenta poorly, fetal thyroxine is necessary to prevent prenatal cretinism. In male fetuses, testicular testosterone has been found by week 11; however, ovarian development seems to favor early gamete production but later hormone synthesis.

The largest endocrine organ of the fetus is the adrenal. Becoming tremendously hypertrophied by midpregnancy and continuing to grow at even greater rates during the third trimester, the fetal adrenal supplies most of the substrate used by the placenta for estrogen production. This hypertrophy takes place in a portion of the cortex not found postnatally, the fetal zone. It is in this fetal zone that huge amounts of dehydroepiandrosterone (DHEA) and its sulfated form (DHEAS) are synthesized. These steroids serve as the precursors for placental production of estradiol and estriol. The hypertrophied cortex is also the site of production of cortisol, which is thought to play a role in initiation of labor. Pregnancies in which the fetus is anencephalic tend to be prolonged, often without spontaneous onset of labor. These fetuses lack both a pituitary gland and the hypertrophied fetal zone.

PLACENTA AS AN ENDOCRINE ORGAN

In addition to serving as the fetal supply line, the placenta is the major endocrine organ of pregnancy. The major hormones produced by trophoblastic tissue are human chorionic gonadotropin (HCG), estrogen (primarily estriol, secondarily estradiol), progesterone, and human placental lactogen (HPL). They are all apparently produced by the syncytiotrophoblast (see Table 3-1 for structural details).

HUMAN CHORIONIC GONADOTROPIN

HCG is produced by the synctiotrophoblast within several days of conception. Maternal serum levels of HCG are detectable shortly after implantation, and in normal pregnancies, double every 48 to 72 hours for the first 6 to 7 weeks after conception. Peak levels, somewhat above 100,000 Mu/ml, are achieved by the end of the third month, after which there is a rapid decline, with stabilization at approximately 2,000 to 10,000 Mu/ml during the second half of pregnancy. Levels are considerably higher in pregnancies characterized by an increase in placental tissue (multiple fetuses, Rh disease, trophoblastic neoplasms).

The only known function for HCG is maintenance of the corpus luteum, although its similarity to LH may enable it to serve as a trophic hormone for fetal testicular development before the fetal pituitary is competent.

ESTROGEN

The estrogen output of the placenta is phenomenal. By the end of pregnancy, daily output is more than 1,000 times greater than that of a normal ovulatory woman. Unlike the ovaries, the placenta produces much more estriol than estradiol. Using an enzyme, placental sulfatase, and its substrate DHEAS from the fetal adrenal that has been hydroxylated by the fetal liver (into 16-hydroxyDHEAS), it produces estriol in prodigious amounts. Smaller amounts are derived from maternal contributions of the same substrate. In lesser amounts, the placenta converts DHEAS directly from the fetal adrenal into estradiol. It cannot covert estradiol directly into estriol and produces no measurable amounts of estrone.

PROGESTERONE

Placental production of progesterone begins by about the eighth week and replaces the corpus luteum. Using maternal cholesterol as a precursor, the placenta produces steadily increasing amounts throughout pregnancy, reaching daily production rates of more than 250 mg/day by term. Being the primary progestational hormone, its major functions during pregnancy appear to be maintenance of uterine quietude and expansion of maternal blood volume, although its effects on maternal physiology are widespread (see other sections of "Maternal Adaptations to Pregnancy," below).

HUMAN PLACENTAL LACTOGEN

Like HCG, HPL is produced only during pregnancy. First detectable in the middle of the first trimester, its production increases steadily until term, when as much as 1 g/day may be generated. Its major actions are apparently metabolic, resulting in increased availability of glucose to the fetus by shifting maternal metabolic processes to a dependence on fat and exerting an anti-insulin-like activity.

MATERNAL ADAPTATIONS TO PREGNANCY

Pregnancy is a time of very rapid change for the mother as well. Although the most notable alterations occur in the

[handwritten margin note: no milk during pregnancy due to ↑↑ Progesterone]

reproductive organs, pregnancy affects all body systems and functions.

UTERUS

The pregnant uterus begins to grow almost immediately after conception. Even though the developing pregnancy does not fill the endometrial cavity until the end of the first trimester, by that time uterine volume has increased manyfold. Extremely high estrogen levels mediate extensive hypertophy of muscle and elastic tissue and rapid dilatation of blood vessels, mostly in the fundal region. By the end of the pregnancy, the uterus will have increased in volume 500 to 1,000 times, having a capacity of over 5 L and a weight of more than 1 kg. Initially, the growth results in much-thickened walls. However, as the fetus grows rapidly after the second month, the increasing bulk of the uterus is stretched even faster so that at term the walls may be only 1 to 1.5 cm thick. Typically, the large uterus is rotated somewhat to the right. This avoids compression of the sigmoid colon. Whether the presence of the sigmoid is causative is unknown.

CERVIX

As early as the uterus shows the changes of pregnancy, so does the cervix. Responding to the same hormonal changes, the cervix experiences an increase in blood flow and a hypertrophy and hyperplasia of cervical glands. These alterations combine to soften the cervix (Hegar's sign) and to make it appear bluer (Chadwick's sign). The glandular hyperplasia results in an eversion of the squamocolumnar junction, and the mucus, responding to very high progesterone levels, becomes thick and forms the mucus plug, which will remain throughout the pregnancy.

VAGINA

[handwritten margin note: during Prs acidic pH; Glycogen → lactic acid]

Many of the same changes that affect the cervix also occur in the vagina. The hyperemia and hypertrophy thicken the walls. In addition, an increase in glycogen is converted by a flourishing *Lactobacillus* population into lactic acid, resulting in a decreased pH.

OVARIES

As previously described, the corpus luteum does not degenerate but persists for approximately 6 to 8 weeks, continuing progesterone production under HCG stimulation from the trophoblast until the placenta takes over. The surface is frequently covered with decidual reaction. By the middle of pregnancy, the ovaries have a quiet appearance, suggested by the absence of follicular development.

BREASTS

Breast development during pregnancy responds to rapid increases in the production of three hormones: estrogen, progesterone, and prolactin. It is characterized by hypertrophy of all elements: glands, ducts, nipples. The nipples also become more erectile, and their pigment increases, resulting in darkening. During the last few months, the breasts produce colostrum, but milk production is suppressed by the high levels of progesterone, which persist until after parturition.

SKIN AND MUSCLES AND SKELETAL SYSTEM

Stretching of the skin and muscle of the abdominal wall occurs in the later months of gestation, often resulting in diastasis recti. In combination with high levels of steroids, the mechanical stretching of the skin often results in striae gravidarum, or stretch marks, especially around the lower abdomen, buttocks, and breasts. Pigmented areas such as the areolae, labia, and linea nigra become darkened secondary to increased levels of melanocyte-stimulating hormone (MSH). Occasionally, a more generalized pigmentation of the skin, chloasma, occurs. Angiogenesis caused by high estrogen levels often results in the formation of vascular spiders, especially on the face and trunk. The major skeletal changes are an increased lordosis and a greater mobility of the pelvic joints.

METABOLIC CHANGES

Most of pregnancy is characterized by the retention of large amounts of water. More than 3 L goes into formation of the products of conception, the fetus, placenta, and amniotic fluid. Blood volume increases by 2 to 3 L, of which more than half is fluid. Still more water is retained in variable amounts late in pregnancy as edema, mostly in the lower extremities.

Approximately 500 g of protein is needed to build the fetus and placenta, while another 500 g is incorporated into the hypertrophied uterus and breasts. Additional protein is used in the formation of blood components.

Fat and carbohydrate metabolism are greatly altered as well. Fasting insulin levels tend to be increased, resulting in lower fasting glucose. However, probably secondary to HPL and progesterone, glucose tolerance is decreased, so that postprandial sugars tend to be elevated. Consequently, normal values for glucose tolerance tests are markedly different during pregnancy. The same hormone changes result in a marked increase in plasma lipids and fat storage.

The mineral needs of pregnancy are centered around iron and calcium. Approximately 300 mg of elemental iron is necessary to build the fetus and placenta, while another 500 mg is used to increase maternal hemoglobin stores. Similarly, large amounts of calcium are required for the production of the fetal skeleton. Dietary needs for these are detailed in the section on prenatal care. Other mineral needs and requirements change little during pregnancy, except that serum levels of protein-bound minerals will fluctuate with changing serum albumin concentrations.

HEMATOLOGY

Maternal blood volume increases 40 to 50%, initially mostly in the plasma fraction, but subsequently in red cell mass as well. Even though the red cell mass increases by up to a third, plasma volume is expanded 50 to 60%, so that throughout most of pregnancy, hematocrit is decreased, resulting in the physiological anemia of pregnancy. Hematocrits as low as 30% and hemoglobin concentrations down to 10 g/100 ml are considered nonpathological. This expansion of intravascular volume is accomplished by the actions of increased **erythro-poietin** production (increased red cell production) and progesterone and aldosterone (relaxation of the vascular tree and expansion of volume).

These changes are not synchronized. By the end of the first trimester, significant expansion of plasma volume has begun, so that hematocrit has begun to fall. This continues and remains ahead of increases in red cell mass until the end of the second trimester, when hematocrit values are at their lowest. In the early third trimester, volume expansion slows or ceases, but red cell production continues at an increased rate, resulting in a partial return toward normal nonpregnant values.

White blood cell (WBC) counts increase slightly, the extra number due mostly to polymorphonuclear leukocytes (PMNL). Normal WBC counts may range up to 12,000/mm^3, whereas normal nonpregnant counts are rarely above 10,500/mm^3. Total lymphocyte concentrations are largely unchanged. Platelet concentrations change little. There may be a slight artifactual decrease due to increases in plasma volume or perhaps a real one due to the mildly hypercoagulable state that exists throughout pregnancy.

In general, pregnancy is characterized by a more dynamic coagulation system. Increased levels of fibrinogen (50% from 200 to 400 mg/100 ml to 300 to 600 mg/100 ml) and Factors II, VII, VIII, IX, and X result in hypercoagulability, while thrombolytic activity is enhanced by rising levels of plasminogen and fibrin split products and decreases in Factors XI and XIII. The net effect is a slightly hypercoagulable state.

Standards for many hematologic tests are altered as a consequence of the above changes. Sedimentation rate is markedly elevated by high fibrinogen levels. Both the prothrombin and activated partial thromboplastin times are shortened. Fibrin split products concentrations are mildly elevated.

PT, APTT shortened
hyper coagulable ← ↑ level, ↓ coag factor

CARDIOVASCULAR SYSTEM

The predominant changes in the cardiovascular system serve to increase blood flow. Heart rate increases 15 to 20% (10 to 15 bpm), as does stroke volume. There is a concomitant decrease in peripheral resistance, which is most marked in the second trimester but is present from early pregnancy until after delivery. Both systolic and diastolic blood pressures may drop as much as 15 to 30 mm Hg, again most markedly during the second trimester. The overall effect is to increase cardiac output by as much as 50%.

In addition, because of the increasing bulk of the uterus and its effect on the central vascular system, maternal position may have a great influence on blood pressure and cardiac output. By the late second trimester, the uterus and its contents are large enough to impede cardiac return through the vena cava when the mother assumes the supine position. To a lesser extent, it may also interfere with output through the aorta. The net effect of this, when it occurs, is to drastically reduce cardiac output and blood pressure (the **aortocaval compression** or **spine hypotension syndrome**), thereby reducing placental perfusion. Late in pregnancy, during labor and in situations when there is fetal compromise, this may be an important factor to reckon with in maintaining fetal health. Conversely, maternal cardiac output and placental perfusion are greatest in the lateral recumbent (left > right) positions.

Numerous findings on physical examination are different in pregnant women. Because of the increased volume of the heart, it appears larger on x-ray. In addition, its position in the chest is shifted upward and to the left by the growing uterus. Increased flow results in systolic murmurs in over 90%, while diastolic (20%) and continuous (10%) murmurs are found in the absence of pathology. Third heart sounds (S3) are also common in normal pregnant women. Aside from positional changes, the ECG is unaltered.

RESPIRATORY SYSTEM

As in the cardiovascular system, so in the respiratory system. Increases in respiratory rate, tidal volume, and minute ventilation result in a greater exchange of oxygen and carbon dioxide. These changes are probably mediated by the high levels of progesterone found throughout the pregnancy and result in a chronic metabolic alkalosis secondary to the decreased PCO_2.

Interestingly, this hyperventilation is accomplished in spite of several anatomic alterations that are actually counterproductive. Because of the increasing size of the uterus, diaphragmatic excursion is limited on the downward side by several centimeters. This is compensated for by greater retraction upward, so that overall movement is increased, and by greater intercostal activity. Functional residual capacity is decreased, while compliance does not change appreciably.

URINARY TRACT

Significant increases in most body functions and the metabolic demands of the fetus both require an increase in waste disposal. Conveniently, the increased cardiac output is accompanied by concomitant and proportional changes in both renal blood flow (RBF) and glomerular filtration rate (GFR) (up approximately 50% by late midpregnancy). Creatinine clearance is similarly affected. Most likely because of increased flow through the kidneys, the thresholds for several substances are exceeded. We therefore see glucosuria in the face of normal blood glucose and albuminuria at twice the normal nonpregnant level (up to 0.3 g/24 hours).

Perhaps because of the increased RBF, kidney size seems to increase slightly. Mild hydroureter is commonly seen on intravenous pyelography (IVP) and is thought to be due to smooth muscle relaxation secondary to progesterone. That this occurs somewhat more often on the right may be related to uterine dextrorotation, but it does not seem to be associated with any functional impairment.

Several changes that occur in pregnancy mimic urinary tract pathology. Urinary frequency is the rule rather than the exception. While this can be, in part, attributed to increased urine production, changes in bladder position contribute. As the uterus grows out of the pelvis, the bladder is stretched upward, causing a relative loss of the urethrovesicle angle and in later pregnancy in a tendency toward stress incontinence.

DIGESTIVE SYSTEM

The GI tract is made of smooth muscle. As one would expect, high levels of progesterone cause a generalized decrease in GI motility beginning early in the first trimester and not abating until after delivery. Additionally, mechanical displacement of organs compounds the problem. Constipation is common in the pregnant woman. Indigestion results from a combination of upward displacement of the stomach, decreased emptying time, and relaxation of the cardiac sphincter resulting in esophageal reflux. Hemorrhoids are products of both the greater incidence of constipation and increased venous pressure in the lower half of the body. They are among the most common minor complications of the second stage of labor. The gallbladder exhibits a similar lassitude, having a tendency toward bile retention and gallstone formation. Although there is no increase in the incidence of appendicitis, its diagnosis is made more difficult by both a shift in the position of the appendix upward and laterally and its inaccessibility behind the uterus after about the 14th week.

Liver function is not truly altered, but many liver function tests are. Elevations of serum alkaline phosphatase suggest liver disease to the unwary but are due instead to large amounts produced in the placenta. Concomitant rises in SGOT and SGPT are not encountered. Even though the gravida is relatively hypoalbuminemic, hepatic production is actually increased. The net decrease is a dilutional effect of the rapid volume expansion. Production of alpha$_2$-globulins, used to bind many minerals and hormones in the serum, is rapidly accelerated in response to high levels of estrogen and accounts for the increased total amounts of many of these compounds, even though the unbound, active fractions remain relatively constant.

ENDOCRINE SYSTEM

The most striking endocrine changes in pregnancy are, of course, those that result directly from the pregnancy itself—that is, placental and fetal production of HCG, estrogen, progesterone, and HPL. These hormones, in fact, cause many of the alterations and seeming alterations seen in the function of other endocrine glands.

PITUITARY

Pituitary production of FSH and LH are effectively suppressed by placental estrogen and progesterone. Similarly, HPL, previously called placental growth hormone, may cause the slight decreases noted in pituitary growth hormone.

Conversely, the spectacular increase in pituitary production of prolactin is probably a response to very high estrogen levels. Serum concentrations of prolactin begin to rise shortly after the missed menses and continue so throughout the course of pregnancy, often reaching 150 to 200 ng/ml (normal non-pregnant levels being 5 to 20 ng/ml). The huge amounts of prolactin produced seem to be necessary for preparation of the breast for lactation but do not cause its initiation until after the progesterone withdrawal that ocurs with delivery of the placenta. Many other functions have been proposed for this hormone based on analogy with lower animals (not limited to mammals), but none has been substantiated.

OVARIES

The ovaries are considered to be quiescent after regression of the corpus luteum sometime late in the first trimester. Theca lutein cysts occasionally occur and persist until delivery, when they may be found at cesarean section. They are thought to be stimulated by HCG and regress spontaneously after delivery.

THYROID GLAND

There are dramatic alterations in endocrine function during pregnancy, but most of the changes in laboratory measurement of thyroid function reflect the increases in alpha$_2$-globulin production previously noted. Total thyroxin (T$_4$), triiodothyronine (T$_3$), thyroid-binding globulin (TBG), and protein-bound iodine (PBI) all are elevated by this mechanism. T$_3$ resin uptake (T$_3$RU) is decreased by the same action. Free T$_4$, free T$_3$, and iodine metabolism, however, all remain unchanged. Although the basal metabolic rate increases, this results from the addition of the fetus, rather than from changes in thyroid function.

Of the thyroid hormones, only calcitonin is significantly altered by pregnancy. Produced in increased amounts, its action is to prevent the resorption of bone. It would seem to be a protective mechanism in the face of the calcium demands that pregnancy places on the mother.

PARATHYROID GLAND   PTH↑

Parathormone, which serves to increase serum calcium by mobilization from bone and by increased absorption from the GI tract, is produced in slightly greater amounts during pregnancy.

PANCREAS

Hypertrophy of the islet cells of the pancreas is associated with increased insulin production during pregnancy. The combined actions of HPL, progesterone, and estrogen lead to a diabetogenic state based on decreased insulin sensitivity. In the fasting state, insulin levels are higher and glucose levels are lower (below 90 mg/100 ml). However, even though the insulin response to a glucose load is exaggerated, postprandial serum glucose concentrations are higher than in the non-pregnant woman.

ADRENAL GLANDS

Several adrenal hormones are affected directly by the tremendous intravascular volume expansion during pregnancy. The natriuretic effects of progesterone and the relative insensitivity to the vasospastic effects of angiotensin II result in higher baseline concentrations of renin, angiotensin I, and angiotensin II. This, in turn, stimulates much greater adrenal production of aldosterone, which leads to salt retention and increased plasma volume.

PREGNANCY TESTING

The recognition of the pregnant state has traditionally been divided into identification of symptoms and probable, presumptive, and definite signs.

Symptoms are sore breasts, nausea (morning sickness), fatigue, and urinary frequency, all very nonspecific. Signs classified as presumptive may be no more specific: amenorrhea, increase in breast size, Chadwick's sign all may occur with anovulation, with prolonged estrogen stimulation.

Probable signs carry a greater likelihood of pregnancy but still do not constitute proof: Uterine enlargement and softening, cervical softening, and increasing abdominal girth in the presence of amenorrhea are highly suggestive. Most of the pregnancy tests in current use (HCG antibody detection and the radioreceptor assay), although very accurate, again do not constitute proof of pregnancy since, with the exception of the beta-subunit assay for HCG, they do not discriminate LH from HCG. They are sufficiently good, however, that someone who acts based on a positive result from a reliable laboratory cannot be faulted. The over-the-counter slide and tube tests are notably less dependable when performed by people inexperienced in their use. The beta-subunit assay for HCG is specific for the hormone of pregnancy and is the most sensitive assay available. With currently available technology, this test is capable of detecting pregnancy several days after implantation, even before the first missed period. The only uncertainty in this method is related to the fact that there are occasionally sources for HCG other than trophoblast, although this is extremely rare.

A definite diagnosis of pregnancy is established by the detection of a fetal heart (by stethoscope at 20 weeks, by Doppler stethoscope as early as 10 weeks amenorrhea) or by ultrasonic identification of the fetus (a gestational sac at 5 weeks amenorrhea, a pulsating fetal heart at 7 or 8 weeks. Also included in the definite category is the detection of fetal movements by the obstetrician. This, however, is sometimes misleading. Previously considered a positive sign of pregnancy, x-ray identification of the fetal skeleton in today's world may be considered a failure of clinical judgment and diagnostic skill. In the real world, the diagnosis of pregnancy is made by the liberal use of HCG detection in any woman with a suspicious menstrual history (amenorrhea or a recent abnormal period) or an enlarging uterus.

Pseudocyesis is a rare condition, usually associated with psychiatric disorder, in which a woman becomes so convinced she is pregnant that it becomes difficult to convince her otherwise. She may develop amenorrhea, nausea, enlargement of the abdomen and breasts, galactorrhea, and an awareness of fetal movement. These manifestations may be related to weight gain, drug use (phenothiazine tranquilizers), obstipation, or abnormal ovarian function. Normal uterine size and consistency mediate against pregnancy. However, in a woman who has an enlarged uterus due to leiomyoma or adenomyosis or even previous childbearing, HCG testing and ultrasonography may be necessary to rule out pregnancy.

ROUTINE ANTEPARTUM CARE

The purpose of antepartum care is to assure an optimal outcome for the pregnancy. In today's world, this includes preconceptual care and counseling to detect and avoid conditions that may be dangerous to the fetus or mother in early pregnancy, as well as antepartum care to achieve similar ends during the prenatal course. The cornerstones of such care are education and communication to alert the prospective parents to things that will affect the pregnancy positively, such as good nutrition and proper physical preparation, as well as to habits and activities that may have negative effects, such as drug use. It is also critical to be sure that the pregnant woman has no underlying conditions that will endanger pregnancy or will be worsened by it.

Preconceptual counseling should include the following:

1. Genetic counseling.
2. Advice regarding drug use and abuse (especially medications, alcohol, and tobacco).
3. Determination of conditions that will endanger the pregnancy, such as lack of rubella immunity or the presence of diabetes, anemia, or human immunodeficiency virus (HIV) seropositivity. Preconceptual testing should, at the least, include all the standard blood work commonly done after the first prenatal examination.

FIRST PRENATAL VISIT

At the first prenatal visit, a complete history should be taken. Special attention should be directed to the following:

1. Menstrual history, including the date and character of the last menses and normal menstrual interval; calculation of the estimated date of conception (EDC)
2. Obstetric history
3. Surgical history, especially gynecologic or obstetric
4. Medical history, especially diabetes, hypertension, or cardiovascular disorders
5. Drug use, prescription or otherwise

A complete physical examination should also be performed, with special attention to the following:

1. Vital signs, including weight and height
2. Breasts
3. Heart murmurs
4. Pelvic exam

Laboratory testing should include the following:

1. Complete blood count (CBC)
2. Blood type and Rh with antibody screening
3. Serology for syphilis
4. Rubella titer
5. Complete urinalysis on a clean-catch specimen
6. Serum glucose
7. Pap smear
8. Cervical culture for gonorrhea
9. Cervical smear for *Chlamydia*, either Microtrak or Chlamydiazyme
10. Many obstetricians now include routine screening for the rest of the TORCH diseases, as well as hepatitis B and HIV

11. Tine test or purified-protein derivate (PPD) for tuberculosis; if positive, a chest x-ray after the first trimester, may be done with abdominal shielding

Also during the first prenatal visit, the obstetrician should discuss nutrition, weight gain, exercise, sex, drug use, amniocentesis, prepared childbirth, seemingly minor details like hygiene and clothing, and certain danger signals to be noted.

NUTRITION AND WEIGHT GAIN

At the end of the average pregnancy, the pregnancy itself will weigh approximately 20 pounds (fetus 7.5, placenta 1.5, amniotic fluid 2, uterus 2.5, extra blood volume 4, breasts 2). Therefore, a woman who at term has gained less than 20 pounds has, in fact, lost weight. Ideally, optimal fetal and maternal outcomes are associated with maternal weight gains between 25 and 30 pounds. Typically, this is distributed as 5, 10, and 10 to 15 pounds in the first, second, and third trimesters, respectively.

To achieve optimal outcomes, the following daily dietary intakes are recommended for an average (50- to 60-kg) woman:

1. Calories: 2,400
2. Protein: 75 g
3. Vitamins: Most vitamin needs are unchanged by pregnancy, the notable exceptions being vitamin D (up 25%, to 500 IU), vitamin C (up 33%, to 80 mg), and folic acid (up 100%, to 0.8 mg).
4. Minerals: Most mineral needs appear to be unchanged except for iron (up more than 100%), calcium (up 30%, to 1,200 mg), and iodine (up slightly).

These needs can largely be met by a diet composed of three meals and a snack daily, suppying the following foods: milk (1 quart), animal protein (two 4-ounce servings), eggs (1), green vegetables (2 servings), fruits (2), and bread (2 slices). There should be no restrictions on salt or water intake. Vitamin and mineral supplementation is common, usually as a prenatal formulation, but a one-a-day type multiple vitamin with iron and minerals is probably sufficient. If extra iron supplementation is necessary, ferrous sulfate, 325 mg on an empty stomach with 250 mg vitamin C, will provide for best absorption and least constipation. If milk products cannot be taken, the cheapest and easiest calcium supplement is an antacid that contains calcium carbonate.

ACTIVITIES OF DAILY LIFE

Moderate, safe exercise is desirable. It should be stressed that pregnancy is a time for maintenance, not for getting into shape. There are no particular forms of exercise that are known to be dangerous to pregnancy, but situations in which physical injury is not unlikely (like skiing) are probably best avoided. Exercise sessions should be tailored to avoid significant overheating, as this may be comparable to having a fever.

If employment involves no physical danger or exposure to toxic substances, there is no reason why the normal woman cannot work throughout her pregnancy. In more stressful occupations, the fatigue associated with pregnancy may necessitate rest periods. This is usually most pronounced in the middle of the first and in the late third trimesters.

Travel carries no known risks for pregnancy, other than exposure to exotic diseases, although prolonged sitting in one position, especially with one's legs crossed, should be avoided. Pressurized aircraft have been shown to be safe.

If there is no associated pain or bleeding, sex may be considered safe.

Clothing should be sensible. Knee-high stockings with elastic bands may predispose to venous stasis and probably should be avoided. High-heeled shoes may become precarious by midpregnancy.

Normal hygienic measures need not be changed. Douching, which is of questionable need under any circumstances, is a definite caveat. Dental work done with local anesthesia poses no danger. Although diagnostic x-rays are acceptable if needed, they should probably not be done as a routine measure.

DRUG USE

All medications should be cleared with the obstetrician. Many can be safely taken, but need should be clearly established. Most obstetricians do not object to their patients taking occasional acetaminophen (Tylenol, Anacin-3) for headache. Certainly, if the pregnant woman has fever, acetaminophen is indicated. For the most part, aspirin has fallen into diuse because of its anticoagulant effects.

Smoking cigarettes is objectionable on purely common-sense grounds. Apart from carbon monoxide, carbon dioxide, nicotine, and tars, cigarette smoke contains many chemicals about which not enough is known. On empiric grounds, mothers who smoke one pack a day have been shown to have smaller babies with higher perinatal mortality rates.

Alcohol has become an increasingly widely recognized teratogen. Since its identification in 1974, the fetal alcohol syndrome has been expanded to include even more subtle signs at still lower alcohol intake levels. It now includes intrauterine growth retardation (IUGR), craniofacial abnormalities, cardiovascular and limb defects, impaired IQ, and increased perinatal mortality. The best advice regarding alcohol is that none is preferable to some.

Illicit drugs generally have effects on the fetus similar to those on the mother. The infant born of a narcotic or cocaine addict may be presumed to be similarly addicted and will go through similar withdrawal at birth. Marijuana and hashish have not been shown to be harmful, but it seems prudent to avoid them.

SPECIFIC WARNINGS

Although most pregnant women tend to be in constant contact with their obstetricians about everything that bothers or worries them, they should be specifically instructed to report certain signs or symptoms:

1. Vaginal bleeding
2. Abdominal pain
3. Leakage of amniotic fluid

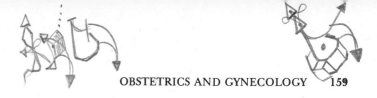

4. Fever
5. Persistent headache or vision changes
6. Severe swelling of the hands or face

SUBSEQUENT PRENATAL VISITS

It is customary to reexamine the pregnant woman at 4-week intervals throughout the first and second trimesters. By the 28th week, visits become biweekly until the 36th week, and weekly until delivery thereafter. An interval history is taken. Also at each visit, weight, blood pressure, urinary glucose and protein, uterine growth, and fetal activity and/or heart rate and position are assessed. Custom has established that cervical status and position of the presenting part should be checked at each visit from 36 weeks on.

If amniocentesis for karyotyping is not to be performed, serum alpha-fetoprotein (AFP) should be measured as soon as possible after the 15th week, to check for the likelihood of neural tube defects.

Hematocrit, RH antibody screening, and VDRL should be repeated at 24 and 36 weeks. If the gravida is Rh− and her mate is Rh+, she should receive Rh immune globulin, 300 μg, at approximately 28 weeks.

Fast becoming standard practice is a so-called mini-glucose tolerance test, consisting of a fasting blood glucose followed by ingestion of 50 g of glucose and a 1-hour postprandial blood glucose measurement, to identify the 8 to 10% of pregnant women who are gestational chemical diabetics. Some perform it early in the third trimester, whereas others do it twice, at approximately 22 to 24 and again at 32 to 34 weeks.

PHYSICAL FACTORS AFFECTING BIRTH

Birth is the process by which a fetus is forced out through a hole usually somewhat too small for it. Labor is the progressive effacement and dilatation of the cervix and descent of the fetus caused by uterine contractions that exert both retractile force on the lower uterine segment and cervix and expulsive force on the fetus. The quality of the individual labor is a function of pelvic architecture, fetal size (especially head size) and position, cervical resistance, and strength of uterine contractions.

PELVIC FACTORS AFFECTING DELIVERY

Aside from supporting the upper body on the legs, the female pelvis serves the additional function of being the bony structure of the birth canal. Under estrogen stimulation at menarche, the pelvic bones of the woman assume a different shape from those of the man. Ideally, they form a canal that is roundish (maximum usable space for a given width or length), that is of relatively constant dimension throughout its length, and that contains no structures protruding inward to obstruct passage.

The pelvis is formed by four bones: the **sacrum, coccyx,** and the right and left **innominate** bones (each formed by the fusion of the **ilium,** the **ischium,** and the **pubic** bone on that side). It is typically divided into the false and true pelves, which are separated by the **linea terminalis.** Above the linea terminalis, the false pelvis is defined by the **iliac fossae** and the **lumbar vertebrae** posteriorly and laterally, and is open

anteriorly. Below the linea, the true pelvis is provided by the **sacrum** (posteriorly), the ischial portions of the **innominate** bones and the **sacrosciatic notches** and **ligaments** (laterally), and the ischial rami and pubic bone portions of the **innominate** bones (anteriorly).

Several dimensions are important in pelvic function as a birth canal. The **true conjugate,** or anterior-posterior (AP) diameter from the sacral promontory to the top of the symphysis pubis, is a measure of the pelvic inlet or entrance to the true pelvis. The **obstetric conjugate,** or AP diameter from the promontory to the closest portion of the pubic bone, is the narrowest point to be passed on the way to the midpelvis. The **diagonal conjugate,** or AP diameter from the promontory to the lower edge of the pubis, is the only one of these three accessible to measurement on pelvic examination and is used to estimate the others. The **transverse** diameter is measured at the level of the linea terminalis.

In the midpelvis, which is usually the narrowest portion of the birth canal, the distance between the ischial spines defines the **transverse** diameter, which is usually considerably less than the AP diameter at the same level.

At the outlet, the AP diameter is measured from the bottom of the pubis to the tip of the coccyx, the **transverse** between the two **ischial tuberosities,** and the **posterior sagittal** diameter from the sacrum to an imaginary line drawn between the ischial tuberosities. The posterior sagittal diameter is of importance because it tends to define the usable space in the pelvic outlet unless the interpubic angle is extremely wide.

The following measurements are considered to be normal for the above diameters. If they are met or exceeded by the pelvis in question, the architectural prognosis for delivery is usually good for the average-size fetus:

True conjugate	10.5 cm
Obstetric conjugate	10.0 cm
Diagonal conjugate	11.5 cm
Transverse inlet	13.5 cm
Transverse midpelvis	10.0 cm
AP midpelvis	11.5 cm
Transverse outlet	10.0 cm
AP outlet	11.5 cm
Posterior sagittal	7.5 cm

As above, the ideal pelvis would be rounded with few obstructions to delivery. In fact, only about half the pelves in this country fit that ideal description. Having a fairly round inlet, with parallel walls, ischial spines that are not prominent, and a wide pubic arch, these pelves are termed **gynecoid.** The gynecoid pelvis of adequate dimension is the most favorable type of birth canal for delivery. In reality, of the 50% of otherwise shaped pelves, most are also adequate, often molding the fetal head to fit into diameters that are proportioned differently. Of these, the **android** and **anthropoid** pelves are most common. The anthropoid shape is elongated in the AP diameter and has somewhat convergent sidewalls and a narrow pubic arch (not very significant because of the long posterior sagittal dimension, allowing for posterior displacement of the head). Like the anthropoid, the android pelvis is narrowed with convergent sidewalls, prominent spines, and a narrow pubic arch, but unlike it, there is no compensatory expansion of the posterior space, so that the likelihood of vaginal delivery here is much smaller unless the overall dimensions are large. A much less common pelvic shape is the **platypelloid,** which is extremely wide but foreshortened from front to back.

FETAL FACTORS AFFECTING DELIVERY

The two fetal factors that are most significant in determining the ease of vaginal delivery are the size and position of the presenting part (most importantly the skull).

Fetal skull

The bones of the fetal skull are not fused, but approximated at **suture** lines. The mobility imparted to the skull by this lack of fusion allows for **molding** during labor to accommodate to less than ideal pelvic shapes and sizes. There are three sets of bilaterally symmetrical bones (frontal, parietal, temporal) and two singular (occipital, sphenoid). The sutures at which they meet are the **frontal** (frontal-frontal), the **sagittal** (parietal-parietal), **coronals** (2) (frontal-parietal), and **lambdoids** (2) (temporal-occipital). In the midline, anteriorly and posteriorly, respectively, the **greater** and **lesser fontanels** allow for more shifting. The greater fontanel is the space created by the failure to fuse of the frontal and parietal bones and is rhomboid in shape. The lesser fontanel is the triangular space bordered by the posterior edges of the parietal bones and the occipital.

The important **diameters** by which head size is gauged are the **occipitofrontal** (from the occiput to the frontal prominence), the **biparietal** (the greatest transverse diameter, between the parietal prominences), the **bitemporal** (the smallest diameter, between the two temporal sutures), and the **suboccipitobregmatic** (from the anterior fontanel to the base of the occiput). In most pregnancies, the fetal skull measurement of most importance is the biparietal diameter (BPD), which ranges from 9 to 10 cm in mature fetuses.

Fetal size

The average size of a term fetus (at EDC) is between 3,200 g and 3,400 g, or between 7 and 7.5 pounds, with normals ranging from 2,500 g to 4,000 g. Its BPD, correspondingly, will vary from 8.5 to 10 cm. Obviously, for any given pelvis and fetal orientation, assuming proportionality between head and body sizes, the 2,500-g fetus will be more easily delivered than its 4,000-g counterpart. As one would expect, cephalopelvic disproportion (CPD) is less common earlier in gestation than later. Since the fetus gains almost 200 g per week in the late third trimester, the average 37-week fetus will weigh almost 2 pounds less than its postdate counterpart.

Fetal orientation

The position that the fetus takes in the uterus is characterized in several steps. First, lie is determined by the direction of the long axis of the trunk. This may be **transverse, longitudinal,** or **oblique.**

Next, one considers the presentation, which is named according to the part of the fetus that is most likely to enter the pelvis first, usually termed **head, breech,** and **acromial** (shoulder). These are further broken down according to the orientation of the presenting part. The head presentations are divided into **vertex** (occiput presents), **face** (anterior face), **sinciput** (portion of the head presenting is one-third anterior to the vertex), and **brow** (portion is one-third posterior to the face or the brow). The breech presentations are modified in accordance with the status of the legs. If the lower extremities are flexed at the hip and the actual presenting part is the rump, the fetus is said to be in either the **frank breech** (legs extended at the knees so that the feet are next to the head) or the **full breech** (legs flexed at the knees) position. If one or both feet extend below the hips so that it (they) will enter the pelvis first, the fetus is said to be in a **footling breech** presentation.

Lastly, the rotational position of the presenting part is described as either **left** or **right** and **anterior, transverse,** or **posterior.** For example, a vertex presentation may be **direct anterior** or **posterior** (OA or OP), **right anterior, transverse** or **posterior** (ROA, ROT, or ROP), or **left anterior, transverse,** or **posterior** (LOA, LOT, or LOP).

At term, 96% of fetuses are headfirst, 3.5% breech, and 0.5% shoulder. Of the head presentations, the overwhelming majority are **vertex,** with only an occasional face. The sinciput and brow presentations are transitory and are converted into either vertex (almost always) or face by labor.

CERVICAL FACTORS

Throughout pregnancy, the cervix provides a barrier between the fetus and the outside world. It must remain uneffaced, closed, and plugged, its collagen matrix resistant to change. However, when labor ensues, it is necessary that all these virtues be abandoned. If this occurs too early, premature delivery may result; if not on time, dystocia during labor. This process of "ripening" is not well understood but is probably prostaglandin mediated, and it may certainly be accomplished by the application of prostaglandin E_2 gel directly to the cervix. The softening or ripening allows for the cervix to be effaced and subsequently dilated. Although cervical dystocia is rarely a reason for failure to deliver, an unripe cervix certainly is a harbinger of harder, longer labor for both the mother and fetus.

Assessment of cervical condition has been quantified as the Bishop score. Assigning point values ranging from zero to three for **cervical dilatation** (0, 1 to cm, 3 to 4 cm, 5+ cm), **cervical effacement** (0 to 30%, 40 to 50%, 60 to 70%, 80+%) and **station of presenting part** ($-3, -2, +0, +1$ etc.) and from zero to two for **cervical position** (posterior, midposition, anterior) and **consistency** (firm, intermediate, soft), Bishop concluded that the higher the score the more "inducible" the cervix. More specifically, a total score of five or less indicated a very resistant cervix, whereas eight or more usually bode well.

DETERMINATION OF FETOPELVIC RELATIONSHIPS

The prospects for delivery are proportional to what might be called the fetopelvic ratio. Simply stated, a small baby will be more easily delivered through a large pelvis than vice versa, all other factors being equal. This ratio may be assessed by determination of pelvic and fetal size.

PELVIC ASSESSMENT

Pelvic assessment may be performed at any time during pregnancy but is best reserved until late in the third trimester, or even in labor. The three pelvic dimensions (inlet, midpelvis, and outlet) are of concern. These may be most accurately measured by x-ray **pelvimetry,** but this procedure has fallen into virtual disuse because of radiation exposure to the fetus. If one needs this information (perhaps for vaginal breech delivery), AP and lateral films of the pelvis are taken with the patient erect and appropriate diameters for all three pelvic planes are calculated and compared with norms (see above). Barring the use of pelvimetry, there is no way to measure either the inlet or midpelvis, but only to estimate. The diagonal conjugate (an indirect measure of the inlet) may be considered adequate for an average fetus if one cannot reach the sacral promontory per vaginam. Better yet, if the leading edge of an unmolded head has descended to the level of the ischial spines, the head is presumed to be engaged, proving that the inlet is adequate.

Midpelvic assessment is even more precarious on clinical grounds, and one can only extrapolate from the prominence of the ischial spines and the degree of convergence of the sidewalls. Only descent of the fetus during labor provides proof of an adequate midpelvis.

Finally, an intertuberous diameter of greater than 8 cm, or roughly the width of a fist, suggests adequacy of the outlet. If combined with a wide pubic arch, outlet dystocia is extremely unlikely.

ASSESSMENT OF FETAL SIZE

Clinical estimates of overall fetal size become increasingly less accurate as the fetus deviates from the ideal 3,000 to 3,500 g. The tendency is to estimate closer to the norm so that the weight of very small babies is overestimated and that of large ones underestimated. Ultrasonography, however, provides safe and quite accurate measurements, especially of head size. BPD is easily measured in unengaged heads (not necessary, if engaged), and, although overall body size is somewhat less accessible, except in extreme cases, it is also less important. If this information is critical, it may be calculated from complex nomograms using thoracic, abdominal, and femoral measurements.

ASSESSMENT OF FETAL POSITION

Leopold's maneuvers, combined with vaginal examination, are the simplest method for determining fetal position. Divided into four steps, Leopold's maneuvers are designed to determine whether the fetus is headfirst or breech, whether it is facing left or right, whether it is engaged or not, and whether it has a flexed or extended presenting part. They are as follows:

1. Feel the fundus with both hands to see if it contains a hard, regular mass (head) or a more irregular one (breech).
2. Feel both sides of the uterus simultaneously to determine which is more regular (back) and which has multiple small projections (hands and feet).
3. Feel directly suprapubically with the thumb and fingers

of one hand to determine if there is a movable mass (unengaged) or not. If no structure can be clearly delineated, the presenting part is presumably engaged.
4. Push down along both sides of the presenting part simultaneously to determine whether the presenting part is flexed or extended.

This information may be supplemented by vaginal examination to assess degree of descent of the presenting part. In addition, the presenting part is often easily felt through the anterior lower uterine segment. If there is any cervical dilatation, position of the head may be more accurately gauged.

Finally, if the examiner is uncertain after performing all these operations, sonography can almost always provide the necessary information.

ANTEPARTUM AND INTRAPARTUM FETAL EVALUATION

KARYOTYPING

Chromosomal anomalies of the fetus are detectable by analysis of fetal cells. These cells may be obtained from those shed into the amniotic fluid by **amniocentesis** or from the early chorion by **chorionic villus sampling** (CVS). Chromosome analysis using modern banding techniques can detect a variety of abnormalities with greater than 99% accuracy. If obtained by amniocentesis, the process is best done between 16 and 18 weeks gestation, which is late enough for there to be adequate amniotic fluid and a sufficient number of shed fetal cells to provide a good culture, and early enough to allow the 3 to 4 weeks necessary to grow the cells and still have time to act on the results. If CVS is performed, it is usually done between 7 and 10 weeks gestation, allowing for early termination of abnormal pregnancies.

Since both the methods for obtaining fetal cells involve some risk and considerable expense, indications for performing these procedures are usually limited to those pregnancies with an increased likelihood of fetal anomaly. These include the following:

1. Maternal age 35 or over, when the risk of abnormality is about 1/180, approximately half of which are Down's syndrome or trisomy 21
2. Chromosomal anomaly in one of the parents
3. Previous pregnancy with known or suspected chromosomal abnormality
4. Known risk of a sex-linked hereditary disorder

AMNIOCENTESIS

Puncture of the amnion with removal of amniotic fluid may be done at various stages of pregnancy. When being performed for chromosomal studies or AFP analysis, it is usually done between the 16th and 18th weeks but may be used as late as the 22nd week. To determine fetal maturity or fetal jeopardy from Rh disease, it is essentially a third trimester procedure. In most cases today, amniocentesis is performed with ultrasonic guidance. By delineating the position of the fetus, placenta, and cord, as well as, in the late third trimester, available

AFP 16 wks - normal - no NTD
↑ if ↑ → repeat if high
amniocentes AFP Lacetylcholinesteras

pockets of fluid, both the efficacy and safety of amniocentesis have been greatly improved.

Risks. Trauma to fetus, cord, or placenta may be minimized by preceding the puncture with ultrasonic evaluation of the uterine contents. Currently available ultrasonographic technology even allows for real-time monitoring of the puncture by inserting the needle through the center of a specially designed transducer, so that the actual course of the needle can be seen in relation to the fetus and cord. In third trimester punctures, if ultrasonography is not available, trauma may be best avoided by a suprapubic tap (after emptying the bladder) after elevating the fetal head out of the pelvis.

Possible maternofetal bleeding may also be minimized by simultaneous ultrasonography. In Rh− mothers, the risk of sensitization should be protected against by the administration of 300 μg of Rh immune globulin. Infection is a real but minor risk if the tap is performed using sterile technique. The overall risk of a miscarriage as a complication of second trimester amniocentesis is commonly quoted as approximately 1/200 when all of the above precautions are taken by an experienced physician. The risk of fetal injury is generally considered to be much smaller.

CHORIONIC VILLUS SAMPLING

A recently devised technique, CVS allows the physician to obtain fetal cells for prenatal diagnosis much earlier than by amniocentesis. By inserting a small suction catheter transcervically into the uterus under direct ultrasonic guidance, one may removal small portions of the chorion without disturbing the fetus. These cells of fetal origin may be grown in tissue culture and then used to karyotype the fetus. Usually done between 7 and 10 weeks gestation, this procedure allows for early genetic diagnosis and first trimester termination of the pregnancy if necessary. Still considered an experimental procedure because of the high loss rate in most hands (up to 5 to 8%), CVS may be most useful for pregnancies with a very high risk of abnormality such as parental translocations. Since only cells are obtained, there is no fluid for analysis, and the procedure cannot be used to evaluate the risk of neural tube defects or other enzyme-deficiency diseases that require chemical analysis.

Fetal sex determination is of primary importance when there is a considerable risk of a sex-linked hereditary disorder such as Duchenne's muscular dystrophy. Today this is usually done by amniocentesis and karyotyping, which are rarely wrong, but good quality sonography may be extremely reliable for visualization of the genitalia after 18 to 20 weeks gestation.

ALPHA-FETOPROTEIN

AFP is made by the yolk sac and then the liver of the developing fetus. It passes from the fetal serum to the amniotic fluid and then to the maternal serum. By analyzing maternal serum for AFP and interpreting the results according to gestational age, an increased risk of numerous fetal abnormalities can be detected. Of critical importance in understanding the screening process is the concept that a normal result is very highly correlated with a fetus free of those conditions that will increase the AFP, but an elevated AFP is only indicative that

one of these abnormalities may exist. Many elevated AFP levels are never explained and are associated with apparently normal fetuses. The most common of these abnormalities, an open neural tube defect (NTD) should be screened for. Curves exist for gestational ages from 15 to 22 weeks, so samples should be done as early as possible in that time range. What is commonly reported as a normal AFP reduces the risks of an open NTD to virtually nil. Serum AFP levels greater than normal are associated with

More advanced gestation
Multiple gestation
Open NTDs
Ventral abdominal wall defects, esophageal and
    duodenal atresia
Pilonidal sinus and sacococcygeal teratoma
Fetal urinary tract disease (congenital nephrosis, renal
    agenesis, bladder neck obstruction)
XO karyotype
Fetal death
Bloody tap (aminocentesis only)

Method. Obtain the first sample as early as possible between 15 and 22 weeks. If this is in the normal range, the fetus is almost certainly without an open NTD (950/1,000).

If the first sample is elevated (50/1,000), repeat the sample. If the repeat sample is in the normal range, this is statistically the same as if the first sample were normal (30/50).

If both samples are elevated (20/1,000), perform ultrasonography. If an explanation for the elevation is discovered (larger, older fetus than suspected, twins, visible defect), either recompute or act appropriately.

If the ultrasonographic examination is not explanatory (15/1,000), perform amniocentesis and analyze the fluid for AFP and acetylcholinesterase.

If the amniotic fluid AFP and acetylcholinesterase are normal, the fetus may be assumed to be normal. If not, there is a presumptive NTD, ventral wall defect, or other anomaly. Acetylcholinesterase in the amniotic fluid may be considered specific for NTD.

FETAL MATURITY STUDIES

When the decision to terminate pregnancy in the third trimester is of importance, the consequences of delivery must be weighed against those of continuing the pregnancy. This entails primarily the determination of fetal maturity, especially lung function, and may be approached in either of two ways. Since neonatal lung function is rarely a problem after 37 completed weeks of gestation (except in pregnancies complicated by diabetes or intrapartum asphyxia), studies that imply fetal age can be of use (amniotic fluid bilirubin and creatinine, ultrasonic determination of fetal size, accurate dating of pregnancy soon after the onset of amenorrhea). However, more specific assessment of lung maturity may be obtained by testing the amniotic fluid for the presence of surfactant (determination of the L/S ratio, phosphatidylglycerol levels, shake test).

Amniotic fluid bilirubin

Amniotic fluid bilirubin may be assessed by any qualified chemistry laboratory. Levels of bilirubin in the amniotic fluid approach zero as the fetus becomes mature. This measurement has been used to imply lung maturity in the past but has been largely replaced by surfactant determinations, which are more specific. If one uses this measurement, one must be aware that levels are influenced by fetal hemolysis (Rh incompatibility) and by elevated maternal bilirubin. It is usually measured by the change in absorbed light at 450 nm and is expressed as the ΔOD_{450}.

Amniotic fluid creatinine

Creatinine levels in amniotic fluid can be assessed by any qualified chemistry laboratory. As the fetus grows and its kidneys mature, creatinine levels in the amniotic fluid increase. Levels above 2.0 mg/100 ml usually indicate a fetus large enough to be mature. Like amniotic fluid bilirubin measurement, however, it is affected by maternal levels and has been largely replaced by amniotic fluid surfactant determinations.

Determination of fetal size and/or gestational age

Except in pregnancies complicated by diabetes, lung function can almost always be safely presumed to be mature at 37 completed weeks. This can be most efficiently and accurately determined by early dating of the pregnancy. In most cases, physical examination in the first trimester that correlates with a known last menstrual period and regular menses are sufficient for accurate dating. Also in the first trimester, ultrasonic measurement of the amniotic sac or of the fetal crown-rump length may effectively date the gestation to within 2 or 3 days. After this early period, environmental and hereditary factors affecting growth progressively loosen the correlation between fetal size and age, so that by the middle of the third trimester, accurate ultrasonic sizing of the pregnancy may determine fetal age to only + or − 2 weeks. Less exact measurements like physical examination are even less useful.

Lung maturity studies

As described earlier, lung maturity in the fetus is heralded by the production of surfactant-like chemicals to prevent expiratory collapse and ease inspiration. These phospholipids are shed into the amniotic fluid during fetal breathing and may be measured in samples obtained by amniocentesis. Tests fall into two categories: direct measurements and inferential tests.

L/S ratio—direct measurement. As the fetus nears maturity, the lecithins phosphatidylinositol and phosphatidylglycerol are produced in increasing amounts. By measuring them and the relatively constant sphingomyelin concentration and comparing the two as a ratio, the L/S ratio, one may measure fetal pulmonary maturity. If the L/S ratio is greater than 2, the fetus will almost never develop RDS unless there is maternal diabetes. With ratios from 1.5 to 2.0, RDS may occur as often as 50% of the time, and below 1.5, 75%. Because of advances in neonatal management, fatal RDS is much less common, so that most fetuses with L/S ratios greater than 1 will usually survive.

Inaccuracy of the test occurs when the amniotic fluid is contaminated with either blood or meconium. Both artificially lower the L/S ratio in proportion to their concentration.

Phosphatidylglycerol—direct measurement. Increasing lecithin production is associated with a shift from phosphatidylinositol to phosphatidylglycerol production. Now that phosphatidylglycerol can be measured directly, its presence is known to be associated with an extremely small risk of RDS, even in diabetic pregnancies. Its detection is not affected by contamination of the amniotic fluid with blood or meconium.

Shake test—indirect measurement. Based on the ability of surfactant, under the right conditions, to support bubble formation, this test may be done in the delivery room but must be performed strictly according to protocol for the results to be reliable. The wrong size tube, small changes in reagent amount, or dirty glassware will invalidate the test.

Prepare two tubes, each 100 mm in diameter. In the first, mix 1 ml amniotic fluid with 1 ml 95% ethanol; in the second, 0.5 ml amniotic fluid, 0.5 ml distilled water, and 1 ml 95% ethanol.

Shake each tube for 15 seconds and stand it upright for 15 minutes.

Read a complete ring of bubbles at the surface as a positive test. Positive tests in both tubes are an extremely good predictor of fetal lung maturity. Negative or intermediate tests are *not* good predictors of immaturity, but rather fail to predict.

FETAL OXYGEN SUPPLY—PLACENTAL SUFFICIENCY

Perhaps the major threat to fetal well-being in the third trimester is the increasing likelihood of placental insufficiency. Even though structural and functional changes in the placenta toward term increase its ability to support the pregnancy, the rapidly growing fetus becomes progressively more likely to outgrow its oxygen and food supply. It is therefore often necessary to evaluate the fetus in utero. Testing procedures available for this include hormone assays (HPL and estriol), electronic fetal monitoring (nonstress test [NST] and contraction stress test [CST]), and ultrasonography (biophysical profile and measurement of fetal growth).

HORMONE ASSAYS

Human placental lactogen

HPL is secreted by the healthy placenta in proportion to its mass and passes into the maternal serum, where its levels continue to increase until approximately the 36th week of gestation. Attempts to correlate HPL levels with fetal well-being have not been as promising as was originally hoped, largely because its presence reflects placental mass more than fetal condition. It, like estriol measurement, has been mostly replaced by electronic fetal monitoring (EFM).

Estriol

Estriol, estetrol, and quinestrol are three estrogen products of the fetoplacental unit that have been measured in an attempt to monitor the health of the fetus. Since most work has been done with estriol, this discussion is limited to it. Made in the placenta from precursors supplied by the fetus, estriol does reflect the competence of the fetoplacental unit. Secreted into the maternal circulation, then conjugated in the maternal liver and excreted into the maternal urine, it is available for assay in both maternal plasma and urine. Seemingly, serial measurement of estriol levels in either the maternal urine or plasma would be a useful tool for evaluating the fetus. In practice, however, it is subject to limitations that make it less than ideal.

Because estriol levels may vary fairly widely, it is necessary to establish a baseline over several days. Subsequent estriol levels must decrease by 50% from this baseline to be significant. Therefore, deteriorating placental condition cannot be diagnosed in less than several days.

Several factors besides fetoplacental condition influence the production of measurable estriol. Sharp decreases in precursors, especially DHEAS from the fetal adrenal, as in pregnancies complicated by anenecephaly, will markedly decrease both serum and urine estriol levels to a point at which they are not useful. A rare hereditary condition, placental sulfatase deficiency, found only in male fetuses, does not affect fetal welfare but results in a complete inability of the placenta to produce estriol. Maternal liver and kidney disease interfere, respectively, with conjugation and renal clearance of estriol into the maternal urine. Many drugs (e.g., ampicillin) block clearance of estriol by the maternal kidney and result in falsely low urine estriol measurements in the face of normal serum values.

For these reasons, estriol determination has largely given way to the more sensitive and readily interpretable EFM.

ELECTRONIC FETAL MONITORING

EFM depends on two principles: (1) that the fetal heart rate (FHR) patterns reflect, in some way, fetal oxygenation and pH and (2) that the FHR will respond to fetal jeopardy before lasting damage is done to the fetus. The FHR may be recorded by any of several technologies incorporated into fetal monitors. External FHR recording may be accomplished by ultrasonography (detection of heart valve motion), phonocardiography (actual heart sounds), or external ECG. Because of various technical difficulties with phonocardiography and external ECG, most monitors employ ultrasound technology. Internal monitoring (appropriate only for labor after rupture of the membranes) is done via an electrode applied directly to the fetal scalp and is most reliable. In all cases, FHR recordings are accompanied by simultaneous monitoring of uterine activity and fetal movement.

Under normal conditions, the healthy fetus has a baseline **FHR between 120 and 160 bpm**. FHR baselines outside this range are categorized as **mild bradycardia** (100 to 120 bpm), **severe bradycardia** (less than 100 bpm), **mild tachycardia** (160 to 180 bpm) and **severe tachycardia** (greater than 180 bpm). In addition, in the normal, healthy fetus, the heart rate responds to both adrenergic and parasympathetic stimuli, resulting in beat-to-beat variability (5 to 15 bpm is considered normal), and the normal sleep-wake cycle of approximately 20 minutes is reflected in increased variability while the fetus is awake and decreased variability while asleep (long-term variability). Furthermore, various stresses are associated with predictable FHR alterations, termed **periodic changes**:

1. Vagal stimulation, usually in the form of head compression, results in a temporary slowing (**deceleration**) of the FHR.

2. Complete cord compression, through an acute baroceptor response to umbilical artery occlusion and fetal hypertension, also results in a deceleration.

3. Partial cord compression, in which the low-pressure umbilical vein is occluded but the higher-pressure arteries remain patent, may cause fetal hypotension and an **acceleration** of the fetal heart.

4. Hypoxia, at a PO_2 below 18 to 20 mm Hg, has a direct toxic effect on the fetal myocardium, resulting in deceleration of the FHR.

5. Acidosis, by interfering with central control mechanisms, results in a loss of variability and, sometimes, sustained tachycardia.

6. Narcotics, tranquilizers, and anticholinergics administered to the mother will decrease FHR variability.

Fetal heart rate

Bradycardia. Mild bradycardia (100 to 120 bpm) without periodic changes is usually benign. Severe bradycardia (less than 100 bpm) usually reflects either fetal hypoxia, in which case it often becomes worse with contractions, or fetal heart block. If a fetal ECG can be obtained via direct monitoring, these can sometimes be distinguished before birth. Occasionally, recording of the maternal heartbeat is mistaken for fetal bradycardia. This almost never happens with direct internal monitoring. Severe bradycardia always deserves investigation.

Tachycardia. Mild tachycardia (160 to 180 bpm) without periodic changes is usually benign but may reflect early fetal distress. FHRs over 180 bpm may result from fetal compromise (anemia, shock, or asphyxia), fetal arrhythmia (e.g., paroxysmal atrial tachycardia), maternal fever, or thyrotoxicosis. Severe tachycardia always deserves investigation.

Variability. Decreased beat-to-beat variability may result from maternal drug therapy (narcotics, tranquilizers, or anticholinergics), fetal sleep, and fetal acidosis. It is also an artifactual accompaniment of tachycardia, since with a faster FHR there is less room for variability. In the absence of periodic changes and maternal sedation, the meaning of decreased variability may be unclear, but a trial of oxygen therapy and hydration or assessment of fetal pH may be indicated.

Early deceleration (type I). The FHR begins to decelerate at the onset of the contraction, reaches it nadir at the peak of the contraction, and recovers as the contraction wanes. Probably resulting from head compression and subsequent increased vagal tone, which are greatest at the peak of the contraction, this pattern forms a mirror image of the contraction and is usually considered benign unless the decelerations are too long or too frequent. Then the decrease in FHR may *cause* fetal problems secondary to decreased cardiac output.

Late deceleration (type II). Characterized by a decrease in the FHR that begins at or beyond the peak of the contraction, is most pronounced as the contraction ends, and recovers after the contraction, the late deceleration reflects fetal hypoxia. The pattern appears as it does because placental blood supply is cut off early in the contraction and is not restored until almost its end. Therefore, by midcontraction, the fetus is "holding its breath" and begins to become hypoxic. It does not begin to recover until placental flow is reestablished near the end of the contraction. The presence of late decelerations, however small, indicates a hypoxic fetus and demands immediate attention.

Variable deceleration (type III).   Type III decelerations, unlike types I and II, are not uniform. Their timing, shape, and intensity may vary from contraction to contraction. Usually the drop and recovery of the FHR are sharp rather than gradual and may be preceded or followed by mild acceleration. These mostly reflect the hemodynamic consequences of cord compression described above and do not, in and of themselves, indicate fetal distress. However, if they are prolonged, very deep, or very frequent, they may represent danger to the fetus, both because of decreased fetal oxygenation and decreased fetal cardiac output. Often, in severe cases, the variable deceleration will appear to have a slow recovery. This represents a superimposed late deceleration (**combined deceleration**) and is an ominous sign. Mild variables may be innocuous and may respond to changes in maternal position (perhaps relieving cord compression) or hydration. Severe and combined variables should always be attended to immediately.

Acceleration.   Transient increase in the FHR is generally considered to be a reassuring sign. It probably represents an appropriate response to mild stresses such as fetal movement or contractions. In addition, it may reflect partial cord compression but is usually not considered threatening.

By interpretation of the baseline FHR and the above changes in relation to various stresses, fetal oxygenation may be evaluated. Although this technique was originally introduced for monitoring the fetus in labor, it has become extremely useful in the antepartum period. It is advantageous in that information is available immediately and there are very few false-negatives. However, the equipment is expensive and false-positives are not rare.

NONSTRESS TEST   NST

Based on the fact that the normal fetus moves with regularity and its cardiovascular response is acceleration of the FHR, the NST is performed by simply monitoring the FHR and marking fetal movements on the strip. The presumably healthy fetus will exhibit a normal baseline with adequate variability, at least two movements in a 20-minute waking period, and acceleration of the FHR by at least 15 bpm (and of 45 seconds duration) in coordination with those movements. A test that fulfills these criteria is called **reactive** and is very good evidence that the fetus is not in immediate jeopardy. A **nonreactive** test is one in which either the fetus does not move for prolonged periods of time or its movements are not associated with accelerations of the FHR. This is suggestive of a compromised fetus but is not sufficient evidence by itself to mandate delivery. It is important to continue a nonreactive NST for at least 40 minutes to be sure of traversing one whole sleep-wake cycle. A nonreactive NST is usually evaluated by performing a CST.

CONTRACTION STRESS TEST

Since the hypoxic myocardium decelerates (see "Electronic Fetal Monitoring," above), the CST may be used to identify the fetus in jeopardy. By applying stress to the fetus in the form of contractions, during which blood flow to the uterus is cut off, we can unmask those who are in such poor condition that they cannot tolerate 30 seconds of "breath holding." Contractions may be spontaneous or induced, either by nipple stimulation or intravenous oxytocin in minute amounts. Sufficient stress to evaluate the fetus has been applied when three contractions, lasting 40 to 60 seconds each, occur in a 10-minute period.

Technique

1. Establish a baseline of 15 to 20 minutes by monitoring the fetus using an external FHR transducer and tocodynamometer. Pay particular attention to maternal position (reclining at about 45° with perhaps a slight tilt to the side), since the production of aortocaval compression and maternal supine hypotension may artifactually decrease placental perfusion and result in a false-positive test.
2. If there are no contractions, or fewer than three contractions per 10 minutes that are not associated with abnormal FHR patterns, begin either nipple stimulation or IV oxytocin drip by infusion pump. If using oxytocin, begin at 1 mU/minute and double every 15 to 20 minutes until three contractions of sufficient duration occur in 10 minutes or an ominous pattern occurs.
3. Monitor the patient after cessation of the oxytocin until contractions have returned to baseline levels.

Interpretation

If three contractions in a 10-minute period occur without late decelerations, the test is called **negative** and the fetus is in no jeopardy from placental insufficiency. If repetitive late decelerations occur with contractions, even if the frequency is less than three per 10 minutes, the test is **positive** and the fetus is presumably in immediate danger and should be delivered. When late decelerations occur with some contractions, but not consistently, the test is called **suspicious** and may either be prolonged or repeated in 24 hours. If uterine contractions are either prolonged (longer than 90 seconds) or more frequent than every 2 minutes, late decelerations may not mean placental insufficiency but rather **hyperstimulation**. Hyperstimulation without FHR decelerations can still be read as negative. Variable decelerations during a CST have the same significance as in labor: either oligohydramnios or cord entrapment.

Unlike the NST, to which there are no contraindications, the CST should not be performed under certain conditions. Most simply, one should avoid the CST when one is afraid of contractions. These circumstances include previous classic cesarean section, placenta previa, and pregnancies at considerable risk for preterm labor (multiple gestation, polyhydramnios, premature labor in this or a previous pregnancy).

USE OF NST/CST

Usually one begins EFM antenatal evaluation when one suspects a condition dangerous to the fetus. However, it may be less reliable in the earliest weeks of the third trimester (28 to 31) because of immaturity of the cardiovascular control mechanisms. After the beginning of the 32nd week, EFM is frequently used to screen fetuses at risk for uteroplacental insufficiency. Usually the NST is the primary screening tool because of its simplicity and safety. If reactive, the NST should be repeated at weekly intervals, at the least, and some advocate as often as every 2 or 3 days. Under most circumstances, a reactive NST is good assurance that the fetus is receiving enough oxygen to survive for another week, but the testing must be tempered by the awareness that conditions in utero may deteriorate more rapidly and should be scheduled accordingly.

If the NST is nonreactive, a CST may be performed. A negative CST following a nonreactive NST is usually considered reassuring for a week but may be repeated in as little as 2 to 3 days by some. A suspicious CST should be repeated in no more than 24 hours. A positive CST mandates immediate delivery after maximizing fetal oxygen supply by placing the mother in the lateral supine position, hydrating her with IV lactated Ringer's solution, and supplying her with supplemental oxygen by mask.

False-negative NSTs and CSTs do rarely occur, as evidenced by occasional fetal demise within a short period (less than 1 week) of negative tests. As noted above, changing intrauterine environment may endanger a fetus thought to be safe, so a false sense of security should not be engendered by either of these tests.

False-positive tests are much more common if one accepts the delivery of a healthy baby as evidence that this has occurred. In some series, as many as 25% of fetuses delivered after a nonreactive NST and a positive CST show no evidence of fetal distress. This is extremely troublesome, especially in cases where immediate delivery may be dangerous for the fetus, so other information such as a biophysical profile or fetal maturity studies may be indicated. However, it is probably extremely difficult to avoid delivery of a fetus after obtaining the combination of a nonreactive NST and a positive CST.

FETAL ACTIVITY DETERMINATION

An outgrowth of the NST, fetal activity determination (FAD) has been proposed as a simple, noninvasive method of determining fetal well-being. Since the criteria for a healthy fetus, as determined by an NST, include an adequate number of fetal movements, it has been suggested that the presence of such movements themselves might be used as evidence of fetal health. By training mothers to become aware of their fetuses' movements and cataloging them, one can often gain information on fetal health cheaply and easily. In reality, in this country, this method has been used mostly in conjunction with other tests discussed above, with a decrease in fetal activity as an additional indicator of the need for further testing.

BIOPHYSICAL PROFILE

Real-time ultrasonography enables the obstetrician to obtain a sort of antenatal Apgar score on the fetus. By assessing fetal tone, reactivity, breathing, and amniotic fluid, an indication of fetal well-being may be obtained. The fetus is observed for 30 minutes, and two points are alloted for

1. An episode of extension and flexion
2. Three body or limb movements
3. Thirty seconds of breathing movements
4. One 1-cm pocket of amniotic fluid

The sum of these scores is combined with either two points for a reactive NST or none for a nonreactive NST. A total of eight or more is indicative of a healthy fetus. Below six indicates fetal jeopardy, and six is equivocal.

MONITORING OF FETAL GROWTH

It has been well documented that the healthy fetus grows at a standard rate when one corrects for different-sized fetuses. By establishing a growth curve for the average fetus and also for the individual, placental supply may be indirectly evaluated by ultrasonography. Also, since head, femurs, chest, and abdomen grow at standard rates in relation to each other in the healthy fetus and are stunted differentially in cases in which placental supply is compromised, discrepancies in the growth rates of one or more of these may indicate particular types of intrauterine growth retardation. Briefly, **symmetrical** growth retardation, in which the entire fetus is proportionally small, may indicate a genetically small baby, appropriate for parental size, a chromosomal or cardiovascular abnormality, heavy maternal drug use (alcohol, narcotics, and tobacco), or intrauterine infection such as cytomegalic inclusion disease. **Asymmetric growth retardation**, on the other hand, in which fetal head growth is spared but the abdominal viscera are not, is more usually associated with decreased placental supply as in maternal vascular disease (e.g., severe diabetes, pregnancy-induced hypertension, and chronic maternal hypertension with kidney disease).

RADIOLOGICAL PROCEDURES

Once commonly used for antepartum evaluation, procedures based on x-rays have been progressively abandoned as newer, safer technologies have become available. Determination of multiple gestation, fetal presentation, and anomalies by x-ray and of placental anomalies (most notably hydatidiform mole) by amniography (injection of radiopaque dye into the amniotic sac followed by x-ray) have been largely supplanted by ultrasonography.

INTRAPARTUM FETAL MONITORING

Although some investigators have shown that, with the proper care, stethoscopic monitoring of the low-risk fetus in labor may be as effective as EFM and may, in fact, result in fewer cesarean sections, the legal climate has pushed obstetric management further and further into the EFM camp. For practical purposes, therefore, intrapartum monitoring starts with EFM. The theoretical foundations of EFM in labor are the same as for antepartum testing. A baseline in the 100 to 180 bpm range, good beat-to-beat variability, and the absence of late or severe variable decelerations indicate that the fetus is receiving adequate oxygen. If one or more of these criteria are not met, further investigation and usually therapy are necessary.

It is usually customary to begin intrapartum EFM with an

external FHR monitor and tocodynamometer. If there are no untoward changes in the FHR and labor is progressing adequately, these may be all that are necessary. However, if an adequate FHR or contraction recording cannot be obtained because of fetal movement or necessary shifts in maternal position, internal recordings may be required. Also, in cases of suspected fetal jeopardy (any repetitive late or severe variable decelerations, severe bradycardia or tachycardia) when rupture of membranes is feasible internal FHR recordings are usually preferable.

DIRECT FHR MONITORING

By attaching a thin wire electrode directly to the fetal scalp and a grounding plate to the mother, one may obtain a direct FHR recording. By subtracting the maternal signal (from the grounding plate) from the combined maternal-fetal signal (from the scalp electrode), the fetal monitor is able to produce a fetal ECG that exactly corresponds to the FHR. This may be printed either as a continuous FHR recording (which has no artifactual variability) or as an ECG (especially useful for the identification of arrhythmias). Obviously, since the electrode is attached directly to the fetal scalp, this method can only be used after the membranes have been ruptured and the cervix is sufficiently dilated (1 to 2 cm) to allow careful placement of the electrode. Since this procedure carries a very small risk of infection at the electrode site, sterile technique is essential during placement. In addition, the obstetrician must know the details of the fetal presenting part, taking care to avoid inserting the electrode into the face, between sutures, or over a fontanel. There is no contraindication to the use of internal electrodes in breech presentations.

INTRAUTERINE TOCODYNAMOMETRY

Internal monitoring of contractions using a fluid-filled catheter connected to a strain gauge at the monitor and inserted beyond the fetal head into the uterine cavity supplies more information than external tocodynamometry. Unlike external recordings, which indicate only timing and duration of contractions, internal pressure monitoring accurately assesses the strength of contractions as well. In cases of poor external recordings secondary to maternal position (e.g., left lateral supine) or when there is a need for information regarding the actual pressure generated by contractions (e.g., frequent contractions of seemingly adequate intensity to palpation in the face of a failure to progress), intrauterine tocodynamometry is helpful. Like internal FHR monitoring, this procedure requires ruptured membranes and adequate cervical dilatation. There is a small risk of perforating the lower uterine segment or damaging a low-lying placenta, so care must be taken to avoid these complications.

FETAL SCALP pH

Because sustained hypoxia causes the fetus to shift to anaerobic metabolism, it eventually results in lactic acidosis. Presumably, hypoxia of short enough duration to *not* cause acidosis will not harm the fetus. Therefore, when the fetus is

considered to be in jeopardy because of oxygen deprivation, a better assessment of its condition may be obtained by analyzing blood obtained from the fetal scalp or buttock, whichever is presenting. When the cervix is at least 3 cm dilated and the membranes ruptured, the fetal scalp may be directly viewed and isolated through a cone-shaped tube. After wiping it dry and coating it with a silicone gel, one makes a small puncture in the scalp with a scalpel (specially designed to limit depth of penetration) and collects the blood (which beads because of the silicone) into a heparinized capillary tube. While one person then applies pressure to the puncture site with a large cotton applicator, another quickly measures the pH of the collected blood. A pH of 7.25 or higher is considered normal, between 7.20 and 7.25 is borderline, and below 7.20 is acidotic. When interpreting pH, one must be aware that factors other than asphyxia can alter it. Maternal acidosis (often seen in diabetics) causes fetal acidosis, with the fetal pH usually being 0.1 to 0.2 units less than that of the mother. Conversely, maternal alkalosis (usually secondary to hyperventilation, seen in patients in pain) may mask fetal acidemia.

The major danger to the fetus from scalp sampling is hemorrhage. Although the fetus with normal coagulation status is unlikely to bleed significantly after this procedure, there have been cases of fetal exsanguination when an unrecognized coagulopathy existed. Therefore, any episode of vaginal bleeding after scalp puncture should be investigated, both by an attempt to visualize the puncture site (which is often difficult if not impossible), and by a Kleihauer-Betke test on the blood to see if it is of fetal origin. Infection at the puncture site is also a risk, so sterile technique should be rigorously observed. Both of the complications become more likely when multiple samplings are required, which is often the case.

Some have advocated measurement of fetal scalp PO_2 and PCO_2 as well, but these vary greatly from minute to minute and are not as useful as pH, which provides a better overall indicator of fetal condition.

APPLICATION OF INTRAPARTUM MONITORING TECHNIQUES

Begin with external FHR and contraction monitoring. As long as FHR and labor are satisfactory, continue. Switch to internal FHR electrode if

1. A good FHR tracing is not obtainable, because of either maternal positioning or fetal activity
2. There are FHR patterns that are not reassuring (late or persistently severe variable decelerations, severe tachycardia or bradycardia, or loss of variability for no apparent reason

Undertake measures to remedy the situation. If the problem appears to be cord entrapment or compression (severe variable decelerations), attempt shifting the maternal position to either lateral recumbent or knee-chest. If the problem appears to be fetal hypoxia (late decelerations, bradycardia, tachycardia, or unexplained loss of variability), attempt to increase fetal oxygenation by

↑ fetal oxygen:

1. Administering maternal oxygen by mask.
2. Increasing <u>placental perfusion</u> through ma<u>ternal hydra</u><u>tion</u> with <u>lactated Ringer's solution and shifting the</u> <u>mother to a lateral recumbent position to avoid</u> aorto-caval compression.

mat. lat. recumbent position to avoid aorto caval compression

If the <u>abnormal pattern persists for more than 20 minutes,</u> obtain a <u>fetal scalp pH.</u>

1. When the fetal scalp pH is 7.25 or greater, labor may continue with all of the above precautions. If the ominous patterns do not resolve, the pH should be retested in 20 to 30 minutes. If it passes, no further sampling is necessary.
2. If the initial pH is between 7.20 and 7.25, even if the pattern resolves, the scalp sampling should be repeated in 20 to 30 minutes.
3. An initial pH lower than 7.20 is an indication for immediate resampling. Confirmation of such a low pH requires immediate delivery.

repeat in 20 min if still acidotic ↓ immediate delivery

Intrauterine pressure monitoring is indicated when the progress of labor has not been satisfactory in the face of contractions of apparently normal intensity. In many cases, a trial of oxytocin stimulation without internal tocodynamometry may be sufficient as long as the situation is low risk for uterine rupture and the FHR shows no evidence of distress. When this does not succeed or there is a suspicion that the contractions are sufficiently strong and that the real problem is cephalopelvic disproportion, intrauterine monitoring may help verify this. Normal uterine contractions are generally considered to vary between 25 and 60 mm Hg in intensity.

LABOR

INITIATION OF LABOR

Labor has been called the "acute process that terminates the chronic condition of pregnancy." It is defined as the occurrence of regular uterine contractions that result in progressive effacement and dilatation of the cervix. Ideally, it should occur after fetal maturity has been obtained but before the placenta begins to deteriorate, usually between 37 and 41 weeks of completed amenorrhea. The causes of the onset of labor are unknown. Although considerable attention has been devoted to this subject in the past two decades and considerable progress has been made in understanding the process, the factors that initiate labor are still obscure.

It has become clear, however, that multiple factors are at work, including the fetus and the amniotic membranes. Although it has long been suspected that the fetus plays a role in terminating its own stay within the uterus, the exact sequence of events has proved elusive. In many pregnancies characterized by anencephaly and its associated adrenal hypoplasia or by fetal adrenal hypoplasia alone, the onset of spontaneous labor is greatly delayed. However, in normal pregnancies, despite much diligent searching, no consistent change in any of the steroids produced by the fetal adrenal has been documented. It is also apparent that at some point the uterus begins to contract

in a more rhythmic and organized fashion, and currently the prime suspect as an inciting agent is prostaglandin E_2 (PGE_2), which, unlike oxytocin, is capable of inducing both cervical ripening and uterine contractions at any stage of pregnancy. The most likely site for production of PGE_2 that induces labor is the amnion/chorion complex, which may explain why both "stripping" of the membranes and amnionitis may precipitate labor.

DIAGNOSIS OF LABOR   *Braxton-Hicks cont*

Labor may be diagnosed with confidence when uterine contractions resulting in progressive effacement and dilatation of the cervix occur. Late in pregnancy, false labor will often occur, with uncomfortable rhythmic contractions but no change in the cervix. These so-called accelerated Braxton-Hicks contractions may represent either prodromal labor or may stop and start for weeks. Conversely, the effacement and dilatation commonly seen late in pregnancy do not represent labor because they are not attended by regular contractions.

UTERINE CHANGES IN LABOR

The contractions of labor are concentrated in the upper two-thirds of the uterus, whereas the <u>lower uterine segment</u> is <u>less active</u> and the cervix remains passive. The effect is to progressively thicken the fundus while thinning out and "drawing up" both the lower segment and the cervix. The cervix is converted from a 2-cm cork-like structure to an extremely thin (100% effaced), easily stretched membrane not distinguishable from the equally thinned lower uterine segment. The combination of the two is separated from the fundus by the physiological retraction ring. The upper segment is capable of doing this to the cervix because of the pressure generated by the descending presenting part or by the bulging intact membranes. Theoretically, once effacement has occurred, the force of the contracting body of the uterus serves to progressively pull the cervix over the presenting part, effecting cervical dilatation. In reality, however, early dilatation usually occurs simultaneously with effacement. Coincident with effacement and dilatation, the force of uterine contractions causes the fetus to gradually descend into the birth canal. Although most of the descent usually occurs after full dilatation and is caused by the combined pressure of contractions and simultaneous maternal "pushing," a considerable portion of this work may be accomplished during the first stage.

PROGRESS OF LABOR

Labor has been divided into stages and normal progress rates established for each. These progress rates are used as guidelines to assess the quality of the labor and to gauge the need for intervention.

Stage I   *cervical ripening / effacement*

From the onset of labor to the attainment of full cervical dilatation, labor may be expected to fall within certain predictable norms. This stage, however, encompasses several phases. The latent phase may vary from nonexistent to as long as 24 hours and is characterized by relatively short contractions

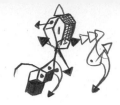

(15 to 30 seconds) of variable frequency, intensity, and discomfort. Typically, cervical softening and effacement are the prime accomplishments of this phase. The **active phase** of labor follows and is usually associated with longer (30 to 60 seconds), stronger, more frequent (every 2 to 3 minutes) contractions that effect cervical dilatation. In normally progressing labors, once the active phase has begun, cervical dilatation will occur at the rate of at least 1 cm/hour in nulliparas and 1 to 2 cm/hour in parous women. Some deceleration of progress is often described as full dilatation is neared, but equally often the reverse may occur.

Stage II
- 1hr multipar
- 2hrs nullipar

After full cervical dilatation has been attained until the birth is completed, the force of the contractions serves to push the fetus through the birth canal. The obstructions to birth at this point are the muscles of the pelvic floor and bones of the pelvis. These cannot usually be overcome by contractions alone but require active maternal participation in the form of pushing. Although many factors may affect the length of this stage (fetal size, pelvic capacity, weakness or strength of the pelvic floor, frequency and intensity of contractions, effectiveness of the mother as a "pusher"), the generally accepted norms are 2 hours for a nullipara and 1 hour for subsequent deliveries. Since the advent of EFM, however, many physicians have allowed parturients longer second stages if fetal condition is good and progressive descent is occurring.

Stage III
5-10 minutes

Immediately after the delivery of the fetus until expulsion of the placenta, the uterus changes shape. As it contracts while expelling the fetus, its surface area decreases, causing the placenta to be separated from it in spots at the level of the decidua spongiosum. This causes hemorrhage at the sites of initial separation, which coalesce to further the cleavage. When separation is complete or at least sufficiently advanced, the placenta is expelled into the vagina through the dilated cervix, pulling the fetal membranes with it. Usually the third stage of labor lasts from 5 to 15 minutes. If the placenta has not delivered spontaneously within this time, it may be expressed manually by transabdominal uterine compression (Credé's maneuver) or removed manually from the inside.

MOVEMENTS OF THE FETUS DURING LABOR

As the fetus is propelled through the birth canal during labor, it is forced to change position several times to accommodate both its own anatomy and that of its mother's pelvis. Failure to follow this course may obstruct labor, or at least retard its progress. Knowledge of these positional changes is of importance to the obstetrician as he or she follows the course of the labor and performs the actual delivery. The ensuing steps are described for an OA presentation with modifications for OP in parentheses. The principal movements are **engagement, descent, flexion, internal rotation, extension, external rotation,** and **expulsion.**

Engagement of the fetal head, or descent into the pelvis so that the widest transverse diameter is past the inlet, may occur any time from several weeks before the onset of labor until late in its course. Typically, in first pregnancies with adequate pelvic diameters for the fetus, the fetal head becomes engaged before labor begins, while in subsequent gestations it usually occurs after the onset of contractions. The usual positon for engagement is transverse (LOT, ROT), with the anterior fontanel presenting (so that the occipitofrontal diameter enters the pelvis). Failure of the head to become engaged suggests a contracted pelvis. Engagement may be diagnosed on vaginal examination by determining that the leading edge of the fetal skull has descended at least to the level of the ischial spines, unless there is considerable molding.

Descent past the point of engagement then occurs until the head meets resistance, which results in **flexion** (extension if posterior) to allow the narrower suboccipitobregmatic diameter to descend further. Upon approaching the pelvic floor, the head undergoes **internal rotation** toward the OA (or OP) position, usually being detectable in an intermediate stage (LOA, ROA, LOP, ROP). Further descent brings the head, usually in either the direct OA or OP position, to the perineum, where it delivers by **extension** (flexion if OP). Once the head has delivered, it undergoes **external rotation** back to the plane of the shoulders, which usually fit best into the AP diameter of the outlet. If it has come from the LOA position, it will rotate back to the left, and if from the ROA, to the right. The birth is then completed by **expulsion,** which rapidly follows after the delivery of the anterior shoulder by downward traction on the head to bring it under the symphysis.

MANAGEMENT OF LABOR

Most labors are managed within a hospital center, so that on diagnosis of labor, by the criteria previously enumerated, the patient is admitted to the labor and delivery area. Most physicians prefer to know earlier rather than later that a patient is in labor, and they use the criterion of contractions every 5 minutes to have her call.

On admission to labor and delivery, the following measures are taken:

1. A brief but appropriately thorough history is taken, including the following: last menstrual period and EDC; the character and timing of contractions; the presence or absence of fluid leakage; significant events of the pregnancy; previous significant obstetric, surgical, and medical history.

2. A brief but appropriately thorough physical examination should include the following: vital signs; abdominal examination for height of the fundus, location and rate of the fetal heart, and Leopold's maneuvers; a sterile vaginal examination for cervical dilatation, state of the membranes (by nitrazine pH testing and microscopic examination for ferning, if there is any question), presentationa nd station of the fetus, and pelvic architecture; and routine examination of the heart, lungs, and neurological status.

3. Laboratory examination includes a hemoglobin/hematocrit and blood type and Rh determination (if not already known); a urinalysis for protein, glucose, and ketones; other tests as mandated by the patient's specific condition.

4. Fetal monitoring, either by EFM or stethoscope, is begun.

Once maternal and fetal well-being have been established, the following procedures may be performed:

Side effect
oxytocin

Oxytocin T½: 90-180 sec
i.e 1-3 min

1. A mild enema may be administered. Although some object to this as uncomfortable and unnecessary, the aesthetic benefits of childbirth without stool, the lower risk of contamination during delivery, and the mother's not needing to have a bowel movement for several days postpartum would seem to outweigh the discomfort. Contraindications to enema include imminent delivery and ruptured membranes with an unengaged presenting part if the cervix is not closed.

2. If epsiotomy is anticipated, removal of hair from the posterior half of the perineum is desirable.

3. An intravenous infusion of lactated Ringer's solution at a rate from 50 to 150 ml/hour may be begun if the patient requires hydration. Since several studies have shown that fetuses tolerate hypoxia better when they are not fed glucose, maternal IV glucose solutions should be used sparingly, mostly to avoid or treat maternal hypoglycemia. Although it is preferable for the mother to avoid consuming solid foods during labor, both because they promote nausea during active labor and because of the possible necessity of anesthesia, most patients in labor tolerate small to moderate amounts of clear fluids.

4. Most patients seem most comfortable in a semireclining position during labor, although early in the process many prefer to walk between contractions. Although external FHR monitoring and tocodynamometry may be best performed in the supine position, this may predispose to aortocaval compression and supine hypotension syndrome. In most cases, it is possible to adjust the machinery so that it does not compromise either maternal comfort or fetal safety. Certainly every effort should be made to this end. It is also worthwhile to note that EFM is not incompatible with periodic ambulation.

5. Unless the mother has been sedated or narcotized or has had epidural anesthesia, there should be no need for bed pans or catheters.

6. Maternal vital signs should be monitored and recorded hourly.

7. Fetal condition should be monitored by either continuous EFM or auscultation of the fetal heart at 15-minute intervals in the first stage of labor and 5-minute intervals during the second stage.

8. Vaginal examinations should be repeated every 1 to 2 hours to assess the rate of cervical change and fetal descent. Proper vaginal examination requires two sterile gloved hands (one to hold the labia open while an antiseptic is applied and one to perform the examination).

INDICATIONS FOR NONINTERVENTION DURING LABOR

If there is no evidence of fetal jeopardy and cervical dilatation is progressing at 1 to 2 cm/hour during the first stage of labor or descent is progressive during the second stage and delivery can be anticipated within 1 to 2 hours after full dilatation, the obstetrician serves the patient best by remaining an observer and providing her with moral support.

INDICATIONS FOR INTERVENTION DURING LABOR

1. **Fetal jeopardy**, at any stage during labor, demands immediate action by the obstetrician to safeguard the fetus. The various threats to the fetus in labor, and appropriate responses, have been outlined in the section on fetal monitoring or will be covered in future sections dealing with specific conditions.

2. **Hypotonic or desultory labor**, characterized by contractions of inadequate intensity or frequency in the presence of an adequate pelvis, should be suspected when cervical dilatation does not occur quickly enough. Appropriate treatment for this is intravenous oxytocin administration by pump. An appropriate solution for infusion is 10 units in 1,000 ml of either lactated Ringer's solution or 0.9% NaCl, resulting in a concentration of 10 mU/ml. There are three major risks associated with the use of oxytocin during labor:

Fetal distress: By beginning the infusion at the rate of 1 mU/minute and increasing the flow by 1 to 2 mU/minute every 15 to 30 minutes until adequate contractions are obtained, the likelihood of hyperstimulation and fetal distress is minimized. However, even while taking this precaution, oxytocin stimulation of labor should not be attempted without continuous EFM, so that if the labor does become too intense for the fetus, it will be detected as soon as possible. When this does occur, because its half-life is very short (between 90 and 180 seconds), prompt cessation of the infusion will offer almost immediate relief. Oxytocin should never be administered during labor without a constant infusion pump to guarantee a continuous and accurate flow rate.

Water intoxication: Because oxytocin has an antidiuretic effect, interfering with free-water clearance by the distal tubule of the kidney, it is possible to produce water intoxication by administering it in amounts in excess of 20 mU/minute if it is dissolved in a salt-free solution (D_5W). This does not occur if it is given in either lactated Ringer's solution or 0.9% NaCl.

Uterine rupture: The risk of uterine rupture due to hyperstimulation with oxytocin infusion is minimal in the previously intact uterus. Even in the patient who has had a previous cesarean section or hysterotomy, in general, if labor is not contraindicated then judicious use of oxytocin is not unreasonable. Some feel more comfortable, in such situations, when monitoring the strength of the contractions with an intrauterine pressure gauge.

3. If failure to progress in labor is due to CPD, as determined by pelvic examination or by failure of an adequate trial of oxytocin to effect progress, cesarean section is appropriate. Although there are still some who advocate x-ray pelvimetry to diagnose CPD, most believe that the radiation exposure to the fetus is best avoided and that a trial of oxytocin is preferable if the obstetrician is not certain that CPD exists.

THE ACTUAL DELIVERY

When the head begins to crown (becomes visible without manually separating the labia), the end of the second stage is near. Delivery may be performed in the dorsal lithotomy position, the lateral Sims' position, or a number of variations on sitting or squatting (birthing chair, birthing bed). In the United States, the dorsal lithotomy is still most common and affords the obstetrician the most control of the delivering fetus. Advocates of birth without episiotomy prefer the lateral Sims', which may place slightly less strain on the perineum. Fans of birthing chair-type positions claim a shortened second stage.

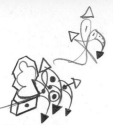

However, in my experience, birthing chairs are associated with more perineal edema and a greater likelihood of laceration.

The size of a normal introital opening may be 3 to 5 cm by 1 to 2 cm, while the diameter of the fetal head is approximately 10 cm. Obviously, there is a mismatch. **Episiotomy**, or incision of the perineum between the vagina and anus, is commonly done in an attempt to prevent uncontrolled or extended tears during delivery. The episiotomy may be either midline or mediolateral. Midline episiotomies have several advantages. They are associated with less blood loss, they heal better, and they are less painful afterward. The only advantage to the mediolateral (usually right mediolateral to avoid the descending rectum) is that it may avoid tears through into the anus if the perineum is very short.

If episiotomy is planned, some sort of anethesia for the perineum is administered. This may be local infiltration or regional (pudendal or epidural) block (see the section on anesthesia). Regional anesthetics generally offer better coverage for repair and have the additional advantage of not distending the perineal tissues, making extension of the episiotomy less likely.

Delivery of the fetus

Once the head is ready for delivery, it may be allowed to exit spontaneously, propelled by either a contraction or maternal pushing. More often, however, manual control of the head is exerted by the obstetrician in an attempt to minimize trauma to the vaginal outlet. This may be either the Ritgen maneuver, which consists of pulling the chin of the fetus through the distended perineum with one hand while pushing upward on the already delivered occiput with the other, aiding with extension and speeding delivery. An alternative is to allow the head to be delivered by maternal force while protecting the perineum by pinching together the perineal skin at the base of the episiotomy (or introitus, if no episiotomy has been done) with one hand while controlling the speed of the delivery by exerting opposing pressure on the occiput with the other.

Immediately upon delivery of the head, restitution occurs and the head rotates back to the lateral position it occupied prior to birth. The nostrils and mouth should be suctioned to remove excess amniotic fluid. This is of special importance if there has been meconium but is desirable in all cases.

Next one must check for the presence of a nuchal cord. If it is present, it can usually be unwound by pulling it over the fetus's head. If the cord is too tightly wound around the neck for this, it should be clamped, cut, and then unwound.

Once all this has been attended to, the external rotation of the head, if it has not occurred completely spontaneously, should be completed. One next delivers the anterior shoulder by downward traction on the head. This should be performed slowly and gradually until the shoulder appears under the symphysis. Reversal of the traction to an upward direction then results in the delivery of the posterior shoulder. The arms may follow spontaneously or may require individual delivery. The delivery of the rest of the fetus almost always occurs immediately. Repeat suctioning of the mouth and nose should now be performed, perhaps with gentle stimulation to encourage breathing.

If the umbilical cord has not yet been cut, now is the time.

Two clamps are placed on the cord, several centimeters from the navel, and it is cut between them. If the infant is breathing normally and needs no special care, it should be covered with a blanket and given to the mother and father.

Delivery of the placenta

A specimen of blood from the umbilical cord should be obtained and the vagina and outlet inspected for lacerations or extensions of the episiotomy while awaiting separation of the placenta. This may be recognized by the following signs:

1. A gush of blood, signaling separation of an edge
2. A change in shape of the uterus, to more globular, signaling a collection of blood behind the placenta
3. Descent of the cord

In reality, examination of the cervix within several minutes after delivery of the infant usually detects the bulging placenta filling the lower cervix or upper vagina. Spontaneous delivery of the placenta often occurs within 5 minutes, but many obstetricians prefer manual expression. By combining *gentle* traction on the cord with a squeezing motion on the shrunken fundus, the third stage may be accelerated. Care must be exercised not to pull hard on the cord while pushing down on the fundus or a uterine inversion may result. Manual removal of the placenta is sometimes necessary. This is indicated in cases of partial separation attended by excessive bleeding and in prolonged third stages (greater than 15 minutes). Preferred technique for this is to feel for the partially separated edge and to dissect along cleavage planes within the uterus.

As soon as delivery of the placenta is complete, uterine contraction, which stops the bleeding, is encouraged by massage or by oxytocic infusion. While we still consider an informal fourth stage of labor to last for an hour after completion of the third, and careful observation for bleeding during this period is mandatory, most cases of postpartum hemorrhage can be avoided by a constant infusion of normal saline or lactated Ringer's solution containing 20 units of oxytocin during this time.

The newly delivered placenta must be inspected for missing pieces or torn edges, indicating retained placental tissue. After the uterus has been emptied, the entire birth canal should be systematically inspected, from the top down. In today's world of aseptic technique and effective diagnosis and treatment of infection, manual exploration of the uterus should be standard. One can be virtually certain there is no retained tissue and will sometimes discover anomalies or uterine rents that are otherwise unsuspected. Following uterine exploration, the cervix and vaginal vault should be visualized. Finally, if not done before, the lower tract must be thoroughly inspected.

Lastly, episiotomy or laceration repair if necessary is performed.

ANALGESIA AND ANESTHESIA

Labor and delivery are usually painful processes that often require pain relief. This may be either an attempt to ease the pain (analgesia) or to eliminate all sensation (anesthesia). It may be necessary for a prolonged period of time (labor) or for relatively short duration (delivery). The basic principle of obstetric pain relief is to afford the mother as much comfort as possible while affecting the following factors as little as possible:

1. Fetal well-being
2. Maternal well-being
3. Progress of labor

Since all pharmacologic agents have potential side effects, the less intervention necessary, the better. Mothers who have taken prepared childbirth classes (Lamaze or other) usually will be less afraid and have various nonpharmacologic tools for coping with labor. They therefore need less analgesia during labor and generally have better experiences.

ANALGESIA

The most commonly used agents during labor are narcotics (meperidine, morphine). All narcotic analgesics are essentially comparable in their effects and side effects. They all

1. Are systemic agents that make the mother oblivious to the pain
2. May be administered IV or IM
3. Have a rapid onset of action (almost instantaneously IV and within 15 to 20 minutes IM) and relatively short duration (2 to 4 hours)
4. Are easily reversible with a narcotic antagonist such as naloxone (Narcan)
5. Have virtually no effect on established labor
6. Cross the placenta to affect the fetus

Undesirable side effects including the following:

1. Maternal nausea and vomiting
2. In large doses, maternal respiratory depression and sedation
3. FHR changes, specifically loss of beat-to-beat variability for up to 4 hours
4. If given shortly before delivery, fetal respiratory depression and sedation, which may be persistent because of poor detoxification by the fetal liver

Usual dosages are 50 to 100 mg of meperidine or 5 to 10 mg of morphine repeated as often as necessary. In general, IV administration is more effective and shorter lived and therefore more desirable. One aims for minimal discomfort during a contraction as a therapeutic endpoint. Overdosage is unlikely if one stays within recommended dosages and awaits patient discomfort before readministration.

If one needs to rapidly reverse the narcotic effect, IV naloxone (0.4 mg adult dosage, 0.02 to 0.04 mg neonatal dosage) is completely effective within 1 to 2 minutes. A pure antagonist, it has no depressive effects of its own. Its effect, however, last only 30 minutes, so repeated doses may be required. Resuscitated babies may lapse into unconsciousness when its action wears off, so careful observation is important.

Narcotic analgesics are often given in conjunction with a tranquilizer of the phenothiazine class, such as promethazine, to potentiate the analgesia and relieve the nausea. Although these are desirable ends, the combination involves more sedation and fetal depression. In addition, there is no way to reverse the effects of the tranquilizer. The usual dosage is 25 mg along with the narcotic. Tranquilizing agents of the benzodiazepine category are extremely long-lived and poorly metabolized by the fetus and so should not be used.

ANESTHESIA

Anesthesia may be used for either labor or delivery. Alternatives for labor are paracervical block (which is much less widely used than before) and lumbar epidural block. For vaginal delivery, perineal anesthesia is desirable and may be obtained by local infiltration, regional block (pudendal, spinal, epidural), or general anesthesia (much less desirable). When cesarean section is necessary, either regional (spinal, epidural) or general anesthesia is used. Aside from general anesthesia, all techniques involve blocking various nerve fibers with local anesthetic agents, all members of the "-caine" family.

Anesthetic agents

For the most part, the members of the -caine family are largely interchangeable. All have similar side effects and toxicities (especially CNS) except for prilocaine (Citanest), which in addition to other effects may precipitate methemoglobinemia. Demonstrated allergy to one may be considered allergy to all. Some are shorter acting, like procaine (Novocaine) and chloroprocaine (Nesacaine); others are intermediate, like lidocaine (Xylocaine) and mepivacaine (Carbocaine); and still others longer acting, like tetracaine (Pontocaine). Choice of agent is usually determined by timing needs.

Anesthesia for labor

The pain of labor arises from two sources. Uterine contractions create fundal pain and, by dilatation, cervical pain. These sensations are carried from Frankenhäuser's paracervical ganglion to the pelvic and hypogastric plexuses and then into the spinal cord from T10–L1. This pain may be blocked either at Frankenhäuser's ganglion (paracervical block) or its entry to the spinal cord (epidural).

Paracervical block. By infiltrating a local anesthetic agent submucosally at the cervicovaginal junction at the 3 to 4 o'clock and 8 to 9 o'clock positions, one may anesthetize Frankenhäuser's ganglion and relieve the pain of uterine contractions and cervical dilatation. Great care must be taken to limit the penetration of the needle (usually a guide is used) and to avoid injection through the lower uterine segment *into the fetus.* Although it is effective, this form of anesthesia has several major drawbacks:

1. Large amounts of anesthetic (10 to 20 ml) are necessary, long before delivery, often in repeated doses.
2. Due to excellent blood supply to the area, large amounts of anesthetic are absorbed by both the mother and fetus, frequently resulting in fetal bradycardia and occasionally in maternal toxicity.

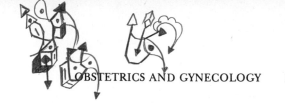

3. Risk of a pelvic hematoma from laceration of a paracervical vein is not small.

Because of its frequent undesirable consequences and because it provides no anesthesia for delivery, paracervical block is less commonly used than before, especially when epidural block is available.

Epidural anesthesia. By injecting an anesthetic agent into the epidural space, the nerve roots that supply the abdomen and pelvis may be blocked at their entry into the spinal cord. Because the space is relatively large, a small catheter may be left in place and repeated doses given, extending the period of anesthesia to many hours. By varying the strength and amount of the agent and the position of the patient, the level of the block may be controlled to supply anesthesia for labor (T10–L2), vaginal delivery (down to S5), or cesearean section (up to T6 or T8). Typically, the block is begun during labor and then extended upward or downward depending on the kind of delivery planned.

The major advantages of this form of anesthesia are as follows:

1. When done correctly, most patients obtain complete relief of pain without changes of sensorium.
2. It may be extended, by indwelling catheter, for the length of the labor.
3. Relatively small amounts of anesthetic are absorbed, so toxicity risks for both mother and child are small.

The major risks of this procedure are as follows:

1. *Most seriously,* if inadvertant spinal puncture is performed and *not realized,* relatively much too much anesthetic is directly into the subarachnoid space, resulting in a "high spinal" and possible cardiorespiratory arrest.
2. If inadvertant spinal puncture occurs but is recognized, since the needle for epidural is much larger than that used for spinal, a postspinal headache is likely. In skilled hands, this occurs approximately 1% of the time. It may be managed either by bed rest or a blood patch.
3. *Most commonly,* because the epidural involves a large sympathetic blockade, there is pooling of blood in the lower half of the body. This impairs cardiac return and may result in severe **hypotension and subsequent fetal distress**. Late decelerations of the FHR and bradycardia are not rare shortly after placement of epidural anesthesia. They are best managed by correction of hypotension (rapid infusion of lactated Ringer's, maternal repositioning, possibly small doses of ephedrine), and **maternal hyperoxygenation**.
4. Epidural anesthesia may interfere with labor, especially early in its course. This, however, is usually not of major importance as pain relief is usually not necessary until labor is well established. In addition, if labor is impeded, oxytocin augmentation may be performed.
5. Second stage labor may be impaired by pelvic anesthesia if the mother cannot feel herself pushing. This is easily overcome by timing the anesthesia so it wears off at about the time of full dilatation and reinstituting it shortly before delivery. This sort of management should eliminate the higher incidence of midforceps deliveries sometimes attributed to the use of epidurals.
6. Rarely, the epidural needle may come to rest in an epidural vein. If the anesthesiologist is unaware, direct IV injection of anesthetic will result, possibly causing convulsions and cardiovascular complications. This may be easily avoided by always aspirating before injecting.
7. Because of the large volumes of fluid infused and the concomitant pelvic anesthesia, bladder distension and subsequent atony may result. Therefore, careful monitoring of the state of the urinary bladder is necessary.

Epidural anesthesia should obviously be performed only by someone very skilled in this procedure and only in settings where emergency life support, resuscitation, and cesarean section are readily available. Even in good hands, however, the above complications may occur, and certain precautions are important to minimize these risks. All patients should

1. Be thoroughly hydrated (at least 1,000 ml lactated Ringer's) and have a running IV from institution of anesthesia until delivery
2. Have continuous electronic FHR monitoring, preferably by internal electrode, since frequent maternal repositioning may be necessary
3. Have frequent blood pressure monitoring

Additionally, certain conditions pose either relative or absolute contraindications to epidural anesthesia. It should never be performed in the face of

1. Local infection
2. Maternal coagulation disorder
3. Maternal hypotension
4. Active fetal distress

Relative contraindications include (1) maternal hypertension or gestational hypertension and (2) neurological or vertebral disorders.

Anesthesia for delivery

Delivery, unlike labor, is of relatively short duration, so that the need to be able to continue anesthesia for long periods of time does not figure into the equation.

Local infiltration. For vaginal delivery, to perform either episiotomy or repair of lacerations, only perineal anesthesia is required. The safest way to obtain this is local infiltration. Only a few milliliters of a -caine are usually necessary, only a few minutes before delivery. Unless one injects directly into a blood vessel or the mother has an unknown allergy to the agent, there are no important or common maternal or fetal complications. This major disadvantage is that the anesthesia obtained, while sufficient for episiotomy and repair, is frequently not complete.

Pudendal block. The pudendal nerves, carrying sensory fibers from the entire lower vagina and perineum, may be anesthetized as they pass behind the sacrospinous ligaments at the tip of the ischial spines on both sides of the pelvis. Using a trumpet guide to limit penetration of the needle to 1 to 2 cm, one can place 10 ml of local anesthetic behind and around each ligament, bathing the nerve and obtaining total perineal anesthesia. Usually done in the delivery room minutes before delivery, pudendal block provides better, more global anesthesia than local infiltration for episiotomy and/or repair and involves little extra risk. The major complications arising from pudendal block are toxicity from IV injection (always aspirate before injecting) and hematoma from laceration of a pelvic vessel. The risks of hematoma may be minimized by making as few punctures as possible with as narrow a needle as possible (22-gauge), never attempting pudendal block after delivery (the fetal head in the pelvis tends to tamponade bleeding before delivery), and avoiding its use in patients with coagulation disorders.

Epidural anesthesia. If begun during labor, epidural anesthesia is usually extended to cover either the perineum or abdomen for delivery. If it is being done strictly for delivery (usually cesarean section), anesthesia will often be produced without the use of an indwelling catheter, although many anesthesiologists prefer the security of knowing that if the delivery takes longer than the initial anesthesia lasts (an unlikely event) they may reinforce it through the catheter. Preparation for and complications of epidural anesthesia for delivery are the same as for labor.

Spinal anesthesia. Used much more frequently before the advent of epidural anesthesia, spinal blockade operates in much the same fashion. However, because the small size of the subarachnoid space makes the use of an indwelling catheter fraught with complications, it is limited to a single event resulting in only 1 to 2 hours of anesthesia. As such, its use is more appropriate for delivery than labor. Depending on whether vaginal or abdominal delivery is planned, the levels are adjusted approximately. Essentially, spinal anesthesia requires the same preparation as epidural anesthesia. It involves similar risks, except that the incidence of spinal headaches is far higher and there is a small but definable risk of arachnoiditis. Contraindications are the same as for epidural block, which is usually considered preferable today.

General anesthesia. General anesthesia consists of making the patient unconscious to perform a surgical procedure. There are two major risks to this. First, what makes the mother unconscious makes the baby unconscious. Second, unconscious people have no gag reflex and are at risk for aspiration of gastric contents. For this reason, many procedures that used to to merit general anesthesia are now performed under regional block. There are, however, certain circumstances under which general anesthesia is still preferable:

1. When anesthesia is needed immediately, such as for repair of cervical laceration or in cases of fetal distress or cord prolapse
2. When regional anesthesia is strictly contraindicated, as in coagulation disorders and in the face of maternal hemorrhage, sepsis, or shock
3. When regional anesthesia fails
4. When the patient is allergic to -caine anesthestics

There are two major forms of general anesthesia—inhalation and intravenous. Of the inhalation agents, only nitrous oxide is widely used in obstetrics. Providing analgesia at concentrations of 40 to 50%, it is sometimes used for vaginal delivery along with local anesthesia. However, because it impairs consciousness, it is not suitable analgesia for patients who desire natural childbirth. At concentrations necessary to provide anesthesia (80 to 85%), nitrous oxide inevitably produces maternal and fetal hypoxia and is therefore not suitable as an anesthetic by itself. It is often used in combination with other agents during cesarean section for what is known as "balanced general anesthesia."

Other commonly used inhalation anesthetics, such as halothane, enflurane, and methoxyflurane, are usually avoided in obstetrics because they induce profound myometrial relaxation and predispose to obstetric hemorrhage. In rare cases, however, when uterine relaxation is needed in a hurry, (e.g., in internal versions), one of these agents may be desirable.

Of the intravenous agents, thiopental is most commonly used. Causing unconsciousness in less than a minute, it is usually the agent with which anesthesia is begun. However, since it does not cause muscle relaxation, it is not sufficient by itself. Anesthesia is most often induced with an ultrashort-acting barbiturate, followed by paralysis with succinylcholine and intubation to prevent aspiration. The unconscious state is then maintained with a combination of intravenous narcotics and inhalation of nitrous oxide, while surgical relaxation results from continued paralysis. If the fetus is delivered within a few minutes of induction, there is little or no anesthesia-related fetal depression. This balanced anesthesia offers the patient a pleasant sleep, minimal fetal effect, and few risks related to the anesthesia drugs.

The one remaining complication, aspiration, usually results either during the induction or reversal. Steps should be taken to minimize both the likelihood and consequences of this. Several measures will reduce the likelihood of aspiration:

1. The patient should be NPO as long as possible, up to 8 hours, before any planned procedure.
2. Oral intake during labor should be restricted to small amounts of clear fluids.
3. Intubation should be performed immediately on loss of consciousness.
4. Extubation should be postponed until the patient has regained her gag reflex.

To minimize the risks of aspiration, should it occur, antacids are used to neutralize stomach acid. Sodium citrate is preferable to particulate formulations of magnesium and aluminum. A dose of 30 ml should be given one-half hour prior to anesthesia, if possible.

CARE OF THE NEWBORN INFANT

The moment of birth requires remarkable adjustments by the fetus. Previously dependent on the maternal circulation for much of its survival needs, it has only a few minutes to begin to fend for itself in several very basic ways. The most critical of these is the need to breathe, which involves alteration in both the respiratory and circulatory systems. Upon delivery of the infant, the placental circulation is compromised by the contracting uterus. Within a minute or two at most, on clamping of the cord, the infant is totally dependent on breathing to supply its oxygen needs.

Breathing of amnionic fluid occurs throughout the second half of pregnancy and is, in fact, necessary for proper lung development. At birth, the fluid is replaced with air, and full expansion of the lungs becomes critical. Much of the fluid is perhaps expressed by thoracic pressure experienced during birth. Some of it is coughed up, and the rest is probably removed over several hours by vascular and lymphatic drainage.

The first breath involves much greater expansion of the lungs than occurred in utero and a concomitant drop in pressure. This is made possible by adequate surfactant, preventing local atelectasis. These pressure changes are accompanied by pulmonary vascular decompression and a relative rush of blood through the pulmonary arteries. Exposure of this blood to the much higher PO_2 of air (remember that, in utero the fetus received placental blood with a PO_2 of 30 mm Hg) results in a rapid increase in fetal PO_2 and vasoconstriction of the ductus arteriosus (oxygen dependent). These two factors, lower pulmonary vascular pressures and constriction of the ductus, virtually eliminate shunting from the pulmonic system to the aorta and improve fetal oxygenation.

The second major transition made by the newborn involves heat regulation. Formerly encased in a warm bath, the neonate, being wet, small, and a poor regulator of temperature, will chill rapidly in room-temperature air. There is little the infant can do to compensate, so drying, blankets, and radiant warmers are critical.

EVENTS IN THE DELIVERY ROOM

On delivery of the head, before completion of birth, most obstetricians suction the mouth and external nares to remove excess fluid.

The delivery is completed, and the infant is held head downward to facilitate further pulmonary tree drainage. Suctioning is often performed again. If there is no meconium, further respiratory exploration is not necessary. If there has been meconium, later visualization of the vocal cords is indicated to be sure aspiration has not occurred.

The umbilical cord is clamped and cut. Delayed clamping of the cord will allow transfer of up to 100 ml of blood from the placenta to the baby or vice versa, depending on the level at which the infant is held. For most healthy full-term babies, this makes no difference. If the infant is likely to be anemic, this transfusion may be beneficial. In general, one holds the infant at approximately the same height as the mother's perineum and clamps the cord as soon as is reasonably convenient.

By this time, the infant has usually begun to breathe and cry and exhibits good tone and reactivity. If this is the case, the infant should be wrapped in a blanket to keep warm and may be given to the mother. If breathing is less than optimal, mild stimulation such as rubbing with a towel, tapping the soles, or light shaking is applied. If, after these measures, breathing is still impaired or tone or color is poor, the infant should be transferred to the radiant warmer, where necessary resuscitative measures may be instituted. Delay here will usually compound the problem, since the nonbreathing infant is becoming progressively more hypoxic. This type of assessment is formalized as the Apgar score (see below).

If the infant is reactive, an antibacterial ointment is applied to eyes to prevent ophthalmitis. Years ago, penicillin and silver nitrate were the agents of choice, because *Neisseria gonorrhoeae* was the most common etiology. Now, because of the increasing incidence of *Chlamydia,* tetracycline and erythromycin are increasingly used.

The infant is footprinted and the mother fingerprinted, on the same paper.

A brief physical examination is performed, checking for major anomalies.

APGAR SCORING

The Apgar scoring system (Table 3-2) evaluates five aspects of neonatal condition. The infant is scored at 1 and 5 minutes. The 1-minute score reflects the need for resuscitation or not, and the 5-minute score has long-term prognostic value. Because of advances in neonatal care and resuscitation, many babies with poor 5-minute scores may be effectively resuscitated. Therefore, many obstetricians have added a 10-minute rescoring, which they feel has greater prognostic significance.

Apgar scores at 1 minute in the 7 to 10 range indicate a healthy baby in need of routine care only. With scores from 4 to 6, mild stimulatory or resuscitative measures are indicated. The infant with a score below 4 is a medical emergency requiring active resuscitation and skilled personnel.

RESUSCITATION OF THE DEPRESSED NEWBORN

Most depressed newborns are either sedated or hypoxic. Initial care, therefore, should consist of oxygenation via mask

Table 3-2.   The Apgar Scoring System

Criteria	0	1	2
Heart rate	Absent	Below 100	Over 100
Respiration	Absent	Irregular	Good; crying
Muscle tone	Limp	Some flexion	Good tone; active
Irritability	None	Grimace	Active crying; sneeze, cough
Color	Blue	Pink body; blue extremities	All pink

after airway obstruction has been ruled out, mild stimulation, and reversal of narcotic analgesia, if any has been given, with 0.02 to 0.04 mg (1 to 2 pediatric ampules) of naloxone IV.

If these measures do not rapidly correct the problem, laryngoscopy and endotracheal intubation should be performed. Once a reliable airway has been established, an umbilical intravenous line should be placed, blood obtained (for hemoglobin and hematocrit, electrolytes, and blood gases), and 3 to 4 mEq of sodium bicarbonate IV given. Life support and resuscitation are then conducted as for anyone else.

PUERPERIUM

The puerperium may be divided into three periods, based on physiological changes and likely pathological processes: the first few hours (immediate postpartum period), the first few days, and the first few (6) weeks (late puerperium).

IMMEDIATE POSTPARTUM PERIOD

In the first few hours after delivery, uterine contractions prevent postpartum hemorrhage. The uterus shrinks to roughly its size at 16 to 20 weeks. Several factors may facilitate this process:

1. Nursing the newborn stimulates oxytocin secretion.
2. Massaging the fundus intermittently also results in reflex contraction.
3. Finally, many obstetricians give exogenous oxytocin, either by IV infusion (20 units/1,000 ml balanced salt solution) or IM (10 units) to cover the fourth stage of labor. If postpartum hemorrhage has not occurred by 1 to 2 hours after delivery and there is no retained tissue within the uterus, it is extremely unlikely to happen.

Immediate postpartum care incorporates the above measures as well as certain precautions, should they not be effective.

1. Vital signs and lochia should be checked at 15-minute intervals for the first hour.
2. Mothers should be kept NPO for an hour, except for clear fluids.
3. Because of the large infusion of fluids and diuresis, bladder function should be monitored carefully. Postpartum atony may result in retention of more than a liter of urine.
4. Ergot alkaloids, 0.2 mg (Methergine, Ergotrate), may be given IV or IM if uterine relaxation seems to be a problem. These agents are hypertensive and should be used with care in patients for whom this may be a problem.

FIRST FEW DAYS

Immediately after delivery, the uterus and cervix begin to undergo involution. By one week, the uterus weighs half as much (500 g) and the cervix, which was only shortly before completely effaced and dilated, has regained its tubular structure (although the canal is still 1 to 2 cm in diameter). This shrinkage is accomplished through loss of cellular material from each cell while maintaining the number of cells constant. This is accompanied by a tremendous decrease in blood flow, with obliteration of many of the larger vessels by hyalinization.

The endometrium begins to regenerate within a few days from the basal layer, which remained behind after placental separation and shedding of the upper layers. The placental site itself shrinks rapidly with the uterus and is eventually undermined and shed, with new endometrium resurfacing the remaining small defect. The combination of blood and superficial endometrium that is shed is known as lochia. In the first few days, containing relatively more blood, it is known as lochia rubra. This gives way to the lochia serosa and in a week or two to the lochia alba, which consists mostly of leukocytes and serous fluid.

The perineum is recovering either from birth or episiotomy.

Redistribution of fluids is significant. During the pregnancy, maternal blood volume has increased by roughly 2 L. Edema may account for another 1 to 2 L. Blood loss at vaginal delivery averages 500 to 750 ml, and for cesarean section 800 to 1,000 ml. The remaining fluid is excreted in a large diuresis in the near postpartum period. Consequently, even though significant blood is lost at delivery, the subsequent hemoconcentration results in hemoglobin and hematocrit levels that change little in most cases.

While the pelvic organs are undergoing involution, the breasts are prepared for lactation. During the pregnancy, high levels of prolactin do not result in milk formation, presumably because of an inhibiting effect by progesterone and possibly estrogen. With the delivery of the placenta, estrogen and progesterone levels fall rapidly. This appears to have a two-stage effect. In the first day or two, colostrum production, which has been present to varying degrees during the last few weeks of pregnancy, increases markedly. A milk-like substance (but very concentrated and produced in far smaller quantities than milk), colostrum contains higher levels of sodium chloride and immunoglobulins (especially IgA) and lower levels of lactose (slightly) and albumin (much lower).

By the third or fourth postpartum day, colostrum gives way to milk. Containing the proteins lactalbumin (α and β) and casein, and lactose synthesized in the alveolar cells, it is virtually the ideal food for the infant. It supplies all necessary vitamins and minerals in adequate quantities, except vitamin K and iron, as well as many immunoglobulins thought to aid in protecting the newborn from enteric and respiratory diseases.

MATERNAL CARE IN THE FIRST FEW DAYS

The most common problems encountered during the first week after delivery are as follows:

1. Endomyometritis
2. Infected episiotomy/sore episiotomy
3. Phlebitis
4. Urinary tract infection/retention
5. Breast engorgement

6. Rh sensitization in an Rh− mother who has had an Rh+ baby
7. Lack of bowel movement

Postpartum maternal care is therefore targeted toward preventing, detecting, and solving these problems.

1. Problems usually present as pain or fever or both, so frequent temperature measurements are useful. Febrile morbidity consists of two temperatures greater than 100.4°F (38°C) in a 24-hour period.
2. Normal lochia has a slight odor, but any pronounced or foul odor or yellowish color in the first few days should be investigated with culture. Uterine tenderness is a frequent but not constant sign of infection.
3. Episiotomy swelling and pain may be controlled by an ice pack for 24 hours, local spray anesthetics occasionally, and liberal use of narcotic and nonnarcotic analgesics. Therapeutic doses of codeine and combinations such as Percodan and Percocet will have little effect on the nursing infant. Infection should be suspected if pain does not begin to abate after 48 hours.
4. Early ambulation (within hours, in most cases) helps to minimize the risk of phlebitis. The use of aspirin or aspirin-containing analgesics may further reduce this risk.
5. Urinary tract infection may be avoided by keeping catheterization to a minimum. Retention should be checked for frequently in the first day or two. If found, liberal early use of a Foley catheter may quickly resolve the problem. Retention is especially likely in patients who have had spinal or epidural anethesia.
6. While breast engorgement has long been considered a cause of fever, this should only be accepted after a careful search for another cause has been fruitless. Mothers who do not nurse may avoid lactation by taking the prolactin inhibitor bromocriptine mesylate (Parlodel), 2.5 mg b.i.d. for 10 to 14 days. It must be begun by the second postpartum day to effectively suppress milk formation.
7. Rh immune globulin, 300 μg (RhoGAM) given within 24 to 48 hours postpartum, will successfully prevent sensitization in Rh− women with Rh+ babies.
8. Return of bowel function, as evidenced by passage of stool, may take several days, especially if the mother had an enema early in labor. Reassurance is probably the wisest course. If intervention is indicated, a gentle laxative such as milk of magnesia, 30 ml, for 1 or 2 days at bedtime is usually sufficient.

THE LATE PUERPERIUM

Most puerperal problems, as those listed above, occur within several days after birth. The period from the first through the sixth postpartum week is primarily one of gradual return to the nonpregnant state. The uterus continues to shrink, eventually being only slightly larger than before conception, with a slightly greater blood supply.

In the woman who does not nurse, ovarian function may resume as early as 2 to 3 weeks after delivery, with resumption of menses in 6 to 10 weeks. Periods will often be heavier than before pregnancy because of the greater residual blood flow to the uterus. The nursing mother may experience prolonged amenorrhea, presumably because elevated prolactin levels (even intermittently) block ovarian function. These women often have menopausal symptoms, including a thin vaginal mucosa and poor lubrication during sex, for much or all of the time they nurse.

The two most common late postpartum complications are uterine hemorrhage due to retained placental tissue or subinvolution of the placental implantation site and mastitis (in nursing women). Late postpartum hemorrhage usually necessitates dilation and curettage. Mastitis, usually caused by staphylococcal or streptococcal infection and signaled by fever, chills, and localized breast erythema and soreness, is best treated with a semisynthetic penicillinase-resistant penicillin or erythromycin, 250 mg q 6 hours for 7 to 10 days.

PROCEDURES TO ALTER LABOR OR DELIVERY

Although the most common and safest method of birth is simple vertex vaginal delivery after spontaneous labor, many pregnancies are terminated by other methods. Oxytocin stimulation, low and midforceps, vacuum extraction, breech extraction, and cesarean section account for most of the manipulations we perform during labor and delivery.

OXYTOCIN

Because of past misuse, oxytocin has acquired a bad reputation. However, carefully administered under the right conditions and with adequate surveillance, it is quite safe and very useful. Its proper use will often enable one to avoid an operative delivery. In general, one may say that if labor is indicated and not present, oxytocin is indicated. It may be used to initiate labor (induction) or to improve otherwise inadequate labor (augmentation or stimulation).

Careful administration presupposes the following:

1. Oxytocin is administered intravenously as a dilute solution (usually 10 units/1,000 ml or 10mU/ml). This results in rapid onset and fine control of action. A half-life in the body of less than 90 seconds enables one to effectively eliminate the drug's action within 5 minutes. Many require that the oxytocin be piggybacked into another IV.
2. The diluent is a balanced salt solution. Since oxytocin inhibits free-water clearance, administration in dextrose solution at high rates exposes the mother to the risk of water intoxication. Using 0.9N NaCl or lacted Ringer's as a vehicle obviates this risk.
3. Oxytocin is adminstered by pump. This guarantees constant flow rate at desired levels.
4. Infusion is begun at very low rates, usually 0.5 to 1 mU/minute, and is increased relatively slowly, titrating labor. Peak effects at any infusion rate are reached within 20 to 30 minutes. Therefore, most advocate that,

for augmentation, rates be increased by 1 to 2 mU/minute every 20 to 30 minutes until satisfactory labor is established. For induction, many will double the rate every 20 to 30 minutes until a nearly satisfactory pattern is achieved, then slow the rate of increases to augmentation levels.

Appropriate surveillance includes

1. Continuous EFM
2. Continuous attendance to monitor strength and frequency of contractions and fetal condition

Contraindications to oxytocin include those factors that make labor either dangerous or useless, including

1. Evidence of CPD
2. Fetal presentations that contraindicate labor
3. Fetal distress
4. Conditions that predispose to uterine rupture

FORCEPS DELIVERY

In some cases, when the expulsive forces are not great enough or the fetal skull is not well oriented, forceps may be used to facilitate delivery. Their use is also sometimes indicated to shorten the second stage because of fetal distress or maternal contraindications to prolonged pushing and to assist with the aftercoming head in a breech delivery. They should *never* be used to overcome suspected CPD, nor should they ever be applied to any fetal part other than the head.

There are several categories of forceps delivery, based on station and position of the head:

1. Low forceps: Head is on the perineum and in direct OA or OP position
2. Midforceps: Head is engaged but higher than the perineum and in oblique or transverse position
3. Low midforceps: Newer, unofficial category; head on the perineum but in oblique (ROA, LOA, etc.) position
4. High forceps: Head not engaged

Low forceps delivery usually amounts to little more than a last-minute assist to guide the head over the perineum or under the symphysis. Low midforceps delivery, although involving the potential additional maternal trauma of rotating the blades in the pelvis, should also be quite safe if the assessment of station is accurate. True midforceps deliveries involve increasing risk to both mother and fetus. High forceps should *never* be performed.

Safe application of forceps requires rigid adherence to several guidelines:

1. The cervix *must* be fully dilated.
2. The presentation *must* be vertex.
3. The head *must* be engaged.
4. The membranes *must* be ruptured.
5. The position of the head *must* be known.

In addition, adequate anesthesia, an empty bladder, and an empty rectum are desirable.

Safe use of forceps also requires an understanding of their mechanics. The **blades** of the forceps have two curvatures: pelvic and cephalic. The pelvic curve allows the blades to reach into the pelvis and follow its curvature upward. Traction on the blades during delivery must be in a direction that allows the inner portion of the blades to traverse the pelvis along this curve. The cephalic curve is the outward curve, which allows the fetal head to nestle between the two blades. The blades may be either solid (better for rotation) or fenestrated. Each blade is attached to a **shank**, onto which is fixed some form of connecting the two blades together, the **lock**. This is usually either a socket or sliding arrangement. Each shank is attached to a **handle**.

The blades are applied, one at a time, to conform to the fetal head (**cephalic application**); however, one must remember that there is a pelvic curve as well, which must be honored during application and delivery. Each application is best guided by the fingers of the obstetrician so that the blades lie alongside the head with the tips just beyond the cheeks. Once the blades have been placed, they are locked. If the left blade is always placed first, the handles will line up for locking. If the posterior blade is placed first (oblique or transverse positions) and is the right blade, the handles will need uncrossing before locking.

The application of the blades *must* always be checked prior to attempting delivery. The sagittal suture should be midway between the blades and perpendicular to them, and the posterior fontanel (anterior fontanel for posterior presentations) should be one finger's breadth above the shanks.

If rotation is necessary and a forceps with a pelvic curve has been used, one must rotate the handles in a wide arc with the center of rotation at the midpoint of the blades, or the tips will describe a wide arc inside, causing maternal trauma. Once rotation is complete, the fetus is delivered by gentle traction along the axis of the pelvis, again keeping a picture in mind of the course of the curved blades. Pulling should be with contractions, therefore intermittent. When the head reaches the perineum, an adequate episiotomy is wise. The head may be delivered, after removing the forceps, by the modified Rigten's maneuver (less bulk through the introitus) or with the forceps in place (more control of the delivery of the head).

The major risks of forceps delivery are generally related to the difficulty of the application and the pull. For the mother they consist of tears in the vaginal vault, rectum, bladder, or perineum and, rarely, damage to the lower uterine segment and symphysis. Potential fetal injuries include facial injuries and brain damage. Intracranial hemorrhage and tentorial tears, accounting for long-term neurological damage in a significant proportion of cases, are the major reason that difficult midforceps deliveries have, in large part, been replaced by cesarean section.

One may attempt a trial of forceps delivery with the knowledge that one may not succeed. If one takes this approach in a questionable case, one should be prepared for immediate cesarean section if the forceps delivery cannot be safely completed.

VACUUM EXTRACTION

Much more popular in Europe, the attempt to deliver by applying suction to the fetal scalp has its proponents here. It offers the advantages of not occupying space alongside the fetal head, making rotations safer, and avoiding misapplications of blades. However, unfamiliarity combined with a fairly high incidence of scalp trauma has limited its use in this country. The advent of a new type of scalp plate made of flexible material rather than metal may help change this.

DELIVERY OF THE BREECH FETUS

Unlike the vertex, the breech delivery is actually three deliveries of successively larger portions of the fetus. In addition, all the sharp edges and articulations (arms, legs, chin) point the wrong way. Consequently breech delivery involves much more active participation by the obstetrician and frequently requires maneuvers to reposition or guide parts of the fetus. Therefore, certain criteria and precautions should be observed if a breech delivery is to be considered.

The major concern is adequate assessment of the relationships of the fetus and maternal pelvis. This may gauged in several ways:

1. Estimated fetal weight should be between 2,500 and 4,000 g.
2. The mother may be judged to have an adequate pelvis if she has previously easily delivered an equally large baby. If not, x-ray pelvimetry may be used to evaluate the inlet and midpelvis.
3. The fetal head should be flexed.

In addition:

1. The labor should be of good quality, suggesting no dystocia.
2. A liberal episiotomy and adequate anesthesia for potential manipulation help considerably.
3. Breech delivery should be considered to be as much an operation as cesarean section, which means that a trained assistant, an anesthesiologist, and a pediatrician should be on hand, equipped for anesthesia and resuscitation.

TECHNIQUE OF BREECH DELIVERY

The breech delivery begins with the descent of the presenting part to the perineum. There should be no attempt to deliver any breech infant from a station higher than +3. In general, the further the delivery proceeds spontaneously, the easier the birth and the lower the associated morbidity. This may be a sort of selection bias, since the easier deliveries will obviously progress further without help; however, it is considered best to allow spontaneous delivery to the level of the umbilicus if possible.

When the obstetrician begins to pull on the fetus, the delivery becomes an **extraction**. In the footling breech, this may begin at or any time after the feet reach the perineum. In the frank breech, it most often begins after crowning of the rump.

Critical to the delivery of the footling breech is to deliver both feet simultaneously. If one foot has descended without the other, the first step is to bring down the upper foot. The fetus is usually in a transverse position, one hip being anteriorly

placed. Both feet are then grasped with a towel, and gentle constant traction is used to deliver the legs to the hips, until the breech has been delivered. The fetus will now rotate to the AP position, back up. Grasping the hips and buttocks (*never* the abdomen), the obstetrician now pulls downward until the umbilicus and eventually the chest are delivered.

If the presentation is frank breech, spontaneous delivery to the umbilicus is, again, most desirable, but usually the legs are delivered by traction on the hips. If this does not succeed, **decomposition** of the breech is necessary, by drawing the legs down separately until the feet can be reached and delivered. Delivery then proceeds to the chest, as above.

The shoulders are delivered, one at a time, either anterior or posterior first, by rotating the fetus back to the transverse position and either lowering (to deliver the anterior) or raising (to deliver the posterior) the body to provide appropriate traction. If the shoulders do not easily deliver, one must deliver the arms (posterior first) by placing one's fingers in the crook of the elbow and applying downward traction while supporting the body in the appropriate position. One must take care not to pull on the humerus, as it may fracture.

Finally, the head is delivered. The critical aspect of this maneuver is to maintain flexion. This is best accomplished by simultaneous suprapubic pressure on the occiput (by the assistant) and downward traction on the body and shoulders until the mastoid bones are visible. The delivery of the head is then completed by raising the body and allowing the chin to deliver. Many facilitate this by placing a finger in the mouth to keep the head flexed by gentle pressure on the lower jaw (Mauriceau maneuver). This should not be used for traction. The rest of the head will follow easily.

If it does not or if the operator prefers, specially designed (longer, curved handles so the baby's body does not interfere) Piper forceps may be used to deliver the head. They should be applied and used in the same way as other forceps and should be readily available for *every* breech delivery.

The major risks of breech delivery, as noted above, are to the fetus and result from either size or positional problems that either delay the delivery or make it traumatic. Most problematic is that these can occur at any time from the beginning to the end of the delivery and are often unpredictable.

Occasinally the head may be trapped by the cervix after passage of the body. This is a life-threatening complication that must be resolved quickly, without excessive traction, and it may necessitate incising the cervix (Dührssen's incisions), an otherwise thoroughly distasteful procedure attended by hemorrhage and damage to the lower uterine segment and sometimes the urinary tract. Fear of this complication is a major reason for avoiding vaginal delivery of breeches weighing less than 2,500 g, in which there is a greater difference between head and body sizes.

Once the head is past the cervix, the major difficulties with delivery, assuming there is no bony dystocia, arise from failure to maintain constant traction on the body and flexion of the head, so attention to these details is essential.

CESAREAN SECTION

Delivery of the infant by incision of the abdominal and uterine walls has become increasingly common in the past 20 years, in many areas accounting for up to 25% of all deliveries. Several factors have contributed to this trend:

1. Increased safety, primarily in the areas of anesthesia, postoperative care, and infection control
2. Increased awareness of the dangers attendant to vaginal delivery in labors complicated by abnormal presentation, fetal distress, difficult midforceps, or herpes simplex infection (also increased incidence of genital herpes)
3. Repeat cesarean section

Indications

In the simplest terms, cesarean section is indicated when it is safer than vaginal delivery for either the mother or the baby. This may occur when there is

1. Cephalopelvic disproportion
2. Abnormal fetal lie
3. Fetal distress
4. Genital herpes simplex infection
5. Umbilical cord prolapse
6. Placenta previa or abruption
7. The need for early delivery (as in some cases of pre-eclampsia or diabetes) in the face of an uninducible cervix
8. Extreme prematurity
9. Previous surgery violating the uterine cavity, including previous cesarean birth, repairs of anomalies, and transmural submucus myomectomy

Repeat cesarean section has become a major reason for current cesarean section. Because of the morbidity inherent in numerous surgical procedures, attempts have been made to delineate criteria under which repeat cesarean section might safely be avoided and vaginal delivery allowed. Current feeling is that labor may be safely undertaken if the following criteria are met:

1. The previous cesarean section was a low transverse incision
2. There was no postoperative infection
3. Labor is carefully monitored with EFM
4. Labor spontaneously progresses well
5. Blood replacement and cesarean section are immediately available

Risks

Indications for cesarean section must be balanced against the risks attendant to the operation, which include the following:

1. Increased maternal mortality: Most studies have shown maternal mortality rates of 5 to 10 times that of vaginal delivery, up to 0.1%, most of which are due to complications of general anesthesia. Recently, however, large series of cesareans conducted primarily under regional anesthesia have indicated mortality rates similar to those for vaginal delivery.
2. Increased maternal morbidity: Certainly much higher than for vaginal delivery, major causes of morbidity following cesarean section include hemorrhage, pelvic

and wound infection, phlebitis, respiratory and urinary tract infections, and intraoperative urinary tract injury.
3. Essentially no risk to the fetus.

Decisions

Once the decision has been made to perform a cesarean section, several choices and then preparatory measures are in order. The first choice is type of anesthesia. Under most circumstances, regional anesthesia, if available, is preferable, since for practical purposes it eliminates aspiration. The circumstances under which general anesthesia is preferable are described in the section on anesthesia.

The next choice to be made is with respect to the types of incision in the abdominal wall and the uterus. The abdominal wall may be incised either vertically in the midline between the pubis and umbilicus or horizontally at approximately the level of the pubic hairline (Pfannenstiel's incision) (see "Techniques," below). The Pfannenstiel's is cosmetically more desirable and less likely to suffer dehiscence, but it is more time consuming, requires more attention to hemostasis, and is more difficult to extend if not initially large enough. The vertical incision is therefore desirable in cases in which a couple of minutes delay in delivery is likely to be dangerous or in which exposure is likely to be a significant problem (e.g., great obesity).

The uterine incision may also be made in a number of different ways. Most today are **transverse lower uterine segment** incisions, since these involve the least bleeding and are least likely to undergo subsequent catastrophic rupture in subsequent pregnancies. This incision is sometimes inappropriate. In cases of placenta previa, transverse lie, or extreme prematurity, a **low vertical** or even a **high vertical (classic)** incision may be preferable because of easy extendability if delivery is technically difficult. The low vertical incision involves more dissection of the bladder than the transverse and carries a risk of extending laceration downward into the cervix. The classic incision involves the most bleeding, mandates subsequent cesarean section because of the high risk of catastrophic rupture, and is associated with a greater risk of postoperative bowel adhesions. It is rarely used today.

Preparations

Cesarean section is major surgery. Preparation should be similar to that for any abdominal surgery:

1. NPO for as long as possible, up to 8 to 12 hours preoperatively
2. Abdominal preparation
3. Antacid, preferably sodium citrate, 30 ml, 30 to 45 minutes preoperatively
4. Running, large-bore intravenous line
5. Foley catheter in bladder
6. CBC, urinalysis, type and crossmatch two units packed cells
7. Serum electrolytes, if time permits
8. Informed, signed consent

Technique

Sterile prepping and draping of the abdominal wall are performed either after institution of anesthesia (if regional) or before (if general). If a Pfannenstiel's is to be performed, the skin incision should be at about the level of the pubic hairline and large enough to allow for easy delivery of the fetus (remember that skin stretches). Similarly, the subcutaneous tissue is incised down to the level of the rectus sheath. Large vessels are usually encountered. Whether they are clamped, clamped and tied, or just pressed on at this point depends on how heavily they bleed and the urgency of the delivery. The rectus sheath is next opened with a scalpel in the midline and incised bilaterally (usually with scissors) transversely from the midline laterally. The two layers should be incised separately to minimize bleeding. It is then dissected free of the rectus muscles in the midline as far up toward the umbilicus as possible and from the pyrimidalis muscles down to the pubic symphysis. Care must be taken here to avoid trauma to (or to ligate) perforating blood vessels. The adequacy of the Pfannenstiel incision is usually determined by its fascial dimensions (fascia does not stretch well); extending it as far laterally and upward as necessary avoids difficult deliveries. The rectus and pyramidalis muscles are separated vertically in the midline, and the posterior fascia and peritoneum are incised, also in the midline. This is done as high up as possible to avoid accidentally entering the bladder and carried downward to the apex of the bladder.

If the initial incision is to be vertical, it should be in or near the midline (paramedian) and of similar length. The subcutaneous fat and underlying rectus sheath are also incised vertically. From this point on, the procedure is the same as described above.

Upon entering the peritoneal cavity, a retractor (we use the lower blade of a Balfour's retractor) is placed in the lower margin of the incision to aid visualization. The junction of the bladder and anterior uterine serosal surfaces is identified (just below where it becomes tightly adherent to the uterine surface), and a horizontal incision is made just above it, from the midline bilaterally (again large enough for the delivery, but staying on the anterior face of the uterus). The loosely adherent bladder is then separated from the lower uterine segment for several centimeters, using one's finger. Caution is advised here, so as not to completely separate the bladder from the cervix.

A horizontal incision is next made in the lower uterine segment through the exposed area. *There are two caveats here.* Typically, the uterus bleeds a lot when one cuts into it, obscuring the surgeon's vision. Second, it is important to cut through the uterus (and perhaps membranes, if they are intact) but *not to cut the baby.* The best way to solve both these problems is to make a small midline incision all the way through, while applying pressure with a lap pad to the upper edge of the incision, tamponading the bleeding. After identifying the uterine cavity, one extends the incision laterally (either with bandage scissors or manually), being careful to make it large enough *without* entending into the large brances of the uterine arteries.

A new technique involving a stapler has recently become popular. After making a stab wound in the desired area, one inserts a stapler that places two rows of hemostatic absorbable staples across the lower uterine segment. One then cuts between the rows, limiting the bleeding. This is most useful if the lower segment is somewhat thinned by labor.

If one is performing a low vertical incision, one must take the bladder down farther to allow as much of the incision as possible to be in the lower uterine segment. For classic incisions, one begins above the vesicouterine junction and so does not take the bladder down at all.

Upon entry into the uterine cavity, the surgeon inserts his hand, locates the part of the baby he intends to deliver, and guides it toward the incision. The infant is then delivered by a combination of **fundal pressure** (substitute for maternal pushing) and traction, as if the opening were a vagina. After appropriate suctioning, the cord is cut and the infant given to the pediatrician. Usually the person carrying the baby changes gloves.

The delivery of the placenta is conducted under direct vision, with care to be sure membranes are not left behind. The inner surface of the uterus is explored, and patency of the cervix is verified. Simultaneously, the assistant massages the uterus and the anesthesiologist rapidly infuses an oxytocin solution (20 units/1,000 ml 0.9 NaCl or lactated Ringer's to assure uterine contraction and minimize bleeding.

At this point, it is usually easiest to deliver the fundus of the uterus through the abdominal incision and complete its closure outside, since visualization is so much improved. Both cut edges are identified to the angles of the incision (and may be grasped with nontraumatic clamps) and sutured. There are many acceptable techniques, usually using one or two layers of continuous large-caliber chromic suture, designed to obtain hemostasis, reapproximation, and inversion of the uterine scar. At the end of this step, the uterine incision should be without bleeding. Using a smaller chromic suture, one then reapproximates the bladder flap to the upper uterine serosa, covering over the uterine incision.

Both the surgeon and assistant often change gloves, inspect the pelvic viscera for abnormality or bleeding, and then reinsert the uterus into the abdominal cavity, taking care not to trap bowel behind it. Some suction spilled blood from the pelvic gutters.

Closure of the abdomen begins with an instrument and lap pad count while the surgeons close the peritoneum using continuous suturing, taking care to avoid the underlying structures. The fascia is then reapproximated using large-caliber suture. Again, routines are extremely varied, including continuous, simple interrupted and figure-eight techniques and using chromic, synthetic, and nonabsorbable sutures. Some leave the subcutaneous fat unsutured, ligating only bleeding points; others suture this layer using plain catgut, either interrupted or continuous, for hemostasis and reapproximation. Last, the skin is closed using staples, nonabsorbable skin sutures, or a subcuticular closure.

At the end of the procedure, one should express excess blood and clots from the vagina by downward pressure on the uterine fundus. One may also notice blood-tinged urine in the catheter, which may be secondary to blunt trauma to the bladder during the delivery. It should usually clear within several hours after surgery.

Postoperative care

Care of the cesarean section patient combines that of the postpartum patient with that of the postoperative.

Immediate care in the recovery room should include the following:

1. Constant attendance until the patient has regained full consciousness, if general anesthesia was used
2. Monitoring blood pressure, heart rate, respiration, urine output, vaginal bleeding, and fundal firmness, every 15 minutes for the first hour then hourly for 2 to 4 hours
3. 1,000 ml lactated Ringer's (D_5RL, 0.9 NaCl) + 20 units oxytocin at 200 to 500 ml/hour × 2 hours
4. NPO
5. Foley catheter
6. Pain relief. If general anesthesia was used, small doses of narcotic analgesic may be used. If epidural was performed, often nothing is necessary for the first few hours

After transfer from the recovery room, orders should include the following:

1. Vital signs q 4 hours (after the first day, this may be amended to q.i.d.).
2. Bed rest until the morning after surgery, then progressive ambulation as tolerated. In general, earlier ambulation is better.
3. NPO until the morning after surgery, then progressive advancement of diet from clear fluids on postoperative day one up to a regular diet.
4. IV fluids, 2,500 to 3,000 ml/24 hours, of either D_5RL or $D_51/2NS$, until adequate fluids are taken PO. After the first day, add 10 to 20 mEq KCl/L.
5. Foley catheter until the morning following surgery, then careful monitoring of urinary function for a day or two, unless there has been bladder trauma.
6. CBC, electrolytes in morning following surgery.
7. Pain relief. Meperidine, 50 to 100 mg (morphine 5 to 10 mg) q 3 to 4 hours as needed is usually sufficient, but individual requirements vary widely. In general, if the patient is awake enough to ask for pain relief, she will not be endangered by it. Remember, postoperative pain does not help healing.

Daily postoperative care should include the following:

1. The usual postoperative examinations (lungs, heart, extremities, bowel function, bladder function)
2. The usual postpartum examinations (fundus, lochia, breasts)
3. Incision checks. Many advocate daily checking of the incision, and certainly there is no harm in this, but in most cases it is not necessary unless the patient is febrile

Complications

The major complications attributable to cesarean section are as follows:

1. Hemorrhage: Most intraoperative hemorrhage is due to laceration of major vessels laterally, which is best avoided by careful extension of the uterine incision before delivery to prevent it during delivery. Hemorrhage not directly related to but occurring during cesarean section occurs with placenta previa and placenta accreta.

2. Urinary tract injury: The bladder may be injured during entry to the uterus or during reapproximation. More serious injury is inadvertant ureteral damage while suturing extensions or attempting to stop bleeding at the edges of the uterine incision.
3. Postoperative infection: This most common complication, including infection of the uterine and abdominal wall incisions, urinary tract, and respiratory tree (associated with general anesthesia), occurs in one of its forms in up to 75% of cases in some studies. This has prompted many to use prophylactic antibiotics in cesarean section complicated by long labor, prolonged rupture of membranes, many examinations, or extreme bleeding. The antibiotics of choice are usually a third-generation semisynthetic penicillin or cephalosporin, beginning with cord clamping and continuing for 24 hours. In penicillin-allergic patients, the combination of clindamycin and gentamicin may be substituted.
4. Bowel injury: Rarely bowel may be injured during surgery, either upon entering the peritoneal cavity or, more commonly, while lysing adhesions from previous surgery or infection. Usually, however, bowel complications involve postoperative ileus and/or obstruction. Careful surgery and meticulous hemostasis are one's best defense.
5. Aspiration: Accounting for more deaths than any other complication in patients who have had general anesthesia, this is most easily avoided by using regional anesthesia whenever possible. If general anesthesia is necessary, precautions noted in the anesthesia section must be taken.

FACTORS THAT COMPLICATE LABOR

Labor has been defined as the progressive effacement and dilatation of the cervix (stage I), followed by the descent and delivery of the fetus (stage II), and finally the separation and delivery of the placenta (stage III). Today, most also consider the fourth stage to encompass the first hour after the third. Many factors may interfere with this orderly progression or endanger either participant during the process.

In general, factors that compromise labor may be classified as abnormalities of uterine contraction, the maternal birth canal, fetal size, or fetal orientation, which may impede birth. Additionally, there may be complications related to fetal supply (cord and placental), which endanger the mother and/or child. Last, third- and fourth-stage abnormalities and complications of placental, uterine, or traumatic origin may endanger the mother.

UTERINE DYSFUNCTION

Normal labor is characterized by contractions that occur every 2 to 3 minutes, last 45 to 75 seconds, and achieve a strength of 25 to 60 mm Hg. Most disorders of uterine contractility involve **hypotonic dysfunction,** which occurs when the contractions do not achieve these levels. Most often, the cause of this disorder is unknown; however, in many cases, it seems to represent the uterus "knowing" that there is another problem and approaching labor tentatively. Commonly encountered associated conditions include CPD, abnormalities of fetal position, and overdistension of the uterus (twins, hydramnios).

Hypotonic dysfunction may present during any stage or phase of labor. When it occurs during the **latent phase,** one must distinguish it from false labor. The preferred method for this is sedation (barbiturate or narcotic). If, after sleep, the mother continues to have labor-like contractions without progressive effacement and dilatation for a period of 20 hours in the nullipara (14 hours in the multipara), hypotonic dysfunction may be diagnosed. One must consider that this represents an early manifestation of CPD or abnormal presentation; but, if they are not evident, oxytocin stimulation is appropriate. If several hours of adequate stimulation does not effect progress, especially if membranes are ruptured, cesarean section should be considered.

Active phase hypotonic dysfunction may involve labor that is too slowly progressive (**prolongation disorders**) or that stops at some point (**arrest disorders**). Prolongation disorders may be diagnosed when the rate of cervical dilatation is less than 1.2 cm/hour in nulliparas (<1.5 cm/hour in multiparas) during stage I after 3 cm dilatation or the descent of the presenting part is too slow during stage II. It may arise secondary to CPD, abnormal presentation, or cervical dystocia but often occurs without any of these. In and of itself, slow progress during labor is not a problem unless accompanied by prolonged rupture of membranes, but it is frequently a prelude to an arrest disorder. Oxytocin is the treatment of choice if CPD is not evident, cesarean section if it is.

Arrest disorders may occur during either the first or second stage of labor. First-stage arrest usually becomes manifest as a failure to dilate after 6 to 8 cm, while second-stage arrest is a failure of descent and rotation during pushing. More often than prolongation disorders, arrests represent either CPD or positional problems. However, if, during first- or second-stage arrest, contractions seem inadequate and fetal condition is good, a trial of oxytocin is indicated. Poor maternal pushing often causes a prolonged second stage. It may be due to maternal exhaustion (allow rest through analgesia), poor technique (stress the diaphragm's role in pushing), or epidural anesthesia (allow it to wear off). While a second stage longer than 2 hours (nullipara; 1 hour, multipara) is considered abnormal, with good fetal condition and some progress, it may be allowed to continue. If CPD is diagnosed or oxytocin fails to improve the situation, operative delivery is indicated.

The complications of hypotonic labor are three:

1. If labor is extremely prolonged with ruptured membranes (usually more than 24 hours), amnionitis and sepsis may occur. This may be avoided by judicious use of oxytocin and/or operative delivery.
2. Overaggressive use of oxytocin or forceps may cause fetal or maternal injury. *Most arrest-disorder fetal trauma in the absence of distress results from attempts to deliver (forceps) rather than from labor.*
3. Materal morbidity, even mortality, may result from cesarean section.

As a general rule, if fetal condition is acceptable, if CPD is not evident, and if there are no maternal contraindications,

oxytocin may be used to improve labor. Cesarean section should be resorted to when progress does not occur with oxytocin or fetal/maternal jeopardy supervenes. Midforceps operations, especially, in arrest disorders, should be approached with great caution and care.

Hypertonic labor is said to occur when the contractions are more frequent than every 2 to 3 minutes or last longer than 75 seconds or there is no return to baseline pressures between. Usually encountered in early labor, the contractions, though painful, are neither coordinated nor terribly effective. Sedation is the treatment of choice. Rarely, in cases of fetal distress, tocolysis is indicated. More usually, if conservative measures are not sufficient, fetal distress early in labor is remedied by cesarean section. In the absence of distress, small doses of oxytocin will sometimes organize the contractions.

When extremely vigorous coordinated labor occurs in the presence of a ripe cervix, **precipitate labor** may occur. Never clearly defined, it is simply extremely rapid labor and delivery. Major complications of this type of labor include fetal distress, cervical and vaginal lacerations, unattended delivery, and postpartum hemorrhage. Therapy consists of fetal support (oxygen, etc.) and attentiveness both during and after labor. If fetal distress is not manageable with the usual measures, tocolysis and cesarean section are options.

ABNORMALITIES OF THE BIRTH CANAL

Labor may be impeded by obstructions within the birth canal. These may be of the bony pelvis or of the soft tissue and developmental or acquired in origin.

Abnormalities of the bony pelvis

There is great variety in the size and shape of the pelvis. The limits of normal have been described in the section "Pelvic Factors Affecting Delivery." These are considered in terms of the delivery of an average-sized fetus in good presentation. In reality, less than desirable pelves often permit the birth of smaller than average fetuses, or even of average fetuses with a little extra difficulty. However, below certain limits, the pelvis is considered to be contracted and a barrier to vaginal delivery, except under exceptional circumstances. A pelvis may be contracted in any or all of its three planes, and in either the AP or transverse diameter.

The most accurate method for pelvic mensuration is x-ray pelvimetry. When combined with sonographic measurement of the fetal skull, precise relationships may be determined. However, because of worries about radiation exposure, x-ray pelvimetry is little used today, and clinical estimates of pelvic size combined with assessment of the course of labor are the methods commonly employed.

Inlet contraction exists when the AP diameter of the inlet is less than 10 cm or the transverse diameter is less than 12 cm. Since these are determinable only x-ray, the diagonal conjugate measurement is used instead and indicates a contracted inlet if less than 11.5 cm. One should suspect an inadequate inlet when the presenting part is unengaged under any of the following conditions:

1. A nullipara has a floating fetal head before labor at term, and the head cannot be pushed into the pelvis by fundal pressure.

2. The membranes have ruptured.
3. There is an abnormal presentation.
4. Cervical dilatation is delayed in the presence of good labor.
5. Hypotonic labor (usually of the prolongation variety) occurs.

Most of the complications of inlet contraction are due to either failure to recognize it or heroic attempts to get past it. The prolonged labors that result are fraught with danger to the fetus and mother, including amnionitis, birth canal trauma, and fetal skull damage. However, most cases are borderline and the likelihood of vaginal delivery hinges on associated fetal factors. Often a trial of labor is appropriate, but one must be alert for prolapse of the cord or the development of a pathological retraction (Bandl's) ring (which represents a lower uterine segment about to rupture) and be careful not to persist in a futile attempt too long. Timely cesarean section prevents morbidity and sometimes mortality.

Midpelvic contraction is present when the interischial spinous diameter is less than 9 cm. However, like inlet contraction, most cases are less clear, with a moderately small midpelvis presenting a relative obstruction to an average or slightly larger fetus. Also, like inlet contraction, determination is usually made based on obstructed labor, although it more often presents as an arrest disorder (especially transverse arrest). Most of the danger in midpelvic contraction arises from attempts at delivery, more specifically midforceps deliveries when the disproportion is not recognized. This can be avoided by cesarean section.

Outlet contraction exists when the intertuberous diameter is less than 8 cm. It becomes clinically significant only when it occurs as an isolated abnormality, which is rare. Associated midpelvic contraction usually obstructs labor before the outlet is reached. It may be rarely a barrier to delivery. More often, since the posterior outlet is unbounded, the head is forced posteriorly, resulting in perineal and coccygeal trauma from the forceps deliveries that are often necessary.

In addition to variations in size, there are also many developmental abnormalities of the pelvis, associated with skeletal abnormalities, vitamin D deficiency during childhood, various infectious illnesses, and trauma. These are usually quite evident and quite rare. Cesarean section is usually indicated.

Soft-tissue obstruction

Very few **anatomic** abnormalities are compatible with conception and yet may compromise delivery: partial vaginal atresia and transverse vaginal septum. Longitudinal septa usually are pushed to one side or torn. Congenital vaginal (Gartner's duct) and vulvar (Bartholin's) cysts likewise are usually only transient impediments.

On the other hand, a number of **acquired conditions** may delay or even preclude vaginal delivery:

1. Low segment and paracervical myomas, if large enough, may block descent of the fetus.
2. Cervical stenosis following surgery or infection may be insuperable, while conglutination usually yields to digital opening after complete effacement has occurred.

3. Neoplasms (benign and malignant) of the cervix, vagina, and vulva occasionally make delivery difficult or impossible.
4. Previous vaginoplasty or urethroplasty may be considered an indication for cesarean section.
5. Rarely, large ovarian cysts or neoplasms will prolapse into the cul-de-sac and pose a barrier to fetal passage.

ABNORMALITIES OF FETAL ORIENTATION

Labor progresses best with the fetus in the vertex presentation and anterior (LOA, ROA) position since all the diameters presented to the pelvis are as small as possible and all the angles point the right way. Variations in lie, presentation, and position therefore pose potential problems. Some of these are often minor, others life threatening, and many in between.

Occiput posterior

A vertex presentation with the face to the maternal abdomen rather than her back, this positional variation changes stage I labor little except that the fetal station is often estimated to be lower than it really is and the mother frequently experiences "back labor." It is **diagnosed** by palpating the anterior rather than the posterior fontanel on vaginal examinations. Cervical dilatation and descent proceed at or near the usual rate. Over 90% of the time, these fetuses undergo rotation to the OA position during the second stage when the head reaches the pelvic floor. If this does not happen, stage II is often prolonged. This, however, may be associated rather than causal since failure of rotation is usually associated with either mild degrees of CPD or hypotonic labor. **Therapeutic alternatives** are time (observation), oxytocin, forceps delivery in OP or rotation (forceps or manual), and cesarean section (usually last resort). One must always have CPD in mind when considering these. Unless one causes fetal injury during a forceps delivery, the only additional **risk** of persistent OP is perineal tearing from the greater skull diameter presented.

Occiput transverse

Usually the head enters the pelvic inlet as OT and promptly rotates to an OA or OP position. If it does not, one must suspect either CPD (often caused by abnormalities of pelvic shape such as platypelloid and android pelves) or inadequate propulsion (hypotonic labor). This **diagnosis** is almost always made after prolongation of stage II. If there is no evidence of CPD, either oxytocin or midforceps rotation may be a solution. If these are ineffective or CPD is likely, cesarean section should be performed.

Face

Hyperextension of the head is usually associated with factors that prevent flexion, including pelvic inlet CPD, large fetal goiter, neck tumors, and multiple loops of cord. It may also occur if the maternal abdomen is pendulous or in association with anencephaly.

If the face presents, the descent portion of labor becomes more difficult since the optimal diameters are increased. If the position is mentum posterior, vaginal delivery is impossible. For mentum anterior positions, the head is delivered by flexion rather than extension. Delivery is either spontaneous or by cesarean section. Forceps should never be used.

Brow

The brow presentation, midway between vertex and face, is unstable. When the forehead presents, one feels the anterior fontanel and perhaps the eyes on vaginal examination. Engagement of the term brow is impossible and is often associated with the same conditions as face presentation, especially inlet CPD. Labor will usually convert it to either a face or vertex, and birth will proceed accordingly. If it does, management is as per that presentation. If it does not, cesarean section will be necessary.

Breech

At term, only 3 to 4% of fetuses remain in the breech presentation, even though at 28 weeks up to 40% are so oriented. Although the majority of term breeches occur in the absence of other pathology, abnormalities that make the head/pelvis ratio less compatible than the head/fundus ratio seem to predispose the fetus to assume this position. They are often seen in association with

1. Prematurity
2. Grand multiparity
3. Hydramnios
4. Multiple gestation
5. Placenta previa
6. Uterine fibroids and congenital anomalies
7. Hydrocephalus

Diagnosis of the breech presentation is suspected by palpating the head in the upper abdomen or by failing to find it on pelvic examination. Confirmation is most easily and safely made by ultrasonography. If this is unavailable, a single x-ray of the abdomen is diagnostic.

Breeches are **categorized** by the presenting part and the position of the lower extremities. In both the **frank** and **full** breeches, the buttocks are the presenting part. **Frank** breeches have the hips flexed and the legs extended, while **full** breeches have flexed hips and legs. If either or both feet extend down below the buttocks, it is a **footling** breech presentation.

The major **fetal risks** of breech presentation, other than the associated pathology described above, are cord prolapse during labor (especially with footling breeches) and trauma during delivery. Perinatal mortality for vaginal delivery is increased two to five times. Morbidity includes intracranial hemorrhage, tentorial tears, birth asphyxia, Erb's palsy, neck injury, and abdominal visceral damage. There is no increase in **maternal risk** for breeches delivered vaginally, but since cesarean section is so commonly employed the associated morbidity and mortality must be considered.

The **management** of the breech delivery includes three options:

1. **Cesarean section:** Most breeches are probably managed this way today. Assuming an adequate incision and reasonable skill, most fetal trauma is obviated by abdominal delivery. However, because there is the possibility of substituting maternal trauma for fetal, numerous studies have sought to define the subgroup in which cesarean section is not necessary (see below).
2. **Labor** and **vaginal delivery**: Today, this is essentially reserved for the frank or full breech between 2,500 and

4,000 g with a flexed head, a great birth canal, and good spontaneous labor. Anything that complicates the situation or requires intervention (including use of oxytocin) is an indication for cesarean section. Labor itself is not markedly different in the breech presentation, except for the risk of prolapsed or entangled cord. With intact membranes, the cervix dilates well. With ruptured membranes and buttocks presenting, it is usually not much different. Vaginal delivery, however, is a complicated and potentially dangerous affair that should be accorded all the respect of any major surgical procedure (see "Alternatives to Vaginal Delivery").
3. **External version:** Caught between the fears of vaginal delivery and the desire to avoid cesarean section, many obstetricians are now considering turning the breech fetus before labor. Studies show success rates of 50 to 75%. The earlier (32 weeks) the procedure, the easier but perhaps more unnecessary as many turn spontaneously. The later the procedure occurs (36 weeks), the more difficult. Most use sonography for placental localization, constant FHR monitoring, and tocolysis when necessary to reduce the risks of cord entanglement, placental separation, and premature labor. Its eventual place in breech management is not yet clear.

Transverse lie

Transverse lie at term is quite rare (<0.5%) and usually associated with inlet contraction, grand multiparity (pendulous maternal abdomen), or placenta previa. It occurs much more commonly in premature fetuses. When the fetus lies horizontally within the uterus, vaginal delivery is impossible. If the back is down, **diagnosis** is usually easy as there is no presenting part in the pelvis and the head is to one side. Alternatively, with **shoulder** presentation, either the acromion or a prolapsed arm may be in the pelvis and the head to one side. Definitive diagnosis is by ultrasonography or x-ray. Aside from the impossiblity of delivery, labor carries a much higher risk of cord prolapse. Severe fetal and maternal injury and even death are likely if labor is left unattended or if intrapartum attempts at version are made. Therefore, prompt cesarean section is the only appropriate action. Some attempt antepartum external version (see "Breech," above).

ABNORMALITIES OF FETAL SIZE

Macrosomia

Larger babies obviously are born through any given birth canal with more difficulty than smaller ones. Fetuses larger than 4,000 g are called **macrosomic**. Predisposing causes include the following:

1. Genetic and constitutional factors
2. Maternal diabetes without vascular disease
3. Excessive prenatal weight gain
4. Postdate pregnancies

Diagnosis is often not made until labor has not progressed well, but careful abdominal examination and liberal use of ultrasonography may be helpful. Macrosomia may pose a **risk** to the fetus in either of two ways:

1. If the head is large enough, engagement will never occur or become stuck in the pelvis, resulting in prolonged or arrested labor in either stage I or II.
2. If the head passes but the shoulders are relatively larger, they may become stuck in the pelvis after delivery of the head (shoulder dystocia).

Shoulder dystocia is an *emergency*. Upon delivery of the head, the umbilical cord is compressed in the pelvis, effectively eliminating blood flow to the fetus. Delivery must be completed within a very short time or the infant may be severely damaged. However, frantic efforts to deliver may cause neurological (brachial plexus) and skeletal trauma. The best alternative is to avoid shoulder dystocia. This may perhaps be done by careful antepartum screening for diseases such as diabetes and by ultrasonic evaluation of fetuses that seem large.

If it does occur, several maneuvers have been suggested:

1. Avoid impaction of the anterior shoulder under the symphysis by rotating the infant to an oblique position. Make a large, preferably mediolateral, episiotomy. Attempt delivery of the posterior arm by outward pressure in the crook of the elbow and, if successful, then the anterior.
2. If not successful, rotate the fetus 180° and repeat.
3. If still not successful, fracture the clavicle of the anterior shoulder. This must be done with outward pressure to avoide puncturing a lung. Although fractured clavicles are undesirable, they usually heal with no permanent injury if properly splinted.
4. If none of this is successful, some have advocated pushing the head back into the pelvis, rotating it back in the direction from which it came, and then delivering the baby by cesarean section.

Hydrocephalus

Accumulation of CSF (often more than 1L) within the ventricles of the brain causes significant enlargement of the fetal skull. Due to obstruction in the spinal cord, it is frequently associated with spina bifida and other abnormalities. The skull is usually thin and flexible. Hydrocephalus precludes vaginal delivery unless one decompresses the head in labor. There usually is very little brain tissue, and the infant will be mentally retarded if it survives.

One should suspect hydrocephalus when there is a large suprapubic mass or large fontanels are palpable through the cervix. However, almost one-third of affected fetuses present as breeches. In the past, many of these were not detected until the body of the infant had been born. However, today we usually subject all of our breech vaginal deliveries to either ultrasonic or x-ray scanning, so they should be discovered earlier. If hydrocephalus is suspected, it may be confirmed most accurately with ultrasonography, which not only measures the BPD but also demonstrates the dilated ventricles. Also adequate in vertex presentations is an x-ray. Diagnosis of hydrocephalus on x-ray in breeches must be made with some caution because of artifactual enlargement of the head.

Hydrocephalus precludes vaginal delivery unless it is decompressed. This may be done transvaginally or transabdominally. Cesarean section is also an option. If it is undetected, lower uterine segment rupture is a significant danger.

OTHER CONGENITAL ANOMALIES

Distension of the fetal abdomen as seen with distal urinary tract obstruction resulting in an enlarged bladder or kidneys is a rare cause of dystocia. The affected organ may be drained or cesarean section performed.

Incomplete twinning is another rare cause of dystocia, which should usually be remedied by cesarean section especially since many of these infants are salvageable today. The diagnosis of twins, complete or otherwise, is almost always made antepartum because of the liberal use of ultrasonography.

HYDRAMNIOS (POLYHYDRAMNIOS)

Quantities of amniotic fluid in excess of 2,000 ml are considered abnormal but usually are not clinically significant unless greater than 3,000 to 4,000 ml. Hydramnios is often associated with fetal anomalies that disturb amniotic fluid circulation:

1. Esophageal atresia and other obstructive malformations of the fetal GI tract prevent fetal swallowing.
2. Omphalocele, spina bifida, and anencephaly may result in hydramnios by allowing for transudation of fetal fluid into the amniotic cavity.
3. Pulmonary hypoplasia prevents fetal breathing of amniotic fluid.
4. Multiple gestation results in greater volumes of placenta for transudation and of fetal urine.
5. Diabetes and erythroblastosis, which are both associated with larger than normal placentas, seem to predispose to hydramnios.

One should suspect hydramnios when the uterus is larger than appropriate for gestational date and the fetus is hard to palpate. **Diagnosis** may be either on clinical grounds or by sonography, which can be used to estimate total uterine volume and fetal size. In suspected cases, one should always search for associated fetal anomalies.

The **risks** are proportional to the total fluid volume, rapidity of accumulation, and severity of associated malformations and usually involve abnormalities of labor. Chronic hydramnios, with gradual increases in amnionic fluid volume, may result in accumulation of extremely large volumes of fluid with surprisingly few maternal symptoms. Acute hydramnios is much more often symptomatic. Likely complications are as follows:

1. Premature labor
2. Hypotonic labor
3. Cord prolapse with rupture of membranes
4. Placental abruption with rupture of membranes
5. Maternal cardiorespiratory compromise
6. Associated fetal anomalies

Therapy for hydramnios is aimed at correction of underlying maternal disease, if any, and prevention of labor complications. Beyond bed rest, which has no effect on fluid volumes but may postpone labor, little can be done to avoid premature delivery. Repeated antepartum amniocentesis with fluid removal (not large volumes) may occasionally be successful. During early labor, however, gradual fluid removal may improve labor patterns and avoid cord prolapse. Trancervical amniotomy through a small-gauge needle between contractions with gradual decompression may also be useful.

OLIGOHYDRAMNIOS

Less than average amounts of amniotic fluid also threaten pregnancy and labor. Oligohydramnios may begin early in pregnancy (most commonly associated with renal agenesis or fetal obstructive uropathy) or late in pregnancy (a common complication of postmaturity). Since the amniotic fluid serves to cushion and lubricate the fetus and cord, lesser volumes are associated with skeletal and cutaneous compression syndromes (abnormal skin, clubfoot, hip abnormalities) if of long duration, and cord compromise (both before and during labor). In addition, since amniotic fluid is necessary for lung development, severe antepartum oligohydramnios often causes pulmonary hypoplasia. Unfortunately, there is not much that can be done antepartum. During labor, one must be alert for cord compromise. Some have experimented with transcervical infusion of saline solutions during labor after rupture of membranes to improve cord compression.

AMNIOTIC FLUID EMBOLISM

Usually an acute event of labor, amniotic fluid embolism (AFE) is thought to be almost always rapidly fatal. Perhaps lesser versions escape our notice. Since the amniotic fluid is sealed within the membranes, it usually has no access to maternal circulation. However, if the membranes are torn within the uterus (perhaps with placental abruption), the pressure of a contraction may force fluid into a uterine vein and then into the maternal venous circulation. The amniotic fluid causes maternal injury in two ways:

1. Particulate matter (lanugo, meconium, vernix) lodges within the pulmonary vasculature to cause acute cor pulmonale and right heart failure.
2. Thrombaplastic substances, found in great quantities in amniotic fluid, initiate disseminated intravascular coagulopathy (DIC).

Symptoms and signs of AFE are those of sudden maternal cardiorespiratory failure (dyspnea, syncope, tachycardia, hypotension, tachypnea) and DIC (bleeding from multiple sites). **Diagnosis** is primarily on clinical grounds, supported by evidence of hypoxia and right heart failure (Swan-Ganz catheter). Definitive diagnosis is usually postmortem, with the demonstration of amniotic fluid debris in the maternal circulation. **Therapy**, only occasionally effective, consists of cardiopulmonary support and resuscitation and delivery.

PLACENTAL AND CORD ABNORMALITIES COMPROMISING LABOR

PROLAPSED CORD

If the umbilical cord slips down in front of the presenting part, fetal blood flow will be compromised. Although it sometimes occurs before labor, it usually becomes symptomatic during. It is associated with conditions in which the inlet is not occluded by the presenting part:

1. Transverse lie, footling breech
2. Premature rupture of the membranes with a floating presenting part or with a very premature infant
3. Inlet contraction with failure of engagement
4. Twins
5. Hydramnios

Cord prolapse may occur in any of three degrees:

1. **Occult prolapse:** The cord has slipped into the pelvis next to the presenting part but not below it and therefore is not palpable. This will present during labor as cord compromise and should be managed as such.
2. **Forelying cord:** The cord has prolapsed beyond the presenting part but, because membranes are not ruptured, may be cushioned somewhat by amniotic fluid. It may be felt through the cervix and intact membranes and will give a typical cord compromise pattern on EFM. Appropriate action is cesarean section before the membranes rupture.
3. **True prolapse:** The cord is below the head and usually out in the vagina. The FHR pattern may be either variable decelerations or bradycardia depending on the constancy of the pressure. It can be felt on vaginal examination. Unless vaginal delivery can be anticipated within 5 to 10 minutes (which is almost never the case except in very premature infants), emergency cesarean section should be performed. While preparing, the presenting part should be pushed out of the pelvis and the patient maintained in deep Trendelenburg's position.

ABNORMAL INSERTION OF THE CORD

The umbilical vessels usually run the length of the cord and insert somewhere near the center of the placenta. Sometimes, however, the cord inserts maginally, often called a **battledore insertion.** This is an incidental finding of no known importance. When the umbilical vessels do not implant directly into the placenta but traverse the amnion, this is termed a **velamentous insertion.** Usually, velamentous insertions have no implications for labor (they *are* associated with a higher rate of congenital anomalies) unless the vessels traverse the amnion that crosses the cervix, (**vasa previa**), and so precede the fetus. With vasa previa, rupture of the membranes carries considerable risk of tearing the umbilical vessels and killing the fetus. If there is any excess bleeding associated with amniotomy or spontaneous rupture, prompt testing by the Kleihauer-Betke acid elution test may identify fetal hemoglobin. If positive, immediate cesarean section with preparation for a severely distressed, shocky baby is essential.

ABNORMAL CORD LENGTHS AND NUCHAL CORD

Although there is much variation in cord length, abnormally short cords (less than 30 cm) may create stage II problems, specifically descent problems, for the fetus. The typical picture is a fetus who descends with pushing and ascends between contractions. Often there are associated variable decelerations. Forceps delivery may be required to bring these fetuses down. Cesarean section may be necessary, depending on fetal condition.

Very long cords are more likely to become entwined around fetal parts and to prolapse. Two and even three loops of cord may be wrapped around the fetus's neck (**nuchal cord**). The likelihood of cord compromise or a short-cord syndrome with nuchal cord is usually proportional to the length remaining unentangled. These complications usually manifest as variable decelerations during stage I and are accentuated during stage II, but if there is adequate uncompromised cord there may be no sign of fetal danger.

Rarely, one will see a true knot in the cord. Unless the knot has been pulled tight, this is of curiosity value only. Tight knots obviously cause fetal compromise when they occur, which may be before or during labor and rarely during actual delivery.

PLACENTA PREVIA

The placenta may implant anywhere in the uterine cavity. Most often it does so in the fundus, but occasionally it implants in the lower uterine segment or even directly over the cervical os. Much of the time, when this happens, poor vascularization results in early abortion. When it does not and the placenta remains low, one of the degrees of placenta previa results:

1. **Total:** The entire cervical os is covered
2. **Partial:** Part of the os is covered
3. **Marginal:** Only the edge of the placenta is palpable through the os
4. **Low-lying:** Not a true previa, but a sonographic diagnosis

Placenta previa is usually **diagnosed** in the third trimester of the antepartum period when cervical effacement begins, because small vessels are torn by the changing lower segment. Typically the first **sign** is painless bleeding, often quite heavy but usually self-limited. The obstetrician who appropriately performs sonography at this point is rewarded with the diagnosis. One should *never* perform vaginal examination after heavy vaginal bleeding without knowing the location of the placenta by sonography unless one is prepared for immediate delivery, and then only under double set-up conditions, for torrential hemorrhage may follow inadvertant placental manipulation.

Management of prenatally diagnosed placenta previa depends on the severity of the bleeding and the age and condition of the fetus. One must weigh the dangers of continuing the pregnancy against those of delivery. If the fetus is severely premature, delivery should be postponed as long as possible unless the life of the mother is threatened by hemorrhage.

Hospitalization is desirable. Bed rest is obligatory. Transfusion may be necessary. Immediate delivery via cesarean section should always be available. If the fetus is mature or shows evidence of distress, delivery should not be delayed. Occasionally, previa first presents during labor, as heavier than normal bleeding. Double set-up examination is appropriate here.

All total previas and most partial previas preclude vaginal delivery for two reasons. Not only does the hemorrhage during labor become life threatening, but the placenta itself obstructs the birth canal, preventing passage of the fetus. Marginal previas and low-lying placentas may permit labor. In these cases, the head, as it descends into the pelvis, may tamponade the bleeding.

Although cesarean section is the desirable route of delivery for most previas, the condition poses certain additional **risks** for abdominal delivery. In anterior low-lying and previous implantations, the transverse low-segment incision may cut directly through the placenta, resulting in torrential hemorrhage of both maternal and fetal blood and difficulty delivering the infant. Therefore, a vertical incision may be preferable.

Placenta previas are also often placenta accretas (see below).

PLACENTAL ABRUPTION

Separation of the placenta after the 20th week of gestation and before the third stage of labor is termed placental abruption. It is associated with bleeding from the separated portion, which usually continues to a greater or lesser degree until delivery. This is because the uterus cannot contract and ligate the bleeding vessels as long as the placenta is attached and the fetus inside. The bleeding may be from the edge (**marginal separation**) or located centrally behind the placenta. The central type is usually more serious for three reasons:

1. The trapped blood tends to cause further separation by dissecting the placenta from its bed. In contrast, when the bleeding is from a marginal site, it tends to dissect between the membranes and the uterus and exit through the cervix.
2. The collected blood may predispose to a coagulopathy (see below).
3. The obstetrician does not see the blood and tends to underestimate the degree of hemorrhage.

The major **etiologic** factor for placental abruption seems to be hypertension, which coexists almost 50% of the time. *A previous pregnancy complicated by placental abruption makes the next extremely high risk.* Other conditions that may predispose to abruption are those that may result in a rapid decrease in intrauterine volume, mimicking delivery of the fetus, such as hydramnios with rupture of membranes and delivery of a first twin. Trauma has occasionally been implicated.

The prominent **symptoms** of prelabor abruption are vaginal bleeding and abdominal pain, associated with (**sign**) localized uterine tenderness. In severe cases, the tenderness may be generalized and may even progress to uterine rigidity. Sometimes, extravasated blood will suffuse the myometrium (**Couvelaire uterus**), which may or may not result in atony. Frequently signs of maternal shock and fetal distress (see

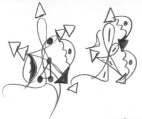

below) accompany severe cases. When separation occurs during labor, fetal distress may be the first sign.

If the separation is marginal and minor (**marginal sinus rupture**), the bleeding may be painless and indistinguishable from that of placenta previa. Ultrasonography, which should be performed in all cases of antepartum vaginal bleeding unless immediate intervention is necessitated by maternal or fetal jeopardy, may demonstrate either placental separation or a retroplacental clot, *but more often nothing*.

Placental abruption creates several **risks** for both mother and fetus:

1. **Maternal shock:** Blood loss with placental abruption may be several liters. This may be true even though there is little or no visible bleeding. **Acute renal failure** and obliguria, sometimes attributed to abruption directly, are due to hypovolemia.
2. **DIC:** DIC is probably secondary to tremendous amounts of placental thromboplastin released. Characterized by hypofibrinogenemia (<100 mg/100 ml), elevated fibrin split products, prolonged prothrombin time (**PT**) and (**APTT**), and thrombocytopenia, it results in generalized bleeding from puncture and wound sites. Spontaneous hemorrhage may accompany platelet counts below 20,000/mm³. Occasionally, a large retroplacental clot may consume enough fibrinogen to cause isolated hypofibrinogemia.
3. **Fetal distress:** A healthy fetus may tolerate up to a 50% loss of placental function. However, when caused by abruption, this is usually compounded by decreased perfusion of the remaining placenta secondary to maternal blood loss. If abruption occurs to a significant degree outside the hospital, fetal death is not rare.

Upon admission to the hospital, the following steps should be taken if placental abruption is suspected:

1. Determine if the fetus is alive or in distress (**EFM**).
2. Assess maternal condition by examination (vital signs, uterine tenderness and/or rigidity, urine output).
3. Start an IV with 0.9N NaCl or lactated Ringer's.
4. Obtain laboratory tests (CBC, electrolytes, fibrinogen, PT, APTT, [FSP], urinalysis). Coagulation status may be roughly assessed by collecting a tube of unheparinized blood and waiting 5 minutes. If a clot forms, coagulation status is satisfactory.
5. Type and crossmatch four units of packed red blood cells and fresh-frozen plasma (whole blood if necessary), plus platelets if necessary.
6. Perform sonography, if necessary, to rule out placenta previa and then perform cervical examination to assess dilatation.

Definitive **therapy** for placental abruption is delivery. This stops the bleeding and DIC. However, if the abruption seems to be minor and the fetus is very premature, careful observation of both mother and child in the hospital is preferable, with the knowledge that the situation can worsen at any moment. If delivery is chosen, avoiding cesarean section, if possible, is desirable for two reasons: Maternal blood loss may be greater and coagulopathy, if present, will significantly increase any operative risks. In addition, labor often progresses quite well in cases of abruption, even if induction is necessary, as a result of associated uterine irritability.

Labor and vaginal delivery may be attempted under the following conditions:

1. Maternal vital signs are acceptable and measured frequently.
2. Ongoing maternal blood loss is limited.
3. Continuous EFM verifies fetal well-being.
4. Labor progresses well, as defined by a good contraction pattern and progressive cervical dilatation.
5. Cesarean section is *immediately* available in case of worsening maternal or fetal condition.

Coagulopathy should be treated only when the patient shows signs of abnormal bleeding or surgery is planned or platelet counts are less than 20,000/mm³. Administration of fibrinogen, 4 g (if below 100 mg/100 ml), or several units of fresh-frozen plasma, and platelets (if count is below 50,000/mm³) shortly before cesarean section will provide adequate hemostasis for the surgery. Termination of the pregnancy usually corrects the process within several hours. Heparin, a common treatment for ongoing DIC of various medical origins, usually only makes things worse.

Obviously, whenever immediate delivery is necessary, cesarean section is the choice. Even if the fetus has died, it may occasionally be necessary to save the mother because active hemorrhage can only be controlled by emptying the uterus.

COMPLICATIONS OF THE THIRD AND FOURTH STAGES

The third stage of labor spans from delivery of the fetus through the delivery of the placenta, the fourth for 1 hour after that. Many of the problems here overlap. Most involve heavier than normal bleeding, or **postpartum hemorrhage**.

UTERINE ATONY

The most common cause of postpartum hemorrhage is failure of the uterus to contract after delivery of the placenta. This process often begins during the third stage, with delayed separation, since uterine contraction plays a major role in this process. Although the cause is sometimes obscure, atony seems much more likely to follow labors complicated by

1. Uterine overdistension (multiple gestation, hydramnios, macrosomia)
2. Prolonged labor, especially with oxytocin stimulation
3. Precipitate labor

One can easily **diagnose** atony by uterine palpation. If the fundus is soft, the diagnosis is made. If it is not, one must look elsewhere.

Most obstetricians try to avoid atony, usually successfully, by rapid infusion of large amounts of oxytocin (20 units/1,000 ml at 200 to 300 ml/hour) over the first postpartum hour.

Should it occur anyway, immediate **therapy** consists of bimanual uterine compression and massage, which may or may not effect contraction but will control the bleeding while trying other things. Ergot alkaloids (Methergine, Ergotrate 0.2 mg) IV or IM or prostaglandin $F_{2\alpha}$ (IV or intramyometrially) should be tried. If these fail, another careful search of the uterine cavity should be performed to rule out retained placenta and rupture. As a last resort, surgical intervention (hypogastric artery ligation, hysterectomy) is available.

Since hemorrhage is usually great by the time the problem is recognized and may be life threatening, if simple measures do not succeed, blood replacement should be early and aggressive. Combinations of packed red cells and fresh-frozen plasma are best, but whole blood may be used if necessary.

RETAINED PLACENTA

The placenta normally separates from the decidua within 5 to 15 minutes after the birth of the baby, allowing for uterine contraction and prevention of hemorrhage. In cases of uterine atony and abnormal placentation (see "Placenta Accreta," below), this may not occur. Other times there is no apparent reason, but the placenta does not spontaneously separate. The problem is often compounded because after several minutes the cervix begins to close, limiting the time one has to act.

Manual removal is indicated if, after 10 minutes, there is no evidence of separation or when partial separation leads to increased bleeding. This is done using the fingers to locate a plane of cleavage and dissecting the placenta off the uterine wall, exerting the pressure inward into the cavity. This must be done with care and the foreknowledge that sometimes one is trying to separate a placenta accreta (so one should not be committed to manual removal).

Sometimes retained placenta only involves a fragment of tissue or a **succenturiate lobe.** This can usually be prevented by careful manual inspection of the uterus after every delivery. If not, this more often presents as late postpartum hemorrhage (several days to several weeks), rather than earlier. If the retained fragments are not too large and the uterus is well contracted, curettage with a horseshoe curette may be useful.

If the cervix has "clamped down," oxytocin stimulation in the delivery room may effect delivery.

What one must *not* do to deliver the retained placenta is to pull on the cord while pushing on the fundus. This may have two undesirable effects: tearing the cord from the placenta and inverting the uterus (see below).

UTERINE INVERSION

If one does pull hard enough on the cord and it does not rip, one may invert the uterus. This is an emergency. The following steps should be taken:

If the placenta has separated in the process,

1. Use a fist to push the fundus back through the cervix immediately.
2. Provide oxytocin stimulation.

If the placenta is intact, try the same maneuver. If not immediately successful,

1. Start a large-bore intravenous line.
2. Begin fluid replacement, including blood, if necessary.
3. Anesthetize the patient.
4. Remove the placenta manually.
5. Use a fist to replace the fundus through the cervix.
6. Provide oxytocin stimulation.

Rarely, laparotomy is necessary to reposition the uterus. Hysterectomy is almost never required.

PLACENTA ACCRETA

The placenta normally implants into the decidua. This serves as a barrier to myometrial penetration so that after delivery, with uterine contraction and retroplacental hemorrhage, a plane of cleavage is easily established and separation readily occurs. When something interferes with decidual formation, this barrier fails and some degree of placental penetration into the uterus itself occurs, termed **placenta accreta.** There are three degrees of penetration:

1. Accreta: Superficial penetration of the myometrium
2. Increta: Deep penetration of the myometrium
3. Percreta: Penetration totally through the myometrium

Placenta accreta is usually **associated** with previous endometrial trauma (curettage, cesarean section, grand multiparity) or placenta previa (poor decidual response in the lower uterine segment).

Most are accretas and may involve varying amounts of placenta. They typically are **diagnosed** after failure of the placenta to separate during an attempt at manual removal (unless associated with placenta previa, when they usually become evident before labor). Percretas often involve antepartum hemorrhage and predispose to uterine rupture, both before and during labor.

The major **risk** posed by adherent placenta is maternal hemorrhage. Appropriate **therapy** can often be determined only by hindsight, since it depends on the degree of penetration and the area of involvement. If the area of adherence is large, attempts at manual removal always result in massive blood loss; therefore, blood replacement is critical. Sometimes curettage followed by uterine packing is effective. More often, hysterectomy is necessary. The real problem is deciding whether to attempt less drastic solutions or to go directly to hysterectomy.

If one knows there is a total accreta, an unusual solution, borrowed from the management of abdominal pregnancy, is to leave the placenta in place and allow involution in situ either spontaneously or via methotrexate. This has occasionally worked but cannot be attempted after partial removal has provoked bleeding.

BIRTH TRAUMA

The birth canal may be injured during labor and delivery. The uterus may rupture during labor or may be injured during forceps delivery. The cervix may be torn by hypertonic labor, attempts at manual dilatation, or application of forceps. The upper and lower vagina and perineum may be similarly injured during either forceps or spontaneous delivery. A thorough inspection, either visually or manually, should be performed after every delivery.

UTERINE RUPTURE

Spontaneous rupture of the previously intact uterus is extremely rare. Most cases involve oxytocin stimulation superimposed on CPD (especially with unrecognized hydrocephalus) or grand multiparity for long periods of time. It is usually catastrophic, presenting with sudden onset of pain, cessation of uterine contractions, maternal shock, and fetal distress or death. The only adequate therapy is immediate abdominal delivery with blood replacement. Sometimes the laceration is reparable; hysterectomy is often necessary.

A much more likely source of spontaneous rupture is the previous uterine scar. If the separation occurs in a low transverse incision from a previous cesarean section, there may be little bleeding or pain. Indeed, these are sometimes noted on routine exploration of the uterus after a seemingly uneventful vaginal delivery. Other times, more bleeding or a cessation of labor will occur, necessitating cesarean section. In these circumstances, repair of the dehiscence is usually sufficient.

If the separation is of a previous vertical incision, from either cesarean section or myomectomy, it more resembles the catastrophic rupture described above in both course and therapy.

CERVICAL TRAUMA

Small cervical lacerations are inevitable during labor. Indeed, the change of the cervical os effected by delivery is testimony to this. Minor cervical tears, unless they cause heavy bleeding, do not require suturing. Sometimes greater tears are caused by hypertonic labor, but the most common source of significant cervical trauma is forceps delivery, either when the head is too high or the cervix is not recognized as being incompletely dilated. Such tears frequently extend into the lower uterine segment, resulting in heavy postpartum bleeding in the presence of a well-contracted uterus. The treatment is surgical repair, usually transvaginally, but sometimes at laparotomy if the tear extends high enough.

VAGINAL AND PERINEAL LACERATION

The most common cause of vaginal/perineal trauma is the episiotomy (intentional second-degree laceration), or lack thereof, meaning that most vaginal deliveries will involve spontaneous vaginal or perineal laceration unless an intentional one (episiotomy) is performed. These tears are categories as follows:

1. First degree: mucosa only
2. Second degree: mucosa and underlying fascia or muscle
3. Third degree: above plus anal sphincter muscle
4. Fourth degree: above plus rectal mucosa

They may involve only the lower vagina, posteriorly or anteriorly toward the periurethral area, or the upper vagina into the vault. They tend to be more severe as a result of forceps delivery. Thorough inspection of the birth canal after delivery reveals the presence and extent of damage. If proper repair is performed, with anatomic reapproximation and good hemostasis, they usually heal without incident. Many obstetricians will use antibiotic prophylaxis if a fourth-degree laceration has occurred.

ABNORMALITIES OF FETAL GROWTH

The normal fetus grows at a certain rate for a certain period of time, achieving a certain size. Abnormalities of growth may occur either by increasing or decreasing the growth rate or the period of time, resulting in smaller or larger and preterm or postterm babies. The following definitions will help to clarify the terms used when discussing these abnormalities:

Term: The length of a normal pregnancy, anywhere between 37 and 42 completed weeks after the beginning of the last menstrual period (assuming a 28-day cycle), or between 35 and 40 completed weeks after ovulation.

Preterm: Anytime before the end of the 37th week (which is the same as the beginning of the 38th week), but after the 20th (before the 20th week, the applicable term is abortion).

Postterm: Anytime after the end of the 42nd week.

Premature: A functional term denoting inadequate development, usually referring to lung function but encompassing other parameters as well.

Postmature: A functional term referring to intrauterine conditions, usually indicating too long a gestation, as evidenced by placental aging and a degenerating intrauterine environment. Characterized by oligohydramnios, fetal wasting, long nails, and parchment-like skin.

Appropriate for gestational age: The right size for fetal age; between the 10th and 90th percentiles in weight for gestational age.

Small for gestational age: Growth retarded; below the 10th percentile in weight for gestational age.

Large for gestational age: Macrosomic; above the 90th percentile in weight for gestational age.

Premature rupture of membranes: Rupture of the membranes at least 2 hours before the spontaneous onset of labor. May be preterm, term, or postterm.

PRETERM LABOR

Preterm labor culminating in delivery is the leading cause of perinatal morbidity and mortality in morphologically normal infants. Primarily due to respiratory distress syndrome and neurological deficits, morbidity and mortality are most effectively prevented by avoiding preterm delivery. Consequently, the remainder of this section deals with preterm labor.

Etiology. The actual cause of preterm labor is unknown. Obviously, what has occurred is that the receptors for oxytocin or prostaglandin that are absent or blocked until term become activated earlier and/or the tocogenic agents themselves are produced in greater quantities earlier. Although the events themselves have not been defined, there are several groups of pregnant women in whom they are more likely to occur. These include pregnancies complicated by

1. A history of preterm labor or second trimester loss

2. A history of cervical conization (increased risk of incompetent cervix)
3. Preterm rupture of the membranes
4. Multiple gestation
5. Hydramnios
6. Uterine anomalies that decrease intrauterine capacity, especially DES related
7. Congenital anomalies
8. Maternal infection, especially pyelonephritis
9. Intrauterine infection, especially TORCH infections
10. Maternal age under 20 or over 35

In addition, many diseases may prompt intentional early delivery, even when they do not induce preterm labor. These include

1. Preeclampsia
2. Diabetes
3. Antepartum vaginal bleeding, especially placenta previa and abruption
4. Medical diseases causing maternal hypoxia or vascular diseases
5. Intrauterine growth retardation and/or fetal distress

Diagnosis.   Most simply, preterm labor is diagnosed when labor begins before term. However, since effective therapy is so dependent on early initiation before labor is well established, the diagnosis of preterm labor is, and should be, a calculated guess that the early contractions will become active labor if not stopped immediately. Consequently, one often diagnoses preterm labor on criteria far less rigid than those used at term. Certainly, when there are regular, painful contractions every 3 minutes and cervical effacement and dilation are in progress, the diagnosis is indisputable. Indeed, in such cases, the question is not should one stop labor, but *can* one stop labor (see "Management," below). On the other end, the criteria become increasingly lax the earlier in the pregnancy one is making the diagnosis. In the second and early third trimesters, contractions every 10 to 20 minutes, even if not painful, should be sufficient to arouse alarm, while by the 35th week they should either be more frequent than every 10 minutes or accompanied by some cervical change. Additionally, any discharge that is even slightly bloody should arouse suspicion of cervical effacement or dilation.

Management.   The first step in the management of preterm labor is to decide whether to attempt to stop it. Usually, one makes this attempt if *all* of the following conditions are met:

1. Membranes are intact.
2. Cervical dilation is less than 4 to 5 cm. (Attempts after this point are usually doomed to failure.)
3. There is no suggestion of amnionitis.
4. There is no fetal distress.
5. There is no fetal anomaly.
6. The fetus is sufficiently premature that intervention is warranted. The usual guidelines for this vary from 33 to 35 completed weeks.
7. Continuation of the pregnancy seems, in sum, safer for both the fetus and mother than does immediate delivery.

For example, if the pregnancy is complicated by severe preeclampsia, its continuance might pose more danger to either mother or fetus than would early delivery.

8. There is no contraindication to the use of the specific tocolytic agent.

Techniques.   **Bed rest** in the lateral recumbent position with hydration often seems to arrest preterm labor if initiated early in its course. Perhaps many of these cases would not have progressed anyway, but nothing is lost in the attempt, if the diagnosis is not clear or the labor seems to be extremely early (minimal cervical effacement or dilation). Sedation with barbiturates or narcotics usually is not useful, and if delivery occurs soon after, may complicate neonatal resuscitation.

Beta-adrenergic agents have become the mainstay of tocolysis. They bind to the $beta_2$-adrenergic receptors in the myometrium and inhibit contractions. Only one, ritodrine (Yutopar) is currently approved for the treatment of preterm labor, but others such as salbutamol, terbutaline, and fenoterol have been used. All are epinephrine derivatives that have preponderantly $beta_2$-adrenergic effects, but significant residual $beta_1$-adrenergic (cardiac) activity. Some are claimed to have fewer side effects, but the relative benefits of one compared with the next have yet to be established. They, like other agents, are most effective when begun early. They may be used intramuscularly, intravenously, subcutaneously, or orally, although the most common regimens seem to begin with intravenous use and progress to oral.

Maternal (and probably fetal) side effects of all the beta-adrenergics include tachycardia and other arrhythmias (which may be experienced as palpitations), secondary myocardial ischemia (chest pain or pressure), pulmonary edema (dyspnea), hypotension, hypokalemia, hyperglycemia, nausea and vomiting, headache, and anxiety. These effects are dose related and form the basis for a list of precautions, contraindications to, and reasons for discontinuance of therapy.

Prior to beginning therapy, the following should be performed:

Ritodrine

1. Complete history and examination
2. ECG
3. Serum potassium and glucose (SMA-8)
4. FHR and contraction strip by EFM

Ritodrine is used according to the following schedule from the package insert:

1. Begin with an IV solution of 150 mg/500 ml 0.9% normal saline or lactated Ringer's solution, yielding a concentration of 0.3 mg/ml.
2. Administer by infusion pump beginning at the rate of 0.1 mg/minute (20 ml/hour) and increase by 0.05 mg/minute every 10 to 15 minutes until contractions cease, a maximal dose of 0.35 mg/minute is reached, or maternal side effects prevent further increases.
3. Continue effective dose for 12 hours of no contractions.
4. Begin oral therapy with 10 mg q 2 hours, 30 minutes before cessation of IV therapy.
5. If well tolerated and effective, switch to 20 mg q 4 hours

PO for maintenance. Effective maintenance doses may be between 10 and 20 mg q 4 hours.

During IV therapy, constant monitoring of maternal and fetal vital signs is essential. Additionally, periodic assessment of maternal serum glucose and potassium should be performed. If long-term oral tocolytic therapy is planned, similar occasional testing is indicated.

Relative contraindications to beta-adrenergic agents include maternal heart disease, diabetes, and hypertension.

Magnesium sulfate ($MgSO_4$) has been used with success to arrest preterm labor. Probably acting as a calcium antagonist to inhibit myometrial contraction by the same mechanism as it prevents convulsions in preeclampsia, $MgSO_4$ is an alternative to beta-adrenergics, especially in those with diabetes and heart disease. The details of its use may be found under "$MgSO_4$ Therapy" in the section on gestational hypertension. The major differences is that to stop labor, after the loading dose of 4 g the initial infusion rate should be 2 g/hour rather than the 1 g/hour used in preeclampsia.

Antiprostaglandin agents, such as ibuprofen, indomethacin, and mefenamic acid, to name a few, have been used sporadically to inhibit premature labor. By blocking the actions of prostaglandin synthetase (and prostaglandin actions, for some of the newer agents), they are capable of stopping preterm labor. However, the widespread activity of these chemicals causes many side effects, not the least of which are maternal coagulation disorders and possible premature with closure of the ductus arteriosus. Their use in the acute situation may be perilous, and they are inappropriate for long-term use.

Alcohol infusion, common before the advent of beta-adrenergics and $MgSO_4$, is no longer used because of its lesser effectiveness and unpleasant side effects.

Delivery. Should the measures discussed above fail, one is faced with the delivery of a premature infant. For the very premature (less than 32 weeks), cesarean section may offer less traumatic delivery, perhaps decreasing the incidence of skull injury. For those delivered vaginally, liberal episiotomy is essential. Certainly, cesarean section is preferable for the premature breech. A pediatrician skilled in resuscitation should be in attendance.

PREMATURE RUPTURE OF THE MEMBRANES

Premature rupture of membranes (PROM) occurs in up to 20% of all pregnancies. Most often, this is a technical distinction since it occurs at or after term and is followed in several hours by the onset of labor. In such circumstances, it poses no management problems other than that the labors are more likely to be longer or complicated by cord compression. However, if PROM occurs significantly preterm or is not followed at term by labor, it involves significant risk for both the mother and child.

Preterm rupture of the membranes in the absence of labor is a major cause of preterm delivery. If labor ensues, one is committed to delivery, as ruptured membranes constitute a contraindication to tocolysis. If labor does not follow shortly, the management becomes more complicated. Most simply, the

question to be answered is, Is the fetus in more danger if delivered than if left in the uterus, or vice versa?

Diagnosis. Continued leakage of clear fluid from the vagina is usually amniotic fluid (AF). Differential diagnosis includes vaginal discharge and urinary incontinence. The surest method of diagnosis is to observe fluid leaking from the cervix. Vaginal discharge and urine are usually acidic, whereas AF is alkaline, and a simple nitrazine test for pH is sufficient to distinguish them. At term, this poses no problem because the nitrazine paper may be applied directly to the cervical os without fear of contamination, since delivery will be imminent. If for some reason this is not clear enough (too little fluid), AF may be distinguished from urine by the characteristic ferning it undergoes when allowed to dry on a glass slide. Vaginal secretions and urine do not fern. Rarely, various other tests, such as vital staining for fetal cells and intra-amniotic instillation of dye, may be used.

If PROM occurs preterm, one may want to postpone delivery, so fear of contamination by examination assumes greater importance. If large amounts of AF are leaking, the diagnosis, as above, will be easy. If not, a single sterile speculum examination (although some question its sterility) may be used to determine status. Digital examination is contraindicated until the actual process of delivery has begun.

Risks. If PROM occurs significantly preterm, the major risks to the fetus are those of early delivery versus those of intrauterine infection. The incidence of amnionitis varies with the population and the bacterial colonization of the lower genital tract, while the morbidity and mortality of prematurity depend, in part, on the quality of neonatal intensive care. Apart from these variables, the longer the membranes are ruptured, the greater the risk of amnionitis, and the more premature the fetus, the greater the morbidity and mortality.

The risk of amnionitis increases sharply after 24 hours and tends to level off after several days. If intrauterine infection does occur, perinatal mortality may be increased up to 25%.

Immediate delivery of the preterm infant may result in minimal morbidity and mortality if the gestational age is over 35 weeks, but may result in increasingly severe respiratory distress syndrome and associated complications before that. However, in many centers, physicians feel more comfortable dealing with prematurity than with the increased risk of infection as early as 32 to 33 weeks. The incidence of respiratory distress syndrome may be reduced by a period of intrauterine existence after PROM of 24 to 48 hours. Many studies have considered the acceleration of pulmonary maturation that may be prompted by prolonged PROM, but have been unable to resolve the question. Each side of the argument has its proponents.

The major maternal risks of PROM are related to amnionitis from delay. There are no maternal benefits from delay in delivery. Although amnionitis, appropriately treated, rarely causes maternal mortality, the morbidity may be considerable.

Management. Since the risks of PROM are related to the stage of gestation at which it occurs, appropriate management must take this into consideration. If PROM has occurred in a term pregnancy, pulmonary maturity may be presumed and there will be no benefit obtained by delay. Induction of labor or cesarean section (depending on obstetric considerations) should be initiated in a timely enough fashion so that delivery will occur within roughly 24 hours of membrane rupture.

If the fetus is premature (cutoffs for various centers will vary from below 32 to below 36 weeks), so-called conservative management is employed. This consists of no vaginal examinations (except for, perhaps, the one sterile speculum examination to establish the diagnosis and obtain an AF culture) and observation in the hospital for signs of labor or amnionitis (maternal fever, increasing WBCs). This is continued until signs of infection, labor, or pulmonary maturity occur. In some centers, an attempt to induce pulmonary maturity (see below) followed by delivery in 24 to 48 hours is the preferred course of action.

In between these is a degree of prematurity in which neonatal mortality or serious morbidity is unlikely, but a stay in the neonatal intensive care unit is virtually assured. The course of action may be less clearly defined. Some will opt for immediate delivery, some for procrastination, others for a little of each (24 hours of procrastination followed by delivery).

Pulmonary maturity

Since pulmonary maturity is the major determinant of the premature infant's morbidity and mortality, its determination or, better, its induction is of considerable concern. In general, in the very premature fetus, lack of pulmonary maturity is presumed. However, in cases where one is less certain, an L/S ratio and prostaglandin assessment may be done on AF obtained either transvaginally or transabdominally (if a suitable pocket can be located on ultrasonography).

In the pregnancy between 28 and 32 weeks duration, pulmonary maturity may be accelerated by corticosteroid administration. Significant increases in L/S ratio and decreases in respiratory distress syndrome have been obtained 24 hours after maternal injection of betamethasone (12 mg IM), a long-acting corticosteroid. Interestingly, the results are transient, wearing off within several days. Therefore, if one attempts to induce pulmonary maturation, one should probably be prepared to effect delivery within 1 to 3 days.

There are, however, potentially serious side effects of this therapy. The risk of sepsis is increased several times, and pre-existent diabetes or preeclampsia may be considerably worsened. Long-term effects on the fetus are unknown, although thus far there are none demonstrated in humans.

POSTTERM PREGNANCY

After the fetus has achieved maturity, it can safely be born. For the most part, what we anxiously await is for the uterus to expel it. continued intrauterine existence can only result in a fetus that continues to thrive and grow (presenting a more difficult delivery) or one that begins to outgrow its placental supply (resulting in a more dangerous delivery). This becomes increasingly common after the due date has passed and is a real danger by the end of the 42nd week. Pregnancies lasting beyond the end of the 42nd week are all **postterm**. Those in which the fetus appears to be compromised are also **postmature** (see definitions above). Because the postmature fetus is one in danger, one would prefer to prevent it rather than diagnose it.

Diagnosis.   The diagnosis of postterm pregnancy is strictly one of dating. A pregnancy cannot be effectively dated in the third trimester, because there is too much variation in size and maturation rates to correlate with age. In other words, the key to the diagnosis of postterm pregnancy is to date the pregnancy as early as possible, preferably in the first trimester, by last menstrual period, early pelvic examination, sonography and perhaps HCG levels.

On the other hand, diagnosis of the postmature fetus is often made at delivery, by observation of the wasted infant with characterstic long nails and shedding skin. This is too late. Earlier detection may be achieved by the biophysical profile (BPP) to detect oligohydramnios and serial ultrasonography documenting failure to grow. Although this is better, it is still later than it should be. As mentioned above, the postmature fetus is best prevented. This is done by expeditious delivery of the term and postterm pregnancy.

Management.   Effective management of postterm pregnancy is designed to avoid postmaturity, placental insufficiency, and CPD by delivering as soon as possible but carefully monitoring the fetus while waiting for safe delivery to become possible. There is considerable variation in protocol to achieve these ends.

Most involve some combination of NSTs, CSTs, and BPPs at intervals of no longer than 1 week after term, but perhaps less (as often as is necessary to ensure fetal health), while awaiting spontaneous labor or inducibility. When the cervix becomes favorable, if the pregnancy has progressed beyond 41 weeks, it is terminated by induction of labor. If the cervix remains unfavorable, one continues careful observation of the fetus as described above. Unfortunately, the longer the pregnancy continues, the less the likelihood of successful vaginal delivery, either because of CPD or fetal distress in labor. The only alternative in these cases, however, is induction in the face of an unfavorable cervix, an unpleasant prospect at best.

Obviously, if fetal monitoring suggests jeopardy (nonreactive NST, +CST, poor BPP), the pregnancy should be ended. This need not automatically be by cesarean section, since a significant minority will tolerate labor with optimization of fetal condition (see "Fetal Monitoring"). Also, EFM obviously is of extreme importance in all such labors.

INTRAUTERINE GROWTH RETARDATION (IUGR)

The fetus that weighs less than 90% (below the 10th percentile) of its gestational-age peers is defined as small for gestational age (SGA). Except for the fetus that is small because its heritage is small (genetic), these fetuses are growth retarded. They are generally at increased risk for morbidity and mortality because something has interfered with their growth.

There are two patterns of IUGR, symmetric and asymmetric. Symmetric IUGR is characterized by a uniformly small fetus, while asymmetric IUGR exhibits sparing of head size (normal BPD) in the face of decreased abdominal circumference. Symmetrically SGA babies typically are constitutionally small, genetically abnormal, or malformed, whereas asymmetric IUGR is more likely due to nutritional or hypoxic deprivation.

Etiology.   Most of the insults resulting in IUGR interfere with oxygen or nutrition supplied to the fetus. This may be a primary deficit or secondary to decreased blood supply. Additionally, fetuses that are genetically abnormal are often SGA. A partial listing of these conditions follows.

Conditions resulting in hypoxia:

1. Severe maternal anemia, especially hemoglobinopathies
2. Cyanotic heart disease
3. Severe pulmonary disease
4. Pregnancy at very high altitude
5. Maternal smoking

Conditions resulting in poor fetal nutrition:

1. Maternal starvation or poor maternal weight gain
2. Maternal drug use (heroin, cocaine)
3. Maternal alcoholism?

Conditions resulting in decreased placental perfusion:

1. Preeclampsia
2. Diabetes with small vessel disease
3. Chronic renal disease
4. Multiple gestation
5. Placental anomalies and infarction
6. Postterm pregnancy

Other conditions:

1. Congenital rubella
2. Cytomegalovirus
3. Chromosomal anomalies
4. Congenital heart disease

Diagnosis. IUGR may be diagnosed by any of these criteria:

1. The fetus is shown to be below the 10th percentile in weight for its age.
2. It has failed to grow in accordance with its own previously established growth curve.
3. Asymmetric IUGR is demonstrated on sonography.

The first presumes an accurate knowledge of gestational age, which may be based on last menstrual period correlated with either early examination, ultrasonography, or HCG level. The second requires a previous accurate measurement of size and a failure to grow sufficiently during a known interval. The last is the only one that can be determined without prior dating or sizing.

Estimates of size are subject to the vagaries of physical examination and the limitations of ultrasound technology. Their interpretation into age depends on the size of the comparison population (black fetuses are smaller than white, Denver fetuses smaller than Californians) and the age at which the measurements are made. Sonography may date a pregnancy to within 2 to 3 days in the first 2 months, but by the early third trimester, a given size may fit into age categories spanning 3 weeks.

In most cases, poor interval growth cannot be demonstrated in a period under 3 weeks. Therefore, sonographic monitoring of growth is typically done at 3- to 6-week intervals, depending on the degree of suspicion.

Management. One presumes that the SGA fetus is nutritionally deprived until proven otherwise. Management, therefore, consists of extremely careful monitoring of fetal well-being and growth. NSTs, CSTs, and BPPs should be performed at least weekly, sonography at least every third week.

If the IUGR is diagnosed many weeks prior to term, the prospects for good intrauterine growth until term are extremely poor. These fetuses, however, frequently tolerate early delivery very well because the hostile intrauterine environment seems to hasten pulmonary maturity. If the fetus fails to grow well as demonstrated by serial sonography, amniocentesis for L/S ratio may be useful.

Oligohydramnios complicating IUGR is an extremely poor sign and is often an indication for delivery, except in cases of extreme prematurity.

The fetal distress one is so carefully watching for obviously is an indication for immediate delivery.

Delivery. Mostly, babies suffering from IUGR, if they are deprived, do not tolerate labor well. Oligohydramnios drastically exaggerates this. Although it is appropriate to maximize fetal condition (hydration, lateral recumbent position, maternal oxygen), cesarean section should be immediately available and will frequently be necessary.

MULTIPLE GESTATION

Pregnancy complicated by more than one fetus occurs spontaneously in slightly more than 1% of cases. In the absence of ovulation induction, almost all of these are twins. Such pregnancies carry far greater risk than singleton pregnancies. Since the problems and complications associated with triplets etc. are essentially those of twin pregnancy, only more so, these will not be discussed separately. The following definitions will help to clarify the terms used in the discussion.

Dizygotic twins: Also known as fraternal twins, these fetuses arise from fertilization of two ova and are, in fact, only simultaneous siblings. Any sex combination is possible. Rates of occurrence vary with population, maternal age, and maternal history.

Monozygotic twins: So-called identical twins arise from a single fertilized egg by cleavage. Depending on the age of the zygote at cleavage, these exhibit various degrees of separation between the fetuses. The earlier the cleavage, the greater the degree of separation. These are always same sex twins, unless there has been chromosomal dropping.

Diamniotic, dichorionic twins: These have separate chorions, amnions, and placentas. They may be either dizygotic or monozygotic. Although there are two separate placentas, they may be physically fused, giving the appearance of only one. If monozygotic, they represent separation before the third day after fertilization.

Diamniotic, monochorionic twins: These have one chorion and placenta but separate amnions and are always monozygotic. Separation of the fetuses occurs between the fourth and eighth postconceptual days.

Monoamniotic, monochorionic twins: These share one

amnion and therefore one chorion and one placenta and are always monozygotic. Separation occurs after the 8th day but before formation of the embryonic disk (9th to 11th day).

Conjoined twins: Separation at any time after the ninth day results in incomplete twinning. The degree of separation depends on the timing and may result in fetuses joined at the head (craniopagus), the chest (thoracopagus), the pelvis (ischiopagus), or the back (pyopagus).

Chimerism: Rarely, two cell lines are present in the same individual. This may be from two sperm fertilizing the same egg or from transplacental exchange of genetic material between dizygotic twins. Most cases of this are blood chimerism (the presence of two blood types), probably due to bone marrow migration between fetuses in utero.

Etiology. Most twinning is dizygotic and results from multiple ovulation. As a spontaneous event, this is more common among women over 35, blacks, and women with a family history of twinning. Also, all twins due to fertility drugs are dizygotic. With clomiphene citrate the incidence is 6 to 7%, and with HMG therapy, over 20%. Almost all cases of multiple gestation involving three or more fetuses are due to gonadotropin therapy.

Monozygotic twinning occurs at a relatively constant rate of 0.4% across various populations and is thought to be due to some sort of insult, whether hypoxic or teratogenic. This has never been proved, however.

Diagnosis. It used to be said that the diagnosis of twins was made more than 50% of the time in the delivery room. Fortunately, since many of the complications are antenatal, this is almost never true any longer, because of the availability of two technological advances: serum AFP screening and sonography. Even in the absence of a larger-than-dates uterus, with the advent of AFP screening for most pregnancies, the diagnosis should be suspected in the early second trimester, since twin pregnancy usually results in higher than normal levels. Confirmation at this point is obtained by ultrasonography.

If this technology is not used, the usual reasons for suspecting twins are the presence of a larger-than-dates uterus, the presence of many fetal parts, or the detection of two fetal hearts (at least 10 bpm different from each other). Regardless of the reason, the diagnosis can usually be made with confidence by careful sonography.

Complications. Pregnancy complicated by more than one fetus is fraught with risk. The overall perinatal morbidity and mortality rates are many times higher than for singleton pregnancy (up to 15% mortality) and even higher for monozygotic than for dizygotic twins. The major causes of morbidity and mortality are discussed below:

Antenatal complications:

1. Prematurity: This is the major cause of morbidity and mortality. It is usually attributed to increased intrauterine volume and premature labor. The average duration of pregnancy decreases by several weeks for each additional fetus. Hydramnios is also much more common in twin pregnancies and contributes to the risk of prematurity.
2. Growth retardation: Twins fetuses grow more slowly than singletons, contributing to the complications of prematurity.

3. Intertwin transfusion: Resulting from vascular communications between fetal circulations in monochorionic twinning, this causes one fetus to become anemic while the other is plethoric. Most commonly associated with artery-vein communications, the result is one growth-retarded twin and the other twin with cardiac hypertrophy and hypertension.
4. Cord accidents: In monoamniotic twins, there is a very high incidence of one twin becoming entangled in the cord of the other. This frequently results in the antenatal death of one fetus.
5. Preeclampsia: Probably due to increased placental mass, this occurs with twice to three times the frequency in twins as in singletons. It also occurs earlier and with increased severity.
6. Spontaneous abortion: Many threatened abortions are now known to be the first trimester loss of one twin, with the survival of the other, apparently unharmed. This has been demonstrated by sonography.
7. Congenital anomalies: More common among monozygotic than dizygotic twins (related to insult?), the rate is two to three times higher than for singleton pregnancies.

Intrapartum complications:

1. Hypotonic labor: Related to increased uterine distension, abnormal labor patterns are far more common.
2. Abnormal presentation: Breech and transverse presentations during labor are exaggerated by prematurity but are more common even when corrected for gestational age.
3. Cord prolapse: Associated with increased incidences of breech, prematurity, and unengaged second fetuses, this is a significant risk in labor.
4. Premature placental separation: This becomes a risk primarily after delivery of the first twin.
5. Postpartum hemorrhage: Like hypotonic labor, this is related to increased uterine distension.

Management. Antepartum management of pregnancy complicated by multiple fetuses is directed at avoidance of complications, primarily prematurity. While tocolytics, cerclage, progestins, and special diets have been tried, the only known action that may decrease prematurity-related morbidity and mortality is bed rest. Although there is some controversy about whether bed rest actually prolongs pregnancy, it is clear that it does increase placental perfusion and enhance fetal growth, improving morbidity and mortality statistics. It probably also decreases the risk of preeclampsia. Careful monitoring of maternal weight gain, blood pressure, and fetal growth will aid in early detection of problems.

Intrapartum management of the mother with multiple fetuses includes careful EFM for all fetuses, an awareness of the potential for hypotonic labor and hemorrhage, and appropriate management of abnormal presentations. A running intravenous line is usually standard procedure. Careful augmentation of labor with oxytocin is acceptable. There are no specific contraindications to any forms of anesthesia/analgesia, but one must be aware of the greater likelihood of hypotension with epidural and the supine position.

Delivery is also fraught with danger. Many physicians are turning increasingly to cesarean section. As with breech deliveries, many elect for cesarean birth unless everything is perfect. Indications for abdominal delivery frequently include the following:

1. Either fetus presenting as other than vertex: The incidence of cesarean section is much higher if twin A is not vertex, but many now prefer it even for a twin B breech.
2. Interlocking twins: If the first is breech and the second vertex and the head of the first lies above the head of the second, the chins may lock as the first descends. This is an absolute indication for cesarean section.
3. Multiple gestation involving more than two fetuses.
4. Growth retardation and labor complications.

Vaginal delivery, however, is commonly undertaken if the first fetus is a vertex and not markedly smaller than the second. The following guidelines are useful for vaginal delivery:

1. Deliver the first infant.
2. Clamp the cord with one clamp. Do not unclamp until after delivery of the second.
3. If the presenting part of the second descends into the inlet, rupture membranes and guide it down.
4. If there is no bleeding and no cord prolapse, allow labor to continue as if this were a first delivery. Continued fetal monitoring is essential. If labor does not spontaneously resume within a few minutes, cautious use of oxytocin is advisable.
5. If the presenting part does not descend into the pelvis on delivery of twin A or if there is placental separation or cord prolapse, immediate action is necessary. Under good uterine relaxation (essential) and adequate anesthesia (both are provided if epidural is already in place), version and extraction should be performed before the cervix has a chance to contract. If one is not skilled at version and extraction, cesarean section and should be performed.
6. The cord of the second twin should be doubly clamped for later evaluation.

Postpartum. The postpartum management is the same as for singleton delivery, except more vigilant, since the incidence of postpartum atony (hemorrhage) and lacerations is greater. A careful examination of the placenta and membranes aids greatly in determining monozygosity or dizygosity.

PREGNANCY-INDUCED HYPERTENSION

Gestation-related hypertension is a significant source of perinatal and maternal morbidity and mortality. Differing from ordinary hypertension in its genesis and behavior, it must be treated as a separate entity. We begin with specific definitions and terms:

Hypertension: Systolic blood pressure higher than 140 mm Hg or a rise of at least 30 mm Hg over first-trimester levels and/or diastolic pressure greater than 90 mm Hg or a rise of at least 15 mm Hg over first-trimester levels.

Gestational hypertension: Isolated hypertension that begins after the 20th week of gestation or during the first 24 hours postpartum.

Gestational edema: Edema sufficient to cause 5 pounds of weight gain within 1 week, with onset during the same time period. Edema sufficient to cause swelling of the feet on arising in the morning or of the hands and face in the evening is also suspect. This must be distinguished from the edema that naturally occurs with pregnancy.

Gestational proteinuria: Proteinuria in excess of 0.3 g in 24 hours, in the absence of other kidney disease, with onset during the same time period.

Preeclampsia: Hypertension coexistent with either proteinuria or edema or both during the same time period. Preeclampsia may be either mild or severe. **Mild preeclampsia** may be diagnosed when

1. Systolic pressure remains below 160 mm Hg
2. Diastolic pressure remains below 110 mm Hg
3. There is no evidence of organ involvement beyond the vascular tree.

Severe preeclampsia is characterized by any of the following:

1. Systolic pressure greater than 160 mm Hg
2. Diastolic pressure greater than 110 mm Hg
3. Proteinuria greater than 5 g/24 hours
4. Hyperreflexia
5. Oliguria
6. Headache, altered sensorium, or visual symptoms
7. Epigastric or right upper quadrant pain (hepatic involvement)
8. Cardiorespiratory compromise
9. Clinically evident DIC or thrombocytopenia

Eclampsia: Preeclampsia with convulsions, not related to other neurological disease.

These are to be distinguished from **chronic hypertension,** which coexists with pregnancy and may be differentiated by its presence before the 20th week of gestation. Exceptionally, preeclampsia and related conditions may occur earlier than the 20th week in pregnancies complicated by multiple gestation or hydatidiform mole. **Superimposed preeclampsia** is the occurrence of preeclampsia in the presence of extant chronic hypertension.

Pathology

Preeclampsia is essentially a disease of vasospasm. Although the etiology of the disease is still undetermined, much of the process is being unraveled. An important factor in maintaining normal blood pressure is the angiotensin-renin system. **Renin,** produced in the kidneys by the juxtamedullary cells, acts on **renin substrate** to produce **angiotensin I,** a decapeptide, which is in turn cleaved by **angiotensinase** in the blood to **angiotensin II,** an extremely potent vasopressor. In addition to producing increased vascular tone, angiotensin II stimulates

Puthognomonic lesion? preeclampsia

aldosterone secretion, which leads via salt retention to increased intravascular volume. During normal pregnancy, increased production of both these hormones combined with refractoriness of the vascular tree to angiotensin II results in an increase in intravascular volume in the face of decreased blood pressure.

For unknown reasons, in preeclampsia the vascular tree exhibits an increased sensitivity to angiotensin II. Even though actual serum levels are lower in preeclampsia than during normal pregnancy, the vascular response is exaggerated. Consequently, generalized arteriolar vasospasm causes simultaneous hypertension, decreased intravascular volume, and decreased end-organ blood flow. There is also generalized endothelial damage (seen most clearly in the glomeruli of the kidney), which allows leakage of protein from capillaries. In the kidneys, this leakage leads to proteinuria; in the extremities, in combination with increased hydrostatic pressure, it leads to edema.

The combination of decreased organ perfusion and organ congestion leads to the compromise of organ function. Most of the pathology and symptoms of preeclampsia can be explained on this basis. The organ systems with which we are most concerned are cardiovascular, renal, hematologic, hepatic, neurological, and uteroplacental.

Although the etiology of preeclampsia is unknown, it is clear that the placenta plays a central role. Preeclampsia does not occur in nonpregnant women, and definitive therapy is delivery, which cures the disease within a few days. Furthermore, pregnant states characterized by increased placental mass (hydatidiform mole, twins, diabetes, erythroblastosis fetalis) predispose to its development.

Some suspect an immunologic reaction to placental tissue as the culprit. Nulliparous women account for most cases, while multiparas who did not experience the disease in prior pregnancy have next to no risk in subsequent ones. However, the recurrence rate among the previously affected may be as high as 15%. Interestingly, some studies have demonstrated that the risk for parous women in pregnancies fathered by a different man is the same as that for first pregnancy.

Another theory implicates a chronic coagulopathy initiated by placental thromboplastins, which generate fibrin split products whose deposition in vascular walls may play a part in changing vascular reactivity. Indeed, there is laboratory evidence for coagulopathy in many but not all cases, but no substantial proof that a coagulopathy is more than a by-product of the disease.

Additionally, many nutritional theories have been proposed, none substantiated.

Cardiovascular. The major cardiovascular changes in preeclampsia are the decrease in intravascular volume, which is central to the disease process, and the increase in blood pressure. Cardiac output usually decreases slightly as a result of decreased intravascular volume, a change that may be marked in the later stages of the disease. The work capacity of the heart is unchanged.

Renal. Decreased intravascular volume and vasospasm lead to decreased renal blood flow (RBF), which leads to decreased GFR, which in severe cases leads to oliguria and, rarely, anuria. The increases in RBF, GFR, and urine output encountered in normal pregnancy return toward nonpregnant

levels and, in severe cases, fall well below. Most cases of anuria are due to **acute tubular necrosis,** from which recovery is the rule, but occasionally RBF will fall to such low levels that **renal cortical necrosis,** a largely irreversible destruction of kidney tissue, may occur. These changes are reflected in blood chemistry as increased creatinine and BUN and decreased creatinine clearance.

The so-called pathognomonic lesion of preeclampsia, **glomerular capillary endotheliosis,** may be seen in the kidney. Fibrin monomer, a fibrin split product, is deposited in the endothelial cells of the capillaries, resulting in swelling, loss of integrity of the wall, and occlusion of the lumen. These changes are thought to be the cause of the proteinuria. Most likely, similar lesions occur in blood vessels throughout the body.

Hematologic. The two major hematologic abnormalities are related to changes in intravascular volume and coagulation. Secondary to a decrease in intravascular volume there is hemoconcentration, since red cell mass is unchanged. This is manifested by an increased hematocrit. Before easy determination of BUN and creatinine clearance, changes in hematocrit were used to monitor the progress of preeclampsia, an increase heralding a worsening of the disease.

A low-grade chronic DIC is thought to be part of the disease process of preeclampsia, although its place in the schema is uncertain. Laboratory evidence is seen with a high incidence of elevated fibrin split products, prolonged thrombin time, thrombocytopenia, and hypofibrinogenemia, especially in severe cases. Certainly, this concept fits with the fibrin deposition seen in vascular walls and may account for the **microangiopathic hemolytic anemia** encountered in some cases of severe preeclampsia.

Hepatic. Elevation of hepatic enzymes (SGOT, SGPT, GGTP) is not uncommon and seems to reflect the combined effects of decreased hepatic blood flow, secondary to vascular spasm, and hepatic edema. Similarly, the epigastric and right upper quadrant pain now considered a symptom of serious disease are caused by hepatic edema and stretching of Glisson's capsule.

More permanent damage, like intrahepatic and subcapsular hemorrhage and **periportal necrosis,** usually only occurs with eclampsia. Indeed, most cases of hemorrhagic liver damage have been diagnosed on postmortem and may reflect terminal events.

Neurological. Cerebral and retinal edema are thought to be the source of the vision symptoms and headache that so often accompany severe preeclampsia. Funduscopic examination will often confirm this. Rarely, vascular spasm will be so severe as to cause retinal ischemia or detachment. The etiology of hyperreflexia is less clear. As with the liver, cerebrovascular hemorrhage probably results from convulsions or death and is not part of the basic process.

Electrolytes. There are no consistent electrolyte changes in preeclampsia. Serum sodium, potassium, chloride, and bicarbonate seem unchanged. Total intravascular sodium is decreased, but this reflects decreased intravascular volume. Similarly, serum BUN, creatinine, and uric acid are increased, but this reflects decreased GFR.

Uteroplacental. The same vascular spasm affects the uterine arteries, resulting in decreased uteroplacental blood flow. The more severe the disease, the greater the decrease. This obviously results in decreased placental perfusion, threatening the fetus. In addition, a similar pattern of placental endothelial damage is noted.

Diagnosis of preeclampsia

An understanding of the disease provides the means for early diagnosis. One must be constantly on the lookout for early signs and symptoms. Much of the standard prenatal checkup is directed to this end (measurement of blood pressure and weight, analysis of urine for albumin, checking for edema). Minor increases in blood pressure should arouse suspicion. One must also be alert for symptoms that may signal other organ involvement (see the definition of severe preeclampsia above), since severe preeclampsia may superimpose itself on mild disease with frightening speed. Indeed, patients may progress to eclampsia with only mildly elevated blood pressure.

The "roll-over test" may be used to prospectively identify nulliparas at risk. Capitalizing on increased angiotension sensitivity, which might result in an exaggerated pressor response, this test is an attempt to provoke such a reaction. By rolling the patient from the lateral recumbent to the supine position, one creates a certain amount of aortocaval compression and supine hypotension, which in turn elicits angiotensin production. Appropriate responses correct the hypotension. Those who exhibit an exaggerated response overshoot and become transiently hypertensive are thought to be at increased risk for preeclampsia. In practice, the test is best performed between 28 and 32 weeks gestation. A significant response is any increase in supine diastolic pressure greater than 20 mm Hg over the lateral recumbent.

Risks

Preeclampsia is a double threat to the pregnant woman and her fetus. By progressively decreasing uteroplacental perfusion, it endangers the fetus. Growth retardation in chronic cases and fetal distress are common. Second, eclampsia may supervene at any time. Eclamptic convulsions outside the hospital, because they do not abate, may result in fetal death up to 90% of the time and frequent maternal death. If they occur under medical supervision, appropriate action may save virtually all the mothers and most of the fetuses. However, worsening preeclampsia may force delivery of a premature infant in an attempt to avoid eclampsia.

Therapy

Treatment is obviously designed to avoid the dangers. The first priority is avoidance of eclampsia. Second, one tries to avoid premature delivery, cognizant that this may be superseded by one's first priority or by fetal distress. The ever present risk of eclampsia mandates that once the diagnosis of pregnancy has been made, the mother be hospitalized.

If the preeclampsia is mild and the fetus premature, watchful waiting with careful constant evaluation of mother and fetus is desirable. If the preeclampsia is severe or the fetus is mature, expeditious delivery, usually by attempted induction, is the best choice. If the mother is eclamptic or the fetus distressed, one must deliver immediately.

Upon admission of the mild preeclampsic to the hospital, certain measures are taken:

1. Complete history and examination
2. CBC, urinalysis, urine culture, SMA (electrolytes, glucose, BUN, creatinine, uric acid, liver enzymes, albumin), coagulation studies (fibrinogen, fibrin split products, thrombin time, prothrombin time, activated partial thromboplastin time), 24-hour urine for protein and creatinine (and calculation of creatinine clearance)
3. Sonogram to assess fetal age
4. EFM (NST, CST) and possibly biophysical profile to assess fetal condition
5. Bed rest in a quiet room in a lateral recumbent position, to help control blood pressure and increase placental perfusion
6. Eclamptic precautions, consisting of airway, injectable anticonvulsant, and tracheostomy set *at the bedside*
7. Vital signs q 4 hours except 2 AM (sleep is important too)
8. Diet providing 2,400 kcal/day, 65 g protein/day, no restriction of salt or fluids

Conservative management should continue until fetal maturity is obtained or worsening fetal or maternal condition forces delivery. In addition to the above, it should include

1. Daily weights
2. Careful intake and output measurements, with maintenance of output at a minimum of 30 ml/hour
3. Urinalysis b.i.d. for protein
4. Daily BUN, frequent coagulation and enzyme studies
5. Assessment of fetal condition by EFM and biophysical profile at least twice weekly and possibly more often
6. Assessment of fetal growth by sonography at 2- to 3-week intervals
7. Assessment of fetal maturity by amniocentesis at 34 to 36 weeks, unless preeclampsia is extremely mild

Measures that are traditionally part of the management of preeclampsia but have been for the most part abandoned are

1. Sedation with phenobarbital, which probably does little to avoid convulsion and may adversely affect the fetus
2. Diuretic therapy for either hypertension or edema, since it can only worsen the underlying disease process of decreased intravascular volume
3. Assessment of fetal well-being by serum or urine estriol measurement (too long a lag time and too much room for error) or by serum placental lactogen (more a measure of placental mass than fetal condition)

Severe preeclampsia mandates the addition of the following measures:

1. IV or IM magnesium sulfate for hyperreflexia
2. Antihypertensive therapy for systolic pressure greater than 180 mm Hg or diastolic greater than 110 mm Hg
3. Immediate delivery for clinical coagulopathy, epigastric or upper quadrant pain, sensorial or vision changes, oliguria, or cardiopulmonary compromise

4. Coagulopathy is usually best treated by delivery rather than medical management. Although heparinization may briefly benefit some patients, it cannot enable one to prolong the pregnancy and makes the physical act of delivery more dangerous. A more sensible policy is to correct whichever abnormalities (hypofibrinogenemia, thrombocytopenia, etc.) one must in order to safely conduct birth, and the rest will usually resolve within 24 hours.

Magnesium sulfate therapy. $MgSO_4$ blocks the myoneural junction and prevents convulsions in therapeutic doses. It is indicated in all cases of severe preeclampsia and during labor even in mild cases. It has little effect on blood pressure or fetal condition, but in overdose may cause cardiorespiratory arrest. Administered either IV or IM, levels must be carefully clinically monitored. Many in addition measure serum levels, which should be between 4 and 7 mEq/L.

The following guidelines ensure safety:

1. If IV, begin with a 4-g loading dose over several minutes (4 g/20 ml); continue with 1 to 2 g/hour (100 to 200 ml/hour of 10 g/1,000 ml solution).
2. If IM, begin with 5 g each buttock (5 g/10 ml) for a total of 10 g; follow with 5 g q 4 hours, alternating buttocks.
3. Maintain running IV and Foley catheter and ensure urine output of at least 30 ml/hour, since $MgSO_4$ is excreted primarily by the kidneys.
4. Observe carefully for signs of magnesium toxicity:
   a. Loss of patellar reflex (8 to 10 mEq/L)
   b. Respiratory depression: Rate less than 8/minute (12 mEq/L)
   c. Cardiac arrest (>15 mEq/L)
5. If signs of toxicity arise or adequate suppression of reflexes is not obtained with above therapeutic doses, measure serum magnesium levels.
6. Have 10 ml of 10% calcium gluconate solution at the bedside, as this is the antidote for magnesium toxicity.

Antihypertensive therapy.   Control of hypertension is indicated when systolic levels surpass 180 mm Hg or diastolic levels reach 110 mm Hg, because the mother is at increased risk for cerebral hemorrhage. However, rapid drops in pressure may threaten the fetus by decreasing perfusion.

The ideal agent for this is **hydralazine** (Apresoline) because it is a vasodilator in addition to its antihypertensive action, so it tends to maintain perfusion of vital organ systems and the fetus. Initial dose should be 5 to 10 mg every 20 minutes until the desired effect is achieved. Maintenance may be PO, IM, or IV. The fetus should be monitored with continuous EFM during this process.

Other agents have been used, as well. **Diazoxide** (Hyperstat), 300 mg IV, is extremely effective but has several undesirable side effects. Pressure drops may be precipitous and profound; it may interfere with uterine contractions; salt retention and circulatory overload are a real risk. If diazoxide is used, it should be administered with furosemide, 40 mg IV, to avoid this last.

Delivery

Delivery is indicated under any of three conditions:

1. The fetus is mature.
2. Preeclampsia is complicated by one of the ominous signs.
3. The fetus is distressed.

The method of delivery will depend on an assessment of several factors. Labor in preeclampsia usually proceeds apace. Uterine irritability seems to predispose to easy inducibility and good progress, even when the cervix may not seem ripe. Therefore, unless fetal distress is present, induction of labor is probably the preferred route. All preeclamptics in labor should be treated as if they were severely preeclamptic, which means a running IV, $MgSO_4$ therapy, and intensive maternal and fetal monitoring.

While many eschew epidural anesthesia in favor of narcotic analgesia and pudendal block for these patients, others feel that with careful, adequate hydration, regional anesthesia may be appropriate. Certainly the risk of superimposing sudden, massive vasodilatation on a contracted intravascular volume resulting in severe hypertension is one that cannot be taken lightly.

Cesarean section becomes preferable when induction fails, fetal distress is present, or severe fetal prematurity and an uninducible cervix coincide with the need for immediate delivery. As for labor, all preeclamptics undergoing cesarean section should be on $MgSO_4$ therapy. Anesthesia is usually balanced general, but some consider regional to be acceptable (see above).

Postpartum

Preeclampsia officially ends 24 hours after delivery, and all precautions initiated during the antepartum and intrapartum periods should be continued until then, including $MgSO_4$ therapy. In reality, although the risk of convulsion decreases almost to zero after 24 hours, many of the other symptoms persist up to several weeks. Antihypertensive therapy should be maintained until blood pressure levels approach normal. Proteinuria should be checked periodically until it has resolved. If symptoms persist beyond 6 weeks postpartum, serious consideration must be given to the presence of underlying hypertensive or renal disease.

ECLAMPSIA

If a preeclamptic gravida has a seizure and there is no underlying neurological disease, this is eclampsia. Eclampsia is a medical emergency characterized by tonic-clonic seizures that are usually recurrent and frequently unremitting. By definition, preeclampsia always precedes eclampsia. Although the interval may be short and the preeclampsia mild, usually some time has elapsed during which the underlying disease has not been recognized.

Most of the permanent injury to mother and fetus is derived from two sources. First, during seizures, the mother does not effectively breathe, so that both she and the fetus are subjected to varying degrees of hypoxia, depending on the length and frequency of the seizures. Second, the risk of cerebrovascular accident is considerable with recurrent seizures. In addition, any of the complications of severe preeclampsia (hepatic dysfunction, renal shutdown, coagulaopathy, cardiopulmonary compromise) may occur.

The first priority of **therapy is to stop the seizures.** This may be done with IV MgSO$_4$ (see above). If this is not effective in a few minutes, diazepam, 10 mg, or amobarbital, 250 mg by IV push will usually succeed. When this has been accomplished, the following measures should be taken *while* preparing for delivery. The concept of "stabilize and deliver" has been amended to "stabilize while preparing for and beginning delivery."

1. Continue MgSO$_4$ infusion at 1 g/hour
2. Vital signs q 30 minutes, with careful attention to respiratory rate to be alert for respiratory distress (pulmonary edema)
3. Intensive fetal monitoring with EFM
4. IV fluids sufficient to maintain urinary output at 30 to 50 ml/hour
5. Foley catheter to measure urine output
6. Oxygen by mask at 5 to 10 L/minute
7. Blood work as for preeclampsia
8. Management of hypertension as for severe preeclampsia
9. Management of other complications as for severe preeclampsia

Delivery

As soon as the eclamptic seizure has been arrested and all of the above measures have been initiated, one must begin delivery. The resolution of the eclamptic process, like its preeclamptic predecessor, is resolved only by termination of the pregnancy. As with preeclampsia, the preferred method of delivery is induction of labor and vaginal delivery. Often, little anesthesia is necessary, and meperidine suffices well. Pudendal block is preferred for delivery. Although some use regional anesthesia for preeclampsia, most, because of the tremendously reduced intravascular volume and often abnormal sensorium, will not in eclamptic patients. Indications for cesarean section are identical to those in preeclampsia.

Postpartum

The postpartum care of eclampsia is the same as that for preeclampsia, except that the risk of having infarcted various organ systems, especially the brain, is much greater. If one of these complications has occurred, the appropriate medical management should obviously be added. Unless there has been permanent injury in the form of infarction, eclampsia completely resolves postpartum, during the same 6-week period as preeclampsia. Follow-up should be essentially the same as for preeclampsia.

CHRONIC HYPERTENSION

Hypertension (blood pressure above 140/90) detected before the 20th week of pregnancy (except in molar or multiple gestations) or in the nonpregnant state is an entirely different disease from gestational hypertension or preeclampsia. It may,

however, be mistaken for it if one has not recorded blood pressures during the early first trimester or nonpregnant state. This is because pressures typically fall during the second trimester and rise in the third, back to baseline levels. If the baseline pressure is hypertensive, the rise back toward it may be mistaken for preeclampsia. Chronic hypertension, however, is not accompanied by proteinuria or edema. It is, in fact, the same disease as in the nonpregnant state.

Several groups of women seem to be predisposed to chronic hypertension during pregnancy: blacks, women over 35, obese women, and diabetics. These are essentially the same groups as in the nonpregnant population.

The major **complications** associated with chronic hypertension are as follows:

1. Superimposed preeclampsia: Although the risk of preeclampsia in the general nulliparous population varies from 2 to 7%, in the previously hypertensive woman it may be between 15 and 50%.
2. Placental abruption: Chronic hypertension is the one true predisposing medical risk factor for abruption (see "Placental Abruption").
3. Fetal growth retardation: In severe cases of hypertension (blood pressure above 160/105 or those associated with vascular disease) there is a significant risk, based on chronic placental insufficiency, for growth retardation and fetal distress.

Management

Pregnancy complicated by chronic hypertension is essentially managed as normal pregnancy, with some exceptions: more careful maternal and fetal surveillance and, for severe hypertensives, antihypertensive therapy.

Additional maternal surveillance includes

1. Careful search for signs of vascular disease (retinopathy, renal involvement, hypertensive cardiac disease)
2. Initiate electrolyte, BUN, and creatinine determinations
3. First, second, and third trimester creatinine clearance determinations, if hypertension is severe or there is any evidence of vascular disease
4. Extra prenatal visits, especially during the second half of pregnancy, when preeclampsia is likely to occur

Additional fetal testing should include

1. Sonographic documentation of fetal growth at 3- to 6-week intervals during the second half of pregnancy
2. NST/CST fetal evaluation at weekly or shorter intervals from 32 weeks

Antihypertensive therapy is usually best done with either hydralazine or methyldopa (Aldomet). In practice, although hydralazine enjoys the theoretical advantage of being a vasodilator as well as an antihypertensive, in reality, methyldopa seems as adequate and is easier to manage.

In mildly hypertensive gravidas, antihypertensive therapy seems to contribute little to fetal or maternal outcome, so that if the blood pressure is less than 160/100, many will not impose the theoretical risks of drug exposure on the fetus. Therapy is indicated for severe chronic hypertension and for women who have conceived while on medication. Salt restriction may occasionally be of use, but diuretics are not indicated.

Labor and delivery should be managed as for any high-risk pregnancy, with intensive fetal and maternal monitoring during labor. Analgesia and anesthesia choices are not restricted by chronic hypertension. In the postpartum period, one should avoid ergot alkaloids because of a potential for acute aggravation of hypertension.

MEDICAL DISEASES AND PREGNANCY

The diagnosis and treatment of medical diseases during pregnancy may be complicated by several factors:

1. Pregnancy changes many physiological parameters. These changes may mimic signs and symptoms of disease, complicating diagnosis.
2. Pregnancy may increase the severity of disease.
3. Pregnancy may be adversely affected by disease.
4. Pregnancy may be adversely affected by treatment.

The following sections will be organized according to system and the parameters above.

DIABETES MELLITUS

Diabetes mellitus is characterized by higher than normal blood sugars, which are due to lower than necessary levels of insulin. It is, in many cases, also a vascular disease. Next to hypertensive disease, it is the most common medical illness encountered in pregnancy. It is also among the most serious.

Diabetes makes pregnancy more dangerous, and pregnancy makes diabetes both more likely and more severe. Under normal conditions there is an interplay between intake of glucose, its absortion into the bloodstream, its use by cells, and its excretion in the urine. For the most part, the body regulates these processes by producing hormones. The most important of these is insulin; however, glucagon, adrenal steroids, thyroid hormone, estrogen, progesterone, and likely others play modifying roles. Pregnancy is diabetogenic because it not only alters the levels of many of these hormones but also adds new ones, as well as a new consumer of glucose.

The major diabetogenic agent of pregnancy appears to be placental lactogen. Secondarily, extremely high levels of estrogen, progesterone, and prolactin seem important. Even though in normal pregnancy fasting and postprandial levels of insulin are increased, insulin half-life is shortened by an insulinase from the placenta and its cellular effects (uptake of glucose by cells) seem to be reduced (peripheral insulin resistance), so that plasma levels of glucose are raised in all but the fasting state, when fetal demand for glucose seems to be a depleting factor. If insulin production is borderline or decreased (diabetes), not only are postprandial sugars elevated even more, but fasting levels also rise. In addition, because of peripheral insulin resistance and a corresponding inability to get glucose into cells, ketosis is more likely to occur. Finally,

exogenously administered insulin is less effective during pregnancy on a unit basis, resulting in a worsening of preexistent diabetes.

The major effects on the fetus seem to derive from the facts that glucose freely crosses the placenta while insulin does not and that the fetus may be adversely affected by ketosis. The fetus is therefore subjected to hyperglycemia, which results in antepartum fetal hyperinsulinemia. Since insulin is an important growth hormone for the fetus, the combination causes increased fat deposition and protein synthesis (macrosomia). Anomalous development may result either from hyperglycemia or ketosis. Postpartum complications such as neonatal hypoglycemia may arise when the glucose supply is abruptly cut off at birth.

Classification

For prognostication and for management, diabetes in pregnancy has been classified in many different ways. The traditional method is the White system, which has been revised several times since its initial formulation:

1. Class A: Chemical diabetes or an abnormal glucose tolerance test (GTT)
2. Class B: Adult-type diabetes, less than 10 years duration, no vascular disease
3. Class C: Onset of diabetes between ages 10 and 19 (C_1) or diabetes of 10 to 19 years duration (C_2)
4. Class D: Onset of diabetes before age 10 (D_1), diabetes present for more than 20 years (D_2), or complicated by benign retinopathy (D_3), calcified leg vessels (D_4), or hypertension (D_5)
5. Class E: Calcified uterine or iliac vessels (no longer considered significant)
6. Class F: Diabetic nephropathy
7. Class G: Recurrent reproductive failure (new category)
8. Class H: Cardiomyopathy (new category)
9. Class R: Proliferating (as opposed to benign) retinopathy
10. Class T: Renal transplant (new category)

A simpler and more functionally oriented categorization is often used:

1. Gestational diabetes: onset during pregnancy
2. Preexisting diabetes: onset before pregnancy

Either type may fit into any of the following categories, although the gestational diabetics tend to cluster in the less severe groups:

3. Diet-controlled diabetes: Those who can regain normal glucose levels with diet (usually only gestational). Tend to have abnormal GTT with normal fasting blood sugar (FBS).
4. Insulin-dependent diabetes, no vascular disease: Require insulin, but sugar management is usually the only problem (either gestational or preextant). Usually have abnormal FBS.
5. Insulin-dependent diabetes, with vascular disease: Require insulin, but have evidence of microvascular

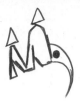

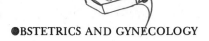

disease, which will often interfere with renal, eye, and placental function. IUGR and fetal death are much increased in this group.

Diagnosis

Diabetes is diagnosed by measuring blood glucose. Measurement of urine glucose is influenced by renal threshold too often to be accurate in either the detection or management of diabetes. In addition, because pregnancy is a dynamic state during which the diabetogenic pressures continually increase almost to the end, someone who is not diabetic earlier in pregnancy may become so later. Therefore, optimal detection of diabetes in pregnancy requires repetitive testing.

FBS should be included among the initial blood studies at the first prenatal visit. One may diagnose diabetes if the FBS is greater than 90 mg/100 ml in whole blood (105 mg/100 ml in plasma). If the FBS is normal, the gravida may still be a chemical diabetic (abnormal GTT). The only method for detecting these women is by some form of GTT. In pregnancy, the most reliable GTT is the 3-hour oral GTT (OGTT), performed after 3 days of carbohydrate-rich (100 g/day) diet.

The 3-hour OGTT is performed by obtaining a FBS followed by administration of 100 g glucose in water solution. Subsequent blood sugars are then taken at 1, 2, and 3 hours. Normal values are up to (about 15% higher for plasma or serum than for whole blood):

1. FBS: 90 mg/100 ml whole blood (105 mg/100 ml plasma)
2. 1 hour: 165 mg/100 ml whole blood (190 mg/100 ml plasma)
3. 2 hour: 145 mg/100 ml whole blood (165 mg/100 ml plasma)
4. 3 hour: 125 mg/100 ml whole blood (145 mg/100 ml plasma)

If the FBS is elevated, insulin-dependent diabetes may be diagnosed. If it is normal but two of the postprandial glucose measurements are high, then one has diagnosed chemical diabetes.

Because the traditional 3-hour OGTT is such a cumbersome, unpleasant, expensive test to perform on all pregnant women even once, let alone several times, obstetricians have traditionally used criteria for selecting those women believed to be at high risk for the disease to screen. The following are indications for 3-hour OGTT testing:

1. Glucosuria
2. Family history of diabetes
3. Maternal age over 35
4. Obesity
5. Excessive weight gain during any stage of pregnancy
6. Grand multiparity
7. Recurrent urinary tract infection
8. Previous macrosomic fetus
9. Previous stillbirth

Many cases of mild gestational diabetes will still be missed. In an attempt to find those, most obstetricians now employ the 1-hour OGTT (mini-GTT), which consists of measurement of FBS, administration of 50 g glucose in water solution, and measurement of 1-hour postprandial glucose. Various standards place normal 1-hour level below 135 to 150 mg/100 ml plasma. If the test is normal, diabetes is ruled out. If it is abnormal, a 3-hour OGTT should be performed for definitive diagnosis. The least aggressive recommendation is to perform the test at 28 to 32 weeks gestation. Many are performing it more often, in an attempt to avoid the complications of mild diabetes by early detection.

Complications

Maternal complications from diabetes in pregnancy are an increased risk of

1. Ketoacidosis: Due to the diabetogenic effect of pregnancy
2. Preeclampsia: Possibly due to underlying diabetic vascular disease
3. Pyelonephritis: Probably related to the increased likelihood of urinary tract infection in diabetics in general
4. Hydramnios: Seems to occur in up to 25% of diabetic pregnancies
5. Postpartum hemorrhage: Possibly related to the increase in difficult labors associated with large fetuses

Fetal/neonatal complications commonly occurring are as follows:

1. Congenital anomalies: Due to hyperglycemia or ketosis in the first trimester; most often cardiovascular or neurological; tend to occur in insulin-dependent but not in gestational diabetics, since abnormal glucose tolerance and hyperglycemia do not develop until later.
2. Macrosomia: Due to a combination of maternal hyperglycemia and fetal hyperinsulinemia; tends to occur more in diabetes without vascular disease since vascular disease causes compensatory growth retardation; may be avoided by careful glucose control.
3. Growth retardation: Due to impaired fetal blood supply; usually associated with placental vascular abnormalities in diabetics with vascular disease or those pregnancies complicated by preeclampsia.
4. Intrauterine death: Cause unknown; much more common in diabetics with vascular disease; probably not sudden, as we used to think, because most are avoidable by careful metabolic management and antepartum fetal testing.
5. Postpartum respiratory distress syndrome: Due to late maturation of lungs caused by the late appearance of phosphatidylglycerol and other lecithins; probably due to hyperglycemia, since it may be largely avoided by careful glucose control.
6. Postpartum hypoglycemia: Due to antepartum hyperglycemia causing fetal hyperinsulinemia, which continues in spite of a sharp drop in glucose supply at cord clamping; may be avoided by careful glucose control.
7. Postpartum hypocalcemia: Etiology unknown.
8. Postpartum hyperbilirubinemia: Etiology unknown.

Management

The proper treatment of the overtly diabetic patient begins before pregnancy. Since the earliest complications are congenital anomalies, which occur mostly within the first 10 weeks, preconception control is critical. This is complicated by the fact that the end points of therapy in the pregnant woman are different from those otherwise, in that during pregnancy we aim for strict metabolic control, which is essentially normo-glycemia. This requires more frequent measurement of blood glucose and usually more frequent administration of insulin. Appropriate therapy for the gestational diabetic begins as soon as she is identified. Management typically may be divided into diet-controlled versus insulin-dependent diabetes and consists of three areas: glucose control, ancillary maternal studies, and fetal evaluation.

Many studies have demonstrated that, class by class, the outcome of diabetic pregnancies is proportional to the degree of glucose control. If maternal glucose is maintained at fasting levels below 105 mg/100 ml (plasma) and postprandially below 140 mg/100 ml (plasma), perinatal mortality rates fall from the 15 to 50% of poorly controlled diabetes to below 2 to 3%.

Diet-controlled (class A) diabetes. Diet, which is of critical importance in the management of all diabetic gravidas, may be all that is necessary to control plasma glucose levels in the chemical gestational diabetic. It should provide all the nutrients necessary for a healthy pregnancy, aiming for a total weight gain of 25 to 30 pounds, almost but not quite that of normal pregnancy. The diet should provide approximately 35 kcal/kg of ideal body weight, with at least 150 g of carbohydrate and 125 g of protein per day. Complex carbohydrates are preferable to simple sugars, which cause rapid fluctuations in glucose levels.

The adequacy of therapy should be monitored by fasting and postprandial glucose measurements at least weekly until delivery. In addition, glycosolated hemoglobin (HbA$_{1c}$), a fraction of hemoglobin that binds glucose and is stable over many weeks, may be monitored to yield an estimate of long-term glucose status. If plasma glucose levels cannot be maintained within euglycemic ranges with this diet, insulin should be considered rather than further calorie restriction. If levels are acceptable, ancillary maternal testing beyond glucose levels is not necessary.

Because perinatal mortality rates in well-controlled class A diabetics approach those of normal pregnancy, some believe that no special fetal surveillance is necessary. Most, however, agree that it should include the following:

1. Sonography: Since the major morbidity of chemical diabetes is macrosomia secondary to hyperglycemia, fetal growth is best monitored by periodic ultrasonography. One should begin on diagnosis and repeat at 4- to 6-week intervals, as necessary.
2. EFM: NST, CST, and biophysical profiles are the major methods of determining fetal well-being. Testing should begin at 35 to 36 weeks and continue at least weekly until delivery.

Insulin-dependent diabetes. Total nutritional needs and protein/carbohydrate breakdown should be the same as for diet-controlled diabetics, providing essential nutrition for fetal growth. However, since a great deal of the insulin management is exogenous, the breakdown of the calorie input my be spaced differently. In general, four or five smaller meals are preferable to fewer larger ones.

Fasting, preprandial, and postprandial glucose levels ideally should be determined at least four times daily using either a glucometer or test strips that are specific for glucose. If this is not feasible, one should approach it as closely as possible. HbA$_{1c}$ measurements should also be obtained at 3- to 4-week intervals. Control of plasma glucose should be maintained at below 105 mg/100 ml plasma (fasting) and below 140 mg/100 ml plasma (postprandial). This is usually accomplished by at least twice-daily administration of combinations of short-acting (regular) and longer-acting (NPH, Lente) insulins. Pumps for subcutaneous administration of insulin have recently become available. Exact dosages depend on individual needs and are adjusted to eliminate undesirable peaks and valleys in plasma glucose concentrations. Needs generally increase throughout pregnancy.

Ancillary maternal testing primarily to detect vascular disease should include

1. More frequent prenatal visits, each with review of blood glucose levels, blood pressure, and urinalysis
2. Creatinine clearance, performed on diagnosis or early in pregnancy and repeated each trimester
3. Funduscopic examination, performed on diagnosis or early in pregnancy and repeated each trimester
4. Urine culture, performed on diagnosis or early in pregnancy and repeated each trimester

Fetal surveillance should include

1. Sonography: On diagnosis or early in pregnancy to detect congenital anomalies and accurately date the pregnacy, and at 3- to 4-week intervals to monitor growth, which may be disturbed by either macrosomia or growth retardation.
2. EFM: NST, CST, and biophysical profiles, on attainment of fetal viability (28 to 30 weeks) and (minimally) at weekly intervals until delivery. In severe cases of vascular disease or growth retardation, they may be necessary as often as daily.
3. Fetal maturity studies: Amniocentesis for L/S ratio and prostaglandins, when elective delivery is contemplated.

Delivery

The practice of arbitrarily delivering the fetus at a certain stage in pregnancies complicated by diabetes has largely been obviated by tight control and antepartum fetal evaluation. In diet-controlled and well-controlled insulin-dependent dia-beticcs, fetal death is rare, and deteriorating fetal condition is usually detectable before permanent damage is done. Therefore, timing of delivery is determined by cervical ripeness, fetal condition, and glucose control. In many areas, gravidas are admitted to the hospital for closer surveillance during the last few weeks.

If fetal condition and glucose control are good, amniocentesis to determine fetal maturity (after 37 to 38 weeks) should be performed when the cervix is ripe, as labor may be safely induced. If the cervix is not ripe and delivery would likely involve cesarean section, as long as fetal condition and maternal glucose control are good, spontaneous labor may be awaited, although most become anxious by term. If fetal jeopardy intervenes, delivery is obviously necessary. Labor and vaginal delivery are usually desirable, with cesarean section chosen for obstetrical indications, most often fetal distress and macrosomia.

Glucose control during labor is critical to avoid neonatal hyperglycemia. It is best obtained by constant of D_5W at approximately 125 ml/hour and enough regular insulin, preferably by IV infusion (1 to 3 units/hour) or subcutaneously to maintain glucose levels between 60 and 120 mg/100 ml, which should be measured at least q 2 hours.

For elective cesarean section, recommendations regarding insulin/sugar management vary from none until after delivery of the fetus (do the cesarean section at the time breakfast would be and give no glucose, and the levels should be acceptable in a well-controlled patient) to one-third to one-half the usual dose on the morning of delivery.

Choice of anesthesia/analgesia for labor, vaginal, and abdominal delivery is largely unaffected by diabetes. Continuous EFM during labor is essential.

Postpartum

Insulin needs decline precipitously with birth. The diet-controlled diabetic requires no further attention; her condition is resolved. The insulin-dependent diabetic, especially if she is NPO after cesarean section, will often require no insulin for several days. Since such tight control is no longer necessary, she may be monitored by either urinalysis with regular insulin coverage or by blood glucose determination. Gradually, over several days, NPH/regular combinations are reinstituted. Many will continue the frequent monitoring they learned during pregnancy. This is to be encouraged, as evidence suggesting beneficial effects from long-term tight control is accumulating.

HEART DISEASE

Diagnosis. The cardiovascular system is the system most affected by pregnancy. As detailed in the section "Maternal Adaptations to Pregnancy," numerous physiological changes would spell pathology in the nonpregnant woman. Cardiac output increases up to 50%, heart rate 10 to 15%, stroke volume accordingly. This high-output state seems to increase the incidence of systolic murmurs to 90%, and even diastolic and continuous murmurs to 10 to 15%, and often seems to create a third heart sound. Dyspnea is not rare. Therefore, the diagnosis of heart disease is, to say the least, more difficult during pregnancy.

The following symptoms are considered to be suggestive: activity-related chest pain or syncope, severe or progressive dyspnea, or orthopnea. Signs suggesting disease are cyanosis, clubbing, loud harsh (3/6) systolic murmurs, diastolic murmurs, arrhythmia, and unquestionable cardiomegaly.

Effects of pregnancy on disease. Pregnancy generally tends to worsen heart disease, since it places an increased strain on an already stressed system. These stresses increase in proportion to cardiac demands, which begin in the late first trimester and continue to increase throughout.

It was previously thought that there was an abatement of this process after the 28th week, but this was because studies on cardiac output were conducted in the supine position so that aortocaval compression falsely lowered it. In fact, cardiac output rises steadily throughout the third trimester, although not as rapidly as earlier. Directly postpartum, the contraction of the uterus with the injection of almost 500 ml of blood back into the vascular system may add additional stress.

The degree of worsening that is likely is adequately predicted by the New York Heart Association classification. Based on functional parameters, this classification is applicable to most kinds of heart disease in nonpregnant patients:

Class 1: No symptoms on ordinary activity
Class 2: Comfortable at rest; symptoms on ordinary activity
Class 3: Comfortable at rest; symptoms on minimal activity
Class 4: Symptoms at rest

Patients who are class 1 or 2 will generally tolerate pregnancy but may find themselves on the edge of decompensation at the slightest complication. Adequate rest, minimal activity, and strict dietary control (calorie and salt) are essential. Early detection and aggressive management of congestive heart failure (CHF) with diuretics and digitalization are necessary, as is meticulous avoidance of respiratory infections.

Women with class 3 are likely to decompensate during normal pregnancy, and therapeutic abortion is considered reasonable. Maternal mortality rates may be as high as 15%, even when patients are on constant bed rest throughout the pregnancy. If a woman with class 3 heart disease insists on continuing her pregnancy, all the measures appropriate for management of less ill cardiacs plus hospitalization for the entire pregnancy should be instituted in an attempt to avoid maternal and/or fetal death.

Class 4 cases are already decompensated and, although hospitalized for the entire pregnancy, experience even higher mortality rates. Therapeutic abortion in these patients is the preferred course. All pregnant cardiac patients should be jointly managed by both a cardiologist and an obstetrician.

In general, vaginal delivery is best for cardiac patients. The hemodynamic stress of cesarean section is far greater than that of the second stage of labor. During labor, these women must be intensively monitored for signs of hypoxia and CHF, using Swan-Ganz catheterization if necessary. Anesthesia/analgesia must be administered carefully, with attention to its effects on cardiac output (especially epidural).

Effects of disease on pregnancy. Heart disease tends to affect pregnancy via two mechanisms:

1. CHF decreases maternal cardiac output, predisposing to growth retardation and fetal distress in labor.
2. Maternal hypoxia increases the risk of both the above as well as congenital anomalies and spontaneous abortion. The rates of these latter are roughly parallel to the degree of hypoxia.

Effects of therapy on pregnancy.   Since therapy varies so much for different forms of heart disease, its effect will be considered under each specific category below.

Valvular disease

Mitral stenosis, largely caused by rheumatic fever, has become far less common in the last decade as the incidence and virulence of the disease have decreased. Cardiac output is decreased, pulmonary congestion increased, right failure is common, and atrial fibrillation and clot formation (with arterial embolization) are the major risks. Rheumatic fever prophylaxis with penicillin (or erythromycin) should be employed throughout pregnancy, with expanded coverage at delivery to prevent endocarditis. Rest as necessary and drug therapy for CHF and arrhythmia (digitalis is the mainstay) are commonly necessary. Anticoagulation, if required, should be with heparin as the warfarin derivatives are associated with teratogenesis. Definitive treatment for severe mitral stenosis is commissurotomy or, secondarily, valve replacement, preferably before pregnancy, but during if absolutely necessary.

Aortic stenosis is much less commonly encountered than mitral but carries a higher maternal fetal and maternal mortality rate. Left ventricular hypertrophy with increased cardiac oxygen requirements makes angina common. Syncope or dyspnea on slight exercise (and during labor) due to inadequate output through a severely stenotic valve poses grave dangers for both the mother and fetus. Although the risk of embolism or arrhythmia is less than with mitral stenosis, the incidence and severity of hypoxia are greater, resulting in a great likelihood of IUGR, fetal distress, and congenital anomalies (mostly cardiac). Antibiotic prohylaxis, as described above, is indicated. Again, definitive therapy is commissurotomy or valve replacement, preferably before conception. If artificial valves are used, anticoagulation through the pregnancy is necessary.

Mitral insufficiency may be due either to disease or heredity. As many as 10% of women have a mild or hemodynamically insignificant form of mitral regurgitation due to mitral valve prolapse. Although some of these have conduction defects resulting in arrhythmias (mostly paroxysmal atrial tachycardia [PAT]), most have no symptoms and require no special attention except for antibiotic prophylaxis with delivery. More severe mitral insufficiency results in decreased cardiac output, left ventricular hypertrophy, left atrial enlargement, a tendency toward right heart failure and, less often, thromboembolism. Since these severe symptoms are not common, pregnant women with mitral insufficiency generally fare well.

Aortic insufficiency is usually a result of rhematic fever and most often occurs in tandem with mitral damage. It may also be of autoimmune or congenital origin. There typically is a decrease in cardiac output because of reflux in diastole, but this is much less significant than with aortic stenosis. Cardiac oxygenation is compromised in severe cases, and then the prognosis is poor. Aortic regurgitation usually causes only minor problems during pregnancy, unless combined with mitral disease.

Pulmonic stenosis is rare. When it is present, right heart failure with chest pain and dyspnea are the rule. If hypoxia is manageable, conservative therapy as for other forms of heart failure is the rule. If not, commissurotomy must be done.

Tricuspid valve disease is rare and usually is not much of a problem unless associated with active endocarditis, when septic emboli may occur. As with other valvular diseases, antibiotic prophylaxis is indicated at delivery.

Prosthetic valves are not rarely found in childbearing women today. If the surgery has corrected the underlying disease, mechanical (most) prosthetic valves pose two risks: embolization and endocarditis. Therefore, anticoagulation throughout the pregnancy and antibiotic prophylaxis at delivery are necessary. If a porcine valve has been used, anticoagulation is not necessary.

Congenital heart disease

Most congenital heart diseases are recognized during childhood and corrected and therefore pose no danger during pregnancy. If they are not recognized and/or corrected, the risk during pregnancy is proportional to the degree of hypoxia or CHF. Those that result in pulmonary hypertension contraindicate pregnancy, since the maternal mortality rate may approach 50% in such cases. Antibiotic prophylaxis is generally indicated at delivery (unless otherwise stated below). Most congenital heart disease, except that from intrauterine infection, when present in one parent or sibling, has a recurrence risk of up to 10 to 20%.

Coarctation of the aorta often results in CHF, demanding aggressive management. Less common but more serious are the risks of dissecting aneurysm and rupture, and of an associated cerebral aneurysm. Hypertension is also a frequent concomitant. Ideally, correction is done before pregnancy. If not, control of hypertension and CHF and limitation of exercise are required.

Atrial septal defects rarely cause symptomatic disease. In fact, they are often not diagnosed. The left-to-right shunt usually has no functional significance and, since the defect is in a low-pressure system, antibiotic prophylaxis is not believed to be necessary.

Ventricular septal defects (VSD) are also well tolerated unless there is associated pulmonary hypertension. In these cases, the left-to-right shunt is reversed, resulting in hypoxia, and associated maternal mortality is high. Most severe cases, however, are recognized in childhood and corrected.

Patent ductus arteriosus, like VSD, is almost always recognized and corrected during childhood. In pregnancy, unless there is pulmonary hypertension, complications are not common.

Tetralogy of Fallot, consisting of pulmonic stenosis, pulmonary hypertension, and VSD, is, like other right-to-left shunts, associated with a poor prognosis. The severity of the disease is proportional to the degree of shunting and is exacerbated by any decrease in venous return.

Eisenmenger's syndrome, with pulmonary hypertension, also carries a grave maternal and fetal prognosis.

Other hereditary heart diseases   IHSS

Idiopathic hypertrophic subaortic stenosis is characterized by hypertrophy of the ventricular septum with occlusion of the outflow tract on vigorous exercise, resulting in a rapid decrease in output with syncope, fetal distress, and occasionally sudden death. Since pregnancy and especially labor are vigorous exercise, these risks are real throughout. The treatment is

R4   Propranolol

propranolol, which has been associated with an increased risk of IUGR. This condition is inherited as an autosomal dominant trait.

Marfan's syndrome is also inherited as an autosomal dominant. Because of a collagen defect, these patients are likely to develop aortic aneurysms and rupture. Pregnancy greatly increases this risk and is contraindicated (maternal mortality up to 50%). If pregnancy occurs and abortion is refused, bed rest in the hospital throughout is the wisest course.

Miscellaneous heart diseases

Cardiomyopathy and myocarditis are virtually indistinguishable except on cardiac biopsy. Management is the same for both. Because of maternal mortality rates approaching 50% and almost equally high fetal losses, pregnancy should be avoided. If it does occur and abortion is declined, management of CHF must be aggressive. If it is of inflammatory origin (diagnosed by biopsy), steroidal and nonsteroidal anti-inflammatory agents are necessary.

Endocarditis, encountered in patients with valvular disease and in IV drug users, is a life-threatening illness during pregnancy. It must be aggressively treated with appropriate antibiotics.

Arrhythmias, mostly tachycardias of the paroxysmal variety (PAT), are not rare. In otherwise healthy mothers, cardiac decompensation is not common and arrhythmias often are asymptomatic. Correction should be attempted with either pharmacologic therapy or cardioversion when symptoms necessitate it. Bradycardias may be treated with a pacemaker when cardiac output is not sufficient.

PHLEBITIS AND PULMONARY EMBOLISM

Phlebitis

The diagnosis of phlebitis is both more difficult and more critical during pregnancy. Superficial phlebitis is usually easily diagnosed when there is a tender, palpable vein near the surface. The diagnosis of deep vein thrombophlebitis (DVT) is, however, much more difficult in all but the most obvious cases. Pain and edema may be due to venous distension caused by the enlarged uterus or may be mimicked by orthopedic diseases secondary to postural changes. Cords are rarely palpable in DVT. Laboratory testing, therefore, assumes even greater importance than in the nonpregnant state.

Venography is the gold standard for diagnosis but involves injection of radiopaque dye and exposure of the fetus to radiation. ^{125}I-fibrinogen scanning is contraindicated. Therefore, one usually begins with the noninvasive tests that do not employ x-rays: ultrasound evaluation, by Doppler, of blood flow through the leg and impedance plethysmography (IPG). Both tests, done carefully, are quite accurate if negative, since normal blood flow through the venous system makes phlebitis extremely unlikely. False-positive results, however, may reflect decreased flow secondary to pressure from the enlarged uterus. Because DVT is potentially life threatening, one often has to decide between making the diagnosis, even though uncertain, and exposing the fetus to the radiation of venography. In the third trimester, one may choose careful venography with attempts to shield the fetus, but earlier this is much less acceptable.

Phlebitis does not affect pregnancy directly. If it progresses to pulmonary embolism, however, the life of the mother is in grave danger. This is rare with superficial phlebitis, which may be treated with local heat, bed rest, and anti-inflammatory drugs (aspirin). The only effective treatment for DVT is anticoagulation, which is combined with strict bed rest for several days until clot fixation and then continued by itself for the remainder of the pregnancy.

Heparin is the agent of choice for anticoagulation of the pregnant woman, because it does not cross the placenta. Warfarin derivatives are usually not used during the first trimester because of a well-documented fetal syndrome, warfarin embryopathy, consisting of nasal hypoplasia and skeletal abnormalities, probably related to multiple small hemorrhagic infarcts. Even with use in later pregnancy, multiple anomalies have been found to occur, again probably related to repeated episodes of fetal hemorrhage.

Heparin, however, is not completely safe. The risk of maternal hemorrhage is considerable, and even though heparin does not cross the placenta, it extends to it, so that placental hemorrhagic infarcts with compromise and abruption are much more likely with heparin therapy. Therefore, careful maternal and fetal monitoring of the heparinized pregnancy are essential.

Anticoagulation is begun with heparin, preferably by constant IV infusion. The usual regimens include a loading dose (3,000 to 6,000 units) followed by 1,000 to 2,000 units/hour. The actual rate is governed by the APTT, which should be maintained at 1.5 to 2 times normal. It is not unusual, in pregnant patients, to require these much greater doses of heparin to maintain this level of anticoagulation because of high Factor VIII and fibrinogen levels. IV heparin is continued for 10 to 14 days and then replaced with subcutaneous heparin q 12 hours (doses range from 5,000 to 15,000), still sufficient to maintain the APTT at 1.5 to 2 times normal. During labor, the patient is switched back to IV heparinization, which is terminated and reversed (with protamine sulfate) 1 hour before anticipated delivery and restarted 1 to 2 hours postpartum. After several days of IV therapy postpartum, anticoagulation is maintained with either intermittent subcutaneous heparin (in nursing mothers) or oral warfarin for 1 to 3 months.

Pulmonary embolism

As with phlebitis, the diagnosis of pulmonary embolism is more difficult during pregnancy. Shortness of breath, tachycardia, and tachypnea are quite common during normal pregnancy, and wheezing, rales, fever, and pleuritic chest pain may be caused by a host of conditions. Hemoptysis is a bit more specific. Therefore, central to the diagnosis is a high index of suspicion followed by adequate laboratory workup.

The first tests done are an ECG, which often only confirms sinus tachycardia, and arterial blood gases (ABG). These typically show hypoxia (PO_2 <80 mm Hg), hypocarbia (PCO_2 <30 mm Hg), and a metabolic alkalosis (pH <7.35). Indeed, it is difficult (but not impossible) to make the diagnosis of significant pulmonary embolism if the PO_2 is greater than 85 mm Hg. Next, one progresses to the chest x-ray, which may show an infiltrate, an effusion, or atelectasis but usually is not specific.

The ventilation-perfusion scan is the usual procedure that

makes the diagnosis. Although it involves a radioisotope, [125]technetium, it has such a short half-life that it is considered safe for use in pregnancy. Matching blood flow patterns against aeration patterns, the ventilation-perfusion scan will ideally reveal an area of well-ventilated lung with no perfusion, suggesting pulmonary embolism. Normal findings on perfusion scans virtually eliminate embolism as a possibility. Overlapping ventilation and perfusion defects may reflect pulmonary infarction, pneumonia, or asthma and so are much less useful.

As with DVT, the gold standard of diagnosis is an angiographic technique, in this case pulmonary angiography. By injecting radiopaque dye into the pulmonary vascular tree, occluded vessels large enough to cause symptoms of pulmonary embolism may be identified. Because of the life-threatening nature of the disease, this procedure may be indicated if one strongly suspects but cannot confirm or eliminate the diagnosis with lesser measures.

The therapy for pulmonary embolism in pregnancy is the same as that for DVT, anticoagulation. Additionally, maternal PO_2 levels must be maintained in order to avoid fetal hypoxia. If the embolic event has been severe enough to cause cardiovascular compromise, various degrees of cardiopulmonary support will be necessary.

HEMATOLOGIC DISEASES

Anemias

Diagnosis. The most common hematologic condition confronting pregnant women is anemia. Its diagnosis is complicated by the so-called physiological anemia of pregnancy. As described earlier, in "Maternal Adaptations to Pregnancy," maternal hemoglobin levels fall late in the first trimester and remain lower throughout pregnancy as a result of hemodilution. Therefore, hemoglobin levels as low as 10 g/100 ml, if accompanied by normal erythrocyte indices, may be normal. Lower levels or abnormalities of erythrocyte shape or size should arouse suspicion of anemia. Since the normal prenatal laboratory evaluation includes several hemoglobin/hematocrit determinations and at least one CBC, the diagnosis of most anemias should occur as a matter of course.

Effects of pregnancy on disease. Anemias are typically categorized as either acquired or hereditary (mostly disorders of hemoglobin production), although some of the former are intermittent conditions based on hereditary abnormalities (e.g., G6PD deficiency). All of these conditions tend to be exacerbated by pregnancy, since hemodilution reduces the effective hemoglobin concentration, regardless of the underlying pathology. Additionally, specific anemias may be adversely or positively affected. These will be discussed individually below.

Effects of disease on pregnancy. The anemias may threaten pregnancy in two ways: All of them, by reducing hemoglobin concentrations, decrease the oxygen-carrying capacity of maternal blood and, at low enough levels, interfere with fetal oxygenation and growth. This may result in prematurity, low birth weight, and increased perinatal mortality. Some of them also precipitate acute events that may injure the fetus, especially the sickling diseases. These will be discussed individually below.

Effects of therapy on pregnancy. For the most part, the therapy of anemias is unaffected by and does not affect pregnancy.

Iron deficiency anemia

Diagnosis. The diagnosis of iron deficiency anemia is complicated by the hemodilutional effects of pregnancy. One does not suspect true anemia until hemoglobin concentrations fall below 10 g/100 ml. Indices, however, do not change much (there is, in fact, a small increase in erythrocyte size during pregnancy), so that microcytosis (MCV<82) and hypochromia lead one to think first of iron deficiency. Unfortunately, serum iron is hemodilutionally low and TIBC artifactually higher. Most accurate among the blood tests is serum ferritin, which is unaffected by pregnancy. If definitive diagnosis is essential, bone marrow aspiration with staining for iron, as in the nonpregnant patient, is necessary. Usually, however, since the therapy is innocuous (and even part of normal prenatal care), if iron deficiency anemia is strongly suspected, therapeutic trial rather than bone marrow aspiration is the usual course.

Effects of pregnancy on disease. Pregnancy increases the likelihood of iron deficiency anemia because of the tremendous iron needs superimposed on the borderline deficiency that many women already have.

Effects of disease on pregnancy. The primary effects of iron deficiency anemia result from poor oxygenation of the fetus. This does not become clinically significant until hemoglobin concentrations less than 8 g/100 ml are reached. The fetus itself is almost never anemic because the placenta actively transports iron from the maternal circulation.

Therapy. The treatment of iron deficiency anemia is iron. Oral administration is preferable and, in almost all cases, is as effective as parenteral. Certainly, it is associated with fewer serious side effects. The usual dose is ferrous sulfate, 325 mg t.i.d. or ferrous fumarate, 200 mg t.i.d., providing, respectively, 190 and 200 mg of elemental iron per day. Ferrous gluconate is popular for causing less GI disturbance, but this is because it contains only two-thirds the elemental iron. Side effects such as constipation, nausea, and abdominal discomfort are related to the dose of iron, not the number of pills swallowed or its form. Many believe that iron is better absorbed on an empty stomach and when taken with 250 mg vitamin C. A prenatal vitamin with 0.8 to 1 mg of folic acid, if not already prescribed, is usually added.

The first response to iron therapy is an increase in the reticulocyte count within 10 days. Hemoglobin levels begin to rise within 1 week after that. If this does not occur, one must question whether the iron is being taken. If it is, the diagnosis of iron deficiency anemia is suspect and bone marrow aspiration is indicated. If the pregnant woman will not or cannot take the required dose orally, parenteral iron dextran (Imferon) may be used. It is, however, painful when administered IM (and may cause tattooing) and dangerous when given IV (anaphylaxis is a real risk), so it should be used with discretion. Transfusion for iron deficiency anemia should almost never be necessary.

Megaloblastic anemia

Most megaloblastic anemia in pregnancy is due to folic acid deficiency. A very small percentage results from B_{12} deficiency, which is almost never of dietary origin unless the patient is a strict vegan (vegetarian with no milk or egg consumption), but rather from the absence of intrinsic factor (pernicious anemia). Since folic acid is present in quantity in leafy green vegetables, salad eaters rarely become deficient. Boiling these vegetables destroys the folic acid.

Diagnosis. One may diagnose megaloblastic anemia when macrocytosis (MCV > 102) and anemia are present, although if there is concomitant iron deficiency anemia there may be two distinct populations of erythrocytes, one large and one small, which may average out to a normal set of indices on automated screening. Therefore, adequate diagnosis depends on a peripheral smear, where in addition to macrocytosis one may see nucleated red cells and hypersegmented polymorphonuclear leukocytes. In severe cases, pancytopenias result.

Serum folate and B_{12} levels are always evaluated in patients with megaloblastic anemia; however, since folate levels may rebound in as little as a day, they are unreliable. Red cell folate levels are more dependable. Definitive diagnosis is, again, made by examination of bone marrow aspirate.

Effects of pregnancy on disease. Pregnancy increases the likelihood of folic acid deficiency because of increased metabolic demands. A good diet is usually sufficient to overcome this, and all the prenatal vitamins have adequate supplementation.

Effects of disease on pregnancy. Many have suspected folic acid deficiency as a cause of fetal anomalies, placental abruption, and preeclampsia. These associations have not been proved. As with iron deficiency anemia, the placenta actively transports folic acid, so that the fetus is rarely anemic.

Therapy. Folic acid, 0.8 to 1 mg/day PO, is the treatment for folic acid deficiency. Reticulocyte counts will rise within 1 week, and the anemia will begin to respond within 2 to 3 weeks. Since women who are folate deficient are almost always iron deficient as well (dietary deficiencies overlap), iron supplementation should also be provided. If the source of the megaloblastic anemia is B_{12} deficiency, this is almost never due to dietary deficiency but to a lack of intrinsic factor. Therefore, the therapy is usually B_{12} IM.

Hemolytic anemias

Diagnosis. Hemolytic anemia may complicate many diseases, including G6PD deficiency, hereditary spherocytosis, preeclampsia, DIC from any cause, thrombotic thrombocytopenic purpura, valvular heart disease, and autoimmune diseases, especially lupus. The diagnosis of these diseases and of the hemolysis itself is largely unchanged by pregnancy.

Initial suspicion is based on anemia, confirmed by peripheral smear examination showing fragmented erythrocytes or, in the case of spherocytosis, microcytic spherocytes. A high reticulocyte count, urine studies for hemosiderin-laden macrophages, decreased serum haptoglobin, and increased bilirubin levels complete the picture, although haptoglobins may be spuriously elevated since they are alpha$_2$-globulins, which are increased during pregnancy. In cases of autoimmune hemolytic anemias, an antibody complex will be detectable on the red cell surface by either the direct or indirect Coombs' test. Identification of the antibodies should be performed. Erythrocyte G6PD levels may be measured if this deficiency is suspected but are often normal after an acute hemolytic event, since it is the older red cells that are more deficient. Once they are lysed, the remaining younger cells may be normal.

Effects of pregnancy on disease. Pregnancy may exacerbate autoimmune hemolytic anemia, especially when it is part of thrombotic thrombocytopenic purpura (TTP). In some cases, it is the inciting event (e.g., preeclampsia). In others, such as G6PD deficiency and spherocytosis, the pregnancy often has no particular effect.

Effects of disease on pregnancy. In addition to the effects of anemia, in cases of autoimmune hemolytic anemia, IgG antibodies may cross the placenta and cause anemia and congestive failure in the fetus, as in Rh isoimmunization. Severe associated thrombocytopenia may cause hemorrhage in both the mother and fetus.

Therapy. The treatment of hemolytic anemias in pregnancy is essentially no different from that in its absence. In cases of autoimmune disease, prednisone or other steroids may be used. The fetus should be monitored as described below under "Rh isoimmunization." Splenectomy may be necessary to control the hemolysis associated with spherocytosis. Underlying diseases must be treated appropriately. In all cases, folate supplementation and probably iron as well should be provided. Transfusion is sometimes required.

Hemoglobinopathies

The hemoglobinopathies fall into two major categories: the sickling diseases and the thalassemias, although there is overlap between them. The sickling diseases are characterized by the formation of abnormal hemoglobin (S, C) which changes shape under low oxygen tension, causing sickling of the red cell. The thalassemias result from a decreased rate of production of one of the peptide chains (a, B) which form the globin molecule. Both are inherited disorders.

Sickle cell disorders

There are a host of abnormal hemoglobins, the most common of which are hemoglobins S and C. These are inherited as pairs, so that one may be homozygous for either, heterozygous with hemoglobin A for either, or heterozygous SC. They are most commonly found in the black population, the gene for S occurring with a frequency of 1 in 12 and for C of 1 in 40. Sickle trait (heterozygous SA) is obviously most common (1 in 12), followed by sickle cell disease (SS) (1 in 500), then sickle cell-hemoglobin C disease (SC) (1 in 2,000), followed by pure hemoglobin C disease (CC).

Diagnosis. Except for sickle trait, these diseases are invariably diagnosed in childhood or early adulthood. All black women who are pregnant or considering should be screened for sickle trait.

Effects of pregnancy on disease. Except for sickle trait, these diseases all are exacerbated by pregnancy. Stress of any sort tends to increase the likelihood of a sickling crisis. In pregnant women with sickle trait, urinary tract infections are more common than normal.

Effects of disease on pregnancy. For SS disease, maternal mortality may be almost 2 to 5% and pregnancy loss up to 40% (half as miscarriage, half as perinatal mortality). Fetal damage is associated with crisis resulting in acute hypoxia, while maternal injury results from infarcts caused by sickling cells, obstructing the circulation of various organs, and congestive failure. These patient often are drug dependent because of the necessity for frequent narcotics to combat the pain of crises. The fetus, even

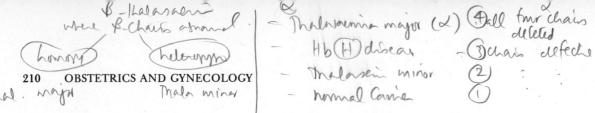

if it has inherited SS disease, will be normal until several months of age, when hemoglobin F is replaced with hemoglobin S.

Hemoglobin SC disease predisposes to the same problems but on a lesser scale, so that fetal and maternal complications, while of the same type, seem to be about half as common.

Sickle trait has no adverse effect on pregnancy.

Equally important is being able to advise the parents of the risk of bearing a child who will be afflicted with the disease. If one parent carries the trait and the other is normal, 50% of the children will have the trait and 50% will be normal. If both parents have the trait, 25% of the children will be unaffected, 50% will carry the trait, and 25% will have sickle cell anemia. If one parent carries the trait and the other has SS disease, 50% of the children will have the trait and 50% the disease. If both parents are sicklers, all the children will be similarly affected. Today, however, each pregnancy can be diagnosed individually. By using enzyme restriction DNA analysis on material obtained at either amniocentesis or chorionic villus sampling, the condition of the fetus can be ascertained.

Therapy. The best therapy for sickling disease is to avoid crisis. Unfortunately, the major method for accomplishing this is prophylactic exchange transfusion to maintain hemoglobin S levels below a certain level, usually around 50%, beginning at various times during pregnancy from the late first to the late second trimester and continuing until delivery. Although this definitely decreases maternal and perinatal mortality, it creates several new problems. The incidence of transfusion reactions increases with each exchange (multiple transfusions are necessary), and hepatitis is a common complication. Acquired immunodeficiency syndrome (AIDS) is a consideration as well. Pregnancy is usually not adversely affected by anemia until hemoglobin concentrations drop below 7 to 8 g/100 ml, but for cesarean section it should be over 10 g/100 ml.

Crises must be aggressively treated with hydration, antibiotics, oxygenation, and pain relief. The value of transfusion after a crisis has occurred is unproved.

Both sicklers and carriers of sickle trait are at increased risk for urinary tract infection. The folate and iron needs of sicklers are far greater than for any other group of pregnant women, and recommendations for supplementation range to 5 g of folic acid and 0.5 g of iron per day.

Thalassemias

Diagnosis. Resulting from a defect in globin synthesis, the thalassemias may be either alpha or beta chain. They all are diagnosed by hemoglobin electrophoresis. Because they cause extreme microcytosis, they are often confused with iron deficiency anemia, which may be ruled out by finding adequate iron stores in the bone marrow.

The alpha-thalassemias result from deletions causing defects in any or all of the four alpha chains, and the severity of the disease is proportional to the number of chains affected. Deletion of all four genes results in alpha-thalassemia major (incompatible with extrauterine life), of three in hemoglobin H disease (associated with severe hemolytic anemia), of two in thalassemia minor (clinically insignificant microcytic anemia), and of only one in the carrier state (normal). The alpha-thalassemias occur mostly in Orientals and to a much lesser extent among blacks.

The beta-thalassemias occur when there is defective beta-chain production and may be present in either homozygous or heterozygous forms, respectively beta-thalassemia major (Cooley's anemia) (usually incompatible with survival past early childhood) and thalassemia minor (mild, often clinically insignificant anemia).

Effects of pregnancy on disease. Pregnancy frequently exacerbates the hemolytic anemia of hemoglobin H disease. Both alpha- and beta-thalassemia minor patients are only minimally affected, if at all. There is an increased tendency toward urinary tract infection, and the normally present anemia is further diluted. The major thalassemias, since they kill before adulthood, are not a consideration.

Effects of disease on pregnancy. One mostly encounters the minor thalassemias in pregnancy. Their effects on the mother and fetus, except for the anemia noted above and the increased likelihood of urinary tract infection, are negligible. They commonly are mistaken for iron deficiency anemia that seems to be iron resistant.

A more important consideration is advising the parents of the risk of bearing a child with a major thalassemia and whether antepartum fetal testing is to be done. If one parent is completely normal and the other has a minor thalassemia, there is a 50% chance of the child having minor thalassemia. If both parents are minor thalassemics, 25% of the offspring will have thalassemia major, 50% will have thalassemia minor, and 25% will be normal. These fetuses can be identified using restriction enzyme DNA analysis techniques on samples obtained at either amniocentesis or chorionic villus sampling.

Therapy. No special treatment is required except careful avoidance of hemorrhage, since these women are anemic to begin with.

Thrombocytopenia

Low platelet counts may result from many conditions. They most commonly are encountered secondary to preeclampsia, DIC, severe folic acid deficiency, or immune thrombocytopenic purpura (ITP). As thrombocytopenia has been discussed in the context of each of the above separately, we will now consider ITP.

Diagnosis. ITP is an autoimmune disease characterized by antiplatelet antibodies that stimulate reticuloendothelial destruction of platelets. Platelet levels consequently are low, but production is high. The source of the antibody is unknown. Diagnosis is by ruling out other causes of thrombocytopenia and is complemented but not certified by the detection of IgG antibodies. This is because, while these antibodies are present in the overwhelming majority of patients with ITP, they also occur not infrequently with other thrombocytopenic diseases. Bone marrow aspiration helps to rule out pancytopenias, since there is active megakaryocytosis with ITP.

Effects of pregnancy on disease. Pregnancy usually worsens this disease. Even if the mother is in a state of relative remission, exacerbation is not uncommon. The reason for this is unknown. Platelet counts tend to fall as the pregnancy progresses.

Effects of disease on pregnancy. Thrombocytopenia itself threatens the pregnancy because hemorrhage is a risk if platelet counts fall below 20,000/mm³. Additionally, there is a considerable risk that antiplatelet antibodies may cross the

[handwritten top margin: Rh independent Antigens inherited from Mo   C / Cc alleb   D / D no d   E / Ee alleb   ∴ if you don't inherit D - you will not have D or d ∴ Rh⁻   15% white Rh⁻   8% black Rh⁻]

placenta and cause thrombocytopenia in the fetus, endangering the baby during vaginal delivery. This appears to happen in up to 25% of cases, but selecting those in which the fetus is at risk is difficult, since maternal and fetal platelet levels do not correlate. Furthermore, the presence of circulating antibodies is not evidence that the fetus will be significantly affected, since the reticuloendothelial system plays a major role in platelet destruction.

Therapy.   Initial therapy is instituted if platelet counts fall below 50,000/mm³. Above this level there is no appreciable risk of hemorrhage. Relatively small doses of prednisone are usually sufficient to raise the platelet count enough to prevent hemorrhage. If this is not effective, splenectomy usually is. Early delivery is sometimes necessary. Platelet transfusions may be resorted to at delivery, but they often are not useful because of their rapid destruction.

A relatively new therapy that shows promise is the intravenous infusion of high doses of IgG, which seems to inhibit reticuloendothelial destruction of antibody-coated platelets. Although this appears to be safe for the fetus so far, long-term effects are unknown.

Management of the fetus poses another problem. Because there is no good way to determine which fetuses are thrombocytopenic before labor and because a good platelet count in the mother, in response to steroid therapy, does not guarantee a similar response in the fetus, one is faced with either blindly allowing the onset of labor or performing cesarean section on everyone. Neither is a good alternative, since intraventricular hemorrhage and brain damage are real risks for the thrombocytopenic fetus delivered vaginally and cesarean section is riskier for the mother with coagulation problems. In an attempt to solve this problem, many obtain fetal scalp blood for platelet count (as for pH in suspected fetal distress) as early as possible in labor. If the fetus is severely thrombocytopenic, cesarean section should be done.

Hereditary coagulation disorders

The major hereditary coagulation disorder affecting pregnancy is von Willebrand's disease. Inherited usually as an autosomal dominant trait, it is most often not a cause of major hemorrhage. Additionally, being due to defective production of part of the Factor VIII complex, it tends to improve during pregnancy. Rarely, if Factor VIII activity is extremely low, cryoprecipitate may be necessary. Its use, however, has declined precipitously since the rise of AIDS. Current practice favors use of a synthetic vasopressin analogue, DDAVP, which stimulates the woman's own production of Factor VIII complex. Avoidance of trauma during delivery is advisable.

Hemophilia A and hemophilia B are extremely uncommon in women since they are inherited as X-linked recessives. The hemophilias are usually present as the asymptomatic carrier state, and their importance lies in predicting whether the fetus will be affected. Assuming that the father is not a hemophiliac, if the mother is a carrier, half the male offspring will be hemophiliac and half the females carriers. The rest will be without the defective gene. Prenatal diagnosis depends on obtaining fetal blood by fetoscopy, if the fetus is determined to be male. If the mother has hemophilia, so will all her sons. All her daughters will be carriers.

MATERNAL ISOIMMUNIZATION TO BLOOD GROUPS AFFECTING THE FETUS

Rh isoimmunization

The mother may develop antibodies to various blood group antigens that may cross the placenta and affect the fetus. The most important of these are related to the Rh system. Inherited independently of other blood type antigens, there are three Rh antigens: C, D, and E. Both C and E have c and e alleles, but there is no d counterpart to D. People who do not inherit D are apparently without any D or d counterpart antigen and are Rh negative (Rh−). They may be sensitized if exposed to the D antigen by transfusion (or pregnancy). People who carry the D antigen are called Rh+ and may be either homozygous (DD) or heterozygous (D[−]). An Rh− mother ([−] [−]) and an Rh+ father will have either all heterozygous Rh+ children (if the father is DD) or half Rh− and half Rh+ (if the father is D[−]). Depending on racial origin, varying percentages of the population are Rh−. In this country, approximately 15% of whites and 8% of blacks are Rh−.

If a woman who is Rh− is sensitized to D, she will produce IgG anti-D antibodies that circulate and will cross the placenta. If the fetus is Rh+, these antibodies will cause fetal hemolysis. If the hemolysis is severe enough, anemia and heart failure in utero result, often killing the child if the process is not interrupted. This hemolytic process is reflected in an increase in amniotic fluid bilirubin concentration, which is the basis for estimation of fetal jeopardy (see below). The fetus itself does not become severely hyperbilirubinemic because the maternal circulation clears it.

Although this used to be a significant cause of perinatal morbidity and mortality, it has been largely eliminated by the use of Rh immune globulin (RhoGAM) in susceptible women at times of exposure to Rh+ blood. The Rh immune globulin binds to the Rh+ cells and prevents them from serving as a source of sensitization. *[handwritten margin: RhoGAM   binds Rh+ cells Prevents them from sensitizing the mother from immune Ab]*

Management of the unsensitized woman.   The management of Rh disease begins with the identification of every pregnant woman as either Rh+ or Rh−. If she is Rh−, her blood is screened for anti-D antibodies. If there are none, she is not sensitized and appropriate management is to prevent sensitization. If the father of her child is also Rh−, the fetus must similarly be Rh−, so there is no risk of becoming sensitized from the pregnancy.

If the father is Rh+, the fetus may be as well, and may serve as a source of sensitizing blood at the time of a miscarriage, abortion, amniocentesis, or delivery. Sensitization typically occurs during one pregnancy but is not likely to present a clinical problem until a subsequent one. Sensitization can almost always be prevented by administering 300 µg of Rh immune globulin IM (which is sufficient to neutralize up to 15 ml of fetal blood) within 72 hours of the event. There occasionally may be silent transplacental fetomaternal transfusion resulting in sensitization. This can be largely prevented by giving the same dose at 28 weeks gestation to all Rh− unsensitized women. Larger fetomaternal transfusion is occasionally suspected. The degree can be estimated from a Kleihauer-Betke stain on maternal blood and the dosage of Rh immune globulin increased proportionately.

There are no known risks to the fetus from this therapy.

Management of the sensitized woman. If the mother has anti-D antibodies at any time before the 20th week of gestation, she should be followed with serial antibody titers. If the titers remain below 1:16, the chances of a severely affected baby are very small and only continued titers are indicated.

If the titer is 1:16 or higher, the risk of a severely affected baby is considerable and further investigation is warranted as soon as effective therapy (see below) may be instituted based on the results. That investigation is via amniocentesis to obtain fluid for analysis of bilirubin levels by the ΔOD_{450} method, which is then plotted on the Liley curve. If the result falls into zone 1, the fetus is unaffected or only mildly affected and is thought to be safe for 2 to 3 weeks, at which time the study should be repeated. In zone 2, the infant is moderately affected, with projected hemoglobin levels between 8 and 11 g/100 ml (upper zone 2) or 11 to 14 g/100 ml (lower zone 2). Amniocentesis should be repeated weekly until fetal maturity is obtained, at which time the fetus should be delivered. A zone 3 result indicates a fetus in danger of death, and transfusion or delivery should be chosen depending on the gestational age.

If one is capable of performing intrauterine transfusion, this may be begun as early as the 22nd week, and amniocentesis for ΔOD_{450} should be begun then. If this is not an option, amniocentesis should be begun as soon as delivery would be performed if necessary (usually 30 to 32 weeks). In addition to following the ΔOD_{450}, the fetus threatened by Rh disease should be monitored with EFM and biophysical profiles as any other fetus in jeopardy. Very early delivery is usually by cesarean section.

After delivery, since the mother will no longer clear the bilirubin formed by the hemolysis that continues for some time, fetal serum bilirubin levels may increase to the point of kernicterus. This requires careful observation and therapy as necessary.

ABO incompatibility

Mothers of blood type O have circulating anti-A and anti-B antibodies, which may cause hemolysis in fetuses who are A, B, or AB. Unlike Rh disease, this may occur in primigravidas and usually does not cause severe hemolysis. Since anti-A and anti-B titers are meaningless, there is no way to know antenatally if the process is happening, but it is rarely necessary. After delivery, however, significant hemolysis may continue, causing neonatal jaundice and possibly kernicterus, if unobserved. If the mother is type O, all cord blood should be screened for circulating antibodies.

Other blood group incompatibilities

There are numerous other blood group antigens that are quite rare, and some of these may cause significant antenatal hemolytic disease of the Rh type. Kell, Duffy, and Kidd are among the more common of these less-common antigens that may endanger the fetus. They are detected by the antibody screens of maternal blood, which should be a part of every Rh type and screen, and are managed in the same fashion as Rh incompatibility.

DISEASES OF THE URINARY TRACT

Infection

Asymptomatic bacteriuria (positive urine culture without symptoms) occurs in 5 to 10% of all pregnant women.

Although it causes no symptoms at the time of diagnosis, the risk that it will progress to symptomatic infection during the course of pregnancy is approximately 25%. For this reason, antenatal screening and appropriate antibiotic therapy are indicated.

Cystitis and acute pyelonephritis are the two urinary tract infections commonly encountered in pregnancy. The symptoms, diagnosis, and treatment of cystitis are the same in pregnant and nonpregnant women, except that during pregnancy certain antibiotics (trimethoprim, tetracycline) are best avoided.

Pyelonephritis is much more likely to occur in pregnant women than in nonpregnant. Urinary stasis and functional ureteral compression probably predispose to ascending infection. Fever, chills, back pain, costovertebral angle tenderness, and pyuria point to the diagnosis. Treatment should be with appropriate IV antibiotics (ampicillin and/or gentamicin are good starting points) until urinary cultures have identified the organism, which is most often *Escherichia coli*.

The major risk associated with pyelonephritis is that of premature labor.

Glomerulonephritis

Poststeptococcal glomerulonephritis has become increasingly rare in the past decade. It is equally rare during pregnancy. Since its course is usually benign, as little therapy as possible is indicated. The symptoms of proteinuria, edema, and hypertension may be mistaken for preeclampsia, which may only be distinguished by renal biopsy, almost never undertaken during pregnancy.

Chronic renal disease with impaired function

Whether from chronic pyelonephritis, glomerulonephritis, or diabetic nephropathy, decreased renal function may seriously imperil pregnancy. If creatinine clearance is less than 50% of normal, the necessary increases in renal function that usually occur during pregnancy may not. Instead, there is usually a decline in renal function as the pregnancy progresses, which abates postpartum. When serum creatinine concentration is higher than 2 mg/100 ml at the start, pregnancy loss rates are significantly higher in all trimesters.

Management of such pregnancies includes meticulous attention to salt and water balance, to blood pressure control, and to management of underlying disease. Dialysis may be helpful. Intensive antepartum fetal monitoring is also necessary.

Acute renal failure

Most often due to hypovolemia associated with either hemorrhagic shock or preeclampsia/eclampsia, acute renal failure usually presents as oliguria. When the cause of oliguria is prerenal, the urine is low in sodium (the kidney is reabsorbing it all) with a high osmolality and creatinine. Sufficiently low renal blood flow results in intrinsic kidney damage, initially renal tubular necrosis, but if severe enough, renal cortical necrosis. The ideal therapy for acute renal failure is to avoid it by rapid correction of the underlying cause of decreased renal blood flow, whether vasospastic, septic, or hemorrhagic. Attempts to maintain urine output with diuretics must be eschewed until one is certain that hypovolemia, the most common cause, is not present.

If renal tubular necrosis occurs, first there is an oliguric phase during which small amounts (<500 ml/day) of hypotonic or isotonic urine are produced. During this phase, which lasts approximately 2 weeks, management of fluid and electrolytes to match intake to output is critical. This has been made much easier by the ready availability of dialysis, which may be safely done during pregnancy. After this period, the diuretic phase begins, with a return of function and initially the output of huge amounts of fluid and sodium. Here the problem is to keep replacement up to losses. Recovery is complete in most cases.

If the renal blood flow is sufficiently compromised for long enough, either from shock or renal artery thrombosis, extensive parenchymal damage, renal cortical necrosis, occurs. This is most often permanent damage with a very gradual return of limited function and ensuing chronic renal failure. Before the era of dialysis, this was frequently fatal.

Nephropathy of vascular diseases

The two most common vascular diseases (other than hypertension) found in pregnant women are diabetes and systemic lupus erythematosus. Each presents grave management problems for the gravida and is discussed under separate heading.

Renal calculi

The incidence, diagnosis, and management of renal calculi during pregnancy are essentially the same as in the nonpregnant patient, except that one is more careful about using diagnostic radiology and certain antibiotics are not used. One tends to substitute sonographic evaluation of the renal tract for IVP, although a single-shot IVP to delineate a blocked ureter is acceptable. Treatment is essentially supportive (hydration, pain relief) until passage of the stone.

RESPIRATORY TRACT DISEASE IN PREGNANCY

Pneumonia

Pneumococcal pneumonia is the most common infection of the respiratory tract during pregnancy. Its diagnosis (chest x-ray, sputum smear) and treatment (penicillin) are the same as in the nonpregnant state, except that more careful attention must be accorded to prevention of high fevers and hypoxia to prevent fetal injury. The diagnosis (x-ray, cold agglutinins) and treatment (erythromycin) are similarly unchanged for mycoplasma pneumonia. For viral infections, the treatment is supportive as at other times.

Asthma

Asthmatic patients who become pregnant can expect a worsening of their disease 25% of the time, no change 50% of the time, and an improvement the remaining 25%. Those with more severe disease usually are the ones who become worse. The oxygen needs of the gravida are 25% higher than before pregnancy (tending to worsen the disease) while the high progesterone (and possibly corticosteroid) levels cause brochiolar dilation (tending to improve the disease).

The management of asthma during pregnancy is not much changed, except for the greater need to avoid hypoxia and caveats regarding some medications. Hydration is critical, as is maintenance of PO_2. Methylxanthines (theophylline, aminophylline) and sympathomimetics (epinephrine, metaproterenol, terbutaline, and albuterol) are central to control of brochospasm.

Although there are theoretical objections to all of these drugs except epinephrine (minor teratogenesis in some animal studies), they have not been shown to be harmful to human fetuses. In some cases, corticosteroids (prednisone) may be necessary, although its use in the first trimester may be associated with a slight increase in the incidence of cleft palate. If it is necessary, its benefits will likely outweigh its risks. Another commonly used agent, cromolyn sodium, blocks mast cell release and prevents brochospasm. Although it appears to be effective, its use during pregnancy is not officially approved.

Tuberculosis

Tuberculosis (TB) is much less common in this country than 20 years ago, although it threatens to increase again. Screening for TB is part of the normal antenatal care (tine or PPD test). If negative, there is no TB. If positive, physical examination and chest x-ray (with shielding) should be performed. If both are negative, no further action during pregnancy is necessary. After delivery, converters may be treated with isoniazid (INH) for 1 year.

If there is evidence of active disease, treatment must be begun during pregnancy. Standard therapy consists of INH and ethambutol for 1 year. Although there is a small concern regarding teratogenesis from IHN and optic neuritis from ethambutol, the risks of these are quite small and outweighed by the risks of nontreatment. Streptomycin may also be used but carries a risk of ototoxicity for the fetus. The newest drug, rifampin, is extremely effective but may be teratogenic (limb reduction defects).

Other respiratory diseases

Patients with **cystic fibrosis** have only recently survived to childbearing age. Their fertility is decreased, so experience with cystic fibrosis during pregnancy is limited. Half the patients seem to become markedly worse, and half remain unchanged. The management of the disease is standard, with control of infection and general respiratory support being the mainstays.

Sarcoidosis is another disease occasionally encountered during pregnancy. Its course seems to improve, with both x-ray and clinical resolution. This may be because the disease responds to steroid therapy and steroid levels are increased during pregnancy. Therapy itself is rarely changed by the presence of pregnancy, unless the need for it is lessened.

ENDOCRINE DISEASES IN PREGNANCY

Thyroid

The diagnosis of thyroid diseases is complicated in many ways by pregnancy. Physical findings may be obscured, many of the blood tests of thyroid function are altered by the hyperestrogenism (see "Maternal Adaptations"), and radioisotope studies are contraindicated. However, measurements of the unbound hormone fractions are now available and unchanged by pregnancy. Thyroid disease itself is not worsened or ameliorated by pregnancy, but therapy is altered.

Hyperthyroidism can usually be diagnosed by detection of goiter and measurement of free thyroxin and T_3. These patients may have exophthalmos, usually exhibit tachycardia, and fail to gain the proper amount of weight. Therapy is undertaken for maternal jeopardy, usually with propylthiouracil (PTU), which blocks thyroxin synthesis. It is begun with 100 mg t.i.d. for initial control, followed by reduction over 1 to 2 weeks, to 100 mg/day or less.

Since PTU crosses the placenta, the major danger of therapy, fetal hypothyroidism, may be best avoided by keeping the dosage as low as possible. To this end, maternal thyroxin levels should be maintained in the high normal to minimally hyperthyroid range. At these doses, fetal hypothyroidism is a rare complication. Attempts to avoid it by administration of thyroxine are counterproductive for two reasons: (1) Thyroxine increases maternal PTU needs, and (2) thyroxine crosses the placenta poorly while PTU crosses it well. There are no known long-term effects on the fetuses who have not been hypothyroid in utero.

An alternate therapy is the beta-blocker propranolol. Effective in controlling the symptoms of hyperthyroidism and first-line therapy in thyroid storm, it may however cause IUGR with chronic use so fetal monitoring is essential. Radioactive iodine is contraindicated as it crosses the placenta. Subtotal thyroidectomy is available but should be avoided if at all possible.

Thyroid storm is an acute exacerbation of all the symptoms of hyperthyroidism, with extremely high fever, tachycardia, dehydration, and a maternal mortality rate of up to 25%. Therapy consists of propranolol, sodium iodide, PTU, and a full range of supportive measures for dehydration, fever, and shock.

Hypothyroidism is relatively uncommon during pregnancy. Most cases, in fact, are diagnosed before conception, as severely hypothyroid women are relatively infertile and conceive after correction of the disease. For these women, the therapy, thyroid replacement, is unchanged by pregnancy. Milder cases may be quite difficult to diagnose and seem to have little effect on either mother or child.

Parathyroid

Both hypoparathyroidism and hyperparathyroidism are extremely rare during pregnancy. Hypoparathyroidism is most likely in patients who have undergone thyroid ablation by surgery or radiotherapy, so these should be screened by measurement of serum calcium (abnormally low) and phosphate (abnormally high). Treatment is with calcium supplements and high doses of vitamin D and is not altered by pregnancy. Their major effects on both mother and fetus seem to be mediated by calcium levels. If these are maintained in the normal range there are no ill effects.

Hyperparathyroidism occurs from an adenoma, a carcinoma, or hyperplasia and is manifested by hypercalcemia and hypophasphatemia. Diagnosis is unchanged by pregnancy. Therapy is usually surgical (second trimester is preferable) but may be postponed if oral phosphate supplements successfully lower calcium concentrations.

Pituitary

The most common pituitary disease in pregnancy is prolactin-producing **adenoma**. These lesions are usually diagnosed earlier while investigating oligo- or amenorrhea and

have been treated with bromocriptine (Parlodel), restoring fertility. The drug should be discontinued as soon as pregnancy is diagnosed. The patient is followed closely throughout for the appearance of headaches or vision symptoms using regular funduscopic and visual field examination, as pregnancy often causes rapid growth of adenomas. Hypocyloidal tomography and CT scans may be performed if necessary. If there is growth and compromise of vision, either bromocriptine (it works; long-term fetal effects are unknown) or surgery (transsphenoidal hypophysectomy) may be necessary. Late in the pregnancy, delivery is advisable.

Sheehan's syndrome, or pituitary necrosis, is a rare but dramatic condition, usually resulting from a hemorrhagic event related to delivery. It rarely complicates ongoing pregnancy. Therapy consists of adrenal and thyroid hormone replacement.

Diabetes insipidus is another extremely rare condition, occasionally coexisting with pregnancy. It is unaffected by and does not affect pregnancy. Treatment is with arginine vasopressin (DDAVP) to prevent diuresis.

Adrenal

Hypoadrenalism (**Addison's disease**) presents the same way during pregnancy as otherwise. Most cases have been diagnosed prior to conception and are being effectively treated. During pregnancy, corticosteroid replacement needs may increase slightly, but usually not much. During delivery and the puerperium, however, stress is acutely magnified and increased replacement is often necessary. Addisonian crisis should be considered in all cases of postpartum shock, especially when accompanied by diarrhea and vomiting. Corticosteroid fluid and electrolyte replacement is critical.

The diagnosis of hyperadrenalism (**Cushing's disease**) is obscured by pregnancy. Weight gain, edema, hyperpigmentation, and striae all are common in normal gestation, while hypertension is much more often a sign of preeclampsia. Increasing hirsutism, however, suggests Cushing's. Since cortisol levels are also altered by pregnancy, their measurement must be interpreted with care (similarly for the dexamethasone suppression test). Elevated serum ACTH levels may help to diagnose Cushing's of pituitary origin, which may be confirmed on CT scan of the pituitary. Since CT of the abdomen involves much radiation to the fetus, if there is strong suspicion of an adrenal tumor, exploratory surgery may be preferable. Therapy is excision of the pituitary or adrenal tumor. If this is not possible, cyproheptadine may be useful.

Congenital adrenal hyperplasia is perhaps the most common adrenal disorder that occurs concurrently with pregnancy. The adult form, usually due to a 21-hydroxylase deficiency, results in elevated levels of 17-hydroxyprogesterone and DHEAS, with associated virilization. This may have similar effects on the female fetus, causing varying degrees of masculinized genitalia. The effects on male fetuses are usually not so noticeable, being simply larger genitals. The treatment is corticosteroid replacement (cortisone acetate) to block feedback and is unchanged by pregnancy. These virilized women often have android pelves, so labor complications are more frequent.

Pheochromocytoma during pregnancy is extremely rare and carries a high mortality rate. It should be suspected when uncontrollable hypertension is present. The treatment is surgical.

GI TRACT DISEASES IN PREGNANCY

Appendicitis

Appendicitis is not more common during pregnancy but is more difficult to diagnose because the gravid uterus tends to lift the appendix upward from its usual location. Additionally, peritonitis occurs later (the uterus acts as a shield) so symptoms seem less acute. Finally, surgeons are loathe to do exploratory surgery on pregnant patients. Diagnosis consequently is often delayed, with ill effects for both mother and fetus. The treatment is appendectomy.

Esophagitis

Esophagitis is probably the most common GI disease during pregnancy. Heartburn occurs in more than half of all pregnant women and is usually attributed to a combination of factors (decreased GI motility, relaxation of the esophageal sphincter, and increased intra-abdominal pressure from the uterus), all of which promote reflux of acid. When there is more than superficial irritation of the esophageal mucosa, substernal chest pain radiating to the back, shoulders, or arms may result, suggesting cardiac, pancreatic, or gallbladder disease. It is often accompanied by chest pain on swallowing. Definitive diagnosis is by esophagoscopy, which is rarely done. Therapeutic trial with antacids is instead the approach of choice. Usually calcium/aluminum-containing preparations work best, when combined with a bland diet and cool liquids. Cimetidine (Tagamet) and related drugs are most useful in nonpregnant patients, but experience with their use during pregnancy is limited.

Peptic ulcers

Ulcers are rare during pregnancy since gastric acid secretion is decreased. Their diagnosis and management are unchanged except that the GI series is avoided and cimetidine and similar drugs, which have become mainstays of therapy in nonpregnant patients, are used in extreme cases only.

Inflammatory bowel disease

Ulcerative colitis and Crohn's disease (regional enteritis) are now often grouped together as inflammatory bowel disease (IBD). Their diagnosis is often difficult in the nonpregnant patient, requiring radiological studies, endoscopy, and biopsy. It is no less difficult during pregnancy. As currently managed, these diseases do not seem to impair fertility much unless they are quite active or surgery has resulted in adhesion formation.

If IBD is quiet at conception, the prognosis for the pregnancy is good. If it is active, flare-ups are likely, with elevated miscarriage rates. The effects of pregnancy on IBD are variable. Almost half improve, but many experience exacerbation.

The therapy for IBD consists primarily of prednisone and sulfasalazine, both of which may be used during pregnancy. Sulfasalazine, being a sulfa drug, should be discontinued a week before delivery to avoid binding to bilirubin receptor sites on fetal albumin, thereby putting the newborn at risk for hyperbilirubinemia. Other drugs commonly used, but not during pregnancy, are mercaptopurine and azathioprine.

Pancreatitis

Pancreatitis occurs rarely during pregnancy and is diagnosed and treated in the usual way, except for the avoidance of radiological tests. It is mostly secondary to alcohol abuse or gallstones and presents with epigastric pain radiating to the back. Serum amylase levels help to distinguish it from esophagitis and unperforated ulcer. In mild cases, therapy is supportive. Rarely, surgery is necessary. Its course is unaffected by pregnancy.

LIVER AND GALLBLADDER DISEASES IN PREGNANCY

Cholestatic jaundice of pregnancy

Cholestatic jaundice of pregnancy usually occurs in the third trimester and is probably related to high estrogen levels, since it often recurs in subsequent pregnancies and in patients who take oral contraceptives. Liver function is decreased so that bile is incompletely conjugated in the liver, and mild hyperbilirubinemia and a marked elevation of bile acids results. It is characterized by jaundice and pruritus. SGOT and alkaline phosphatase are somewhat elevated, and bile acids markedly so. Other liver function tests are frequently abnormal. Diagnosis is usually suspected because of the intense itching and requires ruling out gallstones and hepatitis.

Intense pruritus is the most common and annoying symptom for the mother. Although the reasons are not clear, there is significant fetal morbidity (fetal distress and prematurity in up to one-half of cases) and mortality (up to 10%). Therapy for the mother is to relieve the itching by binding bile salts using cholestyramine (Questran). One must exercise care in its use, however, as it interferes with the absorption of fat-soluble vitamins and may result in depletion of vitamin K-dependent coagulation factors. Intensive fetal monitoring from the time of diagnosis is essential.

The disease resolves spontaneously shortly after delivery.

Acute fatty liver of pregnancy

Another primary liver disease of the mid- to late third trimester of unknown origin, acute fatty liver presents as progressive degeneration of liver function. It usually begins with malaise, nausea, and vomiting and progresses to jaundice and right upper quadrant abdominal pain and finally coagulopathy, hepatic encephalopathy, and death. Laboratory abnormalities include a general derangement of all liver function and coagulation tests. Hypertension sometimes occurs as well, making the distinction between this and preeclampsia with liver involvement difficult. Definitive diagnosis may be made on liver biopsy, which is characteristic.

Maternal mortality in unchecked cases may approach 90%. In well-handled cases, it is still as high as 30%. Fetal mortality rates parallel those of the mother at a slightly higher level.

Therapy is delivery. If permanent damage has not resulted from encephalopathy or DIC, most cases resolve promptly and completely on termination of the pregnancy. All necessary supportive measures before either induction or cesarean section are appropriate.

Hepatitis

Viral hepatitis A (infectious hepatitis) occurs during pregnancy with the same frequency as outside it. If one ingests the infectious particles, one catches the disease. Symptoms are lassitude, malaise, and loss of appetite. There is generalized derangement of liver function tests with markedly high SGOT and alkaline phosphatase. Hepatitis A antigen (IgM) becomes positive early in the course of the disease and may be used for accurate diagnosis. Except in fulminant cases, which are rare, there is no particular effect on the pregnancy. Infants are almost never infected in utero. Treatment consists of bed rest and a nutritious diet. Recovery begins within 2 to 3 weeks. Enteric precautions should be taken.

Viral hepatitis B (serum hepatitis) is spread by body fluids of all types and is most commonly communicated by needle sharing, sexual activity, and transfusion. Health care workers are also at particular risk because of their exposure to blood products. It presents with symptoms and laboratory findings similar to those of hepatitis B, except more indolently and with more myalgia and joint pain. Distinction from hepatitis A is by identification of hepatitis B surface and e (this is actually whole virus) antigens and hepatitis B core antibody. After several weeks, as the infection resolves, these are replaced with hepatitis surface antibody. Fulminant hepatitis is more common than with type A.

The treatment, bed rest and diet, is the same as for hepatitis A, but the course is different: Approximately 10% will develop chronic active hepatitis, with a high incidence of hepatic carcinoma. Also unlike hepatitis A, if the disease occurs in the third trimester, there is a significant risk of transmission to the fetus during the pregnancy, delivery, and postpartum period (nursing). Those most likely to transmit the disease are those who have e and surface antigens. Their infants should receive hepatitis B immune globulin and vaccine at birth, which is highly protective. Additionally, these mothers should not breast-feed. Delivery room personnel must exercise great care in dealing with these patients, as all their body fluids are highly infectious.

Non-A/non-B hepatitis refers to hepatitis that fulfills the serological criteria for neither hepatitis A nor hepatitis B. It is mostly secondary to transfusion, although there is now a large enough reservoir in the population for significant sexual transmission. Its treatment is largely supportive.

Fulminant hepatitis is usually fatal. Distinction from acute fatty liver of pregnancy and from cholestatic jaundice of pregnancy may be difficult (it can be done by biopsy) but is often academic, since delivery of the fetus is necessary in most cases anyway (in the former two, for the health of the mother; in fulminant hepatitis, to save the baby).

Cirrhosis

Posthepatitic, postalcoholic, and primary biliary cirrhosis all tend to create relative infertility. When pregnancy does occur, it may be fairly well tolerated if liver function is reasonable. If liver function is more severely impaired or esophageal varices are present, the prognosis is poor for both mother and fetus. Corticosteroids are the cornerstones of treatment and may be continued during pregnancy. If varices are present, surgery before conception is desirable.

Gallbladder

Some studies show an increased incidence of cholelithiasis and cholecystitis during pregnancy; others do not. Certainly, the effects of pregnancy on the gallbladder (stasis, increased concentration of bile salts) suggest a greater likelihood. The diagnosis is made by the same parameters as in the nonpregnant person except that one relies more on ultrasonography and avoids radiation exposure. The treatment, either conservative or surgical, is unchanged. As with most other surgical procedures, cholecystomy is best done during the second trimester, if necessary.

NEUROLOGICAL DISEASES IN PREGNANCY

Epilepsy

If a woman has seizures for the first time during pregnancy, the diagnosis of epilepsy becomes more difficult, especially in the last 3 to 4 months, when eclampsia and lupus, among other causes, must be considered. Most epilepsy, however, is present before conception, so the question becomes one of management. It is fairly well established that epileptics who have been seizure-free for more than 1 year tolerate pregnancy well, with only a small risk of recurrence, whereas those who have frequent convulsions often become even more difficult to control. There are several factors by which pregnancy affects epileptic ontrol:

1. Blood volume is expanded and creatinine clearance increased, so that constant doses of anticonvulsants result in lower serum levels. Whether this is counteracted by an increase in the unbound fraction is unknown.
2. Estrogen is known to increase seizure threshold, whereas progesterone decreases it.
3. The mild respiratory alkalosis of pregnancy may also predispose to seizure activity.
4. Noncompliance by patients fearful of congenital anomalies may further complicate matters.

There is no antiepileptic known to be completely safe for use in pregnancy. Diphenylhydantoin (Dilantin) is the mainstay of therapy. Some investigators have suggested that it is linked to a syndrome of craniofacial and limb defects and mental retardation, which may affect as many as 10% of exposed fetuses. Others are less certain. Cleft palate and cleft lip may also occur with increased frequency in these infants. It also has been shown to cause depletion of vitamin K-dependent clotting factors in the fetus and to thereby predispose to hemorrhagic disease of the newborn. This can usually be avoided by prompt administration of vitamin K to the infant at birth, or even to the mother in labor.

Other anticonvulsants used in nonpregnant patients include phenobarbital, trimethadione (Tridione), carbamazepine (Tegretol), and valproic acid (Depakine). Except for phenobarbital, which has been weakly associated with cleft lip and palate, all are known teratogens. Trimethadione is strictly contraindicated; carbamazepine has been associated with mild microcephaly, and valproic acid with neural tube and skeletal defects.

The most important question in management, therefore, is whether to continue anticonvulsant medication. The risk of stopping is that the mother may convulse, endangering both herself and her fetus. This must be balanced against the ill effects of the various drugs on the fetus.

Multiple sclerosis

A poorly understood disease that does not impair fertility, multiple sclerosis (MS) has no clearcut effect on pregnancy, nor does pregnancy on it, although the relapse rate is much higher in the puerperal period. Some suggest that it may precipitate latent disease in those destined to suffer from MS. The only therapy available for use in pregnancy is corticosteroid administration.

Cerebrovascular disease

Hemorrhagic stroke is a major cause of maternal mortality. Occurring mostly in women with arteriovenous malformations and berry aneurysms, it may also follow sickling crises, septic and thrombotic emboli, and choriocarcinoma. Bleeding typically is in the latter half of pregnancy. The main concern is the woman who survives an episode of cerebral hemorrhage, either before conception or after. If before, surgical correction is ideal, as these patients tolerate pregnancy and delivery well. If during, there is controversy. Some feel that surgery is well tolerated by the fetus (hypotension and hypothermia are concomitants) and that maternal management should be as if she were not pregnant. Others feel there is danger for the fetus that may outweigh the benefits derived by the mother.

Thrombotic stroke is a much less likely cause of death and appears to be concentrated among women with cardiovascular predispositions such as atrial fibrillation, phlebitis, endocarditis, sickle cell disease, and collagen vascular diseases. Transient ischemic attacks (TIAs) are also clustered in these women. Unless there is systemic hypotension, TIAs do not affect the fetus, but anticoagulation may be necessary.

Headache

Migraine headaches may become less or more frequent and less or more severe during pregnancy. Because of their prodromal visual symptoms, one must distinguish them from preeclampsia headaches. This is best done by careful history and neurological examination. Ergot alkaloids, the most common therapy, are not used during pregnancy. If analgesia with acetaminophen, aspirin, narcotics, or barbiturates is not sufficient, propranolol may be effective.

Much more common than migraine are tension headaches. Exacerbated by the physical and emotional strains of pregnancy, they are usually distinguishable by history and examination. Mild analgesics, sedatives, and massage are usually sufficient.

Myasthenia gravis

An autoimmune disease in which IgG antibodies interfere with acetycholine receptors in striated muscle, myasthenia is characterized by muscle weakness on minimal exertion. It may improve, remain the same, or worsen during pregnancy. It typically worsens during the postpartum period. The first stage of labor is not impaired (the uterus is smooth muscle), but pushing in the second stage usually is. Muscle relaxants such as $MgSO_4$ are extremely dangerous as they may cause paralysis. Aminoglycosides, although less so, have a similar effect. The fetus does not seem to be affected in utero (reason unknown)

but often (>10%) is after birth. Affects may last for several weeks, which may cause a problem with feeding and aspiration of food.

Therapy is with acetylcholine inhibitors (neostigmine, physostigmine) that do not cross the placenta, thymectomy (occasionally necessary), and immunosuppression (prednisone is acceptable during pregnancy; azathioprine, which is clearly teratogenic, is not). Because the disease is due to a circulating antibody, temporary relief may be obtained with plasmapheresis. Neonates are usually treated with anticholinesterase inhibitors.

AUTOIMMUNE AND CONNECTIVE TISSUE DISEASES IN PREGNANCY

Systemic lupus erythematosus

Known as the "great imitator," systemic lupus erythematosus (SLE) is the most serious of the common autoimmune diseases to coexist with pregnancy. It consists of a complex of inflammatory reactions in various organ systems, manifesting most commonly as arthritis, dermatitis, serositis, and renal and neurological diseases. Affecting perhaps as many as one of every thousand people, primarily women between the ages of 20 and 40, its coincidence with pregnancy is not rare.

The diagnosis is difficult enough without pregnancy that the American Rheumatism Association codified the following 11 possible criteria, the presence of any 4 being strongly indicative of SLE:

1. Butterfly rash on cheeks
2. Discoid rash
3. Photosensitivity
4. Oral ulcers
5. Arthritis
6. Serositis
7. Renal disease, consisting of proteinuria or casts
8. Neurological disease, consisting of seizures or psychosis
9. Hematologic disease, consisting of hemolytic anemia, leukopenia, lymphopenia, or thrombocytopenia
10. Immunologic disease, consisting of + LE prep, positive anti-DNA or anti-Sm antibodies, or false-positive VDRL
11. Positive antinuclear antibody (ANA)

Once the diagnosis is made, the progress of the disease is followed primarily by serum C3 and C4 complement levels (falling levels ae ominous; "falling" is critical here, as opposed to low, because baseline complement levels are elevated during pregnancy) and the presence of anti-DNA antibody, both of which correlate closely with flare-ups and renal disease. Frequent monitoring of renal, hematologic, and hepatic function is also necessary. The sedimentation rate, used extensively in nonpregnant patients, has no use during pregnancy, since it is markedly elevated in all gravidas. A major diagnostic decision is called for during what appears to be a lupus flare-up, since the hypertension, renal disease, convulsions, thrombocytompenia, and hemolysis that may be seen all are equally suggestive of severe preeclampsia/eclampsia, which is also more common in SLE patients.

Effects of pregnancy on SLE.   Pregnancy apparently does not have an adverse effect on SLE that has been quiet for at least several months before conception. It also has less of an effect on well-controlled disease that remains under therapy, as long as there is no renal involvement. In patients who are poorly controlled or who discontinue their steroids or have severe renal disease at the start of the pregnancy, deterioration is not unlikely.

Effect of SLE on pregnancy.   SLE is a vasculitis. As such, it can be expected to imperil the fetus, which depends on an intact vascular supply for growth. In fact, there is danger in all three trimesters. Spontaneous abortion rates may be as high as 25%. IUGR, prematurity, and perinatal mortality rates all may be up to 30%, even in cases without severe renal disease, which further worsens the prognosis.

Also problematic have been direct effects on the fetus. Congenital heart block appears to be highly correlated with SLE to the degree that all infants born to mothers with SLE should be evaluated for it, and the mothers of all infants born with heart block should be evaluated for SLE. Neonatal SLE may also occur, apparently from transplacental transfer of a circulating antibody, anti-Ro. This is a self-limiting disease lasting less than 1 year.

Therapy.   Primary treatment for SLE is with corticosteroids. These should not be discontinued during pregnancy. The small risk of teratogenesis is greatly outweighed by the risk of exacerbation of the disease. Flare-ups are treated with increasing doses. The immunosuppressive azathioprine (Imuran) is probably teratogenic in humans (definitely in animals), but some consider it worth the risk in cases unresponsive to corticosteroids. Therapeutic abortion is no longer commonly performed and may not be beneficial. Obviously, because of the great likelihood of fetal compromise, cesarean section is more common, but this is on obstetric grounds.

Rheumatoid arthritis

Rheumatoid arthritis is the most common of all autoimmune diseases, especially in women. However, even though there are circulating immune complexes, major involvement is apparently limited to joints so there is little if any effect on pregnancy. Similarly, pregnancy does not adversely affect rheumatoid arthritis. In fact, in more than half the cases it actually improves the disease, although most become worse postpartum. The major treatment is large doses of aspirin, which may cause coagulation problems, delay the onset of labor, and cause premature closure of the ductus. Other nonsteroidal anti-inflammatory drugs, such as ibuprofen (Motrin) and indomethacin (Indocin), are less well tolerated and more likely to adversely affect the fetus. Gold and penicillamine are both potentially quite toxic and are generally avoided during pregnancy.

Polyarteritis nodosa

A rare multisystem vasculopathy that has only rarely been reported in pregnant women, polyarteritis is associated with frequent maternal death in the postpartum period from kidney failure and hypertensive crisis. The few cases extant have been difficult to distinguish from preeclampsia. Although fetal survival is better than maternal, a significant number of

antenatal deaths also occur. Therapy is with high-dose corticosteroids and intensive fetal surveillance.

Scleroderma (progressive systemic sclerosis)

Scleroderma is a rare disease causing progressive sclerosis of various systems. Initial presentation is usually vascular compromise of the extremities manifesting as Raynaud's phenomenon. Musculoskeletal and GI involvement are common, causing arthritis and motility disorders (dysphagia and diarrhea). Renal involvement with malignant hypertension is the most common cause of death. Diagnosis is on clinical grounds and may be supported by muscle biopsy.

Like most other connective tissue diseases, scleroderma is usually unaffected by pregnancy in the milder cases and takes a turn for the worse if it is active at the time of conception. Esophagitis usually worsens, as it does in normal pregnancy. In the absence of renal disease, scleroderma has little effect on the fetus. When present, renal involvement bodes ill. There is no known treatment for this disease, so therapy is aimed at minimizing complications: antacids for esophagitis, corticosteroids for myositis, and physical therapy for joint and skin sclerosis.

Dermatomyositis

Another rare inflammatory disease with primary muscle and skin involvement but secondarily affecting multiple systems, dermatomyositis may be either acute and fulminant or chronic. Unlike scleroderma, it rarely is associated with renal damage. Diagnosis is on clinical criteria, electromyography, and muscle biopsy. It has only coincided with pregnancy a handful of times, so data are uncertain, but associated fetal mortality appears to be high. Preferable therapy for dermatomyositis during pregnancy is high-dose corticosteroids.

INFECTIOUS DISEASES IN PREGNANCY

SEXUALLY TRANSMITTED DISEASES

Syphilis

Syphilis is one of the most easily prevented and/or treated sexually transmitted diseases (STD) and one of the most destructive to the fetus if not. For this reason, the VDRL (STS) is part of every prenatal screening program, usually during both the first and third trimesters.

Diagnosis.   The diagnosis is made the same way as in the nonpregnant state, based on identification of a chancre several weeks after infection and confirmed by dark-field examination of material from the chancre, which should reveal treponemes. The VDRL should be done immediately but may not become positive for several weeks after infection. If initially negative, it should be repeated a maximum of 6 weeks later. The VDRL is a nonspecific but easily done test that is highly accurate if negative but may be falsely positive in a variety of conditions. Positive VDRLs should be verified with the fluorescent treponemal antibody-absorption test (FTA-ABS), which is extremely specific.

If the infection is not detected early, secondary syphilis in the form of condylomata lata appears but may be transitory and often is not noticed. Lesions of secondary syphilis may recur

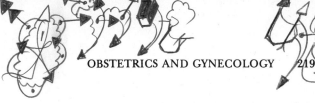

over several years, during which the patient remains infectious. Afterward, a latent period of up to 20 years ensues, during which the VDRL often becomes negative. The FTA-ABS remains positive forever. Following the variable latent period, approximately one-third will develop tertiary syphilis. Although the infectivity of patients is much reduced after secondary syphilis, some patients remain so forever, unless treated.

Since syphilis is so easily missed during so much of its course and potentially so serious for the fetus (not to mention the mother), screening with the VDRL is mandatory.

Effects on pregnancy. Although the course of syphilis is not affected by pregnancy and has little effect on the mother, it may be catastrophic for the fetus. Early infection with a large inoculum may cause abortion. It was previously thought that the spirochete did not cross the placenta during the first trimester. More likely, tissue reaction to it is minimal, making detection difficult. Infection with a smaller inoculum may result in stillbirth or in congenital syphilis in a surviving neonate. Typical pathology includes invasion by the spirochete of the liver, spleen, lymphatic, skeletal, and neurological systems. All infants born to mothers known to have had syphilis should be evaluated at birth.

Therapy. The prescribed treatment for syphilis, penicillin in variable doses, has been established by the Centers for Disease Control and depends on the duration of disease. Treatment is the same for pregnant and nonpregnant patients except that tetracycline is not commonly used during pregnancy.

For disease present less than 1 year, treatment is benzathine penicillin G, 2.4 million units IM (one dose) or aqueous procaine penicillin G, 600,000 units/day IM for 8 days. For disease present more than 1 year (latent or tertiary, except neurosyphilis), treatment is benzathine penicillin G, 2.4 millions units IM/week for 3 weeks, or procaine penicillin G, 600,000 units/day IM for 15 days. Neurosyphilis requires more aggressive therapy, usually with IV penicillin G up to 20 million units/day for up to 2 weeks, followed by benzathine penicillin weekly for 3 weeks. For patients who are allergic to penicillin, erythromycin, 500 mg q.i.d. is substituted for 15 days (less than 1 year duration) or 30 days (more than 1 year duration). All consorts must be identified and treated as well.

Gonorrhea

In the first trimester, gonorrhea (GC) may cause salpingitis, but after the 12th week, the uterine cavity is eliminated as a pathway to the fallopian tubes. It is, therefore, most often present as cervicitis during pregnancy. As such it does not endanger the fetus during its intrauterine stay but may infect it at birth, the most common sequela of which is gonococcal ophthalmitis. If present at birth, GC is also likely to cause ascending maternal infection. Systemic infection may also occur at any time. Neither the transmission, nor the course (except as above), nor the diagnosis is affected by pregnancy.

Screening for GC, as for syphilis, is considered standard prenatal care. The use of effective transport media (Transgro) and the advent of immunologic slide tests (Gonozyme) have made this process much more accurate, cheaper, and easier. When detected, preferred treatment for gonorrheal cervicitis is procaine penicillin G, 4.8 million units IM (or ampicillin 3.5 g PO or amoxicillin 3 g PO) plus probenecid, 1 g PO, to prolong

high tissue levels. The oral therapies are not effective against pharyngitis, so throat cultures should be performed. Additionally, the procaine regimen covers incubating syphilis. For patients who are penicillin allergic or for GC that is penicillin resistant, spectinomycin (Trobicin), 2 g IM, or 1 to 2 g of one of the newer cephalosporins, cefoxitin, or cefotaxime may be substituted. Tetracycline and doxycycline, which are alternatives in nonpregnant patients, are avoided during pregnancy. Simultaneous treatment of sexual partners is also essential.

Chlamydia trachomatis

Now much more common than gonorrhea (with a prevalence of up to 15% in some U.S. populations), chlamydial infection in many ways parallels it. Present mostly during pregnancy as a cervicitis (as with gonorrhea, if the pathway is clear it may ascend to the upper tract), the primary risk for the fetus is acquisition at birth, usually as ophthalmitis, which may cause blindness. For the mother, postpartum pelvic inflammatory disease is a real risk. There is also question about whether premature labor may be induced by infection. Like gonorrhea, the transmission, course, and diagnosis of the disease do not appear to be affected by pregnancy.

The diagnosis is by tissue culture of infected cervical cells (difficult and expensive) or by immunologic slide test (Chlamydiazyme, Microtrak) on the same material. The sensitivity and specificity of these newer tests approach those for culture, and their lesser cost is significant. Although it is not yet considered standard to screen for chlamydia at the first prenatal visit, it seems likely that it will become so in the near future.

The preferred treatment of the nonpregnant individual is tetracycline or doxycycline. During pregnancy, erythromycin, 500 mg q 6 hours PO, is used for a period varying from 10 days to 3 weeks. Longer periods of treatment are associated with lower rates of recidivism. As with all STDs, treatment of the partner is essential to prevent recurrence.

Herpes simplex

In the general population, next to AIDS, herpes is probably the most feared of all STDs. There are two major groups of viruses, types I and II. Type II has traditionally been associated with genital lesions and type I with disease elsewhere, especially in the oropharynx. This has been largely an accident of transmission, and as sexual practices have changed and the virus has become more widespread, a significant proportion of genital herpes has become type I and oral lesions may be type II.

The initial infection is spread by direct contact with a lesion or the shed virus and has an incubation period of 3 days to perhaps 2 weeks. It first manifests as clusters of vesicles, which then ulcerate. If they are on dry skin, they usually crust within a day or so and then heal over a week to 10 days. On mucous membrane, they remain ulcers until healed. Minor secondary infection with skin organisms is not rare. Local lymph nodes are frequently enlarged and sometimes tender. Typically, because there is no preexisting immunity, the clusters appear in several generations over a 2- to 3-week period. Viremia is not rare with primary infection, often resulting in a flu-like syndrome and occasionally disseminated herpes, the most serious form of which is encephalitis.

During the course of the initial infection, the virus somehow takes up residence in the nerve cells supplying the area of exposure. A variety of stimuli, which have not been clearly delineated but which include local irritation and possibly systemic disease and stress, may at any time in the future cause recurrence by awakening the dormant virus in the nerve cell. It then somehow travels to the skin and causes new lesions to be formed. Unlike primary infection, recurrences usually last only 7 to 10 days and are most often singular events. However, *recurrences may be extremely minor, even clinically inapparent, and still result in shedding of the virus.* Although the estimates vary, up to 70% of those infected may experience recurrent disease. The frequency of recurrence may vary from every few weeks to less often than yearly.

Diagnosis. The diagnosis of herpes, unchanged during pregnancy, is by identification of the vesicles and ideally by viral culture from the lesion. Slide and tube tests using monoclonal antibodies may soon be clinically available. Serology for IgM and IgG antibodies is less than ideal for diagnosis of any one event because previous disease is confounding.

Effects on pregnancy. Primary infection during pregnancy, with viremia, may infect the fetus. It is unclear whether transplacental transmission in the first trimester results in abortion. Since there is no associated viremia, recurrences during the antepartum period are of no danger. They do, however, endanger the fetus during passage through the birth canal at delivery or by ascending infection after rupture of the membranes. Shedding may be either from a visible vulvar lesion or from unseen (and unfelt) vaginal or cervical disease. If the fetus is infected, a spectrum of diseases from localized pustules to generalized herpes with brain damage and death may result. In the era before acyclovir, as many as 80 to 90% of infected fetuses were severely damaged.

Therapy. Since recurrent genital herpes is of no danger to the mother, all therapy is aimed at avoiding transmission of the virus to the fetus. Acyclovir (Zovirax), which may be used to treat primary infection or frequent recurrences in the non-pregnant individual, is generally not used during pregnancy. Instead, the woman in the last few weeks before anticipated delivery is counseled to avoid genital irritation (especially sex) in the hope of avoiding a recurrence and to be alert for symptoms. Additionally, since viral shedding may occur in the absence of symptoms, careful weekly examination and viral cultures from the external genitalia, cervix, and vagina (and, obviously, from any suspect lesions) should be performed.

If neither the mother nor the obstetrician has any suspicion of recurrence within 10 to 14 days of delivery, labor and vaginal delivery are allowed. Internal electrodes for FHR monitoring should be eschewed, if possible, since scalp puncture may be a portal of entry for the virus. If lesions are evident or positive cultures are obtained in this period, cesarean section is usually the route in an attempt to avoid contamination of the baby. If abdominal delivery is opted for, it should be performed within 4 to 6 hours after rupture of the membranes. Managed in this fashion, genital herpes rarely infects a fetus and results in a cesarean section rate of approximately 25%. Babies who are inadvertently exposed (perhaps a positive culture returns after delivery) may be watched very carefully for the potential incubation period or prophylactically treated with acyclovir.

The above measures are not so clearly indicated for the woman who is primarily infected during pregnancy, since transplacental infection may occur with viremia. Along the same lines, women who have never had genital herpes but who have afflicted partners might do well to use condoms throughout pregnancy to minimize the risk of infection during this period.

Human immunodeficiency virus (HIV)

AIDS, the result of infection with HIV, is now a significant cause of infant mortality. A viral infection transmitted primarily through infected body fluids (blood, semen, vaginal secretions), HIV selectively destroys parts of the immune system, most notably T4 lymphocytes. As with all other body fluid diseases, it has spread most rapidly through the groups with the greatest exposure: homosexuals (extreme promiscuity was a significant part of much homosexual behavior until recently), IV drug abusers (needle sharing), and hemophiliacs (multiple cryoprecipitate transfusions). Until recently, with effective screening of the blood supply, transfusion was similarly dangerous. Sexual partners of infected people are also at considerable risk. Most pregnant women with HIV are either IV drug users or partners of high-risk men.

Estimates of the number carrying the virus in the United States today range from 500,000 to 2,000,000, most in the so-called high-risk categories above. However, as HIV is spread throughout the population by sexual intercourse and needle sharing, the infection will gradually spread into low-risk groups.

Many statements made about AIDS confuse morality with biology and speculation with fact. Much of what is known is of epidemiologic origin, subject to patient recall and selective divulgence of life-style information, perhaps often unreliable. What can be said with a fair degree of certainty follows:

1. HIV can be spread by exposure to blood and semen (either rectally or vaginally). Transmission in either direction between men and women during sex is definitely possible, although it *may* be more efficient from men to women. HIV is probably not easily spread by casual contact. Spread via oral sex, deep kissing, and other intermediate forms of contact is uncertain.

2. Infection with HIV seems to be for life. To date (7 years, since the identification of AIDS as a disease) no one has recovered.

3. During a follow-up period of 7 years, approximately 50% of infected people develop full-blown AIDS, 30% develop the less serious AIDS-related complex (ARC), and 20% remain asymptomatic carriers of the virus. However, the longer the follow-up period, the more these numbers shift to the left (more AIDS, fewer carriers). Why some remain asymptomatic carriers and what may precipitate clinical disease are unknown.

4. Full-blown AIDS is, to date, uniformly fatal within 3 years.

5. There is significant risk (although not 100%) of transplacental transmission to the fetus, who, if infected, seems to have a more fulminant course than adults.

Diagnosis. AIDS and ARC are suspected on clinical criteria, including a number of opportunistic infections, wasting diseases, and Kaposi's sarcoma (see CDC guidelines). Definitive diagnosis is by identification of antibody to HIV. Initial testing is via an ELISA test, which is easy, cheap, and extremely reliable if negative. The ELISA test, however, is falsely positive up to 5% of the time, with concentrations in women on oral contraceptives, perhaps in pregnancy, and among certain HLA types. All specimens testing positive by the ELISA method are then retested with another more specific assay, usually the Southern blot. False positives are rare. False negatives are slightly less so.

Effects of pregnancy on disease. Not enough is known at this point to say whether pregnancy increases the risk of progression, since the course of the disease may be so poor anyway.

Effects of disease on pregnancy. The risk relates to transplacental infection of the fetus. These babies are often growth retarded and born prematurely, although attribution to the virus or maternal disease may be difficult since most experience with these pregnancies has been with drug-addicted mothers. The infants have abnormal reticuloendothelial and immune function, hepatosplenomegaly, generalized lymphadenopathy, decreased numbers of T4 lymphocytes, and proneness to the same constellation of opportunistic infections, especially oral candidiasis and pneumonias. Definitive diagnosis, as with the adult, is by identification of the HIV antibody. Failure to thrive is the rule, with death within 1 to 2 years.

Therapy. Although there are many experimental trials in progress, there is no known effective treatment for AIDS. At the moment, efforts must be directed to identifying those who carry the virus and advising them against becoming pregnant. HIV screening, at the very least for all women who are IV drug users or whose partners are in high-risk categories (hemophiliacs, bisexuals, or IV drug users), is currently advisable. With time, screening will probably become more the rule than the exception for all women considering pregnancy.

If a woman known to be positive for HIV becomes pregnant, careful avoidance of exposure to infection, good nutrition, and vigilant prenatal care are desirable. Since transmission to the fetus seems to be transplacental, cesarean section is not indicated, except on obstetric grounds. Obviously, delivery room personnel exercise great care to avoid exposure to the body fluids of these women and infants.

Human papillomavirus (HPV)

HPV is, in fact, a collection of 55 viral subtypes, and new types are being discovered every year. They are transmitted by skin-to-skin contact, often involving sexual contact (genital skin). They are the cause of warts (condylomata, papilloma, flat condylomata) on all skin surfaces, including the cervix, vagina, vulva, penis, hands, feet, and larynx (and perhaps others like the esophagus). Conventional wisdom is that certain viral types infect certain skin surfaces, (although this may be a parallel to the thinking about herpes types I and II 20 years ago) and produce characteristic lesions. Perhaps the appearance of the lesions, which may be flattish but slightly raised, papilliform, pedunculated, or invisible except after staining with acetic acid, depends on the skin surface infected as much as or more than on the viral type. In addition, certain viral serotypes are now clearly linked to the development of genital malignancy (cervix, vagina, and vulva). Using sophisticated DNA hybridization techniques, HPV can be isolated from virtually all cervical neoplasia.

Like AIDS, genital condylomatosis is a disease that has been spreading rapidly through the population during the past few years and is becoming more important in the pregnant woman.

Diagnosis. Most genital HPV infection during pregnancy is diagnosed by seeing the characteristic lesions of the vulva or vagina. Confirmation is by biopsy and the findings of koilocytosis and nuclear atypia. A significant number of HPV infections are now also being first detected by abnormal cervical cytology, although this is less reliable before the onset of cervical intraepithelial neoplasia (CIN). Suspected cases are investigated by colposcopy and biopsy. These procedures are essentially unchanged in the gravid woman, although cervical biopsies tend to bleed more.

Effect of pregnancy on the disease. Many cases of HPV infection seem to progress during pregnancy. The most visible of these are the cauliflower-type lesions of the vulva and labia, which may grow enough to obstruct delivery. Significant itching and/or pain may accompany these lesions. More often the intravaginal lesions, noticeable as papillary or cobblestone type configurations, do not pose significant problems for the mother. There is no evidence that pregnancy adversely affects the course of either cervical HPV or CIN.

Effect of disease on pregnancy. The major concern with maternal genital HPV infection is transmission to the fetus at delivery, the most serious consequence of which is giant laryngeal papillomas. Although this seems to happen once in several thousand deliveries, the risk of transmission to the neonate is unknown.

Therapy. In the nonpregnant individual there are many treatments, none wholly acceptable. Recurrence rates are very high, mostly because eradication of the lesions does not include asymptomatically infected adjacent areas (in the vagina, this probably includes the entire intravaginal surface) or infected partners. All methods involve destruction of the infected skin and include application of podophyllin, trichloracetic and bichloracetic acids, electrocautery, cryosurgery, laser evaporation, 5-fluorouracil cream (Efudex 5%), and various interferons. In the pregnant woman, podophyllin, 5-FU, and interferon are not used. The obliteration of vulvar and vaginal lesions by various methods can be done safely during pregnancy. Additionally, cryotherapy and laser have been used, apparently safely, to treat cervical disease.

Since the risk of transmission to the neonate during vaginal delivery is unknown, sensible recommendations regarding the advisability of cesarean section to avoid it cannot be made. In cases where the lesions are large enough to obstruct delivery, cesarean section should obviously be performed.

Other sexually transmitted diseases

Trichomoniasis has been suggested, although not confirmed, as a cause of premature rupture of the membranes. More certainly it is an annoying cause of vaginitis. Diagnosed by visualization of the flagellate on wet smear examination of vaginal secretions, the usual treatment in the nonpregnant individual is metronidazole (Flagyl) orally, either 250 mg t.i.d.

for 7 days or a single dose of 2 g. Since metronidazole has been shown to be mutagenic in bacteria, it is not used during the first trimester. Indeed, many physicians avoid it entirely during pregnancy. In these cases, symptomatic relief may be obtained with careful vinegar douching. Definitive treatment is undertaken after delivery.

Public lice and **scabies** both are parisitic skin diseases whose incidence, transmission, and diagnosis are unchanged by pregnancy. Their treatment is with benzene hexachloride (Kwell) ointment, lotion, or shampoo. The use of this insecticide is controversial during pregnancy. Secondary agents such as crotamiton cream (Eurax) may be used.

Chancroid has become rare in this country. Caused by *Hemophilus ducreyi* and resulting in painful genital ulcers and lymphadenopathy, it is mostly encountered in urban areas among prostitutes and those who frequent them. Diagnosis is by culture of the organism from the lesion, and treatment during pregnancy is with erythromycin, 500 mg q.i.d. until healed.

Granuloma inguinale, caused by *Donovania granulomatis*, is rare in this country. It causes painful genital ulcers. It may be spread by autoinoculation to various sites on the body and may result in elephantiasis of the lower extremities or vulva by lymphatic obstruction. Treatment in the nonpregnant individual is tetracycline, in the gravid woman erythromycin, 500 mg q.i.d. for 2 to 3 weeks.

Lymphogranuloma venereum (LGV) is caused by a strain of *Chlamydia* and is characterized by the formation of buboes, proctitis, urethritis, and fistulae. Diagnosis is by culture of drainage. Treatment is with erythromycin, 500 mg q.i.d. until resolution. Scarring of involved areas with stricure is common and may necessitate surgical correction in unattended cases.

RUBELLA

Rubella (German measles) is a minor disease if contracted any time after birth and a potential disaster if it infects a fetus. Infection usually confers lifelong immunity. The fetus can only be infected by transplacental passage of the virus during the viremia that attends initial infection. The seriousness and likelihood of intrauterine infection vary with the stage of pregnancy. In the first month, 50% of fetuses are severely damaged; in the second, only 25%; and in the third month, 15%. Infants with congenital rubella most commonly suffer from blindness, deafness, multiple cardiac abnormalities, hepatosplenomegaly, and neurological deficits. Other systemic involvement may also occur.

There is no treatment for rubella infection. If maternal infection occurs during the first trimester, the family should be counseled regarding potential fetal sequelae. This is often followed by therapeutic abortion.

Ideally, one should identify women who are not rubella immune and vaccinate them 3 months before conception. To this end, rubella screening is part of most premarital testing. If the already pregnant woman is found to be susceptible, she must be counseled to avoid exposure during the pregnancy and should be vaccinated immediately postpartum. The vaccine poses no threat to a neonate and usually confers lasting immunity.

CYTOMEGALOVIRUS (CMV)

A virus of the herpes group, CMV is the most common cause of congenital infection in the United States. Perhaps as much as 50% of the population carries the virus, and up to 2% of all neonates are infected. Like rubella, it is usually a minor infection, most often subclinical; but like herpes simplex, lifelong carriage with potential reactivation and viral shedding is the rule. Severe forms of the disease, usually among the immunosuppressed (including fetuses and neonates) include hepatitis, pneumonia, and encephalitis. It may be transmitted orally, sexually, transplacentally, at birth, via breast-feeding, and through transfusion. The urine and oral secretions of those infected frequently contain live virus.

Diagnosis. Diagnosis is based on clinical findings supplemented by antibody identification. Most often, the disease is retrospectively diagnosed after the infant is found to be damaged.

Effects of pregnancy on disease. Pregnancy seems to favor reactivation of viral shedding and, in fact, cervical shedding progressively increases with each trimester. Clinical disease does not usually recur.

Effects of disease on pregnancy. Presumably, the fetus may be infected in the course of a viremia that occurs with primary infection or by direct transmission during birth. Some may also be exposed from breast milk. Up to 2% of all babies born in this country are infected. However, only a small percentage of these become ill, so that the incidence of congenital cytomegalic inclusion disease is probably only 1 per 1,000 live births. These babies, however, are often severely damaged. Mortality rates for symptomatic infection range up to 30%, with over 50% of the survivors being severely mentally retarded or neurologically impaired. Most of the rest suffer lesser degrees of impairment. Those who are normal at age 2, however, are likely to remain so.

Therapy. There is no therapy for CMV and not much can be done in the way of prevention. Most primary infection is undetectable at the time of its occurrence, and most cervical shedding does not result in symptomatic infection of the fetus delivered vaginally.

TOXOPLASMOSIS

Like rubella, toxoplasmosis is usually an inconsequential infection, sometimes resembling a viral syndrome, often asymptomatic. Caused by the parasite *Toxoplasma gondii*, it is contracted by eating inadequately cooked, infected beef, lamb, or pork or from the stool (hand-to-mouth) of an infected cat. Again, like rubella, infection confers lifelong immunity.

Diagnosis. The diagnosis of toxoplasmosis begins before conception. If the woman is known to have antibodies prior to pregnancy, she is not at risk for future infection. If screening has shown her to be susceptible and she develops a suspicious illness, subsequent titers determine if she has been infected. IgM will appear within 2 to 3 weeks, IgG several weeks later. If no preconception titers are available, the presence of IgM is suggestive but not diagnostic as low levels may persist for long periods of time. High levels of IgM by the ELISA method are extremely suggestive of recent infection, as are rising IgG titers at 3- to 4-week intervals.

If maternal infection is confirmed, fetal infection may be diagnosed by obtaining amniotic fluid and fetal cord blood via fetoscopy and testing it for IgM and the presence of the organism. This is usually performed between the 20th and 22nd weeks. Positive results are diagnostic; negative results may be spurious. All these pregnancies should be followed with serial ultrasonography to detect hydrocephalus.

Effects of the disease on pregnancy. The fetus is only at risk if the mother becomes infected during pregnancy, when transplacental transmission of the organism may occur. The earlier in the pregnancy the infection, the more likely is fetal damage. This may include spontaneous abortion or, in those who survive, chorioretinitis, microcephaly, hydrocephaly, intracranial calcifications, hepatosplenomegaly, anemia, and low birth weight. Not all those infants infected show clinical evidence at birth, so careful observation of the exposed neonate for several years is indicated.

Therapy. If fetal infection is confirmed, one has the options of treatment with antibiotics to limit the disease or to terminate the pregnancy. Pyrimethamine (Daraprim) in combination with a sulfonamide is effective but has been found to be teratogenic in animals.

VARICELLA

Chicken pox is a common childhood illness with few serious complications. Most adults have had the disease and are immune. For the minority who have not, however, varicella can be dangerous, especially if complicated by pneumonia, sometimes resulting in death. This is at least as true, and perhaps more so, during pregnancy. Although serology to identify susceptible individuals is not routinely done, it is available for those exposed who are not sure if they have ever had the disease.

Maternal varicella infection also poses certain risks for the fetus. Although infection during the first trimester rarely, if ever, is teratogenic and later it is even more benign, the fetus who is born within 4 days after or 2 days before the mother evidences the disease is in considerable danger. Generalized varicella with neurological damage and a high mortality rate is likely. These infants should at birth receive varicella-zoster immune globulin (VZIG), which is highly effective in preventing neonatal damage. Whether it should also be used to treat susceptible pregnant women who have been exposed is less clear.

OTHER INFECTIOUS DISEASES

Both measles and mumps are quite rare during pregnancy. They may cause abortion, premature delivery, stillbirth, and neonatal infection. Teratogenesis is unlikely. If a susceptible mother is exposed to measles, she should be treated with hyperimmune globulin. It has not been shown to be helpful for mumps.

SKIN DISEASES IN PREGNANCY

HERPES GESTATIONIS

Herpes gestationis is a rare immune complex skin disease occurring only in association with pregnancy and characterized by intense itching and an erythematous bullous rash that vaguely resembles herpes lesions. Definitive diagnosis may be made by finding characteristic immune complexes in lesional biopsies. It typically presents during the second or third trimester and resolves within several weeks postpartum. Blistering and itching require treatment with systemic corticosteroids, which are usually quite effective. It may be attended by higher rates of prematurity and perinatal mortality. The newborn will occasionally exhibit similar lesions. Recurrence with subsequent pregnancy is common.

PRURITIC URTICARIAL PAPULES OF PREGNANCY (PUPP)

An urticarial rash of unknown origin, PUPP usually occurs in the late third trimester, seems to be benign, responds well to topical corticosteroids, and resolves postpartum. Diagnosis is usually on clinical grounds but is confirmable on skin biopsy.

MELANOMA

Pregnancy seems to increase the likelihood of malignant degeneration of pigmented skin lesions, perhaps because of high melanocyte-stimulating hormone levels or altered immunity. Melanoma also has a worse prognosis during pregnancy. The most mentionable fact about this skin cancer is that it is the most common malignancy to metastasize to the placenta.

FAMILY PLANNING

The purpose of family planning is to assist individuals in achieving their reproductive goals. Family planning is population control reduced to the individual rather than to the national or global level.

Demographers report that the low reproduction rate and the inordinately high death rate of the human allowed for a stable population from the beginning of time until about the year 1850, when the first billion population was reached. Since that time, it has risen to 5 billion people.

Methodology determines how the patient's method of choice should be prescribed unless there are medical contraindications.

ABSTINENCE

Couples should be queried about their moral and ethical views concerning sexual practices. It is important to counsel them on alternate methods of sexual fulfillment other than sexual intercourse, if they are averse to using contraception. It is rare that this situation will exist, but it must be dealt with when it does.

COITUS INTERRUPTUS (WITHDRAWAL)

In coitus interruptus, the man withdraws his penis from the vagina just prior to ejaculation. This technique is widely practiced. The failure rate is approximately 15 to 25 pregnancies per 100 women years exposure in all users. Since withdrawal at the time of ejaculation is unnatural, it may diminish the sexual satisfaction of the couple.

RHYTHM METHOD (SAFE PERIOD)

At present, the rhythm method is one of two methods officially permitted for Roman Catholics. The method is based on the assumption that the ovum is capable of being fertilized for only 24 hours after its release and that the sperm can fertilize the ovum for only 72 hours after they are deposited in the vagina. If ovulation occurs between days 12 and 16 of a 28-day cycle, the potential fertile period during which intercourse should be avoided is therefore between day 9 and 17 of the cycle. The failure rate is 38 per 100 women years of use.

SHEATH (CONDOM, FRENCH LETTER)

A rubber sheath or a lamb's cecum is placed over the erect penis. It should be used with chemical spermicide for additional contraceptive security. The sheath is drawn or rolled over the penis after erection has occurred. The failure rate is 18 to 20 per 100 women years of use. The failure is due in most instances to rupture of the condom with deposition of the entire ejaculate into the vagina.

VAGINAL DIAPHRAGM (DUTCH CAP)

A rubber diaphragm smeared with spermicidal cream serves as a barrier to sperm.

The diaphragm is inserted into the vagina in such a way that it covers the cervix. The failure rate is 15 pregnancies per 100 women years of use.

CHEMICAL METHODS (AEROSOL, FOAMS, JELLIES, CREAMS, SUPPOSITORIES, SPONGE)

The spermicidal ingredient used in chemical contraceptives is usually p-triisopaprophylphenolopolyetoxy-ethinol. Nonoxynol 9 is the most commonly used spermicide. The failure rate is between 15 and 40 per 100 women years of use.

INTRAUTERINE DEVICE (IUD)

A polyethylene spiral or coil inserted into the uterine cavity effectively prevents conception, although the mode of action is not known. The failure rate is 2.3 per 100 women years of use. IUDs are currently being withdrawn from the market in the United States.

ORAL CONTRACEPTIONS

Contraceptive drugs taken by mouth permit the patient to indulge in normal coitus without the risk of conception. The efficacy of the pill in preventing pregnancy is the greatest of any form of contraception short of permanent sterilization. The failure rate is less than 1 pregnancy per 100 years of use in combination method.

NATURAL FAMILY PLANNING

Natural family planning is accepted by the Catholic Church. A woman determines if she is in her fertile period by examining the consistency of her vaginal secretions. The method has not been widely accepted, nor is it highly effective.

STERILIZATION

Female sterilization provides permanent interruption of the fallopian tube. Vasectomy is the only popular method of male sterilization.

THE MORNING-AFTER PILL

It has been estimated that approximately 60% of first sexual experiences among young, unmarried women on university campuses are unprotected, whereas 40% of subsequent intercourse is insufficiency protected. The need for some form of postcoital contraception clearly exists. This is provided by giving diethylstilbestrol (15 mg), ethinyl estradiol (5 mg) or a conjugated estrogen (30 mg). This combination will effectively prevent pregnancy if given within 72 hours of unprotected midcycle ovulatory exposure and continued for 5 days.

METHODS UNDER INVESTIGATION

Synthetic analogues of Gn-RH are being investigated for use as contraceptives. If these are given continuously, rather than impulsively, they become fixed to pituitary receptors and block the action of Gn-RH so that the output of gonadotropin falls and ovulation ceases.

Immunization against pregnancy has also reached the stage of clinical trial. It depends on immunization against the beta subunit of chorionic gonadotropin and might provide a simple and long-acting method of contraception.

Gossypol is being investigated by the Chinese to serve as a male contraceptive.

GYNECOLOGIC ENDOCRINOLOGY

The gynecologic patient can exhibit any endocrinopathy found in either men or women. However, the female patient possesses an unique, overtly responsive mechanism that readily informs the physician of the possible presence of an endocrine disorder, that is, alteration of the regular menstrual pattern.

ABNORMAL PATTERNS OF MENSTRUATION

Amenorrhea is absence of menses; in primary amenorrhea, menstruation has never occurred; in secondary amenorrhea menstruation has occurred but has stopped.

Oligomenorrhea refers to less frequent menstruation occurring at intervals longer than 5 to 6 weeks.

Polymenorrhea refers to more frequent menstruation occurring at intervals of less than 3 weeks.

Hypomenorrhea is menses at regular intervals (approximately every 28 days) but with significantly reduced amounts of flow; the number of days of flow is of the same duration or less than the patient's usual menses.

Hypermenorrhea is regular menses of approximately 28-day intervals that has the usual 4 to 6 days that are excessive in amount.

Menorrhagia is menses that may come at regular intervals but the bleeding is either profuse, excessive in duration (8 days or more), or both.

Metrorrhagia is unexpected bleeding between menstrual periods. If prolonged, it may manifest itself as totally irregular menses.

Normal menstrual function requires an intact pituitary-ovarian-uterine axis, which in turn may be influenced by the thyroid, adrenals, and hypothalamus.

FEEDBACK CONTROL

Reproductive function is controlled by steroids from the gonads. These are produced by specific cells in the ovary and testes which respond to pituitary gonadotropin, LH, and FSH. As with many other hormones, sex steroids inhibit secretion of their trophic hormones (negative feedback). Under a specific set of circumstances, estrogen may stimulate secretion of gonadotropins (positive feedback).

Receptors are now identified. Hormones exert their effect on target cells by combining with receptors on the cell surface (protein hormones) or in the cell cytoplasm (steroids and thyronines) or nucleus (steroids). The biologic activity is maintained only for as long as the receptor is occupied by the hormone. Thus steroids such as estrogen, whose receptors have long half-lives, are present in lower concentrations than others, such as progesterone and cortisol, whose receptors have short half-lives.

Second-messenger systems demonstrate that there are larger protein hormones, such as the trophic hormones, that cannot enter the cell. They combine with a specific surface receptor that activates adenylcyclase and their cell membrane. This catalyzes production of a second-messenger cyclic adenosine 3,5 monophosphate (cyclic AMP), from ATP. Excessive buildup of these substances is prevented by another enzyme, phosphodiesterase. Cyclic AMP activates protein kinases that cause phospholation, and thereby activation of specific enzymes.

There is also the biosynthesis of protein and peptide hormones and protein binding of hormones.

Current research has demonstrated the clinical roles that Gn-RH and prolactin play in the orderly functioning of the female reproductive tract.

Gn-RH, sometimes described as LHRH, is a peptide that is degraded if taken by mouth but is active by injection or a nasal spray. Gn-RH is a decapeptide hormone, produced in the arcuate nucleus region of the hypothalamus. Pulse release of Gn-RH by the hypothalamus (1 pulse per 1 to 2 hours) permits anterior pituitary production and release of FSH and LH (normal). However, continuous, excessive, absent or more frequent Gn-RH release inhibits FSH and LH production and release (down-loading). Decreased pulse release of Gn-RH decreases LH secretion but increases FSH secretion (slow-pulsing model).

The ovarian feedback modulation of pituitary gonadotropin production and releases produce negative and positive feedback. The presence of pulse Gn-RH and low estrogen and progesterone levels results in increased levels of pulse LH and FSH (negative feedback). The presence of pulse Gn-RH, rapidly increasing levels of estrogen, and small amounts of progesterone, results in high-pulse LH and moderately increased FSH levels (positive feedback). The presence of pulse Gn-Rh and high levels of estrogen and progesterone results in decreases of LH and FSH levels (negative feedback). Therefore, it is evident that the pulsatile release of the proper amount of Gn-RH controls the function of the anterior pituitary.

PROLACTIN

The anterior pituitary hormone is responsible for the initiation and maintenance of lactation after the breasts have been under the previous influence of estrogen and progesterone. A polypeptide is secreted in a pulsatile manner by specialized anterior pituitary cells (lactotropes). Unlike the release of other anterior pituitary hormones, that of prolactin is inhibited, not stimulated, by a hypothalamic factor, dopamine. During lactation, prolactin levels rise after stimulation of the nipple, when dopamine levels fall.

Prolactin may be involved in the control of ovulation and may be an agent that prevents further ovulation once fertilization of the oocyte has occurred. When prolactin levels are raised, ovulation ceases. Hypoprolactinemia may occur with pituitary adenoma.

THE POSTERIOR PITUITARY

The posterior pituitary (neurohypophysis) is a neurosecretory gland. The cell bodies lie in the hypothalamus, and the axon terminals make up the stalk and the gland itself. The axon terminals are closely associated with capillaries as a neurohemal origin. The hormones are the nine peptides (nine amino acids), oxytocin, and vasopressin.

Oxytocin has two main actions: (1) stimulation of the uterus and (2) stimulation of the myoepithelial cells of the breast that cause milk ejection. In human pregnancy, maternal oxytocin is released in spurts during the active and expulsive phases of labor, probably as the result of a neural reflex originating in the cervix and the lower genital tract (Ferguson's reflex). Oxytocin is also released by the fetal pituitary during labor. The maternal circulation contains a placental enzyme, oxytocinase, which can split oxytocin, though this action is not thought to be of any physiological significance. During suckling there is a spurt release of oxytocin as a result of a reflex from nerve endings in the nipple. Oxytocin is found in high concentrations in the human corpus luteum and may be involved in luteal lysis.

ESTROGEN

Estrogens are secreted by the granulosa-theca cells of the ovarian follicle and subsequently by the same cells after they have been luteinized to form the corpus luteum. Estrogens are also secreted in smaller quantities by the suprarenal cortex. The ovaries produce 17_β-estradiol from cholesterol and progesterone. Estradiol undergoes degradation chiefly to estrone and estriol. In clinical practice, only these three classic estrogens are usually considered, although at least 16 other estrogens are found in small quantities in human urine.

The second secondary characteristics are greatly influenced by estrogen. Hypertrophy of the breasts, the appearance of pubic and axillary hair, secretion of apocrine glands, changes in the voice and appearance of the face and figure, with the disposition of fat on the hips and thighs are examples of secondary sex characteristics. Estrogen controls the monthly proliferative phase of the endometrium. The motility of the

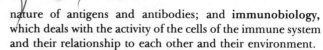

fallopian tubes is increased by estrogen. The cervical glands respond to circulating estrogen by secreting an abundance of clear alkaline mucus, which protects spermatozoa from vaginal acidity, and estrogen causes proliferation of the epithelial cells of the vagina. Estrogens bring about proliferation of the duct system in the breast.

PROGESTERONE

Progesterone is the hormone secreted (together with estradiol) by the corpus luteum. It is responsible for the luteal phase of the menstrual cycle. Progesterone is converted in the liver to pregnanediol and other metabolites, which are excreted in the bile and in the urine.

The physiologic action on the endometrium occurs during the luteal phase of the endometrial cycle. The action of progesterone will only occur if the endometrium has previously been primed by the action of estrogens. The part played by progesterone in bringing about menstruation is not certain. The blood concentration of progesterone in a normal cycle falls at the same time as that of estrogen, but some women bleed regularly each month in a way clinically indistinguishable from normal menstruation, without ever ovulating, forming a corpus luteum, or secreting any progesterone. However, in such anovular cycles the degree of endometrial disintegration may be less than in normal cycles. Progesterone causes growth of the alveolar tissue of the breast, provided that there has been previous estrogen stimulation.

ANDROGENS

Androgens are metabolic precursors of estrogen, and they are found in small amounts in the blood and urine of normal women. They are secreted by the suprarenal cortex and in the stromal cells of the ovary. The part they play in normal female physiology is probably slight, although they may have some effect on libido. In cases of estrogen deficiency, acne and oily skin may be manifestations of androgenic activity.

Adrenal virilism, or the adrenogenital syndrome, may be caused in adults by hyperplasia or a tumor of the suprarenal cortex, when the 17-oxosteroid excretion in the urine is increased. In the fetus and child, adrenal pseudohermaphroditism may occur because of a metabolic disorder of the cortex.

Testosterone is secreted by a rare ovarian tumor, androblastoma, and testosterone levels are increased in polycystic ovary syndrome.

BASIC AND CLINICAL IMMUNOLOGY

Immunology is a relatively new discipline of medicine and has been described as the study of resistance to infection. Immunity has been recognized for centuries, and it has now taken on an expanded role and is the property by which the lymphoreticular system makes a memorized response to an antigenic stimulus. This may result in a state of positive reaction kown as sensitization or a negative reaction known as immunologic tolerance, enhancement, or immunosuppression.

As a scientific discipline, immunology encompasses immunity, dealing with the adoptive response to infective agents; immunochemistry, concerned with the chemical nature of antigens and antibodies; and immunobiology, which deals with the activity of the cells of the immune system and their relationship to each other and their environment.

Antigens are any molecules that are recognized by the immune system and induce an immune reaction. An immunogen is an antigen that elicits a strong immune response, particularly in the context of protective immunity to pathogenic organisms.

Antibodies are a class of serum proteins that are induced following contact with antigen. They bind specifically to the antigen that induces their formation.

Immunoglobulin (Ig) is a synonym for antibody. Most antibodies are weakly charged, have neutral pH, and are found in the gamma-globulin fraction of serum.

T cells are lymphocytes that develop in the thymus. This organ is seeded during embryonic development by lymphocyte stem cells from the bone marrow. Immature T cells occupy the thymic cortex, while more mature cells are seen in the medulla. There is considerable T-cell proliferation and cell death within the thymus, such that the majority of developing T cells die before leaving this organ. T cells acquire their antigen receptors in the thymus and differentiate into a number of subpopulations, which have separate functions that can be recognized by their direct cell surface molecules (markers). These subpopulations include the T helper cells, T inducer cells, T delayed hypersensitivity cells, T cytotoxic cells, T suppressor cells, and the memory cells.

In addition, there are K (killer) cells, or monocytes that can kill target cells sensitized with antibody, which they bind via their Fc receptors; the majority are L cells. NK (natural killer) cells are capable of killing a number of virally infected and transformed target cells to which they have not been previously sensitized. They have not been separated from K cells, although K-cell activity and NK activity develop independently.

B cells are lymphocytes that develop in fetal liver and subsequently in bone marrow. Birds have a specialized organ, the bursa of Fabricius, in which B cells develop. Mature B cells carry surface immunoglobulins, which act as an antigen receptor. They then move through the circulation to secondary lymphoid tissues, where they respond to antigenic stimulation by dividing and differentiating into plasma cells under control of lymphokines released by T cells.

IMMUNE REFLEX ARC

The immune response is divided into three phases. The first begins with the administration of antigen and ends when the antigen encounters antigen-reactive lymphocytes; this phase is termed the afferent limb. The afferent is the means by which the stimulus (the antigen) is delivered to the central processing mechanism (the lymph nodes), which in turn manufactures the effectors of the immune response (antibodies and specifically sensitized cells). The dissemination of the effectors throughout the body compromises the efferent limb of the immune system.

MACROPHAGES

Macrophages are large phagocytic cells found in most tissues; they also line the serous cavities in the lung. They are

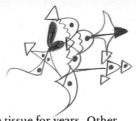

long-lived cells and may remain in the tissue for years. Other macrophages recirculate through the secondary lymphoid organs, spleen, and lymph nodes, where they may function as antigen-presenting cells. The macrophage is the basis for the development of an immune response. In the blood, the macrophage is called a **monocyte**; in connective tissue, a **histiocyte**; and in spleen, lymph nodes, and thymus, a sinus-lining macrophage or a **reticulocyte**. The macrophage is widely distributed.

HUMORAL AND CELL-MEDIATED IMMUNE RESPONSES

The immune response takes two forms. A humoral response results from transformed lymphoblasts being converted to a plasma cell. It is a cell-free fluid containing antibodies that are circulating freely in the bloodstream as well as in other body fluids. Also, a cell-mediated immunity is carried out by sensitized lymphocytes.

Humoral response

The humoral response (B-cell) is mediated by immunoglobulins. It is cell free and is made up of immunoglobulins IgG, IgM, IgA, IgD, and IgE. To have a killing or cytotoxic effect, the cell-free antibody must always have a third substance, **complement,** present. The humoral response offers a defense against most bacteria and some foreign proteins. Bacterial vaccines inoculated into the organism result in the production of antibodies (immunoglobulins).

Cell-mediated response

The cell-mediated response (T-cell) is mediated by sensitized lymphocytes. In the cell-mediated immune (CMI) response, the antibody remains an integral part of the cells that produce it and is a cell-associated antibody. The sensitized lymphocytes carrying such antibody are carried in the lymph to the tumor cells, where their antibody combines with the antigen determinant on the surface of the tumor cell. The cell-bound antibody then becomes capable of rupturing and killing tumor cells. It also produces potent mediators of cell immunity, including transfer factor, lymphocyte transforming activity, lymphocyte blastogenic factor, migration inhibition factor, lymphotoxin, and interferon. The cell-mediated response is particularly important in graft rejection, eliminating viruses as well as intracellular bacteria and cancer cells.

COMPLEMENT

Complement is one of the serum enzyme systems. Its functions include mediating information, opsonization of antigenic particles (including microorganisms), and causing membrane damage to pathogens. The system consists of 19 separate proteins, which may be activated either via classic or alternative pathways. Molecules of the classic pathway are designated C1, C2, etc. Alternative pathway molecules have letter designations—for example, factor B (or Fb, or just B), factor D, etc. The physical chemical properties and functions of the complement components include an enzyme cascade, which is the classic pathway, and the alternative pathway (properdin pathway or amplification loop). Complement is necessary for the B cell to damage or kill a target cell.

AUTOIMMUNITY

Autoimmunity is the reaction of the immune system against the body's own tissue. Autoimmunity may arise whenever there exists a state of immunologic imbalance, in which B-cell activity is excessive and suppresor T-cell activity is diminished. This imbalance occurs as a consequence of genetic, viral, and environmental mechanisms acting singly or in combination. A central mechanism in this concept involves a disturbance of the delicate balance between suppressor and helper activity of regular T cells. Either an excess of helper T-cell activity or a deficiency of suppressor T-cell activity can lead to the development of autoimmunity. The mechanism by which such a balance may be upset may involve both viral factors and abnormal production of thymic hormones.

Burnet proposed the theory of **forbidden clones** to explain the way the body is normally tolerant to its own tissue. He believed that autoreactive cells were effectively forbidden and so were clonally deleted during embryologic development. It is now known that autoreactive B cells are present, but they are not normally active.

Autoimmune diseases occur when autoimmune reactions result in pathological tissue damage. In general, they are either organ specific or organ nonspecific.

IMMUNODEFICIENCY

Immunodeficiency is often identified by the increased frequency of infection in patients. Impaired immunity is a consequence of many pathogenic infections, but primary immunodeficiency is inherited and may affect any part of the immune system, including complement components, granulocytes, macrophages, and lymphocytes.

Deficiency of cell-mediated immunity (T-cell)

In the DiGeorge's syndrome, there is dysplasia or hypoplasia of the thymus and often absence of the parathyroid glands. These patients have no resistance to virus or to other agents that are controlled by CMI, such as tuberculosis, brucellosis, leprosy, fungal infections, and parasitic diseases. They do not have the capacity to develop a delayed hypersensitivity reaction or to reject grafts or foreign tissue. They can produce circulating antibodies and have the ability to respond to bacterial vaccines by developing circulating antibodies (immunoglobulins). T-cell numbers usually rise to normal levels over a 1- to 2-year period.

Deficiency of humoral immunity (B cell)

Patients with B-cell deficiency have normal T-cell function and CMI to viral infections but have very low immunoglobulin levels and cannot make antibody responses. They are particularly susceptible to bacterial infections. The disease was described by Colonel Bruton and is called Bruton's disease.

Combined deficiency of T and B cells

In Swiss-type agammaglobulinemia, which is an X-linked disease of male children, both cell-mediated and humoral mechanisms are deficient. There is a block of the stem cell mechanism. Afflicted children cannot make humoral antibodies (immunoblobulins) or develop CMI reaction. They suffer from progressive bacterial and/or viral infections and die within the first 2 years of life. Some highly selected patients have been treated with bone marrow that has been matched for major histocompatibility antigens. The preliminary work has been promising, and some success has been reported. More than 30 phenotype patterns of immunodeficiency have currently been recognized in human beings.

HYPERSENSITIVITY

Hypersensitivity is a state of the previously immunized (to alter the activity of a host to an antigen by exposing it to that antigen in such a way that produces an immune response) host that results in tissue damage from an immune reaction to a further dose of antigen. It may be antibody or humoral mediated, as in immediate hypersensitivity, or it may be a reaction of CMI, as in delayed hypersensitivity. The term hypersensitivity implies a heightened reactivity to an antigen, but it is difficult to define all hypersensitivity reactions, particularly cell-mediated reactions, in such terms.

Hypersensitivity describes an immune response that occurs in an exaggerated or inappropriate form. These reactions have been classified into four types by Gell and Coombs, according to the speed of the reaction and the immune mechanisms involved. Although they are classified separately, in practice they do not necessarily occur in isolation from each other. Furthermore, several different immune reactions may be found in the single type.

They are now listed under five types, described below:

Type 1 (immediate hypersensitivity), which is manifested in allergic asthma, hay fever, and eczema, develops within minutes of exposure. It is dependent on the activation of mast or basophilic cells and the release of mediators of acute inflammation.

Type 2 (antibody-mediated) hypersensitivity is caused by antibody to cell surface antigens. These can sensitize the cells for antibody-dependent cell-mediated cytotoxicity by K cells or complement-mediated lysis. Type 2 hypersensitivity is encountered in the destruction of red blood cells and transfusion reactions and in hemolytic disease of the newborn.

Type 3 (immune complex mediated) hypersensitivity is due to the disposition of antigen/antibody complexes in tissue and blood vessels. These activate complement and attract polymorphonuclear leukocytes to the site, causing local damage.

Type 4 (delayed) hypersensitivity arises more than 24 hours after encounter with an antigen and is mediated by antigen-sensitized T cells that release lymphokines, attracting macrophages to the site and activating them. This type of hypersensitivity occurs in skin contact reactions and in the response to some chronic pathogens such as *Mycobacterium tuberculosis* and *Schistosoma* sp.

Type 5 (stimulatory) hypersensitivity describes the reactions in which autoantibodies stimulate host tissue, such as the stimulation of thyroid by autoantibody binding to the thyroid-stimulating hormone (TSH) receptor, thus mimicking TSH.

HISTOCOMPATIBILITY LOCI

The major histocompatibility complex and/or system (MHC/MHS) is a cluster of genes important in immune recognition and signaling between cells of the immune system. The gene complex was originally identified as a locus in coding molecules present on cell surfaces, such that animals that differed at this locus would rapidly reject each other's tissue grafts. All mammals have a MHC. H2 is the mouse MHC, and HLA is the human MHC.

Also known as the human leukocyte antigen (HLA) system, the MHC is a group of genes located on the short arm of chromosome 6. These genes code for a surface antigen on many kinds of cells. They are critical to recognition of self versus nonself, since the MHC defines what is self. Thus, HLA antigens are important in tissue crossmatching procedures and are partially responsible for tissue transplant rejection, which occurs when donor MHC and recipient MHC do not match. They also have been associated with more than 60 diseases, such as ankylosing spondylitis, insulin-dependent diabetes, nontropical sprue (celiac disease), and rheumatoid arthritis.

The MHC genes occupy five recognized positions (loci) on chromosome 6: HLA-A, HLA-B, HLA-C, HLA-D, and HLA-DR (HLA-D-related).

GRAFT-VERSUS-HOST DISEASE

In graft-versus-host disease, immunocompetent donor cells (e.g., from a bone marrow graft) recognize and react against the recipient's tissues, either because the recipient is immunosuppressed or cannot recognize the allogenic cells. Sensitized donor T helper cells can recruit the recipient's macrophages to organs to cause pathological damage. The skin, gut, epithelium, and liver are most frequently affected.

BIOLOGIC RESPONSE MODIFIERS

The body's inherent biochemical capacity for killing cancer cells plus the new genetic technology gives biologic response modification, or biomodulation for short. Biologic response modification is the new wave in cancer treatment.

The use of biologics and biologic response modifiers in the treatment of cancers is new. Biologics may be defined as any product of the mammalian organism, and biologic response modifiers are those agents and approaches that alter biologic responses in the tumor-host interaction. The field encompasses traditional immunotherapy but also encompasses the use of molecular biology, recombinant genetics, and hybridoma technology, all of which produce highly purified biologic substances with anticancer activity. The recognition of growth, differentiation, and maturation factors, as well as the possibility of making antagonists or competitive inhibitors to factors that support neoplastic growth, provides an additional biologic approach in this area.

Genetic engineering has brought about a revolution in the field of biology. It will continue to be the front and center of research. Genes will be implanted into bacteria, resulting in the production of any desired protein or enzyme in large quantities. Medicine has already reaped many rewards from recombinant techniques that manufacture proteins in quantity by moving human genes into microorganisms. These genes can program the production of commercial quantities of human insulin, interferon, and human growth factor, as well as genetically engineered vaccines. It is possible that cancers of the reproductive tract will be controlled by the turn of the century. DNA probes and recombitant DNA experiments will change obstetrics and gynecology as they are known today. The biologic response modifiers include interferon, tumor necrosis factors, lymphotoxin, and monoclonal antibodies.

PATHOLOGICAL CONDITIONS

SEXUALLY TRANSMITTED DISEASES

The list of STDs is long, and the number is increasing. These diseases include, in rough order of frequency of occurrence, chlamydial infections, gonorrhea, trichomoniasis, herpes, syphilis, chancroid, lymphogranuloma venereum, and granuloma inguinale. Other diseases that are sometimes transmitted by sexual contact are now included, including candidiasis, genital warts, hepatitis, AIDS, pediculosis, scabies, and molluscum contagiosum.

These diseases have very important public health implications. It will often be best to refer a patient suspected of having a STD to a special department of GU medicine that has a full range of facilities for laboratory investigation. Social workers help in follow-up contacts.

Chlyamydial infections

During the past decade, as the result of availability of specific culture techniques, the obligatory intracellular parasite *Chlamydia trachomatis* has been shown to be a common sexually transmitted pathogen and the cuase of many genital tract infections. In males, it is the causative agent of many cases of epididymitis and at least one-third of the cases of nongonococcal urethritis. In fact, in developed countries, urethritis due to this organism appears to be the most common STD.

The most common manifestations of chlamydial infection in women are mucopurulent cervicitis and salpingitis. The endocervix is the most frequent site of infection, which results in the hypertrophic appearance of the cervix and a mucopurulent discharge. Chlamydial infections appear to be common in women with cervical activity; since oral contraceptives produce ectopia, this may account for the association between oral contraceptives and *C. trachomatis*. The second principal chlamydial infection is salpingitis. A less common manifestation is the acute urethral syndrome. In addition to these infections, chlamydiae are also associated with the Fitz-Hugh–Curtis syndrome, postpartum endometritis, and infertility. Tetracycline and doxycycline are the antibiotics most commonly used to treat chlamydia.

Syphilis

Syphilis is now far less common than nonspecific infections, gonorrheal and herpesviruses, but it may accompany any of them. It has a double importance: First, if it is untreated, it can cause serious lesions of the heart and blood vessels, the nervous system, the eyes, and the bones; second, during pregnancy it may cause fetal death or the birth of an infected child. The Veneral Disease Research Laboratory (**VDRL**) test is a nonspecific flocculation test for antibody (reagin). Transient false reactions may occur after some viral infections, after immunization against typhoid and yellow fever, and in some autoimmune diseases. Specific tests for treponemata include the fluorescent treponemal antibody-absorption test (FTA-ABS) and the *Treponema pallidum* hemagglutination test. These tests may remain positive for many years, even after the disease has been effectively treated. The best combination of screening tests is the VDRL test and the hemagglutination test.

Treatment is with penicillin, but tetracycline or erythromycin can be substituted if the patient is allergic to penicillin.

Gonorrhea

Gonorrhea is caused by infection with *Neisseria gonorrhoeae*. The gram-negative organisms are kidney shaped and are seen under the microscope in pairs with their long axes parallel; they are often intracellular. Culture is not easy, and the inoculate must be incubated immediately.

Since 1975, the number of reported cases of gonorrhea has remained at about one million cases reported annually.

In 1976, penicillinase-producing gonorrhea (PPNG) was first recognized. The resistance of PPNG strains to penicillin is based on the acquisition of a resistant plasma factor that directs the gonococcus to produce penicillinase, an enzyme that destroys penicillin. In 1983, the first U.S. outbreak of penicillin-resistant gonorrhea that did not produce penicillinase was reported; this resistance is presumably chromosomally mediated.

Gonorrhea can remain localized or can ascend to the upper genital tract (salpingitis or pelvic inflammatory disease) or spread through the circulation (systemic gonococcal infection). Treatment of gonorrhea in adult women is with a single dose of ampicillin, 2 g with oral probeiecid, 1 g. If the patient is allergic to the penicillin group of drugs, a single dose of spectinomycin, 2 g, is given by IM injection. Bacterial tests should be repeated after 7 days.

Herpes genitalis

There are two types of herpes simplex virus. Herpes simplex virus type 1 (HSV-1) causes herpes labialis. Herpes simplex virus type 2 (HSV-2) is the usual cause of herpes genitalis, although HSV-1 causes occasional cases through orogenital contact. The virus invades cells, which it disrupts and in which it reproduces.

Primary infections tend to be longer and more severe than recurrent infections. Involvement of multiple anatomic sites is common, with both local and systemic symptoms. Patients who seek attention usually have numerous vesicular or ulcerated lesions that can be very painful. Fever, malaise, myalgia, and photophobia occur in about 40% of the patients. The symptoms in primary genital herpes last about 2 weeks, and healing requires another 1 to 2 weeks; thus the entire episode lasts about 4 weeks. Complications of viral meningitis and encephalitis have been reported.

Treatment with saline baths may relieve the local symptoms. Application of iodoxuridine, 40% solution, and dimethyl sulfoxide is expensive and probably useless. Acyclovir, which inhibits the intracellular synthesis of DNA by the virus, has recently been found to reduce the severity of the attack during the time when the virus is shed, but unfortunately it does not prevent recurrence.

Chancroid (soft chancre)

Chancroid is primarily a venereal infection caused by gram-negative bacillus *Hemophilus ducreyi* (Ducrey's bacillus).

The ulceration is irregular and the base is granulomatous and purulent. There is little or no surrounding induration, but there are erythema and edema, especially if the lesion is in the labia majora. Pain is a common symptom, and the inguinal nodes may enlarge and may separate.

The diagnosis is confirmed by the recovery of *H. ducreyi* from the lesions or from the aspirates of the nodes.

Management is with sulfisoxazole, 4 g initially, followed by 1 g, which may be given 4 times a day for 10 days or longer. Tetracyline may be used, and resistant cases may require kanamycin.

Granuloma inguinale

Granuloma inguinale is a chronic granulomatous and ulcerative lesion that is caused by *Calymmatobacterium granulomatis* and is probably venereal in origin. It is usually first seen as a papular lesion in the region of the small labia. It is primarily a nodule that ulcerates and joins with other papules that ulcerate, forming a large raw area with rolled edges. The disease progresses by fibrous healing, so scarring and ulceration are present together.

The diagnosis is established by demonstrating the presence of Donovan bodies in biopsy specimens. Donovan bodies will appear as red or purple rods within polymorphonucleocytes when stained with Giemsa reagents.

Administration of tetracycline usually cures the lesion, but gentamicin is occasionally required.

Lympogranuloma venereum

Lymphogranuloma venereum is a veneral disease acquired by direct sexual contact. The causative virus is related to *C. trachomatis*. The pathology involves primarily the inguinal, genital, and anorectal regions.

The diagnosis is by Frei intradermal test. The test is negative until several weeks after infection and, once positive, remains so for life.

Tetracyline and sulfisoxazole are the treatment of choice.

Vaginal trichomonas

Trichomoniasis may be expressed as an infection of the vagina, vulva, less commonly the urethra, and rarely the endocervix. Patients usually have a bubbly, greenish-yellow discharge. Speculum examination shows an associated vaginal and cervical mucosa hyperemia. Not infrequently, hemorrhagic stippling of the posterior vaginal fornix and cervix occurs, resulting in the strawberry cervix.

Microscopic examination is of a fresh, wet preparation of vaginal discharge in normal saline for evidence of actively motile flagellate protozoa. Flotility is necessary for examination on microscopic examination.

Metronidazole is the drug of choice. Treatment should also be prescribed for the patient's male sexual partners, although the majority are asymptomatic.

Candidiasis (monilial infection)

Candidiasis or monilial infection, either acute or subacute, is caused by the yeast-like fungus *Candida albicans* or by other species of *Candida*.

The symptoms are those of pruritus vulvae and leukorrhea.

Speculum examination typically reveals a thick, white, patchy or cheesy vaginal discharge, and the vagina and vulva vary from a normal appearance to a state of acute inflammation.

Miconazole cream is the management that is usually chosen.

Condylomata acuminata (venereal warts)

Condylomata are the visible manifestation of a viral venereal disease (venereal warts). These are the common form of vulva papilloma but are granulomatous rather than true neoplasias. The human papillomavirus is the infecting agent.

Biopsy should be performed. Concominant vulvar cancer may be present and has to be ruled out.

Small, isolated condylomata can be treated with 20% podphyllin and tincture of benzoin. Trichloroacetic acid can also be used. Isolated condylomata can also be treated by cryocautery. The carbon dioxide laser is even more effective in removing the lesions.

Gardnerella infections

The diagnosis of *Gardnerella* infection is based on the presence of a pH of 4.5, fishy amine odor with the addition of potassium hydroxide, and clue cells. Microscopic examination after Gram staining reveals a predominance of vaginal epithelial cells and an almost complete absence of polymorphonuclear leukocytes.

Ampicillin, 500 mg PO 4 times a day for 7 to 10 days, usually cures the condition. Appropriate tests for gonorrhea and syphilis should precede this treatment regimen so as not to overlook a concomitant infection.

Mycoplasma

Mycoplasma hominus and *Ureaplasma urealyticum* have been associated with nongonococcal urethritis, acute salpingitis, repeat abortion, prematurity, and postpartum endometritis.

All of the *Mycoplasma* strains are sensitive to tetracycline and resistant to penicillin and other antimicrobial agents that act on the cell wall.

Acquired immunodeficiency syndrome (AIDS)

AIDS is a disease in which natural immunity is defective, helper T cells are deficient, and victims are vulnerable to serious opportunistic infections. It is uniformly lethal.

AIDS has reached epidemic proportions and is causing panic among the public. Currently available commercial assays for antibody to HIV are reasonably accurate, with high positive and negative predictive values in populations or in individuals at increased risk of HIV infections.

There currently is no treatment, and only education and preventive measures will control the spread of this monstrous disease.

BREAST DISEASES   10% of women

One out of every 10 women will develop cancer of the breast sometime in her life. In 1988, there will be 130,000 new breast cancers in women and 41,000 deaths. Among women in the United States who are 25 to 74 years of age, breast cancer is the leading cause of cancer mortality. It is the leading cause of death from all causes in women 39 to 44 years of age.

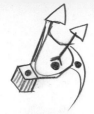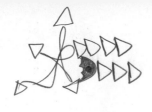

Cancer of the breast usually occurs on the left side and outer quadrants, in women without children, and in women who have not breast-fed. It is often bilateral and is successive in 4% or more of cases. Two first-degree blood relatives who had breast cancer constitute a familial history, constituting a fivefold increase.

Patients at high risk include women over 40 years of age, those with family histories of breast cancer, nulliparous women or those with first parity after age 34, those with previous histories of cancer in one breast, those with precancer masto-pathic fibrocystic changes, those with adverse hormonal milieu, those with lower immunologic competence, patients with excessive breast exposure to ionizing radiation, those exposed to carcinogens, those with endometrial or ovarian cancer, women with a high fat intake, patients with chronic psychological stress, those living in the Western Hemisphere, those in the upper socioeconomic groups, and Causasians.

Radiographic studies of the breast are advised on a yearly basis for all patients who are over 50 years of age, who have symptomatic breasts that are difficult to diagnose clinically, who have an abnormal thermogram, who have predisposing factors relating to increased risk of breast cancer, who required surgery for a breast lump (except when the patient is under age 25), who have had cyst aspiration, who have multinodular breasts, who have large pendulous breasts, who have areas of thickening without a true mass, who have breasts with thin scar formation caused by previous biopsies or trauma, and who are in the higher risk group for breast cancer.

Staging (clinical observations)

Stage I: Breast mass localized; all nodes negative.
Stage II: Breast mass localized; axilla positive.
Stage III: Breast mass locally extensive; axilla, supraclavi-cular, and internal mammary nodes positive.
Stage IV: Distant metastases.

The International Union Against Cancer (IUAC) and the American Joint Committee for Cancer Staging (AJCCS) have provided a classification based on tumor site, nodal stations, and metastatic sites (TNM classification) for cancer of the breast.

Differential diagnosis and characteristic symptom complexes

Fibrocystic changes

1. Symptoms are commonly bilateral and multiple.
2. Characterized by dull, heavy pain; sense of fullness and tenderness.
3. Changes with menses are common.
4. Tenderness is common.
5. Axillary nodes should be normal.
6. There is no venous engorgement.
7. Occurs in women between 20 and 50 years of age.

The term **fibrocystic changes** is more accurate than **fibrocystic disease,** although the latter term may be used by the third-party insurance companies to deny patients coverage for inclusion in their insurance plan.

Fibroadenoma

1. Lesions are very mobile, solid, firm, and well delineated.
2. Fibroadenoma is the classic rubbery, slippery mass.
3. Lesions are multiple and bilateral in about 14 to 25% of patients.
4. A fibroadenoma grows slowly and does not change with menses.
5. Women between the ages of 15 are 40 years are commonly afflicted.

Cystosarcoma phylloides

1. Cystosarcoma phylloides is a rare variant of fibroadenoma.
2. It may cause massive enlargement of the breast.
3. The skin is seldom involved, and the axillae are usually clear.
4. Venous engorgement and skin inflammation may be present.

Galactocele

1. Galactocele typically occurs following lactation.
2. It is usually found beneath the areola.
3. It is occasionally tender.
4. A milky discharge is sometimes found.

Cysts of the Montgomery's glands

1. This is essentially a sebaceous cyst involving para-areolar glands, and it presents under the areola. It is usually very small.
2. It may be fixed to the skin but not the chest wall.

Fat necrosis

1. Fat necrosis usually results from trauma.
2. Skin dimpling and a firm, indistinct mass are characteristic.
3. It may be very difficult to differentiate from cancer.
4. The lesion is occasionally tender.

Mondor's disease

1. Mondor's disease is caused by superficial thrombosis of veins overlying the breast and may produce skin dimpling.
2. Typically, tenderness is present in early cases.
3. The lesion is self-limited and disappears with time.

Intraductal papilloma

1. Intraductal pappiloma presents with a serious (yellow), serosanguineous (pink), sanguineous (bloody), or watery type of discharge.
2. Usually no lump can be palpated.

Mammary duct ectasia (comedo mastitis)

1. Mammary duct ectasia is usually subareolar.
2. It commonly manifests with nipple discharge.
3. The discharge is usually multicolored and sticky, bilateral, and from multiple ducts.
4. The patient may experience a burning, itching, or dull, pulling type of pain around the nipple and areola, and there may be palpable, tortuous, tubercular swelling under the areola.
5. Nipple retraction, skin retraction and a diffuse mass may be present.

6. There may be edema and axillary adenopathy.

7. It may be very difficult to differentiate from cancer.

Treatment

Unless the diagnosis is obvious or there is regression of the lesion within a short period of time, a biopsy is indicated and appropriate therapy is selected. If any malignancy is found, tissue should be sent for estrogen and progesterone receptor assays.

There has recently been a trend to scale down the surgical procedure, and if a radical mastectomy is indicated, it is usually a modified radical mastectomy in which the underlying muscles are left intact. There is a great trend for limited procedures, and these have received a variety of names, including lumpectomy, local excision, partial mastectomy, and tylectomy (comparable to lumpectomy). In each instance, the tumor is surgically removed along with a varying amount of surrounding tissue. The patients are then given radiation therapy and/or chemotherapy as indicated.

Conclusions on management

Adjuvant chemotherapy and hormonal therapy are effective treatments for breast cancer patients. Although significant advances have been made in the past 5 years, optimal therapy has not been defined for any subset of patients. For this reason, all patients and their physicians are strongly encouraged to participate in controlled clinical trials.

Outside the context of a clinical trial and based on the research data presented at the 1985 Consensus Development Conference, the following statements can be made:

1. For premenopausal women with positive lymph nodes, regardless of hormone receptor status, treatment with established combination chemotherapy should become standard care.

2. For premenopausal patients with negative nodes, adjuvant therapy is not generally recommended, but for certain high-risk patients in this group, adjuvant chemotherapy should be considered.

3. For postmenopausal women with positive nodes and positive hormone receptor levels, tamoxifen is the treatment of choice.

4. For postmenopausal women with positive nodes and negative hormone receptor levels, chemotherapy may be considered but cannot be recommended as standard practice.

5. For postmenopausal women with negative nodes, regardless of hormone receptor levels, there is no indication for routine adjuvant treatment. For certain high-risk patients in this group, adjuvant therapy may be considered.

URINARY INCONTINENCE

Incontinence of urine means that the urine escapes involuntarily. The urine may escape continuously, both by night and by day, or it may escape intermittently, and the causes of each variety need to be understood if treatment is to be successful. Uncontrolled leakage of urine is a most distressing and degrading disability, and failure of treatment is often the result of inadequate investigation.

There are several types of true incontinence, which may be of two varieties. One may be caused by a fistula of the bladder or ureter. There are rare congenital lesions that cause incontinence—namely, ectopia vesicae, an ectopic opening of the ureter into the urethra. There is constant loss of urine during the day and at night. Another type of incontinence seen in general medical practice is that in which the patient empties the bladder from time to time without regard to social convenience, either because of cerebral changes or neurological changes.

Overflow incontinence, which is called false incontinence, may occur in cases of retention of urine from any cause, especially in elderly patients with loss of bladder sensation, when the bladder becomes grossly distended and urine may dribble away.

Urgency incontinence is a term that is applied when the patient has an urgent desire to micturate that cannot be controlled by voluntary contraction of pelvic floor muscles. The patient becomes acutely conscious of an urgent need to void, and this is followed by the uncontrolled passage of urine. It is often associated with frequency of micturition and a sensation of incomplete emptying caused by trigonitis or urethritis. Cystometry shows that the bladder reflex is unusually excitable and detrusor tone is unduly high (detrusor instability).

Stress incontinence is a common disorder. The patient complains that a small quantity of urine escapes involuntarily whenever the intra-abdominal pressure is suddenly raised by any exertion, such as coughing, sneezing, laughing, or even walking.

Normal control of micturition

The mechanisms responsible for urinary incontinence in the female are still not completely understood. Three factors may be considered. These include muscle control, external pressure on the urethra, and reflex control.

The muscle control comes from the interlacing, smooth muscle fibers of the involuntary detrusor muscle. The internal sphincter is supported by striped muscle fibers from the medial edge of the pubococcygeal part of the levator ani, which also forms a sling around the bladder neck posteriorly. Below this, between the two layers of the urogenital diaphragm, is the deep transverse perineal muscle (compressor urethra), which can compress the urethra strongly at that level.

The external pressure on the urethra is assisted by external pressure on the intra-abdominal part of the urethra (above the pelvic diaphragm), which is equal to the pressure on the fundus of the bladder. If the pressure in the urethra is less than in the bladder, there will be loss of urine.

Reflex control occurs when the bladder fills with urine. It accommodates the increasing volume with a gradual rise in intravesical pressure until the sensory stretch receptors are stimulated to trigger detrusor contraction and relaxation of the internal sphincter. The sympathetic and parasympathetic control is delicately balanced: In the fundus and bladder neck regions, there is a reciprocal arrangement of adrenergic alpha and beta receptors, which act so that when one area contracts the other relaxes and vice versa.

Stress incontinence

The exact mechanism of urinary incontinence is still not documented. There are many causes of urinary incontinence, only some of which can be treated by surgery. Accurate diagnosis of the cause of stress incontinence requires some consideration of the problems of bladder physiology. The physiology of micturition is summarized as follows: The bladder stores urine at a low pressure. The bladder wall relaxes its tone, and pressure rises very little until over 400 ml of urine accumulates. The pressure does not exceed 20 cm H_2O until the bladder is full (600 ml). The urethra can normally resist pressures between 20 and 50 cm H_2O, which is much higher than the bladder exerts until it is full. The pressure in the urethra is maintained by the urethral wall as well as the sphincter muscle function, which is served by the entire urethra. Urine is contained in the bladder as long as the entire intraurethral pressure is greater than the intravesical pressure.

The nervous control of micturition is not completely understood. Micturition can be described as an autonomic reflex that can be consciously inhibited or facilitated in trained individuals. A desire to void reaches consciousness when about 300 ml of urine fills the bladder. The stimulus passes via the parasympathetic, and reflex detrusor contractions can be inhibited until about 700 ml accumulates. The urethra is strongly contracted. Relaxation of the urethra (which is smooth muscle extending from the detrusor to the end of the urethra) is usually a conscious act at the onset of micturition. It may be psychologically inhibited, as in a patient who is not used to using a bed pan or when another person is present. At the end of micturition, the urethra contracts and forces the last drops of urine back into the bladder (the urethra is normally empty). The disturbed bladder function may be due to urgency incontinence, fistula, overflow incontinence, neurological disease, frequency, noctural frequency, dysuria, or hematuria.

It is agreed that the basic problem in the etiology of stress incontinence is inadequate support of the bladder base, vesical neck, and proximal urethra. If the urethra is properly supported, the proximal two-thirds are intra-abdominal. It is believed that stress incontinence results from dilatation of the urethra and the urethrovesical junction with funneling. About 30% of the patients with stress incontinence do not have funneling.

Breen reports that the posterior urethrovesical junction and urethral axis are crucial factors in the etiology of stress incontinence and its successful correction. He reports that the posterior urethrovesical angle in the continent female is usually about 90 to 100°. The vertical urethral axis is equally important. A vertical line drawn posterior to the urethrovesical junction is used as a base of an angle drawn to the urethra. Normally, the angle should be 15 to 30°. Management varies for abnormal anterior and posterior angles or a combination.

There is not total acceptance of the role that the posterior urethrovesical angle and the loss of a normal urethral inclination play in producing stress incontinence. Ninety-five percent of significant stress incontinence occurs in multiparas. It is found more frequently in Caucasian women who have delivered vaginally and is exaggerated by the erect position with the Valsalva's maneuver.

Fifty percent of nulliparous college women will experience stress incontinence at some time or other. Only about 25 to 30% of symptomatic cystoceles have concomitant stress incontinence. There is no correlation between the degress of cystocele and the frequency of stress incontinence. In the presence of a cystocele, if the herniation is posterior, most patients do not have stress incontinence. Occasionally there may be a combination of these two.

The concept that a short urethra is a primary cause of urinary stress incontinence has not been confirmed. Marked periurethral adhesions with distortion of the normal urethra may interfere with urinary continence. The urethra may be a stiff tube through which urine flows. When this occurs, it is necessary to release all adhesions before normal function can be restored.

It is generally agreed that if vesical funneling, bladder neck descent, and the like are present, it is because of inadequate support of the bladder neck by components of the levator ani in the erect position as well as loss of adequacy of attachments of the urethra to the symphysis pubis. This permits the bladder neck to be the target point in the transmission of force from the dome to the base of the bladder. The chief cause is trauma that may not show up until the postmenopausal years. With the patient in the upright position, straining and coughing should not result in urine loss. Another method of evaluation that may be helpful is asking the patient to void and to voluntarily stop urine flow.

Diagnosis

It is important to differentiate stress incontinence from urgency incontinence, irritable bladder secondary to infection, or neurological disorder. The psychological stability of the patient must be evaluated. On physical examination, there should be a general overall physical evaluation. It is important to evaluate the tone of the levators, the tone of the vagina, and the sensation of the perineal area.

Evaluation

The initial step in evaluation is a urinalysis and urine culture. The second phase includes a urogynecologic history and physical examination, neurological examination, uroflometry with residual urine, urethrocystoscopy, carbon dioxide cystometry, urethra calibration, and cotton swab test. Water cystometry is performed to rule out false-positive bladder instability found with carbon dioxide cystometry. The final triage, reserved for approximately 10% of the patients, includes multichannel urodynamic recordings, water cystometry, urethral closure pressure profiles, cough profiles, instrumented uroflow to determine voiding mechanism, and vesical contraction inhibition. Other specialized testing may also be included.

Management

Nonsurgical-medical. Medical treatment may include the following:

1. Flavoxate (Urispas), 1 tablet t.i.d.
2. Propantheline (Pro-Banthine), 15 mg t.i.d. 30 mg at bedtime
3. Estrogens

Estrogens may help alleviate the symptoms of stress incontinence associated with postmenopausal atrophy. Excessive use of estrogens, on the other hand, may produce or aggravate the problem of stress incontinence.

Exercises. Perineal exercises can help restore bladder control.

1. Perineal exercises (Kegel) increase pubococcygeal muscle control as well as urogenital diaphragm control.
2. A well-trained voluntary sphincter mechanism alleviates the distress of stress incontinence by permitting a quick forceful contraction of these muscles, thus reducing the involuntary loss of urine under stress.
3. These muscles should be voluntarily contracted for 3 or 4 minutes four times a day.

Surgery. The only type of incontinence that is helped by surgery is stress incontinence. A cystocele is rarely associated with stress incontinence. Overvigorous correction of a cystocele may lead to stress incontinence. The operation should be tailored to the pathological findings and to the physiological and anatomic imbalance. The initial result is often good. However, within 5 to 10 years, only about 60% prove to be successful. The failure rate with repeat operations is high, and the number judged successful drops considerably.

Types of operations. The major surgical categories include the following:

1. Vaginal and urethroplasty
2. Marshall-Marchetti-Krantz procedure
3. Sling operations

The best overall treatment is a retropubic surgical approach to replace the urethra within the abdominal cavity, with minimal urethral fixation or periurethral dissection so as to avoid effects on the otherwise normal urethral sphincter mechanism. Suspension is accomplished by placing sutures in the perivaginal fascia, 2 cm lateral to the urethra. These sutures are then anchored at the Cooper's ligament.

Adjuvant measures are sometimes helpful, including a strict diet for women who are overweight and instruction by a physiotherapist in pelvic floor exercises. After menopause, the muscles of the pelvic floor are atonic and the submucosal venous plexus is less vascular; some benefit has been claimed for treatment with estrogens.

CYSTOCELE, URETHROCELE, RECTOCELE, AND ENTEROCELE

It is generally agreed that the support of pelvic structures depends on the endopelvic fascia, the uterosacral and cardinal ligaments, and the levator muscle. This intact fascial system with its attachments to the vaginal fornices and upper two-thirds of the lateral vagina provides a well-supported vaginal tube, which in turn is the most important supporting structure for the uterus and vaginal vault.

In **uterovaginal prolapse,** there is damage to and weakness of the structures that support the pelvic organs, so that some of these descend from their normal position and finally herniate through the vaginal opening.

Prolapse of the bladder and anterior vaginal wall is known as a **cystocele.** Descent of the urethra and bladder neck may occur separately, or it may accompany a cystocele; when sagging of the urethra occurs alone, it is sometimes known as a **urethrocele.**

Prolapse of the rectum and posterior vaginal wall is known as a **rectocele.** It is usually accompanied by some deficiency of the perineal body.

Uterine prolapse is accompanied by descent and inversion of the vaginal vault. Three degrees of uterine prolapse are described: (1) The uterus become retroverted and descends in the axis of the vagina, though the cervix does not reach the introitus. (2) The cervix appears at the introitus from the vaginal orifice. (3) The vaginal walls are everted to such a degree that the uterus lies outside the vulva; this complete form of uterine prolapse is known as procedentia.

Cystocele or rectocele or both may occur without uterine descent, but uterine prolapse is accompanied by descent of the bladder because of the close attachment of the bladder to the anterior aspect of the supravaginal cervix. Descent of the rectum does not necessarily accompany uterine prolapse, because the prolapsing vaginal wall usually becomes separated from the rectum.

A hernia of the rectovaginal peritoneal pouch through the posterior vaginal fornix is known as an **enterocele.** Elongation of the rectovaginal pouch invariably accompanies uterine prolapse, and the small intestine may be found in the peritoneal sac, behind the uterus in cases of procedentia. Enterocele may also occur without uterine prolapse and cause a bulging of the upper part of the posterior vagina, which must be distinguished from a rectocele. Enterocele may occasionally occur after the uterus has been removed by abdominal or vaginal hysterectomy and is usually combined with some degree of vaginal prolapse.

Urethrocele

Urethrocele is a downward protrusion of the urethra from its attachment just beneath the pubic symphysis. This results from the inability of the muscular fibrous tissue to give the urethra normal support. Childbirth injuries to the urogenital trigone and the pubovesical cervical fascia are chiefly responsible for this condition. When it occurs in a nulliparous woman, a metabolic and/or neurological disease should be ruled out.

Management. A urethrocele may be repaired at the time of cystocele repair. The stress incontinence that may accompany it should be corrected by a suitable operation after careful urologic evaluation.

Cystocele

A cystocele is a herniation of the bladder causing the anterior vaginal wall to bulge downward. It is usually the result of childbirth. The baby's head may stretch the pubococcygeal fibers of the levator ani muscle, permitting gradual sagging of the vaginal wall. Probably the most important factor in the development of cystocele is the incompetency of the pubo-vesicocervical fascia. A cystocele very rarely gives rise to stress incontinence but occasionally gives rise to overflow incontinence because of inability to empty the bladder. A large cystocele may pull on the trigone and give a sense of urgency.

Indications for surgery. Surgery is indicated in the following situations:

1. Large cystocele that causes discomfort on sitting and walking.

2. Inability to void without pushing up the anterior vaginal wall manually.
3. Marked stretching of the trigone, resulting in urinary frequency and urgency.
4. Overflow incontinence and/or rarely stress incontinence.
5. Difficulty with intercourse.
6. Bleeding and ulceration secondary to trauma from the bleeding mass.
7. Repeated bladder infections secondary to retention of urine.

Management.   The most important and essential step in the cure of a cystocele is restoring support to the urethra and/or bladder by proper use of the pubovesical cervical fascia. Care must be exercised not to advance the bladder excessively, or the urethra vesicle angle may be increased with resulting stress incontinence.

Rectocele and enterocele

A rectocele is a protrusion of the rectum into the vagina, and an enterocele is a high posterior vaginal herniation of the small bowel, peritoneum, and fascia bulging forward at the apex of the vagina. It usually dissects down between the rectum and the vagina. Unlike a rectocele, it is a true hernia.

Management.   Repair of a relaxed vaginal outlet and repair of a rectocele are two distinct operative procedures. They are frequently undertaken together, but perineal repair is often performed when a rectocele is not present. Rarely a rectocele may be present and require repair in a woman whose outlet is not relaxed. An enterocele is repaired by a high ligation of the sac and closure of the endopelvic fascia.

Prolapse of the uterus

Uterine prolapse is a herniation through the pelvic diaphragm, resulting in protrusion into the vagina and even beyond the introitus.

Management.   Pessaries occasionally give the patient some relief. However, the treatment is usually surgery, and the type of surgery depends on the local findings. The surgery may be a Manchester operation, vaginal hysterectomy, abdominal suspension operation, or a Le Fort's procedure.

A vaginal hysterectomy is the procedure of choice for a uterus with pathology. For a young woman who wishes to maintain menstruation and preserve childbearing, vaginoplasty and abdominal suspension may be indicated. If vaginal repair is undertaken in this patient, the cervix should not be amputated nor the cardinal ligaments plicated. In women who work in industrial jobs and who lift heavy objects, the Manchester operation gives the best results.

ECTOPIC PREGNANCY

In an ectopic pregnancy, the products of conception develop outside the uterus. By far the most common site is the fallopian tube. Combined heterotopic pregnancy is characterized by the existence of a simultaneous intrauterine and extrauterine pregnancy. Cornual pregnancy develops in the cornua, and a pregnancy may develop in a rudimentary horn of the uterus (rudimentary horn pregnancy). It is a most serious problem of ectopic pregnancy.

The adage that anyone in the childbearing years with lower abdominal pain has an ectopic pregnancy until proven otherwise serves as an excellent guideline. Ectopic pregnancy has become epidemic in the United States and is the leading cause of death from pregnancy. It is closely associated with the *Chlamydia* epidemic.

It is impossible to compute the number of ectopic implantations per conception, but in practice the incidence seems to be more than 1 case for every 300 deliveries. The etiology includes pelvic inflammatory disease, intrauterine devices, endocrine disorders, genital anomalies, and a variety of other causes.

Ectopic pregnancies may occur in the ampulla, isthmic, interstitial, or fimbrial part of the tube or in the ovary, cervix, or in the peritoneal cavity.

The two most dangerous are those occurring in a rudimentary horn and in the cervix, and as abdominal pregnancies.

Investigation of suspected tubal pregnancy

When the diagnosis of tubal pregnancy on clinical grounds is in doubt, the following investigations may be performed:

Pregnancy test.   The standard immunologic pregnancy test that demonstrates the presence of HCG in the urine is not helpful: A tubal pregnancy may not produce enough HCG to give positive results. Estimation of the concentration of the beta subunit of HCG in the serum is of greater value, especially when used in conjunction with ultrasonic scanning. If the level of beta-HCG is above 6,000 mIU/L, the patient is likely to have a normal intrauterine pregnancy, especially if the level rises rapidly. Absence of beta-HCG virtually rules out pregnancy, but levels below 6,000 mIU/L are suggestive of tubal pregnancy or missed abortion.

Ultrasonic scanning.   In an early pregnancy of 4 or 5 weeks, the decidua reaction of the endometrium in an ectopic pregnancy may be hard to distinguish from an intrauterine gestational sac. Ultrasonic demonstration of fetal cardiac activity within the uterus is the undeniable evidence of a uterine pregnancy, but this can rarely be certain until the eighth week.

Laparoscopy.   With laparoscopy, a certain diagnosis of tubal pregnancy can be made, but it involves giving the patient an anesthetic, which is undesirable if the pregnancy is intrauterine. Estimation of HCG levels and the use of ultrasonography, as described above, may help to avoid this. When the clinical evidence is clearcut, laparoscopy should not be advised as it will only delay laparotomy, but if the diagnosis is in doubt, it may be valuable in preventing laparotomy being performed on patients with conditions such as salpingitis, which should be treated medically.

Management

The ectopic pregnancy can be removed by salpingo-oophorectomy, salpingectomy, or salpingostomy. If the ectopic pregnancy is ruptured and only one tube is remaining, the ruptured segment may be resected with a view to reanastomosing the two segments of the tube at a later date. Even if both tubes are totally destroyed, the ovaries and uterus should not be removed, because recent successes with in vitro fertilization offer hope to the patient that she may carry a pregnancy in the future.

ACUTE AND CHRONIC PELVIC INFLAMMATORY DISEASE

Pelvic inflammatory disease (PID) is a generalized term describing acute, subacute, recurrent, or chronic infection in the cervix, uterus, tubes, and ovaries with or without involvement of adjacent supportive tissues as well as the peritoneum and intestines. These infections may be bacterial, fungal, parasitic, or viral. Though commonly used in diagnosis for any pelvic complaint, the term should be replaced by specific descriptive terms as to the type of involvement and causative agent of the infection, if known.

PID is diagnosed approximately 800,000 times per year in the United States. It has as its presenting symptoms abdominopelvic pain, fever, vaginal discharge, and less commonly nausea, vomiting, and urinary symptoms. The pelvic examination usually reveals tenderness, especially of the adnexa, and often a palpable mass. Because the signs and symptoms are nonspecific, additional diagnostic procedures may be indicated. These techniques include culdocentesis, sonography, and laparoscopy. A number of microbes appear to be involved in PID: *N. gonorrheae, C. trachomatis*, other anaerobic and aerobic bacteria, and occasionally genital mycoplasmas. Appropriate workup includes CBC, urinalysis, blood cultures (though these are rarely positive), and cervical culture (for *N. gonorrhea* only on selected media). If peritoneal exudate is obtained by culdocentesis or laparoscopy, the specimen should be cultured for aerobes and anaerobes.

C. trachomatis, an obligate intracellular organism due to its inability to produce ATP, has only recently been associated with PID, although it is the most common cause of nonspecific urethritis and is usually the cause of PID when a gonorrheal culture is negative. It is responsible for up to 40% of cases and is epidemic in the United States. It makes a significant contribution to the increased incidence of ectopic pregnancies. Previously, it was difficult to identify in the laboratory. However, a monoclonal antibody slide test has recently been developed that can detect this organism within 48 hours.

Diagnosis

PID is usually a problem of young and low-parity females. Pelvic infection has always been a formidable problem in obstetrics and gynecology. With the present rapid rate of increase of venereal disease, this problem has become more formidable and widespread despite current advances in antibiotic therapy.

The signs and symptoms of PID are relatively nonspecific. Thus, a high degree of suspicion is essential for the diagnosis. It is possible, too, that only very mild symptoms will appear in spite of serious infection. Common findings are adnexal tenderness, fever, dysuria and urethritis, a foul-smelling discharge, adnexal masses, and elevated WBC count and sedimentation rate.

The **differential diagnosis** includes appendicitis, diverticulitis, torsion of the pedicle of a cyst, and tubal pregnancy.

Therapy

Treatment must be individualized. Surgical emergencies such as appendicitis or ectopic pregnancy must be ruled out. A pelvic abscess is suspected. Severe illness precludes outpatient management when the patient has failed an outpatient course of management.

The treatment of choice has not been established. There is no single agent that is effective against all of the possible pathogens. Several combination antibiotic regimens that cover the three major pathogens (gonorrhea, chlamydiae, and anaerobes) include doxicillin, clindamycin, and doxicycline.

Surgery must be considered if there is no response to antibiotic therapy in 48 to 72 hours. This may require colpotomy or laparotomy.

Chronic PID

The patient complains of pelvic pain made worse during menstrual periods, which are regular and heavy. Dyspareunia is common.

Some swelling may be felt, but often there is little to find except tenderness in the fornices. An exact diagnosis and estimate of the degree of PID cannot be made without laparoscopy.

All degrees of inflammation are met, from salpingitis alone to a widespread inflammatory reaction involving all pelvic tissues. It is rare to recover any organism in PID other than in the case of tuberculosis. The ascending infection first attacks the tubes, which are sealed off by edema and adhesions. The tubes either swell up with watery exudate, forming a hydrosalpinx or pyosalpinx, or they become very thickened and adherent to the ovary. The ovary may also be the seat of abscess formation, and the uterus and adnexa, normally mobile, become fixed by adhesions. Since the ovary is often infected, in most cases the term **salpingo-oophoritis** is usually applied.

Treatment

The course of chronic PID is not predictable, and mild degrees may resolve spontaneously. In such cases, the patient should be treated by rest, and, although the infected organism may not be identified, a broad-spectrum antibiotic is usually given. Hydrosalpinx and any abscess formation may be relieved by laparotomy and drainage, and dyspareunia may be relieved by correcting the uterine retroversion. In advanced cases, however, the only effective treatment is an operation to remove the uterus, tubes, and perhaps the ovaries as well.

PELVIC TUBERCULOSIS

The causative organism of pelvic tuberculosis is the acid-fast tubercle bacillus. The majority of cases are secondary to a tuberculosis infection of other organs. It may be transmitted through the bloodstream from a primary lesion in the lungs, kidneys, or peritoneum. Rarely it is transmitted by the male partner who has tuberculosis of the GU tract. About 8% of women dying of pulmonary tuberculosis are found postmortem to have tuberculosis of the genital tract. The diagnosis is often made while investigating infertility problems. The physician inadvertently discovers tubercular lesions in the endometrium by biopsy or curettage. It is the cause of about 5% or more of women seeking help in sterility clinics. When tubercular lesions are found in the endometrium, it can be assumed that the patient has tuberculosis of the fallopian tube.

Diagnosis

Histological evidence is obtained from curettage specimens. This is the most common method, and it is assumed that the tubes are also infected. Biologic evidence from guinea pig inoculation is carried out, and if the guinea pig should show signs of illness in a month, the guinea pig is sacrificed at 6 weeks and examined for evidence of tuberculosis infection. A biopsy from any suspicious, ulcerated area in the vagina or vulva is helpful, and laparoscopy inspection and biopsy may be needed. Once the genital tract infection is identified, the respiratory and urinary tracts must also be investigated.

Pathology

This infection is bloodborne, usually from a primary focus in the lung or kidney, and it infects the tubes, spreading from this source to the fallopian tube and secondarily infecting the endometrium. The tubes may appear normal (endosalpingitis) but usually display the distortion and swelling of chronic infection, and small pinhead tubercles appear on the serosa. The endometrium also shows tuberculous follicles, best demonstrated in the premenstrual and menstrual phase.

Treatment

A combination of rifampicin, isoniazid, and ethambutol has been used effectively in recent years. Dosage is based on body weight, and the first two drugs are given in combination for a year. The ethambutol is withdrawn after 90 days. Cure may be assumed if the endometrium shows no signs of tubercle bacilli and the patient's menstrual cycle is normal.

Surgery

Surgery involves removal of the uterus, tubes, and ovaries, although conservation of one ovary is permissible in a young woman. Surgery is indicated when chemotherapy has failed (about 5% of cases) or in combination with chemotherapy in the older woman. All infected tissue must be removed to avoid subsequent fistulous openings in the bowel or bladder.

Tuberculosis and infertility

Failure to conceive is probably the most important consequence of genital tuberculosis, and 90% of women presenting with the disease would never have had a pregnancy. Pregnancy after successful treatment may be looked for in about 10% of patients, but there is considerable chance of ectopic gestation.

ENDOMETRIOSIS

Definition

Endometriosis is a disorder characterized by the presence of functioning endometrial tissue outside the uterine cavity. It often results in significant pelvic adhesions. It is primarily a pelvic disease. Aberrant tissue may be found in many locations, including the ovaries, uterosacral and other pelvic ligaments, rectovaginal septum, pelvic peritoneum, umbilicus, laparotomy scars, hernia sac, bowel or bladder, lower genital tract, tubal stumps, and lymph nodes.

Basic principles

Endometriosis implies proliferating growth in the function (usually bleeding) in an extrauterine site. An **endometrioma** may be defined as an area of endometriosis, usually in the ovary, that is enlarged sufficiently to be classified as a tumor. When the endometrioma is filled with whole blood (resembling tarry or chocolate-colored, syrupy fluid), it is commonly known as a **chocolate cyst**. Although the complaint of infertility should be sufficient to alert the physician to the possibility of endometriosis, the index of suspicion is elevated if the woman has progressively severe dysmenorrhea and dysparenunia or pain on defecation.

Endometriosis has been noted with increasing frequency and is found in about 15% of pelvic operations. Whether the widespread use of steroidal contraceptives over the past 20 years has reduced the incidence of endometriosis by reducing menstrual flow and thereby preventing tubal reflux remains to be answered.

It is encountered among women of higher socioeconomic groups and is correlated with delayed or deferred motherhood. It has been called a disease of civilization.

The median age of patients at the time of diagnosis is approximately 37 years, but approximately 15% of the patients are under 30 years of age. The typical patient with endometriosis is nulliparous, in her late 20s or early 30s, intelligent, egocentric, overanxious, and perfectionistic.

Histogenesis

Histogenesis has been suggested by several theories: the transplantation or tubal regurgitation theory, coelomic metaplasia doctrine, lymphatic spread, hematogenous root, and the composite or unified concept. Recently a great deal of attention has been directed to the genetic and immunologic influences involved in the pathogenesis of endometriosis. Siblings have a higher risk of developing endometriosis than does a control group. Monkeys with spontaneous endometriosis were found to have a cell-mediated response to autologous endometrial tissue that was significantly lower than controls. Less common, a genetic influence could be manifested through a deficient immunologic system.

Classification

The American Fertility Society uses four categories: stage I (mild), stage II (moderate), stage III (severe), and stage IV (extensive) based on the degree of involvement of the peritoneum, ovaries, and tubes. Involvement is categorized as active endometriosis and/or adhesions. Points are assigned based on dimensional spread in three categories: less than 1 cm, 1 to 3 cm, and over 3 cm.

Maneuvers to avoid

Avoid pelvic examination during the menstrual period or after diagnostic dilatation and curettage, as well as at the time of menstruation or just premenstrually. Uterotubal insufflation should not be done. Pelvic examination after endometrial biopsy should be avoided because of the possibility of endometrial spillage inside the peritoneal cavity. Cryotherapy may lead to a higher incidence of subsequent cervical stenosis, which might result in retrograde flow.

Diagnosis

Diagnostic triad.   In endometriosis, there is usually a triad of (1) a period-related symptom that gets progressively worse,

(2) an interval of 5 years since the last delivery despite the number of previous deliveries, and (3) tender nodules in the cul-de-sac, uterosacral area, and the ovaries, particularly noticeable during menstruation. A fixed retroversion of the uterus may be present.

Diagnostic aids. Laparoscopy, barium enema, intravenous pyelogram, cystoscopy, and examination under anesthesia can aid in the diagnosis.

Differential diagnosis. The differential diagnosis includes the following:

1. Chronic pelvic inflammatory disease
2. Ovarian tumor or cancer
3. Rupture of an ovarian endometrial cyst

Rupture of an endometrial cyst may simulate an attack of pelvic peritonitis, appendicitis, ectopic pregnancy, ovarian cyst with twisted pedicle, ruptured dysfunctional ovarian cyst, or carcinoma of the rectosigmoid.

Medical management

Asymptomatic endometriosis may be safely dealt with by close observation. Mild pain can be controlled by analgesics. For more pronounced symptoms, surgery or hormone treatment still constitutes the only available therapy.

Patients with minimal disease may be followed with expectant therapy. It is especially appropriate in young women with short-term infertility. The pregnancy rate is about the same for this group followed expectantly as it is in those treated with conservative surgery.

Pregnancy has often been suggested as the optimum prophylactic and therapeutic treatment for endometriosis. Regression of endometriosis following suppressive hormone therapy is probably due to the combination of anovulation and amenorrhea brought about by adenohypophyseal suppression. The improvement in the symptoms of endometriosis treated with hormones may be due in part to a transformation of the functioning endometriotic tissue into decidua by increased levels of progesterone.

Hormones that have been given subjective or objective relief of signs or symptoms are estrogen, androgen, progestogens, combined estrogen-progesterone pill, hydroxyprogesterone caproate, medroxyprogesterone, and danazol (Danocrine). The pill creates a pseudopregnancy with amenorrhea. The pseudopregnancy causes deciduation, macrobiosis, and resorption of the ectopic endometrium. Danazol creates a so-called pseudomenopause.

Surgery

Endometriosis is probably best treated primarily by surgery, and this is mandatory if an adnexal mass is present. Hormone therapy over a long period of time is expensive and often unsatisfactory, and the result is not predictable. When the disease is very extensive and there are adnexal masses, particularly in older women, hysterectomy and bilateral salpingo-oophorectomy are indicated.

In young women with less extensive disease than described above, it is possible to preserve an ovary, since hysterectomy alone will relieve most if not all of the symptoms. In young women desirous of pregnancy, conservative surgery should be carried out if possible. It should include resection of an endometrial cyst, unilateral adnexectomy if required, fulguration of implants, suspension of the uterus, and presacral neurectomy.

If a recurrence of the endometriosis following conservative surgery requires a second operation, it should probably include castration. Following castration surgery, subsequent hormonal therapy in the premenopausal woman is an accepted practice.

Treatment by irradiation of the ovaries in cases with extensive bowel or bladder involvement should not be employed as a method of treatment, as pain may not be relieved, and modern surgical methods can overcome most technical problems of excision. Short-term hormonal therapy often makes the surgery easier to perform.

Contraindications to hormone therapy

Unproven endometriosis, especially in the presence of adnexal masses as well as large myomata that may be stimulated to grow during hormone therapy, should contraindicate the hormone therapy. The other contraindications include excessive side effects (either physical or psychological), hepatic disease, previous thrombophlebitis or embolic phenomenon, previous mammary cancer, age over 35 years, and excessive cigarette smoking.

Prolonged therapy

Prolonged therapy is applicable in (1) unmarried patients with maximal symptoms and minimal palpable findings in whom a biopsy diagnosis has been established and (2) patients with persistent or recurrent disease after previous conservative surgery. Short-term hormonal therapy is indicated prior to conservative surgery and subsequent to conservative therapy. It must be emphasized that before any hormonal treatment for endometriosis, a firm diagnosis must be established.

Result

Only 25 to 30% of successful pregnancies are reported after hormonal therapy that results in pseudopregnancy. Between 50 and 60% of successful pregnancies are reported after surgery. Surgery not only eliminates endometriosis but also corrects factors relating to tubal distortion or uterine fixation.

Complications

Endometriosis, untreated, is rarely a fatal disease, and the complications arising from it are few. There will occasionally be some obstruction of the rectosigmoid at the level of the cul-de-sac or obstruction of the small bowel, which usually occurs at the ileocolic junction. Intestinal obstruction is more likely due to adhesions between loops of intestine, which may produce kinking and obstruction. The ureters may be invaded, although it is rare.

Ovarian endometriosis may rupture, may become infected, and occasionally is associated with malignant change.

Malignant changes occurring in endometriomas are very rare and usually of a low-grade adenoacanthoma. Although 10% of endometrioid ovarian carcinomas are associated with ovarian endometriosis, it is unusual for malignant transformation of the endometriosis to be demonstrable. However, endometriosis has a cancer-like characteristic in the insidious, invasive way it spreads, terminating in fibrosis and scarring of any and all pelvic structures.

Endometriosis and infertility

In those cases with extensive endometriosis, the alteration of tubal and ovarian physiology provides an answer for the relationship to infertility. However, in the early cases with minimal disease, it is more difficult to explain. Prostaglandins may play a role in such patients. It has been suggested that degeneration of ectopic endometrial tissue releases prostaglandin, resulting in local vasospasm, hypoxia, tissue destruction, and uterine contraction. Physiological levels of prostaglandins have been shown to be necessary for ovum release, normal tubal motility, uterine relaxation and contractility, and steroidogenesis. An increased concentration of prostaglandins and peritoneal fluid may result in alterations in tubal motility, ovum release, and steroidogenesis.

DYSFUNCTIONAL UTERINE BLEEDING

Dysfunctional uterine bleeding (DUB) is a term that is applied to abnormal bleeding of endometrial origin that occurs in the absence of detectable organic lesions of the uterus and systemic conditions. DUB is a diagnosis of exclusion—that is, it can be made only after complete investigation has ruled out a wide variety of organic lesions. It can be stated that DUB is abnormal bleeding caused by endocrine dysfunction and not organic causes.

Causation

DUB may be caused by alteration in the output or balance of gonadotropic or ovarian hormones, and probably also of endometrial prostaglandins.

Bleeding from the endometrium is controlled by vasoconstriction, myometrial contraction, and local aggregation of platelets, with deposition of fibrin around them, processes that all are influenced by prostaglandins. The endometrium and to a lesser extent the myometrium are able to synthesize prostaglandins from arachidonic acid by the action of the enzyme cyclo-oxygenase. The endometrium contains PGF_2 alpha, which causes myometrial contraction and vasoconstriction; PGE_2, which causes myometrial contraction but is a vasodilator; and prostacyclin (PGI_2), which causes myometrial relaxation and vasodilatation and also inhibits platelet activity.

Etiology

DUB can be either ovulatory or anovulatory.

Ovulatory abnormal uterine bleeding is associated with ovulatory menstruation, which is characterized by regular cycles of approximately the same duration.

Anovulatory abnormal uterine bleeding is bleeding that occurs in the absence of cyclical hormonal changes that determine the menstrual cycle. It has been estimated that 90% of all DUB is anovulatory. It is most commonly encountered in the postpubertal and perimenopausal age-groups. Aberrations of the hypothalamic-pituitary-ovarian axis result in anovulatory uterine bleeding.

Anovulatory DUB is most common at both extremes of the reproductive life: immediately following menarche and just preceding menopause. About 50% of patients with DUB are over 45 years of age, about 20% are adolescents, and the remaining 30% are in their reproductive years.

Ovulatory DUB, on the other hand, is most common during reproductive years and, when not associated with altered corpus luteum function, is related to local endometrial causes such as overreactive endometrial fibrinolysin and/or alteration in the production of prostaglandins by the endometrium or myometrium.

Diagnosis

A careful history differentiates cyclic from acyclic bleeding. In addition, a CBC, a sensitive pregnancy test, and, except in the very young, a fundal endometrial biopsy should be performed. It is important to identify systemic diseases, blood dyscrasia, trauma, or other factors that may be responsible for the anovulation leading to the bleeding. In the history, it is important to find out about the use of aspirin, which often is the cause of bleeding.

The pelvic examination should be normal in DUB. Any enlargement of the uterus or adnexa indicates a diagnosis other than DUB.

Laboratory investigation should include the following tests or measurements: (1) CBC and platelet count, (2) a pregnancy test, (3) thyroid function tests, (4) serum prolactin levels, and (5) serum and androgen (dehydroepiandrosterone and testosterone) levels to rule out adrenal or ovarian disease.

Treatment

Expectant treatment may be followed as the patient presents herself at the first episode of DUB, the bleeding is minimal or moderate, and the hemoglobin is normal. Isolated incidents of DUB are not infrequent in the course of any woman's life. In women in the reproductive age, under age 35, it is important to chart the basal body temperature to find out whether ovulation is occurring. A short course of progestins can restore normal cycles to certain patients. In those with recurrent episodes of bleeding, a biopsy of the endometrium is indicated.

In women over 35 years of age, it is important to do an endometrial aspiration, and currently hysteroscopy or direct visualization of the endometrial cavity is helpful in identifying the cause of persistent uterine bleeding.

Having ruled out an organic cause for the bleeding and having confirmed the diagnosis of DUB, a 10-day course of Provera, 10 mg a day, can be given each month to control the unopposed estrogen. In addition, the patient can be cycled for 7 months with one of the low-dose birth control pills.

BENIGN TUMORS OF THE OVARY

Eighty-five percent of all ovarian tumors are benign. The overall incidence approximates 7% for all females.

Classification of benign cystic ovarian tumors

1. Nonneoplastic
   a. Follicle
   b. Lutein

c. Stein-Leventhal (polycystic ovary)
d. Germinal inclusion
e. Endometrial
f. Tubo-ovarian inflammatory
2. Neoplastic
   a. Epithelial
      (1) Serous
      (2) Mucinous
      (3) Endometrioid
   b. Germ cell
      (1) Benign cystic teratoma (dermoid)
3. Solid
   a. Fibroma
   b. Brenner tumor
   c. Other associated rare lesions

Diagnostic symptoms and signs

Often no symptoms or signs are present, and in many, the first symptom noticed is a palpable mass or an abdominal enlargement. As for the lack of any specific symptoms, uncomplicated tumors are often large by the time the physician is consulted. The symptoms are usually related to the complications that occur.

Differential diagnosis

The differential diagnosis includes a full bladder, ascites, pregnancy, myomata, PID, diverticulitis, appendiceal abscess, distended cecum, pancreatic cyst, mesenteric cyst, broad ligament cyst, and pelvic, kidney, and retroperitoneal tumors.

Complications

Complications include torsion of the pedicle, rupture of cysts, infection of the cyst, hemorrhage, and malignant changes.

Follicle cysts

Persistence of an enlarged follicle may lead to temporary enlargement of the ovary. The patient is usually asymptomatic but may complain of fullness or pain in one adnexal area.

Observation and reexamination after two periods constitute the usual management. Surgical intervention is only indicated if a complication arises.

Corpus luteum cyst

The cyst develops from abnormally excessive secretion and accumulation of fluid associated with the involution process.

Corpus luteum cysts usually are larger than a follicle cyst and may increase to 8 cm in size. Helban's syndrome is characterized by a persistent corpus luteum cyst, amenorrhea followed by irregular uterine bleeding, unilateral pelvic pain, and a tender, small, movable adnexal mass. It is obvious that in most cases the disease is diagnosed after ectopic pregnancy has been ruled out.

After accurate diagnosis by laparoscopy or sonography, conservative management is carried out.

Nonphysiologic, nonneoplastic ovarian cyst

Stein-Leventhal syndrome may also be called polycystic ovary syndrome. It is characterized by amenorrhea or oligomenorrhea, infertility, and usually clinical evidences of excess androgenicity.

The diagnosis is usually made on clinical grounds, but the LH and testosterone levels are often elevated.

Unless the patient is interested in becoming pregnant, Provera is given at monthly intervals to interrupt the constant estrogen stimulation. If pregnancy is desired, clomiphene usually is given, and occasionally Pergonal and HCG may be used.

Neoplastic ovarian cyst

Benign cystic teratomas (dermoids) are rarely large and are bilateral in about 15% of the cases. The malignancy rate is low and has been reported to be from 1 to 3%. The complications that occur are torsion, hemorrhage, rupture, and infection.

Resection of the cyst and, if this is not possible, excision of the ovary are carried out. The other ovary should be bisected and inspected. In the patient who is more than 35 years of age, the treatment of choice is total hysterectomy and bilateral salpingo-oophorectomy.

Neoplastic epithelial cyst

The simple serous cyst represents 15% of all benign ovarian tumors. They are usually unilateral and not larger than 6 cm.

In the younger age-group, the cyst is resected; in the age-group over 35 years, a total hysterectomy and bilateral salpingo-oophorectomy are carried out.

Serous cystadenoma and mucinous cystadenoma are usually unilateral and do not cause symptoms unless they twist or rupture. The management is dependent on the age of the patient, and in the young patient a conservative approach is employed.

Fibroma

Fibromas are composed of fibrous tumors and resemble fibromas found elsewhere. They are common in the elderly and account for about 5% of all ovarian tumors. They may be associated with Meig's syndrome. When hydrothorax is present, the right side is involved 70% of the time and the left side 10% of the time, and both sides are involved in only 15% of the cases. The differential diagnosis includes malignancy with pulmonary metastases, cardiac or renal disease with fluid retention, hepatic cirrhosis, and tuberculous peritonitis.

In the peri- and postmenopausal patient, hysterectomy and bilateral salpingo-oophorectomy are carried out, whereas in younger patients a conservative operation is employed.

Brenner tumor

Brenner tumor is a rather uncommon type of ovarian neoplasm. It grossly is identical to a fibroma. It may cause Meig's syndrome.

Microscopically, the epithelial cells show a coffee bean pattern due to the longitudinal grooving of the nuclei. The management is the same as that for fibroma.

Pregnancy luteoma

Pregnancy luteoma is not a true neoplasm even though it may attain a diameter of 15 cm and have numerous mitoses. It is best interpreted as a focus of reversible nodular lutein-cell hyperplasia, since it depends on HCG stimulation for its structural and functional integrity.

The management is conservative, since it is reversible in most instances, and surgery is only employed for the complications that arise.

Benign uterine tumors

Endometrial polyps are a common type of benign uterine tumor. The term **polyp** is a clinical rather than a pathological one, referring to a growth that is attached by a pedicle or stem and not indicating in any way its histological characteristics. The polyp has a structure like the endometrium itself, consisting primarily of the localized proliferation of endometrium. Most reveal only estrogen response—that is, proliferation of hyperplasia. They are usually benign growths that occur after age 35 and may be single or multiple. The endometrial polyp may give no symptoms or it may give spotting or irregular bleeding.

Removal of the polyp with a tonsil snare or twisting it off with the polyp forceps is the usual method of treatment. A fractional curettage and cervical biopsies should be carried out. The base of the polyp must be carefully curetted.

Endometrial hyperplasia

Endometrial hyperplasia is a uterine condition in which the endometrium remains in a proliferative phase for many weeks or years, resulting in the hyperactivity and growth of both glandular and stromal elements of the endometrium.

Most patients are afflicted between the age of 35 years and menopause. Functional uterine bleeding presents without causative uterine lesions such as tumor, infection, or a complication of pregnancy. Although there frequently may be associated follicle cysts, this diagnosis must be ruled out. Endometrial hyperplasia is usually associated with anovulation or extended periods of amenorrhea. It may be secondary to ovarian unresponsiveness, disturbed pituitary gonadotropin secretion, Stein-Leventhal syndrome, adrenal cortical hyperplasia, functioning ovarian tumors, and administration of estrogen.

In the **management** of the patient who is postpubertal and younger than 30 years, it is important to rule out cancer. Having established the diagnosis of endometrial hyperplasia, treat the patient with either intramuscular progesterone or Provera. In those patients over age 30 to 45, fractional curettage is indicated. It is then repeated. In the postmenopausal period, it is important to rule out pathological conditions such as carcinoma of the endometrium. Hysterectomy may become necessary for recurrent vaginal bleeding.

Adenomatous hyperplasia

Adenomatous hyperplasia, a typical precancerous lesion, may be a focal or general change with its greatest prevalence in women of perimenopausal age with DUB. Those patients presenting with atypical adenomatous hyperplasia are probably at greatest risk.

In young women, they can be followed very carefully by using Provera, progestational agents, clomiphene, and whatever is needed to bring on a period each month. In the perimenopausal and postmenopausal periods, treatment with progesterone is not indicated, but after curettage a decision must be made about whether a hysterectomy will be carried out.

Leiomyomata (fibroids)

The benign, well-circumscribed tumor of nonstriated muscle with supporting fibrous tissue is called leiomyomata. When not encapsulated, it may be shelled out from the uterine muscle. It may arise from immature or undifferentiated cells in the myometrium or possibly from cells in the blood vessel walls. It has been definitely shown that the tumor arises from the muscle cell, probably an undifferentiated myoblast. Rarely it is found in the ovary or in the broad ligament.

Management depends on the associated symptoms, size and location of tumor, age of the patient, and childbearing status. In those perimenopausal patients exhibiting marked symptoms, hysterectomy probably with bilateral salpingo-oophorectomy is the treatment chosen. In the earlier stages, conservative treatment should be carried out.

Plexiform tumorlets

Plexiform tumorlets found in the endometrium are benign. They are incidental lesions of stromal cell origin that are noted microscopically and are associated with a high incidence of uterine fibromas.

Hemangiopericytomas

Hemangiopericytomas are cellular tumors, rarely malignant, and are found in the uterus as well as in other parts of the body. They are vascular lesions not unlike glomus tumors and may be distinguished by a tendency toward concentric arrangement of parasites around capillaries. The malignancy rate is reported as 20 to 25%. The differential diagnosis includes endometrial stromatosis and sarcoma.

GESTATIONAL TROPHOBLASTIC NEOPLASMS

Gestational trophoblastic neoplasms (GTN) comprise a spectrum of diseases that have, at one extreme, a benign hydatidiform mole and, at the other, a highly malignant choriocarcinoma.

A presumptive diagnosis of GTN is made in any postmenarchal woman with an elevated serum (or urine) HCG titer in the absence of pregnancy. For practical purposes, the only other consideration is the rare ovarian germ cell tumor containing trophoblastic tissue. The majority of cases of GTN result from molar pregnancy, and they are detected by serial serum HCG levels using a radioimmunoassay specific for the beta subunit.

Hydatidiform mole

The incidence of hydatidiform mole is approximately 1 per 1,500 to 2,000 pregnancies in the United States. It is more common in other parts of the world. It has been stated that it is caused by deletion or inactivation of all the female chromosomes in the ovocyte, with duplication of the male chromosomes from the fertilizing sperm.

It is important to distinguish between the two different types of hydatidiform mole, which have been called the **complete** and **partial** or **incomplete** types. The complete hydatidiform mole is a classic form of the disease, with dilated avascular villi in the absence of membranes or fetal parts and with at least some degree of trophoblastic proliferation. Patients with hydropic placental villi are occasionally seen also to have an associated fetus (usually malformed) or membranes. These patients do not have trophoblastic proliferation, and they are classified as having a partial mole. This lesion is almost always benign. The classic complete mole has a 46,XX chromosome complement, whereas partial moles usually demonstrate cytogenic abnormalities such as triploidy.

There is a higher incidence of hydatidiform mole before age 20 and after age 40. Vaginal bleeding occurs in all patients and is generally noted between 6 and 8 weeks following the missed period. The bleeding may range from dark brown to bright red and may lead to marked anemia. More than half of the patients have uterine enlargement beyond the expected gestational age. When the uterus enlarges, it does so rapidly and at a nonuniform rate. The uterus feels boggy and, despite its size, no fetal parts can be felt. Amniotic fluid is absent, and ballottement cannot be elicited. Massive enlargement of the ovaries may occur because of the thecal lutein cyst formation. About 20% of the patients with molar pregnancy develop signs of preeclampsia, including hypertension, edema, and/or albuminuria. Eclampsia may rarely occur in association with molar pregnancy. Because it occurs in the first trimester or early second trimester at a much earlier time than toxemia usually does, it should alert the physician to the possibility of a molar pregnancy.

The clinical signs of hydatidiform molar pregnancy are as follows: vaginal bleeding, 100%; uterine enlargement, 50%; hyperemesis, 30%; toxemia, 20%; hyperthyroidism, 10%; and trophoblastic emboli, 2%.

Most hydatidiform moles are recognized by their gross appearance, but some are small and may seem, grossly, to be ordinary abortions. This is particularly true when molar change is seen on the curettage from early therapeutic abortion. Three changes are found in the villi and are typically identified with the hydatidiform mole: trophoblastic proliferation of cytotrophoblasts (Langhans' cells) and syncytiotrophoblasts, hydropic changes in the stroma, and absence of blood vessels.

Diagnosis. Diagnosis is usually made by the use of pelvic sonography. The sonogram picture resembles a snowstorm. There is no fetal heart movement, and the fetal skull and thorax are absent.

HCG is the best method to evaluate and follow the prognosis and progress of a patient with GTN.

Initial evacuation. Once the diagnosis has been made and the patient has been worked up thoroughly and evidences of hyperthyroidism have been eliminated, evacuation is best done by section curettage. Once evacuation has been started, a dilute solution of oxytocin should be given intravenously to maintain uterine contractions and minimize bleeding.

Hysterectomy may be an acceptable method of managing the women with hydatidiform mole who does not desire more children. It should be considered in all patients over 40 years of age with a molar pregnancy.

Follow-up care. Once the mole has been evacuated, the patient should be carefully followed. About 15% of women will require chemotherapy. The patient should be counseled against another pregnancy for the next year, and oral contraceptives are recommended.

Serum beta subunits should be obtained every week until the levels have fallen back to undetectable values. A quantitative serum assay should be used for follow-up, and the usual pregnancy tests are not sensitive enough for accurate evaluation. Routine chest x-rays or other tests are not indicated as long as the beta-HCG levels are falling, the patient has not previously demonstrated a metastatic lesion, and there are no new findings on history and physical examination.

Plateaued arising beta-HCG levels are levels that have not returned to baseline values within 12 weeks. They require chemotherapy, and this will be outlined later. Once the beta-HCG level has returned to normal, the serum levels are checked at monthly intervals for 1 year. After this time, contraception may be discontinued and pregnancy permitted.

Management of gestational trophoblastic disease

About 15% of patients with true hydatidiform moles will require chemotherapy. Those patients having an abnormal HCG regression curve following molar pregnancy have either invasive mole or choriocarcinoma, the ratio being 3 to 5 cases of invasive mole to every 1 case of choriocarcinoma.

GTN after any pregnancy other than a molar pregnancy is always choriocarcinoma. These cases usually present with symptoms caused by bleeding from metastasis to the lung, brain, liver, or genital tract. When there is choriocarcinoma in the uterus, the presenting symptoms may mimic threatened abortion or ectopic pregnancy. The diagnosis of GTN must be confirmed or ruled out by means of HCG testing in any woman in the reproductive age-group presenting with clinical evidence of stroke, brain tumor, hemoperitoneum, GI bleeding, pulmonary infiltrates, or threatened abortion.

Nonmetastatic trophoblastic neoplasm

Patients with nonmetastatic GTN include those who have evidence of persistence of molar tissue and elevated HCG 8 weeks after evacuation of a mole and those patients who have choriocarcinoma limited to the uterus following a molar pregnancy, spontaneous abortion, or a full-term normal delivery.

For a patient to be classified in this category, metastatic disease must be ruled out by chest x-ray, brain scan, liver scan, and a measurement of HCG in the CSF. The possible methods of therapy that can be used in patients with nonmetastatic malignant trophoblastic disease are as follows: single alkylating agent; combination hysterectomy and chemotherapy (the hysterectomy should be done during the first course of chemotherapy on the third day, provided that the patient does not desire further reproduction and that the disease is known to exist in the uterus); and arterial infusion chemotherapy for selected patients.

Choriocarcinoma

Choriocarcinoma is a highly invasive, destructive, hemorrhagic, necrotizing tumor made up mainly of markedly anaplastic trophoblasts and vascular elements and lacking any residual villi structures. Choriocarcinoma is the *enfant terrible* of the family of trophoblastic diseases. In some cases, a presumed interval between conception and the first clinical manifestation of disease may extend for several years.

Choriocarcinoma is a rare disease. The incidence has been given as 1 in 14,000 to 1 in 40,000 pregnancies in the United States. In Hong Kong, the incidence is 1 in 114 pregnancies. It may appear many years after the last pregnancy. Some cases have occurred after the menopause. A diagnosis of choriocarcinoma should be suspected in any patient in whom persistent bleeding occurs subsequent to termination of normal pregnancy, hydatidiform mole, or an abortion.

Deceptive diagnosis

GTN is not only a great masquerader—it is an enigma. The symptoms may appear as nongynecologic manifestations. In patients in whom a diagnosis cannot be established or in whom the primary site of tumor cannot be determined, an HCG level should be obtained. Because choriocarcinoma has been reported in the postmenopausal years, it is no longer advisable to limit HCG assays only to women in the childbearing years.

Histopathology

The chief characteristic is a hemorrhagic mass with a necrotic center and an active periphery. Villus formation is usually absent. The tumor consists of masses of syncytia and cytotrophoblasts. It invades and destroys the surrounding tissue and causes gross hemorrhage because of its ability to erode blood vessels. A histological or microscopic picture of necrosis and marked hemorrhage should alert the examiner to the possible diagnosis of GTN.

Classification of metastatic disease according to risk

Low-risk metatastic disease.   These patients have metastatic disease, most commonly to the lungs or vagina or both. They have an HCG titer under 100,000 IU/day and a duration of disease under 4 months from the termination of the antecedent pregnancy or the onset of symptoms. This group constitutes about 80% of all cases.

High-risk metastatic disease.   High-risk metastatic disease constitutes 20% of all cases. Patients have an HCG titer more than 100,000 IU/day and a duration of disease over 4 months from the termination of the antecedent pregnancy or the onset of symptoms. Patients are also at a high risk if they have had previous unsuccessful chemotherapy for other neoplasms. Metastatic disease is found in multiple sites, including the liver, brain, or both, as well as in the small bowel. The reason for dividing the patients into low- and high-risk metastatic disease categories is to supply the optimum therapy.

Treatment

In women with a favorable prognosis, a single agent, either methotrexate or actinomycin D, gives excellent results. The treatment of the high-risk patient demands combination chemotherapy.

Role of gestational trophoblastic centers

One of the difficult problems in the management of women with trophoblastic neoplasms is determining at what point they should be referred to a specialized center. GTN is probably best handled in a center. At such centers, HCG titers are available and are accurate. The techniques of chemotherapy and the management of side effects and toxicity are understood and managed correctly, and supporting consultative assistance and laboratory and ancillary services are available.

Unless these services are locally available, the patient should be referred to a center. It seems.reasonable that a high-risk patient be referred to a specialized center for the expertise necessary in treatment and for the management of the toxic reactions that most hospitals are inequipped to handle.

On the other hand, patients with nonmetastatic disease or low-risk metastatic disease can probably be treated locally, depending on the expertise of the clinician and the availability of consultative help.

CARCINOMA OF THE UPPER GENITAL TRACT

Cancers of the upper genital tract include those of the endometrium, ovary, and breast. They have a great deal in common with each other epidemiologically, as well as in their possible hormonal relationships. Since the breast has been discussed elsewhere, it will not be included in this discussion.

Endometrial carcinoma

The incidence of endometrial carcinoma has increased. The majority of patients are postmenopausal; 20% are pre- or perimenopausal.

The high-risk factors include obesity, nulliparity, low parity, late menopause, hypertension, diabetes, hormone-secreting tumors of the ovary, polycystic ovary syndrome, exposure to ionizing radiation, exogenous estrogens, and sequential oral contraceptives.

The most common presenting symptom is abnormal bleeding. It is usually bright red and is very distressing to the patient. Watery vaginal discharge is an uncommon presentation. The cervical-vaginal smears are unreliable, and the false-negative rate is greater than 50%. The methods of sampling the endometrial cavity have a diagnostic accuracy of 50 to 80%. Firm diagnosis is obtained by fractional uterine curettage. Parametrium may be encountered at the time of the curettage, in which case drainage should be established and intensive curettage should be discontinued but should be carried out 2 or 3 weeks later, after the drainage has been completed.

Adenocarcinoma is the most common type of endometrial carcinoma, followed by adenoacanthoma and adenosquamous carcinoma. The papillary serous adenocarcinoma is beginning to appear more frequently and, like adenosquamous and grade III, has a very poor prognosis.

Clinical staging of carcinoma of the endometrium.   In January, 1971, a new classification was adopted and will be outlined because this discussion follows the new classification. A case should be classified as carcinoma of the corpus uteri when the primary site of the growth is the corpus. Cases of mixed mesenchymal tumors and so-called carcinosarcoma should be excluded. This staging is as follows:

Stage 0: Carcinoma in situ. Histologic findings suspicious of malignancy. Stage 0 should not be included in the therapeutic statistics.

Stage I: The carcinoma is confined to the corpus. Subdivisions of stage I are
  G1. Highly differentiated adenomatous carcinoma
  G2. Differentiated adenomatous carcinoma with partially solid areas
  G3. Predominantly solid or entirely undifferentiated carcinoma
Stage II: The carcinoma has involved the corpus and the cervix. (Simultaneous presence of normal cervical glands and cancer in the same field will give the final diagnosis.)
Stage III: The carcinoma has spread outside of the uterus but not outside of the pelvis.
Stage IV: The carcinoma has extended outside the true pelvis or has seriously involved the mucosa of the rectum, bladder, or both. A bullous edema does not permit allotment of a case to stage IV.

Three out of four patients will have stage I involvement. Prognostic factors other than clinical stage are important if treatment is to be individualized. These include histological differentiation, myometrial penetration, lymph node metastases (pelvic and periaortic), occult involvement of the cervix, unexpected adnexometastases, and positive peritoneal cytology.

Management.   Stages I through IV are managed by surgery followed by postoperative x-ray therapy except in stage Ia, *G1,* in which external x-ray therapy is not given. However, the external x-ray therapy in the others is combined with intravaginal irradiation. The alternate plan of therapy is to give preoperative x-ray therapy followed by surgery.

Intracavitary irradiation is effective in decreasing the incidence of vaginal metastases. There is less evidence, however, that the 5-year survival is improved, either by vaginal radiation or external megavoltage radiation therapy.

Sixty percent of recurrences occur within 2 years and 90% within 5 years. Undifferentiated tumors tend to recur earlier. Recurrences may be in the vagina (uncommon if radiotherapy has already been given), pelvis, or distally. Plasma carcinoembryonic antigen (CEA) levels may be of use in predicting recurrence. Pretreatment CEA values have been raised in 22% of well-differentiated, 29% of moderately differentiated, and 67% of undifferentiated tumors.

Follow-up.   After treatment of any stage of endometrial carcinoma, follow-up should be at 3- to 4-month intervals for the first year, at 4-month intervals for the next year, and at 6-month intervals following that. A Pap smear should be taken at each visit. A plasma CEA and chest x-ray should be done once a year. Ultrasonography, CT scans, and needle aspiration biopsy should be carried out as indicated.

Ovarian cancer

Ovarian carcinoma is the sixth most common female cancer and the most common fatal gynecologic cancer. Unlike other gynecologic malignancies, ovarian cancer is not diagnosed until laparotomy and histologic examination, either intraperitoneally (frozen section) or postoperatively (definitive histopathoogic examination) of the tumor.

Generally speaking, the older the patient the more likely is her tumor to be epithelial in origin. Germ cell tumors, on the other hand, are more likely to be found in girls and young women, and this should be taken into account when planning the overall management of the patient.

Early diagnosis is a matter of chance rather than a scientific method. Although it is stated that there are no early symptoms of ovarian cancer, a careful history will reveal vague abdominal symptoms and mild digestive disturbances that may be present for months before the diagnosis is made. In women who are older than 40 and who have a history of ovarian dysfunction and bouts of dyspepsia, indigestion, and abdominal pain and in whom no definite diagnosis can be made, it is important to rule out ovarian cancer.

What is interpreted as a normal-size ovary in a premenopausal woman represents an ovarian tumor in the postmenopausal woman.

Staging of primary carcinoma of the ovary.   Staging is based on findings at clinical examination and/or surgical exploration. The histological characteristics are to be considered in the staging, as are results of cytological testing of effusions. It is desirable that a biopsy be performed on suspicious areas outside the pelvis.

Stage I: Growth limited to the ovaries.
Stage IA: Growth limited to one ovary; no ascites. No tumor on the external surface; capsule intact.
Stage IB: Growth limited to both ovaries; no ascites. No tumor on the external surfaces; capsules intact.
Stage IC*:   Tumor either stage IA or IB but with tumor on the surface of one or both ovaries; or with capsule ruptured; or with ascites present containing malignant cells; or with positive peritoneal washings.
Stage II: Growth involving one or both ovaries with pelvic extension.
Stage IIA: Extension and/or metastases to the uterus and/or tubes.
Stage IIB: Extension to other pelvic tissues.
Stage IIC*:   Tumor either stage IIA or IIB but with tumor on the surface of one or both ovaries; or with capsule(s) ruptured; or with ascites present containing malignant cells; or with positive peritoneal washings.
Stage III: Tumor involving one or both ovaries with peritoneal implants outside the pelvis and/or positive retroperitoneal or inguinal nodes. Superficial liver metastasis equals stage III. Tumor is limited to the true pelvis but with histologically verified malignant extension to the small bowel or omentum.
Stage IIIA: Tumor grossly limited to the true pelvis with negative nodes but with histologically confirmed microscopic seeding of abdominal peritoneal surfaces.
Stage IIIB: Tumor of one or both ovaries with histologically confirmed implants of abdominal peritoneal surfaces, none exceeding 2 cm in diameter. Nodes negative.
Stage IIIC: Abdominal implants >2 cm in diameter and/or positive retroperitoneal or inguinal nodes.

Stage IV: Growth involving one or both ovaries with distant metastasis. If pleural effusion is present there must be positive cytological test results to allot a case to stage IV. Parenchymal liver metastasis equals stage IV.

Treatment of the common epithelial ovarian cancer.   Treatment of stage I cancers involves aspiration of fluid for cytology, careful exploration of the abdomen and pelvis, total hysterectomy and bilateral salpingo-oophorectomy, omentectomy, appendectomy, with installation of P32 and chemotherapy optional.

Stages II, III, and IV are treated the same as stage I if possible, with combination chemotherapy playing a significant role as adjuvant treatment.

Treatment of nonepithelial tumors.   Germ cell tumors. If dysgerminoma in the presence have spread beyond the ovary, treatment requires total hysterectomy, bilateral salpingo-oophorectomy, omentectomy, and biopsy of the paraaortic nodes. Postoperative x-ray and/or chemotherapy should be given as indicated. However, in a young woman with a unilateral, encapsulated dysgerminoma, acceptable treatment includes a unilateral salpingo-oophorectomy, biopsy of the other ovary and of the paraaortic nodes, as well as cytological examination of peritoneal fluid.

Endodermal sinus and choriocarcinoma.   These are considered extraembryonic tumors, and the management is generally unilateral salpingo-oophorectomy followed by combination chemotherapy unless they have spread, in which case total hysterectomy and bilateral salpingo-oophorectomy are carried out.

Granulosa cell tumors.   In women over 35 years of age, treatment includes total hysterectomy and bilateral salpingo-oophorectomy. In children and adolescents, the tumor is usually unilateral and encapsulated, and therefore unilateral salpingo-oophorectomy is sufficient treatment.

Gonadoblastoma.   This is a rare tumor composed of germ cells and gonadal stromal elements. Most occur in patients who are intersexual with phenotype habitus; they are amenorrheic and may virilize. The malignancy rate is near zero, but the gonads are useless and both ovaries should be removed. The gonads should definitely be removed in the presence of an XY chromosome pattern, even though the gonads are not enlarged.

Second-look operation.   The question is often raised whether second-look operations should be performed. It is generally accepted that after 6 to 9 months of intensive combination chemotherapy, if there is no evidence of disease clinically or by CT scan or ultrasonography, a second-look operation should be carried out.

CARCINOMA OF THE LOWER GENITAL TRACT

The vulva, vagina, and the cervix constitute the lower genital tract. They share many epidemiologic factors and many hormonal relationships.

Cancer of the vulva is not common; it is the fourth most common malignant tumor of the female genital tract. It accounts for only 3 or 4% of all gynecologic malignancies and 0.7% of all female cancers, a rate of 1.8 per 100,000 females.

There are about 500 deaths annually in the United States due to vulva cancer, and the death rate is about 0.3 per 100,000 women, or about 0.3% of all female cancer deaths.

Little is known about the etiology of vulva cancer. Parity, marital status, and racial differences do not have any etiologic relationship to this cancer. It is common among the poor in various parts of the world. It is usually encountered in women who seldom bathe, but it may also occur in those who bathe daily but whose vulva toilet habits may be inadequate.

The vulva is a very complex structure, consisting of labia majora and minora, the clitoris with its prepuce, the Bartholin's duct, and the distal urethra. The structures are pressed against each other and form folds where dirt and smegma can lodge. In addition, the vulva is subjected to numerous physiological assaults, such as menstruation, micturition, vaginal discharge, and fecal contamination from incorrect anal toilet habits.

Certain skin conditions are associated with this cancer. Chronic irritative states are usually present. Leukoplakia, kraurosis vulvae, granulomatous disease, pruritus, pigmented lesions, chronic ulcers, and syphilis have been identified with cancer of the vulva.

Vulva dystrophies and atypias

The International Society for the Study of Vulva Diseases (ISSVD) has described several types of dystrophies: hyperplastic dystrophy, lichen sclerosis, mixed dystrophy atypias, mild atypia, moderate atypia, and severe atypia. Varying degrees of hyperkeratosis may be seen in all grades of dysplasia, and a granular layer may also be present. In all of the conditions listed above, abnormalities of the cytoplasm, including individual cell keratinization, may be seen.

Vulva carcinoma in situ

There are two varieties of vulva intraepithelial neoplasia—squamous and the rare adenocarcinoma (Paget's disease).

Squamous cell carcinoma in situ is being encountered in younger age-groups. Condylomata acuminata are associated with increasing frequency and occur in 7 to 31% of cases. The human papillomavirus has become the prime suspect in vulva neoplasms. Whatever the initial treatment, recurrences or new intraepithelial lesions are not uncommon.

Localization of biopsy site.   Localization of the biopsy site employs three techniques:

1. Colposcopy
2. Toluidine blue staining (a nuclear stain) washed with 1% acetic acid
3. 5% acetic acid

The biopsy is usually made by multiple punch biopsies, for which the Keyes dermatologic punch instrument is usually used.

Treatment.   Treatment alternatives include the following:

1. Wide local excision
2. Simple vulvectomy
3. Skinning vulvectomy
4. Carbon dioxide laser

5. Cryosurgery
6. Nonsurgical methods such as topical 5-fluorouracil massaged gently into the lesion

Since these lesions are often multifocal and multicentric and occur in very young women, the carbon dioxide laser is the method presently preferred. With local infiltration, it is possible to eradicate all of the lesions with good cosmetic results.

Paget's disease of the vulva

The mean age at which women are afflicted with Paget's disease of the vulva is 63 years. The lesion characteristically presents clinically as white islands of hyperkeratosis over a bright red base. It is usually confined to the apocrine gland (sweat gland) regions of the vulva. Histologically, it is characterized by the presence of Paget's cells. One-third have underlying sweat gland carcinoma (can only be diagnosed after excision). Twenty-five percent are associated with prior malignancy elsewhere, either currently or previously. The breasts are the most frequent site.

Treatment. Wide excision (down through the fat to the fascia and extending at least 2.5 cm beyond visible margins is the primary treatment. The lines of excision must be checked histologically for Paget's cells. If no invasion is found, the patient will be treated as for an in situ lesion; if there is invasion, treatment is as for an invasive lesion.

Microinvasive vulva carcinoma

When squamous cell carcinoma is 2 cm or less in diameter, with 5 mm or less stromal invasion, it is termed microinvasive. The presence of vascular confluency, vascular channel permeation, and cellular anaplasia does not exclude the case from this category.

Vulva condylomata precede or coexist with more than 10% of microinvasive vulva lesions. The lesion may present as a condyloma. The true incidence of lymph node metastases remains to be determined. If penetration is less than a millimeter, metastatic lesions are rare; if there is lymphatic invasion or vascular space invasion, the incidence may rise to as high 30%.

Treatment. Options vary, from wide local excision to radical vulvectomy with or without superficial (inguinal and femoral) and with or without deep (pelvic) lymphadenectomy. Sexual function should be conserved whenever possible.

Invasive tumore of the vulva

Malignant lesions of the vulva are usually squamous carcinomas. Twenty percent of patients have inguinal node metastases, and one-quarter of these have pelvic node metastases.

Staging of Carcinoma of the Vulva. Cases should be classified as carcinoma of the vulva when the primary site of growth is in the vulva. Tumors present in the vulva as secondary growths from either a genital or extragenital site should be excluded from registration, as should cases of malignant melanoma.

Stage O: Carcinoma in situ (e.g., Bowen's disease, noninvasive disease, noninvasive Paget's disease).
Stage I: Tumor confined to the vulva, 2 cm or less in largest diameter. Nodes are not palpable or are

palpable in either groin, not enlarged, mobile (not clinically suspicious of neoplasm).
Stage II: Tumor confined to the vulva more than 2 cm in diameter. Nodes are not palpable or are palpable in either groin, not enlarged, mobile (not clinically suspicious of neoplasm).
Stage III: Tumor of any size with adjacent spread to the urethra and any or all of the vagina, the perineum, and the anus, and/or nodes palpable in either or both groins (enlarged, firm, and mobile, not fixed but clinically suspicious of neoplasm).
Stage IV: Tumor of any size infiltrating the blader mucosa or the rectal mucosa, or both, including the upper part of the urethral mucosa and/or fixed to the bone or other distant metastases. There it also is more extensive and involved TNM classification.

Treatment. The standard operation is extended vulvectomy with bilateral inguinal and pelvic lymphadenectomy. More recently, individualization of surgical therapy has been recommended. Pelvic lymphadenectomy is permitted on occasions (unless histology shows metastases in inguinal glands), and more conservative surgery has been advocated for certain stage I lesions. It has been recommended that hemivulvectomy and ipsilateral lymphadenectomy be carried out in some stage I tumors. There is a tendency to be more conservative in carcinoma of the vulva, and most are radiating the deep nodes now instead of excising them.

Cancer of the vagina

Cancer of th vagina is extremely rare. It accounts for less than 1% of all genital cancers. It usually occurs after age 70, and there are about 300 deaths from squamous cell cancer of the vagina each year. The usual treatment is radiation therapy, and the 5-year survival is about 45%. Persistent bloody vaginal discharge, at first relatively painless, is the initial sign of primary vaginal cancer. It is important to rule out metastatic cancer from other organs.

Vaginal intraepithelial neoplasia

Vaginal intraepithelial neoplasia most often occurs in those 4% of transformation zones that extend from the cervix on to the vaginal wall. This site may be missed at hysterectomy so that the lesion persists, with the erroneous diagnosis of recurrence. In the diethylstilbestrol (DES)-exposed patient, the transformation zone reaches the vagina in over 80% of the patients.

Diagnosis is by biopsy, and treatment is by biopsy excision or carbon dioxide laser therapy, cryotherapy, electrocauterization, local chemotherapy such as 5-fluorouracil, surgical excision, and rarely radiation therapy.

Staging of carcinoma of the vagina. Excluded from this classification are secondary cancers in the vagina, cervical cancers involving the vagina, and malignant lesions extending into the vagina from the urethra or vulva.

Stage 0:   Carcinoma in situ; intraepithelial carcinoma.
Stage I: The carcinoma is limited to the vaginal wall.
Stage II: The carcinoma has involved the subvaginal tissue but has not extended to the pelvic wall.

Stage III: The carcinoma has extended to the pelvic wall.

Stage IIIA: No extension to the pelvic wall.

Stage IIIB: Extension to the pelvic wall and/or hydronephrosis or nonfunctioning kidney.

Stage IV: The carcinoma has extended beyond the true pelvis or has involved the mucosa of the bladder or rectum. Bullous edema as such does not permit a case to be allotted to stage IV.

Stage IVA: Spread of the growth to adjacent organs.

Stage IVB: Spread to distant organs.

Treatment of carcinoma of the vagina. Individualized radiotherapy by a combination of intravaginal and external irradiation is generally used. External therapy is usually given first to reduce the tumor volume. The usual dose is 5,000 rads in 5 weeks. This is followed by intravaginal or interstitial irradiation. This is individualized, but an additional 2,000 to 3,000 rads is given, if possible.

Lesions less than 3 cm in the upper third of the vagina may be treated by radical hysterectomy, bilateral pelvic lymphadenectomy, and vaginectomy. If pelvic lymph nodes are involved, chemotherapy and/or external irradiation should be considered as adjuvant therapy.

Other posterior wall lesions may be suitable for posterior pelvic exenteration, preferably with coloanal anastamosis using the stapler.

Stages III and IV. Three courses of platinum, vinblastine (Velban), and bleomycin are recommended prior to combined external pelvic, interstitial, and intracavitary irradiation.

Stage IVa. Surgically good-risk patients with rectal or bladder involvement alone are suitable for anterior, posterior, or total exenteration, provided pelvic and aortic node biopsies are negative at laparotomy. However, radiation therapy is the treatment usually chosen.

Clear cell adenocarcinoma (müllerian type)

A study at Massachusetts General Hospital revealed a highly significant association between the treatment of mothers with DES during pregnancy and the later development of adenocarcinoma in their daughters.

The incidence rate for the development of clear cell carcinoma of the vagina or cervix is approximately 0.1% in the female fetus whose mothers took DES. About 80 to 90% of these patients develop adenosis of the vagina or have a congenital anomaly of the cervix and/or vagina. From these observations, it was suggested that DES acts as a teratogen rather than a carcinogen. All teenage girls with irregular periods should receive a thorough pelvic examination, including palpation and direct visual inspection of the cervix and vagina plus cytological studies.

Diagnostic signs. The anterior fornix often appears shortened and is less elastic than usual. A cervical hood may be present and gives the appearance of a coxcomb. The cervix appears red, and there is often a red, granular mucosa, small cyst, or papillary lesion that may be multicentric in appearance. On palpation there is a sandy irregularity, and the involved area takes Schiller's or Lugol's stain poorly, if at all. The same findings may exist in patients with adenocarcinoma. The findings usually are more marked, and polypoid, nodular, or papillary lesions are often present.

After a firm diagnosis of clear cell adenocarcinoma of the cervix is made, radical hysterectomy and pelvic node dissection are usually chosen for stages I and IIa. The criteria for prognosis depend on the degree of mitotic activity (one or more mitoses per high-power field carries a bad prognosis), involved regional lymph nodes, and the stage of disease.

The recent observation of pulmonary and/or supraclavicular lymph node metastases indicates that prolonged follow-up of treated individuals is essential.

Carcinoma of the cervix

Carcinoma of the cervix is the disease of the inner city. About 1.6% of newborn girls, or 1 out of 63, will develop invasive cancer of the uterine cervix at some time during their lives.

Cervical carcinoma in situ and dysplasia

The term cervical intraepithelial neoplasia (CIN) denotes all precursors of squamous cervical cancer and embraces a continuous spectrum through CIN 1 (minor dysplasia), CIN 2 (moderate dysplasia), and CIN 3 (major dysplasia and in situ carcinoma). Adenocarcinoma in situ is uncommon.

The age distribution is from middle adolescence to the mid-80s, with the median in the third decade. The condition usually presents as an abnormal Pap smear. Intraepithelial lesions in most cases occur within the transformation zone, which is usually visible in its entirety with colposcopy. Failure to diagnose CIN on colposcopy may be due to (1) a lesion high in the cervical canal, which this is more likely to occur in postmenopausal women, or (2) intercurrent acute cervicitis, often with contact bleeding. Warty atypia due to subclinical human papillomavirus infection can complicate the colposcopic interpretation. Invasive cancer can usually be ruled out by colposcopically directed punch biopsies without having to resort to conization.

Diagnosis. Diagnosis is made by biopsy and by endocervical curettage. Conization is occasionally indicated.

Treatment. After ruling out invasive cancer by combined colposcopic histological study, the management of CIN becomes an academic matter.

Selection of treatment depends on the topography of the lesion, the size of the lesion, the histological diagnosis, the patient's age, parity, desire for more children, desire for sterilization, other gynecologic problems, other medical problems, and social and economic factors. The treatment consists of physical destruction with electrocoagulation diathermy under anesthesia or the use of cryotherapy or carbon dioxide laser surgery.

Adenocarcinoma in situ and adenosquamous carcinoma in situ

Adenocarcinoma in situ is an uncommon entity being recognized more recently by distinctive changes in the Pap smear. The colposcopic appearance of lesions when visible closely mimics the villous outgrowths of normal columnar epithelium. The distinguishing feature of the villi after application of acetic acid is their striking whiteness. The lesions are frequently multifocal. Invasive cancer may coexist deep in the cervical clefts or glands. Cone biopsy is necessary to rule out invasive cancer. In younger patients, this procedure can act as definitive therapy. Careful follow-up is necessary.

Microinvasive and occult invasive carcinoma

Diagnosis by biopsy. Colposcopically directed punch biopsy often supplemented by endocervical curettage is the first approach to histological diagnosis. Wedge resection is indicated in the presence of the colposcopically overt carcinoma. In the postmenopausal woman with a positive smear, a small uterus and negative result for clinical cancer from endocervical curettage, vaginal hysterectomy is sometimes performed as a substitute diagnostic measure for cone biopsy.

Therapy. There are many therapies, and they have to be adapted to the patient. These include (1) radical hysterectomy with bilateral pelvic lymphadenectomy, (2) a conservative approach, (3) conservative hysterectomy, (4) therapeutic conization or amputation of the cervix, and (5) routine hysterectomy with pelvic lymphadenectomy.

Clinical invasive carcinoma of the cervix

The average age is 45, with a trend toward a young age. Postcoital, intermenstrual, and postmenopausal bleeding is the usual presenting symptom. Offensive vaginal discharge is common. The Pap smear in most laboratories is negative in 5% of the cases. The lesions may be exophytic or excavating and ulcerative. With endocervical lesions, the cervix may appear normal or expanded and bell shaped. Parametrial or vaginal spread may be obvious. Bladder and rectal involvement and distal metastases occur with advanced disease.

Clinical staging of carcinoma of the cervix. Stage IA microscopically evident stromal invasion, as well as small cancerous tumors of measurable size. Stage IA should be subdivided into those lesions with minute foci or invasion visible only microscopically as Stage IA-1 and the macroscopically measurable microcarcinomas as stage IA-2 in order to gain further knowledge of the clinical behavior of these lesions. The term IB occult should be omitted.

The diagnosis of both stage IA-1 and IA-2 should be based on microscopic examination of removed tissue, preferably a cone, which must include the entire lesion. As noted above, the lower limit of stage IA-2 should be that it can be measured macroscopically (even if dots need to be placed on the slide before measurement), and the upper limit of IA-2 is given by measurement of the two largest dimensions in any given section. The depth of invasion should not be more than 5 mm taken from the base of the epithelium, either surface or glandular, from which it originates. The second dimension, the horizontal spread, must not exceed 7 mm. Vascular space involvement, either venous or lymphatic, should not alter the staging but should be specifically recorded, as it may affect treatment decisions in the future.

Lesions of greater size should be staged as IB. As a rule, it is impossible to estimate clinically whether a cancer of the cervix has extended to the corpus. Extension to the corpus should therefore be disregarded.

Stage I: The carcinoma is strictly confined to the cervix (extension to the corpus should be disregarded).

Stage IA: Preclinical carcinomas of the cervix—that is, those diagnosed only by microscopy.

Stage IA-1:   Minimal microscopically evident stromal invasion.

Stage IA-2:   Lesions detected microscopically that can be measured. The upper limit of the measurement should not show a depth of invasion of more than 5 mm taken from the base of the epithelium, either surface or glandular, from which its originates; a second dimension, the horizontal spread, must not exceed 7 mm. Larger lesions should be staged as IB.

Stage IB: Lesions of greater dimensions than stage IA-2, whether seen clinically or not. Preformed space involvement should not alter the staging but should be specifically recorded so as to determine whether it should affect treatment decisions in the future.

Treatment. Treatment modalities that are available include radical surgery, radical radiation, and chemotherapy or combinations thereof. Stages IB and IIA are usually treated with radical hysterectomy and pelvic lymphadenectomy unless there is a medical contraindication. Stages IIB, III, and IV are usually treated with radiation therapy as the primary method of treatment. There is a rare case of stage IV in which there is a bladder or rectal fistula that may be considered for pelvic exenteration. The usual plan is to employ pelvic exenteration for central lesions that have not responded to any other method of treatment.

Follow-up. The patient should be carefully followed, and all symptoms, weight change, leg edema, supraclavicular nodes, evaluation of the abdomen, vaginal examination, rectal examination, and rectovaginal examination should be carried out. CEA should be evaluated, and from time to time pelvic and abdominal ultrasonography or CT scan, chest x-rays, and pyelograms should be carried out. The patient should be seen in three monthly intervals for 2 years, at 6-month intervals for 3 years, and annually thereafter.

Carcinoma of the fallopian tube and sarcoma of the genital tract

Primary carcinoma of the fallopian tube is a rare tumor and constitutes 0.3% of all gynecologic malignancies. Sarcoma has also been reported, but it is truly infrequent.

The mean age is 55 years, with a range from 18 to 88 years. The disease is seldom diagnosed before laparotomy. Twenty percent are bilateral. When it is confined to the tube, clinical diagnosis of hydrosalpinx or pyosalpinx may be made.

Only half the cases show the classic triad of bleeding, abdominal pain, and pelvic or abdominal mass. The most common presenting symptom is abnormal bleeding or discharge; the Pap smear is rarely abnormal. Uterine curettage specimens are usually negative or rarely show adenocarcinoma. Diagnosis may follow measures for unknown pelvic mass, such as pelvic ultrasonography, CT scan, or laparoscopy.

Spread is similar to that of ovarian cancer (transperitoneal migration, lymphatic dissemination, and, less commonly, bloodborne). The fimbriated ends of the tube may be open or closed.

Five-year survival rates from collected series range from 27% overall to 60% for stage I tumors. There are at this point no data available on the value of radiotherapy, hormone therapy, or chemotherapy.

The clinical staging is similar to that for ovarian cancer.

As a guideline to a confused topic, **therapy** should follow that recommended for ovarian cancer.

1. Staging laparotomy with peritoneal washings, biopsy.
2. Total hysterectomy, bilateral salpingo-oophorectomy with debulking when indicated in advanced cases, including an omentectomy.
3. Postoperative chemotherapy.
4. Pelvic radiation therapy in stages IIB with bulky residuum. This should be combined with postoperative chemotherapy.

Embryonal rhabdomyosarcoma (botryoid type) of the vagina

Embryonal rhabdomyosarcoma is an uncommon, highly malignant neoplasm that is encountered in infants and young children and has a very poor prognosis. It may be encountered in adults. This tumor, often referred to as **sarcoma botryoides,** is locally invasive and has a rapid growth pattern. It recurs commonly, and a rapidly fatal course follows when improperly treated. This is a radiosensitive tumor at conventional doses; however, it is radiocurable only at high doses beyond 5,000 rads. The lesion arises most frequently from the lower two-thirds of the anterior vaginal wall. The proximity of an anterior vaginal wall lesion to the vesicovaginal septum and posterior bladder wall makes these areas particularly vulnerable to infiltrating tumor. Embryonal rhabdomyosarcoma of the vagina grows rapidly and cause death within 3 months after the onset of symptoms. If left untreated, most patients die within 9 to 18 months.

Formerly, pelvic exenteration with pelvic node dissection and vulvectomy was the most effective **treatment** for this tumor. Surgery (usually less than exenteration) is currently being followed by sequential combination chemotherapy, given cyclically over a 2-year period. Survival depends on the extent of disease present. Almost all patients with tumors limited to the subepithelial connective tissue layers of the vagina can be cured by this method of management.

Uterine sarcoma

Sarcomas constitute about 5% of all malignant uterine tumors. They arise from any mesodermal elements such as smooth muscle, endometrial stroma, blood, and lymph vessels. The histology is variable: (1) leiomyosarcoma, (2) müllerian mesodermal mixed tumor, (3) endometrial stromal sarcoma, and (4) other sarcomas including müllerian adenosarcoma and lymphoma.

The patterns of spread are similar to those of adenocarcinoma but more extensive. The spread is direct to myometrium, cervix, and contiguous structures and is also lymphatic and vascular (i.e., lungs and liver). Preliminary data indicate that in stage I disease (confined to the corpus), 35.7% of cases had pelvic lymph node metastases and 14.3% had para-aortic node metastases. The most reliable prognostic indicator is extension of the tumor behind the uterus at the time of operation.

Histologically, the number of mitoses per 10 high-power field, although subjective, is important. If more than 10 mitoses are present, the tumor is regarded as highly malignant. If less than 5, the tumor may behave in a benign fashion. The tumors with 5 to 10 mitoses per 10 high-power field are less predictable.

Recurrences occur in over 50% of the cases, even if the disease is apparently localized to the uterus. Over 50% will be outside the pelvis. Unfortunately, there are no characteristic symptoms of sarcoma. Early bleeding does not commonly occur, unless polypoid lesions project into the endometrial cavity. On physical examination, the uterus may be enlarged and there may be a suggestion of fibroids. Rapidly enlarging masses in the uterus, especially of soft consistency, suggest sarcoma, but histological study must be carried out to establish a firm diagnosis.

The **treatment** is total hysterectomy with bilateral salpingo-oophorectomy. Radiation therapy has been effective in only about 25% of the cases but is effective for lymphoma. Combination chemotherapy has shown promise, but the final answer is not available. Estrogen and progesterone receptors have been demonstrated in uterine sarcoma, and preliminary results with the use of antiestrogens such as tamoxifen have been encouraging. Since the uterine sarcoma is a stromal type of tumor, it has been found that the progestational agents have been of benefit in their management.

RADIATION THERAPY IN GYNECOLOGY

A working knowledge of the physics, basic radiation biology, permissible radiation exposure, and the application of radioactive isotopes is important in the evaluation and management of clinical problems in oncology. Because of the great advances made in radiophysics, radiation therapy has become too complex for the average gynecologist. Proficiency in radiotherapeutic techniques demands teamwork between the different specialists and competent radiotherapists and physicists. It is not within the province of this short discussion to create radiotherapists, but certain fundamentals are emphasized so that the gynecologist may be an efficient member of the third therapeutic team.

All matter is made up of chemical substances that can be divided into two kinds—elements and compounds. An element is a distinct kind of matter that cannot be decomposed into two or more simpler kinds of matter. A compound is formed when two or more elements combine together chemically to produce a more complex type of matter. Atoms are the smallest particles of an element that can exist without losing the chemical properties of the element. Molecules are the smallest particles of a compound that can exist without losing the chemical properties of the compound. The atom is an electrical structure having three basic units—the **proton,** the **neutron,** and the **electron.**

This concept is adequate for an understanding of most phenomena in radiological physics. The nucleus contains the protons and neutrons, and the orbits—circular or elliptical—contain the electrons. The simplest atom is one of the elements, hydrogen. This consists of a central nucleus comprising one proton, around which one electron moves in a

H₂ < 1 Proton / 1 electron   helium < 2 Proton / 2 electron — v. light 1/1840 mass g electron

Neutron → Proton + electron

atomic no : no. of Protons i.e no. g electron
mass no.   Protons + neutron.

250   OBSTETRICS AND GYNECOLOGY

shell or orbit. The proton is a heavy particle carrying a positive charge, and the electron is a very much lighter particle with a negative charge with exactly equal magnitude (but of opposite signs) to that of the proton. Therefore, almost all of the nucleus is balanced by the negative charge of the electron to make the atom as a whole electrically neutral.

The next simplest atom is that of the element helium. Its nucleus comprises two protons and two neutrons, and there are two orbital electrons moving around the nucleus. A neutron is a particle with a mass approximately equal to that of a proton but with no electrical charge. The electron is a much lighter particle than a proton, having a mass only 1/1,840 of the mass of a proton, and it has negative charge of exactly equal magnitude (but of opposite sign) to that of the proton. Positrons have the same mass as an electron but with a positive charge existing only while in motion.

The nucleus of a helium atom therefore has a positive charge of two units (due to two protons) and a mass of approximately four units. The two positive charges of the nucleus are balanced by the two negatively charged electrons around the nucleus. Every element has a mass number and an atomic number (Z). The **atomic number** of an element is the number of protons in the nucleus (which is equal to the number of electrons around the nucleus) of an atom of that element. The **mass number** of an atom is the total number of protons and neutrons in the nucleus. It is a measure of the mass of the nucleus, or its **atomic weight**. Protons and neutrons are known collectively as **nucleons** because they are found in the nucleus.

The atomic number is written to the left and below (subscript) the symbol for the element. For sulfur, it is $_{16}$S. The atomic mass is written above (superscript) and to the right—that is, S^{32}. It may also be written with the mass number being placed above the atomic number—that is, 32/16.

An **isotope** is a chemical element having the same atomic number as another (i.e., same number of nuclear protons) but possessing a different atomic mass (i.e., different number of nuclear neutrons). **Isobar** is a term applied to two or more substances that have the same atomic weight but different atomic numbers.

Radionuclide is an atomic nucleus that will decay spontaneously into some other nuclear species, accompanied by the liberation of energy—a nuclear species that is radioactive.

Bremsstrahlung is the name applied whenever high-speed electrons, regardless of their source, are abruptly slowed down and their energy is converted into electromagnetic radiation. If the energy is great enough, the electromagnetic radiation is in the x-ray region. High-energy beta particles, passing close to atomic nuclei and undergoing deceleration, also give rise to bremsstrahlung radiation.

TYPES OF RADIATION EMITTED

These radiations, whether natural or artificial radioisotopes, are of three kinds, named after the first three letters of the Greek alphabet: (1) alpha rays (or particles), (2) beta rays (or particles), and (3) gamma rays (energy). **Alpha** particles are streams of high-speed helium nuclei (two protons and two neutrons packed tightly together) that have been ejected from the radioactive substances. **Beta** rays are streams of fast-moving electrons (particles) ejected from radioactive substances with velocities that may be as high as 0.98 of the velocity of light. In soft tissues, beta rays can travel distances ranging from small fractions of a millimeter up to 1 cm, producing ionization in their path. Beta particles come from a neutron in the nucleus. Neutrons change into a proton and an electron. The electron is then ejected from the nucleus. The emission of the beta particle from the nucleus (beta decay) does not change the mass number (the total number of particles in the nucleus) but does increase the atomic number by 1:

$$_{15}P^{32} \rightarrow {}_{16}S^{32} \pm \beta^\circ$$

Gamma rays come from radioactive substances. When they are produced by electrical machines, we call them x-rays. They differ fundamentally from alpha and beta radiations, as they are not particles but waves of the same type as light and radio waves but with different properties of their very much shorter wavelength.

RADIATION QUANTITIES AND UNITS

1. Units for activity are measured by curie.
2. Units of exposure are measured by roentgen.
3. Units for absorbed dose are measured by rad.

DEFINITIONS

1. Roentgen (R) is a measurement of radiation exposure. It is defined as that amount of x- or gamma radiation such that the associated corpuscular emission per 0.001293 g of air produces in air ions carrying one electrostatic unit of electricity of either sign. A milliroentgen is 1/1,000 of an R.

2. Roentgen-equivalent-man (rem) is defined as that quantity of radiation that produces the same biologic effect in a human as 1 R.

3. The rad is a unit of absorbed dose. It is defined as the energy absorption of 100 ergs per gram of any material (roughly equivalent to the roentgen).

4. Curie (Ci) is the quantity of any radioisotope that disintegrates at the rate of 3.7×10^{10} disintegrations per second. The subunits of the curie unit are as follows: millicurie (mCi) = 0.001 Ci; microcurie (μCi) = 0.001 mCi; millimicrocurie (mμCi) = 0.001 μCi.

5. mgRa (milligram radium) is used for radium only (1 mg of radium = 1 mCi of radium = 8.2 rhcm).

6. mgRaeq (milligram radium equivalent) is used for gamma-emitting radioisotopes, which are applied in radiation therapy as substitutes for radium or radon. It is defined as the activity that produces the same ionization in the air by gamma radiation as 1 mg of radium (1 mgRaeq = 8.25 rhcm).

7. Linear energy transfer (LET) is the energy released (usually in keV) per micron of medium (tissue) along the tract of any ionizing particle.

CHARACTERISTICS OF RADIATION

Radiation can be defined as the propagation of energy through space or matter. In radiology, radiation can be divided into two main groups, corpuscular and electromagnetic.

[handwritten annotations at top:]

Radiator α - high speed helium nuclei (2 protons / 2 electrons) → ejected from radioactive substance

β rays - fast moving electrons in tissue (1mm - 1cm)

velocity 0.98 that of speed of light

like light + radio waves although much shorter wavelength

γ ray - come from radioactive substance (energy - not particles but waves)

when produced by machine, they are called X-rays

Radiations produce their effect principally by the process of ionization—the ejection of outer orbital electrons from atoms.

Corpuscular radiation consists of moving particles of matter. **Electromagnetic** radiation consists of transport of energy through space as a combination of an electric and magnetic field, both of which change in magnitude as a function of time and space.

X-rays and gamma rays are examples of these types of energy. Cesium, radium, cobalt, and x-irradiation are examples of this type of energy.

X- and gamma rays lose their energy in matter by three principal processes (1) photoelectric absorption, (2) Compton scattering, which results in the ejection of an orbital electron, and (3) pair production, which involves a change of the photon energy into mass (a positive and a negative electron are formed).

The radiobiologic effects on cells may be inhibition of cell division, chromosome mutation, or gene mutation. The energy of x-rays or gamma rays may cut through a chromosome, allowing the severed ends to join together with little change of function. The use of potentiators such as hydroxyurea or actinomycin D inhibits the chromosome from reforming.

PHYSICAL ASPECTS OF HIGH-LET PARTICLES :–

Protons, helium ions, and heavy ions are heavy-charged particles. The particles pass through matter and travel in nearly a straight line and come to a stop after passing through a certain depth of absorber, depending on their initial energy.

The rate of energy loss increases sharply near the end of the range. There the dose reaches a peak, known as the **Bragg peak**. The dose falls off very rapidly behind the Bragg peak.

Pions, unlike other heavy, charged particles, are unstable and have a very short half-life. They have not been used in treating gynecologic malignancy. Neutrons interact with tissue and release highly ionizing, heavy, charged particles; most of the dose is controlled by recoiling protons from hydrogen and tissue. Current research with neutron therapy has promised but has not added any significant survival in the treatment of gynecologic cancer.

UNITS OF MEASUREMENT

One electron volt equals 1 eV; 1,000 eV equals 1 kiloelectron volt (1 keV); 1 million eV equals 1 million electron volts (1 meV); 1 billion eV equals 1 beV.

OUTLINE OF STANDARD PELVIC FIELD FOR EXTERNAL RADIATION FOR GYNECOLOGIC CANCER

1. Superior border: A transverse line at the upper end of L5. It is centered on the midline of the vertebral body.

2. Inferior border: A transverse line at the lower edge of the obturator foramen (or pubic symphysis). It is centered on the midline of the pubic symphysis. In stage IIIa (disease extending to the lower vagina), the lower edge of the pelvic field should be extended to include all disease, with at least 1 cm margin.

3. Lateral border: Perpendicular lines on each side, through the center of the acetabulum (it is to be emphasized not the head of the femur).

Using this field, approximately 4,000 to 4,500 rads are given for cancer of the endometrium; for cancer of the cervix, up to 5,000 or 5,500 rads.

Except for stage IaG1 carcinoma of the endometrium, intravaginal radiation is given so that between 3,000 and 4,000 rads are delivered 1 cm below the mucous membrane of the vagina.

In cancer of the cervix, a tandem is placed in the uterus and ovoids in the vagina. The position of the application is checked with x-ray, and the amount of radiation is determined to different points in the pelvis. The usual dose is 6,000 mg hours of radium or cesium.

DIAGNOSTIC RADIOLOGY IN OBSTETRICS AND GYNECOLOGY

The use of radiology in obstetrics has almost been phased out by the increased acceptance of the use of ultrasonography. Radiological studies in obstetrics are reserved for rare cases in which ultrasonography has not provided a positive diagnosis.

The limited use of radiology in obstetrics is a result of (1) fear of radiation injuries to the fetus and to the ovaries of women of childbearing age, (2) the fact that no threshold for gene mutation is known, and (3) the fact that the risk for doubling the rate of spontaneous mutations in humans occurs at exposures from 10 to 140 rad.

ULTRASONOGRAPHY IN OBSTETRICS

Ultrasonic scanning has brought a new dimension to obstetric diagnosis, and its use is now widespread and increasing. Ultrasound is technically defined as sound of higher frequency than that audible to the human ear but in clinical practice is limited to frequencies in the range of 1 to 10^7 cycles per second—that is, 1 to 10 MHz. Obstetric ultrasonic scanning is usually performed in the range of 3 to 5 MHz.

Current methods of examination employ reflected ultrasound to produce an image. The image is built up by energy reflected back from the transmitted beam from the transducer. The reflections come from organ interfaces, vessel walls, and parenchymal tissue. The amount of energy reflected depends on the orientation of the reflecting interface and the difference in acoustic impedence of the tissues at the interface. The beam as it passes is attenuated through tissue, and the degree of attenuation determines the amount of energy reaching a given organ or interface. The ultrasonographic image is the result of the interplay of these two acoustic properties of tissue, reflection and attenuation.

A tissue may be reflecting or nonreflecting, attenuating or nonattenuating. The same transducer is used for both transmitting and receiving; several different methods are used for detecting and displaying reflected echoes. These include A mode or scan, which represents the echo amplitude along a single scan line and is the most accurate method of measuring biparietal diameter. In the A mode, the echoes are displayed as vertical spikes along the baseline of a cathode tube, with the height of the spike related to the amplitude of the detected echo.

D mode or scan represents a cross section of a single slice of the body. A bright spot indicates the position of the echo as the probe moves across the surface of the abdomen. These spots coalesce to give an anatomic outline of the plane of the scan. By scanning a number of overlapping areas, a compound picture is built up on the screen, each arc image being stored by the cathode ray tube (storage scope).

Real-time scanner

A real-time scanner is a machine that gives a moving picture of the fetus. The probe, a rectangular block, contains a large number of transducers (up to 64), which are progressively triggered off at the rate of 30 impulses per second so that the movement of the fetal limbs and trunk may be observed. The real-time scanner is easier to use than the static scanner. It is smaller, mobile, and much cheaper, but at present the picture quality is inferior and the measurements not always totally reliable.

Acuson

The Acuson has unparalleled image quality. It has earlier diagnostic capability, so fewer referrals to other modalities are necessary. It requires fewer examinations per patient. It records not only the fetal appendicular skeleton but also the nonoseous structures of the fetal limbs. Prior to the middle of the second trimester of pregnancy, adequate size and intrinsic subject contrast enable distinction among numerous limb structures.

The Acuson employs a 128-channel phased-array real-time scanner. It gives the best in high-resolution sonographic assessment of the fetal extremities.

Measurements using ultrasonography

With care and experience, very accurate measurements can be made of the fetus from early to late pregnancy. The accuracy of the measurements is restricted by the physical limitations of the instrument as well as by observer error. At 3.5 MHz, the resolution is no better than 1 mm. For practical purposes, this means that the measurements can only be made to the nearest whole millimeter. Electronic calipers on the display screen are now commonly used. Although they make measuring easier, the same limitations of accuracy of measurements apply.

Clinical applications of ultrasonography

The greater availability of ultrasonography machines has led to the widespread use of diagnostic ultrasonography in clinical obstetrics. In addition to ultrasonic fetal monitors of varying degrees of complexity, a simple linear ray real-time scanner is fast becoming part of the normal equipment for both the antenatal clinic and the labor ward.

Ultrasonic scanning in the first and second trimesters

In all ultrasonic examinations in pregnancy, the best image is obtained when the patient has a fully distended urinary bladder. Ultrasonography can be used to (1) diagnose pregnancy, (2) evaluate abortion, (3) detect ectopic pregnancy, (4) diagnose hydatidiform mole, (5) disclose multiple pregnancies, (6) detect congenital anomalies, (7) guide amniocentesis, and (8) direct chorion biopsies.

Ultrasonic scanning in the third trimester

The portability of modern real-time scanning machines allows them to be used in the antenatal clinic and labor ward. They are helpful in evaluating malpresentation and multiple pregnancy, localizing the placenta in cases of antepartum hemorrhage, determining placenta morphology, and assessing the fetal growth pattern. There are other uses of ultrasonography in pregnancy. Fetal respiratory and other movements can be studied by using real-time scanning, as can blood flow in the fetal main blood vessels by making use of the Doppler effect. In general terms, fetal movements and good blood flow are indicators of fetal well-being, which can be modified by external influences. For example, fetal breathing slows considerably with hypoxia or after maternal ingestion of alcohol but is stimulated when the maternal blood glucose level rises. In the future, measurements of blood flow may be used to investigate placental function.

Ultrasonography has been widely used as a diagnostic tool in clinical medicine for more than 25 years. To date, studies have not shown any deleterious effects of ultrasound on the fetus or mother. Considerable research has been carried out on animals and tissues, but the adverse affects that have been reported from some of these studies have occurred with ultrasound intensities, pulse lengths, and exposure far in excess of any that is currently used or likely to be used in obstetric diagnostic ultrasonography. The search for possible hazards will continue, but in the meantime there is no reason to withhold the proven benefits of diagnostic ultrasonography.

RADIOLOGY IN GYNECOLOGY

Ultrasonography has replaced most of the radiological tests that used to be employed in gynecology.

Whenever possible, radiological studies in the female of childbearing age should be performed prior to ovulation (first half of the menstrual cycle). Radiological studies in gynecologic patients have generally related to the evaluation of an infertility problem, evaluation of preoperative patients, GI studies and cholecystograms, and the metastatic workup of patients with pelvic malignancy. This workup should include an intravenous pyelogram, upper and lower GI series, bone surgery, and a liver-spleen scan.

PELVIC ARTERIOGRAPHY

Pelvic arteriography, a method of demonstrating pelvic tumors directly, is based on observation of the displacement of the normal arterial system, the presence of abnormal vessels, and the formation of communications to adjacent arterial systems, attesting to the invasiveness of such a tumor. It has very limited usefulness for assessing tumors of the pelvis exclusive of gestational trophoblastic neoplasms. Arteriography that is properly timed may help diagnose a molar pregnancy. There is early bilateral filling of the uterine veins in the presence of mole or choriocarcinoma, presumably on the basis of arterial venous shunt, which may be present. The test cannot be applied except in rare cases because it may expose a normal pregnancy to excessive radiation.

COMPUTERIZED TOMOGRAPHY

The CT scanner can demonstrate the presence of lymph node metastases not detectable even by laparotomy, and it will increase the accuracy of staging ovarian cancer and of assessing the response of treatment.

The scanner takes repeated pictures of a cross section of the body (nearly 300 pictures within 5 seconds) as the x-ray tube is rotated around the patient. Some absorption of the x-ray takes place, and the amount depends on the density of the tissue through which x-rays pass. Thus, the difference between the amount of radiation entering the body and the amount measured by the detectors is equivalent to the density of the tissues. These measurements are passed through a computer, which performs millions of calculations within a few minutes and reconstructs from the detector findings a cross section of the viscera.

IMMUNOLOGIC SCANNING

Immunologic scanning takes advantage of two facts. First, certain strains in mice are prone to develop malignant myeloma. The cells of these tumors can be fused with mouse antibody, producing cells to form hybrid cells that continue to form antibodies. Second, most human tumors produce substances either peculiar to the tumor or normal but in excessive quantities. These substances can be used as antigens to raise antibodies.

This immunologic scanning has clinical use. The antibody is tagged with a small amount of radioactive substance, such as iodine 123. This is injected intravenously into the patient. After a short time, the tagged antibody will be concentrated in tumor cells of the main growth and secondary deposits. The radioactive tumor masses can then be visualized using a gamma camera. A further development may be the combination of an antibody with an antineoplastic drug. Such a combination would hopefully concentrate in tumor cells and kill them.

CYTOLOGY

Cytological screening of women for the cancer of the vagina, cervix, and endometrium may represent the most important advance in gynecology in this century. Cytology probably makes its greatest contribution as a screening method for the detection of cancer of the cervix. It is also used as a diagnostic method in detecting cancer in other organ systems. In addition, it has been employed as an index of hormonal levels.

BASIC PRINCIPLES

Because of the action of estrogen and progesterone, cyclical changes occur in the vaginal mucosa. These can be identified by examining a stained smear. Such smears can, to some extent, be used as a rough guide to the hormonal status of the patient (Table 3-2).

The maturation index, which expresses the level of cellular maturation attained at the time of exfoliation, is expressed as a ratio of the percentages present of parabasal, intermediate, and superficial cells in that order.

Table 3-2. The Normal Cytohormonal Patterns of the Endocrine Periods

Endocrine period	
Childhood	50/50/0
Perimenarchal	45/45/10
Reproductive period ovulation	0/40/60 to menstruation 0/70/33
Pregnancy	0/95/5
Postpartum	100/0/0
Postmenopausal	0/100/0 or 100/0/0
Atrophic pattern	100/0/0 followed by estrogen therapy will approach 0/50/50
Progestogens	0/100/0
Androgens	100/0/0
Cortison	0/100/0
Ovarian granulosa-cell tumors that produce estrogen produces a shift to the right	0/0/100
Vaginal inflammation	31/35/34
Turner's syndrome	0/100/0, which may shift with age to 100/0/0
Simmonds' disease	100/0/0

There will be 16,000 new cases of invasive cancer of the cervix and an additional 36,000 cancers of the endometrium in the United States in 1988. There has been a decrease in the incidence of invasive cervical cancer in the past 40 years. One of the main reasons for the relative decrease in the incidence of invasive cancer of the cervix is the fact that many lesions were discovered by exfoliative cytology before invasion. Exfoliative cytology (Pap test) is primarily a screening test. It is imperative that a diagnosis be made by biopsy prior to the start of treatment.

The presence of endometrial cells detected on a routine Pap smear demands reevaluation and endometrial aspiration. A routine Pap smear is not adequate to screen the endometrium. Cervical scrapings give a low yield of positive cytology for endometrial cancer, with an average return of about 50%. Posterior fornix scrapings would yield about 65%, and endocervical aspiration about 75%. With the jetwasher or similar method or with Novak suction curettage, the accuracy of diagnosis should exceed 90%. Collection of specimens for screening the cervix may include swabbing, scraping, or aspiration of the cervical canal. A combination gives a higher yield.

PAP TEST

In addition to meeting the criteria for an accurate screening test, the Papanicolaou cytology smear (Pap smear or test) is rapid and inexpensive, involves no apparent morbidity, and the sample is easily obtained. The only disadvantage is the number of false-negative and false-positive results that may be reported. However, a clinician who truly understands its use and a cytologist who is well trained can detect the indications for a repeat test without reporting an inordinately high proportion of false-negative or false-positive results. It is estimated that two or three (some report up to seven) unsuspected cases of cervical cancer per thousand women are usually found by this method.

Collection of Pap smear specimen

A lubricant should not be used on the glove or speculum. The finger and the speculum can be covered with normal saline or water prior to insertion into the vagina. The cervix should be visualized and the excess secretion removed with a cotton swab. A cotton-tipped applicator moistened with saline is introduced into the external os and twisted. The cellular specimen is deposited on the slide by rolling and not by rubbing. The external os should be scraped with a spatula. The end that is shaped to conform to the cervix is inserted into the external os. The spatula is rotated, and again the specimen is deposited on the slide by passing the tip of the spatula and its slanted edges slowly and firmly against the surface of the glass. A glass pipette about 15 cm long and 0.5 cm in diameter, with a strong rubber bulb at one end and a slight curve at the other end, will allow the physician to obtain a good endocervical aspiration.

The laboratory request slip, in addition to the usual identifying data, should include the following information: date of last menstrual period, possible pregnancy, present use of oral contraceptives and intrauterine devices, history of hormonal imbalance or dysfunction, current diagnosis, previous surgery (e.g., conization, biopsy), radiation therapy, the time of the last treatment, and a history of previous cancer.

Reporting results

The cytological diagnosis may be reported using a numerical classification system, a narrative description, or both. A numerical classification introduces a great deal of subjective interpretation. Therefore, many laboratories report the results as positive, negative, or borderline.

A numerical classification based on Papanicolaou's original five-class system or its modification is most often used to report results:

Class I: Negative. Only normal cells are present.
Class II: There are no signs of malignancy; some atypical cells are present.
Class III: Doubtful. The smear contains cells with atypical features suggestive but not diagnostic of malignancy.
Class IV: Positive. Isolated atypical cells are present.
Class V: Positive. Numerous atypical cells or cell groups are present.

The principal use of the method is for the discovery of carcinoma in situ of the cervix and the early diagnosis of cervical and uterine cancer. Much less often, malignant cells from carcinoma of the vagina, fallopian tube, ovary, or metastases in the genital tract may be found. Pap test may be used in the follow-up clinic to detect recurrence of a treated carcinoma.

The concept of a higher-risk population is related to the controversy concerning the optimal frequency of cytological screening. Following the release of the Walton report in 1976,

considerable confusion has surrounded the issue of how often a woman should have a Pap smear. The choice of any screening interval is arbitrary and is usually determined by cost-effectiveness considerations. Lengthening the screening intervals will reduce the overall cost but will increase the number of cancers and higher-grade precancerous lesions whose detection will be delayed.

ENDOMETRIAL SCREENING

The routine cervical-vaginal smear is less effective for detection of endometrial carcinoma than of cervical malignancy. Screening methods applying cytology to detect endometrial abnormalities have been elusive. Screening programs by cytology carried out to identify early changes in cervical abnormalities have not yielded the same results in identifying which patients with early changes in the endometrium will be at risk. The detection rate on routine screening for asymptomatic patients is only about 3% or less of all endometrial cancers. Negative cytological findings do not have the same accuracy in prognosticating, but the development of cancer is highly unlikely because on cytological evaluation the preinvasive lesions are not diagnosed with the same accuracy as is obtained in cancer of the cervix.

The cytologist can diagnose benign and malignant conditions of the endometrium with a high degree of accuracy but has trouble detecting the in-between groups with adenomatous hyperplasia, dysplasia, or cancer in situ. Endometrial hyperplasia develops into endometrial cancer in only 1.5% of patients. Endometrial cancer patients do not have a higher estrogen titer; therefore, factors other than simple prolonged estrogen stimulation must be at work. It is believed that estrogen is not a cell transformer and does not play a role in initiating a cancer of the endometrium but is a cell stimulator that acts as a promoter.

The most optimistic detection rate is 75 to 80%. Taking a vaginal smear from the pool of secretion in the posterior fornix has a relatively better chance of detecting endometrial cancer than does scraping the exocervix. In screening for endometrial cancer, uterine aspiration or washing should be added to the routine Pap smear. The rate of positive returns in asymptomatic women is low, and the discomfort is significant. In women who have symptoms of endometrial cancer or even if there is significant suspicion, fractional curettage is indicated.

The incidence of endometrial carcinoma is increasing. The majority of patients are postmenopausal; 20% are pre- or perimenopausal. The high-risk factors include obesity, nulliparity and low parity, late menopause, hypertension, diabetes, hormone-secreting tumors of the ovary, polycystic ovary syndrome, exposure to ionizing radiation, exogenous estrogen without additional progesterone, and sequential oral contraceptives. In these patients, it is most important to have careful screening and cells must be obtained from within the endometrial cavity.

More work utilizing epidemiologic methods in conjunction with metabolic and animal studies is needed to define the relationship between nutrition and cancer of the endometrium in various populations. The role of nutrition as it may affect production and storage of hormones and the interaction of hormones with cellular receptors are difficult to unravel, particularly because these factors may operate differently in various age-groups. Although research in these areas should be continued, it would seem opportune—from the view of public health—to suggest dietary changes for women on a Western type of diet to one that has less fat and cholesterol.

Recent studies of endocrine status suggest that diet may be an important determinant of endogenous prolactin and estrogen production. Postmenopausal vegetarian women have lower plasma prolactin levels and lower excretion of estrogens in their urine than do nonvegetarian women. Estrogen excretion is also strongly associated with total body weight. Estrogen production in immediately postmenarchal girls has also been shown to correlate strongly with total body fat. These observations suggest that it may be possible to explain the geographic variation in the incidence of breast and endometrial cancer through the influence of dietary factors and endocrine status. If true, this observation has important preventive implications.

CYTOLOGICAL SCREENING

Cytological screening programs carried out to identify early changes in cervical abnormalities have not yielded the same results in identifying early changes in the endometrium in patients who will be at risk. The case identification has been routine by screening of symptomatic patients and is probably less than 75% of the incidence. Negative cytological findings do not have the same accuracy in prognosticating that the development of cancer is highly unlikely, because cytological evaluation of preinvasive lesions has not obtained the same accuracy that is obtained in examination for carcinoma of the cervix. Therefore, it is highly unlikely that screening programs directed at detecting cancer of the endometrium will have a major impact on morbidity and mortality rates in the forseeable future. Recent work by Koss may prove that this statement is not totally valid. He has initiated the study of several thousand asymptomatic, postmenopausal women at the Montefiore Hospital. The study started in January of 1979. He hopes that this study will provide objective evidence as to whether or not endometrial detection is applicable on a large scale and if any of the existing methods do contribute to the salvage of patients. His choices for endometrial cancer detection are twofold: (1) vaginal pool smears and endocervical aspiration smears, with both procedures being within reach of most practitioners; and (2) aspiration of the endometrium, obtained by means of one of the many available instruments, a procedure that necessitates penetration of the internal os and thus causes the patient considerable discomfort. He has identified nine endometrial cancers in the first thousand asymptomatic women screened by his protocol. The cytologist can determine whether the endometrium is benign or malignant but has trouble detecting the in-between groups of adenomatous hyperplasia, dysplasia, or cancer in situ; however, this can be done with a high degree of accuracy if tissues are obtained for paraffin block histological examinations.

ENDOMETRIAL BIOPSY

The Novak or Randall curette is used for endometrial biopsy by Hoffmeister. Others have found that a sharp curette

such as the Kervorkian or the Meigs is easy to use, and the only other equipment needed is a tenaculum. Using negative pressure from the syringe and bringing the curette back with a long, steady stroke gives a strip of tissue that can be easily removed with the fine forceps and placed in a specimen jar. Hoffmeister uses 4 ml of sterile, 5% lidocaine hydrochloride introduced into the uterus through the curette and allowed to bathe the endometrial cavity for 60 seconds; he found that it will afford almost complete topical anesthesia without causing any tissue distortion. It is obvious that negative or inconclusive biopsy findings in a symptomatic patient necessitate further evaluation with fractional dilatation and curettage.

A properly performed fractional dilatation and curettage not only provides diagnostic information about the presence of cancer but also aids in determining the extent of spread.

NOTES REGARDING STAGING AND TREATMENT

The extension of the carcinoma to the endocervix is confirmed by fractionated curettage. Scraping of the cervix should be the first step of the curettage, and the specimens from the cervix should be examined separately. It may occasionally be difficult to decide whether or not the endocervix is involved by cancer. In such cases, the simultaneous presence of normal cervical glands and cancer in the same fragment of tissue will give the final diagnosis.

The presence of metastases in the vagina or in the ovary is sufficient evidence as such to designate a case as stage III.

The 5-year survival reported in the Annual Report on Results of Treatment in Gynecologic Cancer (18th volume) are as follows: stage I, 74.2%; stage II, 57.4%; stage III, 29.2%; stage IV, 9.6%; no stage, 60.8%; and the total overall 5-year survival is 66.6%.

An alternate plan of management for carcinoma of the endometrium is to perform surgery as the primary treatment. Having obtained the specimen, if disease extends to the endocervix or through more than one-third of the myometrium, external x-ray therapy is given. This is carried up to 4,000 rads that is distributed from L5 to the symphysis and laterally through the head of the acetabulum (*Note*: not through the head of the femur). No matter what histological grade or myometrial penetration is reported, all patients receive a vaginal applicator 1 month after surgery. The technique is designed to deliver 3,000 to 4,000 rads at 1 cm below the vaginal mucosa. This has cut down the incidence of vaginal recurrences from 15 or 16% to 1% or less.

HORMONE RECEPTORS

CELLULAR MECHANISMS OF HORMONE ACTION

A new era in cancer endocrinology started with the discovery that breast cancer cells retain the ability to incorporate and retain estrogens, both in vitro and in vivo. The road has been uphill, held back at first by the use of outmoded methodology, but has now progressed through the use of more sophisticated techniques.

At the cellular level, hormones increase the activity of certain enzymes selectively, thereby predictably modifying the cellular function. Although the polypeptide hormones and the steroid hormones initiate their action after they have made contact with the cellular membrane, there are differences in their overall action in bringing about the end result.

CYCLIC AMP

Most of the polypeptide hormones affect cellular metabolism through the adenyl cyclase system. Simply, the circulating hormones bind rapidly and reversibly to a hormone-specific receptor on the surface of the cell membrane. This binding results in activation of the enzyme adenyl cyclase, which converts ATP to cyclic AMP. Phosphodiesterase rapidly converts cyclic AMP to inactivated AMP. Before its inactivation, cyclic AMP activates adenyl cyclase, which modifies cellular function. The hormone disassociates from its receptor site as the hormone concentration outside the cell decreases. The specific hormone as "first messenger" and cyclic AMP as a "second messenger," as outlined above, may be similar for hormones such as insulin and growth hormone, which have not been shown to activate adenyl cyclase but may work through a yet undetermined second messenger.

STEROID HORMONE ACTION

The ability of tissue to bind hormones is secondary to specific hormone receptors located within or on the surface of cells. These receptors apparently interact with a given hormone by combining with hormone, thereby initiating biochemical events characteristic of the function of the particular hormone.

The steroid hormone enters the cell, presumably by passive diffusion, and combines with the specific receptor protein. This reaction is labeled **uptake**. The steroid hormone receptor complex is next activated so that it can enter the nucleus. Entrance of the activated complex into the nucleus is labeled **translocation**. Once inside the nucleus, the steroid hormone-receptor complex associates with the nuclear chromatin, and this event is labeled **retention**. The interaction of the steroid hormones with nuclear chromatins stimulates RNA synthesis, which in turn leads to the synthesis of certain cell proteins. To describe the mechanism of action of estrogens in more detail, it has been shown that estrogens, whether administered pharmacologically or whether secreted by endocrine-active tissue, are carried bound to a plasma transport protein. Estrogens are able to enter the cytoplasm of all cells whether they are target tissues or not. However, in the cytoplasm of target tissues are found specific protein molecules that are termed **receptors**. These proteins combine biologically active estrogens with grade affinity and grade specificity. Following this initial binding step, the steroid receptor complex undergoes a temperature-dependent activation. This activation allows the steroid receptor complex to enter the nucleus of the cell and bind to the chromatin, the location of the genetic information of the cell. Once bound to the chromatin, by a process that is poorly understood, the interaction of the steroid receptor complex with the genetic information of the cells leads to an elaboration of a new species of messenger RNA. These messenger RNA molecules then pass into the cytoplasm of the cell, where they can be usefully translated on polysomes to program amino acids into new protein. It is these new proteins that lead to the induced effects of the steroid hormone.

HORMONE RECEPTOR IN ENDOMETRIAL CANCER

Studies of receptors in endometrial tissue have proved that there are receptors for estradiol and progesterone. In addition, it has been demonstrated that concentration of these receptors varies throughout the menstrual cycle. It has been observed that in the menstrual cycle, estradiol is secreted by the developing follicle and the concentration of estradiol receptors and proliferative endometrium is high. Following ovulation is the development of the luteal phase, which is maintained by the corpus luteum and accompanied by the onset of significant ovarian secretion of progesterone. The estradiol secretion, which was high in the proliferative phase, begins to diminish markedly at this point. Measurement of the estradiol receptors reveals that there is a decrease in not only the cytosol but also in the nucleus. Conversely, there are a few progesterone receptors in the early proliferative phase, but these increase to a maximum at the time of ovulation. Since estradiol secretion is maximum at this point, it is believed that the progesterone receptors increase as a result of estrogen stimulation. Additional studies have shown that receptors are present in both the glandular and stromal cells of the human endometrium.

The next logical step is to use the findings of receptor in the normal endometrium and to apply them to hyperplastic tissue such as adenomatous hyperplasia, also including the various stages that lead up to and include invasive cancer of the endometrium.

CHEMOTHERAPY

Chemotherapeutic (antineoplastic) agents for the treatment of neoplastic diseases are varied in their mechanisms of action; however, they all have the common endpoint of cell destruction. This is accomplished by interfering with one or more of the sequences of replication that all cells undergo. Because, without exception, agents used in cancer chemotherapy all are cell poisons without particular specificity for malignant cells, their toxic effect will extend to normal cells.

In contrast to surgery or radiation, which is considered to be the definitive therapy for cancer, chemotherapy—the treatment of cancer with drugs and hormones—can be used effectively for disseminated as well as localized disease.

CELL KINETICS OR CELL DIVISION

Cellular reproduction (cell division cycle or cell kinetics) is divided into five phases: (1) growth I (GI), which is postmitotic and accounts for at least one-half of the cell division cycle; (2) synthesis (S), in which the DNA content is doubled and accounts for about 20 to 30% of the life cycle of the cell; (3) growth II (GII), which occurs just before mitosis and accounts for about 19 to 20% of the life cycle of the cell; (4) mytosis (M), which accounts for about 1% of the cell's cycle; and (5) growth 0 (G0), the resting of nondividing phase of the cell. This cell phase is variable and depends on the type of cancer.

RESPONSE CRITERIA

Complete response is the complete disappearance of all demonstrable disease. Partial response is 50% or more reduction in the sum of the products of the longest perpendicular diameter of discrete measurable disease, with no demonstrable disease progression elsewhere. No change in the size of any measurable lesion or less than 50% reduction in measure of disease as defined above is considered **no response**. **Progression** is defined as greater than 50% increase in the sum of the products of the largest perpendicular diameter of any measurable lesion.

The term **cure** indicates that the life expectancy of a treated cancer patient is the same as normal life expectancy—specifically, the same as that of a matched cohort in the general population.

PRINCIPAL GROUPS OF ANTICANCER DRUGS

Purine
Antimetabolites (folic acid antagonists)

The **mechanism of action** of antimetabolites is to block folic acid reductates to prevent availability of single carbon fragments. This blocks purine ring biosynthesis. By lesser action, they inhibit methylation of deoxyuridylic acid to thymidylic acid, thus blocking pyrimidine synthesis.

These agents are used in the **treatment** of (1) choriocarcinoma, (2) cancer of the ovary, (3) cancer of the breast, and (4) in combination with other anticancer drugs for treating cancer of the cervix.

Pyrimidine
Pyrimidine antimetabolite (fluorouracil; 5-FU)

Mechanism of action is to block the thymidylate synthetase and inhibit methylation of deoxyuridylic acid, thus blocking pyrimidine synthesis.

5-FU is used in the **treatment of** bladder carcinoma, breast cancer, colorectal cancer, gastric cancer, hepatoma adenocarcinoma, ovarian carcinoma, and pancreatic adenocarcinoma.

Polyfunctioning akylating agents

The **mechanism of action** of alkylating agents is by alkylation (insertion of an alkyl group), interfering with synthesis of cross-linking in a number of places. H-bonding between change of DNA is prevented. A monofunctional compound produces nuclear energy by a sheet mass effect. Polyfunctional agents are 50 to 100 times more active than a monofunctional group. They are cross-linking agents, reactive atoms that bridge two chromosome strands that react at two points on a chromosome.

These agents are used in the **treatment** of carcinoma of the ovary, Hodgkins' disease, lymphomas, Burkitt's tumor, multiple myeloma, cancer of the breast, neuroblastoma, carcinoid, and leukemias.

Other antibiotics

The **mechanism of action** of antibiotics is to form a complex with DNA, involving selective binding at the guanine-cytosine segments, with a specific block in the DNA-dependent synthesis (inhibits formation of messenger RNA).

Antibiotics are used in the **treatment** of lymphomas, leukemia, solid tumors and embryonal tumors, trophoblastic disease, and carcinoid and are used to lower calcium levels (mithramycin).

Doxorubicin hydrochloride (Adriamycin)

Doxorubicin acts by the intercalation between base pairs of DNA, inhibiting DNA-dependent RNA synthesis. It is used in the **treatment** of brain carcinoma and sarcomas in the pelvis.

Mitotic inhibitors

Vinca alkaloids.   The vinca alkaloids arrest mitosis in metaphase by the destruction of spindles. They are used in the **treatment** of choriocarcinoma, lymphoma, leukemia, Hodgkin's disease.

Cis-diamminedichloroplatinum (cis-platinum, platinum diamminodichloride, cisplatin [Platinol]).   This alkylating agent also seemingly acts through an immune mechanism. It is used in the treatment of ovarian cancer in particular but has been employed in all gynecological cancers and a variety of other cancers.

TOXICITY

All antineoplastic drugs are extremely toxic when given in effective dosage, and there is invariably some depression of the **bone marrow and of the cells of the GI tract**. *Cis*-platinum is particularly neurotoxic and nephrotoxic and must be preceded by intravenous hydration and accompanied by mannitol or a diuretic to ensure diuresis. Hexamethylenamine is very neurotoxic. Doxorubicin is cardiotoxic and also causes severe alopecia that requires a wig. Prior to treatment, the patient should always have an ejection factor to test the status of the heart. Other complications include tissue necrosis of the veins and liver failure. Patients taking antineoplastic drugs must be kept under continual supervision, with regular checks on marrow, liver, and kidney function.

RATIONALE IN ANTINEOPLASTIC DRUGS

It is believed that after assault by an antineoplastic drug, tumor cells replace themselves more slowly than normal cells. Treatment is therefore interrupted by rest periods (pulse therapy) to allow the normal tissues to recover.

BIBLIOGRAPHY

Barber HRK, Fields DH, Kaufman SA: Quick Reference to OB-GYN Procedures, 3rd ed. JB Lippincott, Philadelphia (in press).

Burrow GN, Ferris TF: Medical Complications During Pregnancy. WB Saunders, Philadelphia, 1988.

Carlson BM: Patten's Foundations of Embryology. McGraw-Hill, New York, 1981.

Creasy RK, Resnick R: Maternal-Fetal Medicine. WB Saunders, Philadelphia, 1984.

Pritchard JA, MacDonald PC, Gant: Williams Obstetrics. Appleton & Lange, East Norwalk, 1985.

SAMPLE QUESTIONS

Each question below contains five suggested answers. Choose the **one best** response to each question.

1. Which of the following statements is true?

    A. Ova complete the first meiotic division before birth
    B. The second meiotic division occurs at puberty
    C. Primary oogonia are haploid
    D. The second polar body is formed during meiosis II
    E. All ova formed by the mother are genetically equivalent, so variation is supplied by the sperm

2. In electronic FHR monitoring, which of the following indicates hypoxia?

    A. Poor beat-to-beat variability
    B. Accelerations with contractions
    C. Type I decelerations
    D. Type II decelerations
    E. Type III decelerations

3. Vaginal delivery should NOT be attempted in subsequent pregnancies after

    A. maternal eclampsia in previous pregnancy
    B. cesarean section for CPD in previous pregnancy
    C. maternal surgery for berry aneurysm
    D. classical cesarean section for placenta previa in previous pregnancy
    E. intramural myomectomy

4. Increased maternal mortality is associated with

    A. thalassemia minor
    B. severe Rh disease
    C. cytomegalic inclusion disease
    D. sickle cell disease
    E. preeclampsia

5. Fractional dilatation and currettage reveal endometrial carcinoma involving the cervix. This finding is

    A. of no prognostic significance
    B. of minor prognositc significance but does not require change in management
    C. significant only if the cervical tumor is clinically obvious
    D. significant even if the disease is present only microscopically
    E. contraindicative for hysterectomy

6. The cardinal symptom of endometrial cancer is

    A. abnormal uterine bright red bleeding
    B. bloating
    C. change in bowel habits
    D. cramps
    E. swelling of the abdomen

7. Dysfunctional uterine bleeding is frequently associated with

    A. endometrial polyps
    B. anovulation
    C. cervicitis
    D. systemic lupus erythematosus
    E. von Willebrand's disease

8. What is the most accurate method of diagnosing an ectopic pregnancy?

    A. Pelvic ultrasonography
    B. Culdocentesis
    C. Measurement of serial HCG
    D. Laparoscopy
    E. Endometrial biopsy

9. The major portion of the blood supply to the pelvis is derived from the

    A. internal iliac arteries (hypogastric)
    B. external iliac arteries
    C. uterine arteries
    D. iliolumbar arteries
    E. internal pudendal arteries

10. The uterovaginal canal contacts the posterior wall of the urogenital sinus, producing the

    A. urogenital bud
    B. urogenital tubercle
    C. müllerian tubercle
    D. genital bud
    E. sinovaginal bulb

11. Characteristics of a hydatidiform mole include all of the following EXCEPT

    A. enlargement of the villi
    B. absence of fetal tissue
    C. proliferation of the lining trophoblast
    D. presence of villous blood vessels
    E. edema of the villi

12. All of the following have been implicated as negative side effects of the barrier methods of contraception EXCEPT

    A. toxic shock syndrome
    B. urinary tract infection
    C. pregnancy rate between 5 and 15%
    D. congenital anomalies
    E. salpingitis

13. Ovarian cancer is of increasing importance because

    A. newer chemotherapeutic measures are more effective
    B. newer diagnostic methods are detecting earlier stages
    C. it is a disease of the adolescent period
    D. death rates from other pelvic malignancies are dropping
    E. it is usually secondary to cancer of another organ

14. Germ cells migrate into the gonad from

A. the germinal epithelium of the gonad
B. the ovarian cortex
C. the müllerian duct
D. the mesonephros
E. none of the above

15. Approximately what percentage of women with tubual tuberculosis will have concurrent endometrial involvement?

A. Less than 10%
B. 25%
C. 50%
D. 75%
E. Over 90%

16. All of the following signs or symptoms have been associated with danazol treatment for endometriosis EXCEPT

A. acne
B. weight gain
C. hot flashes
D. mucoid vaginal discharge
E. decreased breast size

17. The most important etiologic abnormality in the anatomy of the urethra and bladder that leads to stress incontinence is

A. loss of estrogen in the postmenopausal period
B. loss of normal urethral length
C. loss of normal urethral position when supine
D. loss of posterior urethrovesical size and angle of inclination
E. rapid weight loss

18. The neoplasm most sensitive to appropriate chemotherapy is

A. gestational trophoblastic disease
B. ovarian dysgerminoma
C. Burkitt's lymphoma
D. endometrial carcinoma
E. ovarian serous carcinoma

19. All of the following statements regarding ovarian carcinoma are true EXCEPT that

A. it is the most common gynecologic cancer
B. it has the highest mortality rate among the common gynecologic cancers
C. it tends to be asymptomatic until it has reached an advanced stage
D. its development may be influenced by environmental, cultural, or socioeconomic factors
E. Pap smears are ineffective for routine diagnostic screening

20. If a woman presents with a chronic yeast infection, it is important to elicit a history of all of the following EXCEPT

A. diabetes
B. pregnancy
C. use of antibiotics
D. use of oral contraceptives
E. use of vinegar douches

21. A history of acute pelvic inflammatory disease is most commonly associated with which of the following events?

A. Intrauterine device insertion
B. Sexual intercourse
C. Dilatation and curettage
D. Endometrial biopsy
E. A recent menstrual flow

22. The most common cancer among females in the United States is that of the

A. lung
B. ovary
C. breast
D. stomach
E. large bowel

23. Among female, the cancer that causes the most deaths is that of the

A. lung
B. ovary
C. breast
D. stomach
E. large bowel

24. After age 50 years, all women should have a mammography

A. twice a year
B. once a year
C. every 18 months
D. every 2 years
E. only if they have a breast lump

25. Breast carcinoma cannot be palpated until its diameter reaches

A. 1 cm
B. 2 cm
C. 3 cm
D. 5 cm
E. 6 cm

26. All of the following statements about endometriosis are true EXCEPT that

  A. evidence of malignant changes is rare
  B. diagnosis usually can be established by history and physical examination
  C. although present in postmenopausal women, it is most common in women in their reproductive years
  D. affected women may present with infertility
  E. the most common site of involvement is the ovary

27. The best landmark for determining where to separate the rectus muscles in a midline incision is the

  A. urachus
  B. umbilicus
  C. linea nigra
  D. pyramidalis muscles
  E. midline of the symphysis pubis

28. The main health hazard of the menopause is

  A. cardiovascular disease
  B. pelvic relaxation
  C. endometrial cancer
  D. depression
  E. osteoporosis

DIRECTIONS: Each question below contains four suggested answers of which **one** or **more** is correct. Choose the answer:

  A if 1, 2, and 3 are correct
  B if 1 and 3 are correct
  C if 2 and 4 are correct
  D if 4 is correct
  E if 1, 2, 3, and 4 are correct

29. Progesterone has significant effects on

  1. cervical mucus
  2. vascular tone
  3. intestinal motility
  4. ureteral motility

30. Open neural tube defects may be detected by

  1. maternal serum alpha-fetoprotein testing
  2. level 3 ultrasonography
  3. amniocentesis
  4. chorionic villus sampling

31. Laboratory studies that may be used to help document the menopause include

  1. maturation index
  2. serum estriol
  3. FSH assay
  4. urinary pregnanediol

32. Prerequisites for forceps use include

  1. vertex presentation
  2. fully dilated cervix
  3. station of presenting part at least +2
  4. ruptured membranes

33. Multiple gestation is associated with an increased risk of

  1. prematurity
  2. gestational diabetes
  3. breech presentation
  4. preeclampsia

34. Intrauterine infection is common in a pregnant woman who develops

  1. AIDS
  2. syphilis
  3. rubella
  4. toxoplasmosis

ANSWERS

1. D		18. A	
2. D		19. A	
3. D		20. E	
4. D		21. E	
5. D		22. C	
6. A		23. A	
7. B		24. B	
8. D		25. A	
9. A		26. B	
10. C		27. D	
11. D		28. E	
12. E		29. E (all)	
13. D		30. A (1,2,3)	
14. E		31. B (1,3)	
15. C		32. C (2,4)	
16. D		33. E (all)	
17. D		34. E (all)	

4

PEDIATRICS

Audrey K. Brown

THE MAJOR DISEASES OF THE NEWBORN

Diseases of the newborn can be thought of as occurring because of certain unique characteristics of this age-group:

1. Diseases attributable to varying degrees of **immaturity of organ systems**, such as respiratory distress syndrome (immaturity of the lung), susceptibility to sepsis (immaturity of several aspects of immune defense), and hyperbilirubinemia (immaturity of hepatic conjugating function).
2. Diseases related to **congenital defects**, such as cardiac defects, neural tube defects, and tracheoesophageal fistula; these defects become manifest early.

A third group of illnesses unique to the newborn are those related to the **maternal-fetal interactions**, such as Rh and ABO isoimmunization and neonatal thrombocytopenic purpura. In both of these conditions, the mother develops antibodies to the red cells or platelets of the fetus because antigens on these cells are different from the mother's own. These antibodies cross the placenta and destroy the infant's cells.

Special consideration must be given to the lack of usual clinical findings in patients in this age-group. One must rely on the **general signs presented by the infant**, in particular the infant's general appearance, degree of activity, pattern of feeding, and color. Major clues may be obtained by discerning whether the infant is **cyanotic, pale, plethoric, or jaundiced.**

In addition, the maternal history is a most important part of the past history of the newborn infant. A complete history must be obtained of the events during pregnancy as well as a past history of the mother's health, in order to ascertain what is likely to be going on in the infant. Maternal habits such as the use of alcohol, drugs, and cigarettes have a profound effect on the size of the infant, as well as the development of specific disorders.

RESPIRATORY DISTRESS AND CYANOSIS

Respiratory distress and cyanosis are common signs of severe illness in the newborn. The neonate is subject to a variety of disorders, many of which are related to anatomic and biochemical developmental phenomena. Examples of **anatomic derangements** are described in the paragraphs that follow.

Infants with **esophageal atresia** with tracheoesophageal fistula have copious secretions, which may obstruct the airway and lead to respiratory distress. The diagnosis can be made when a nasogastric tube fails to pass into the stomach. X-ray reveals the tube coiled in a blind esophageal pouch.

Choanal atresia is obstruction of the posterior nasal airway by a membranous or bony septum, representing developmental failure of the bucconasal mucosa to rupture. Since newborn infants are obligate nose breathers, bilateral atresia presents soon after delivery as airway obstruction, apnea, and cyanosis. Diagnosis is made by inability to pass the suction catheter through the nostrils into the oropharynx. Emergency management consists of establishing an airway until definitive surgical reconstruction can be performed in the neonatal period.

Pulmonary hypoplasia, with decreased numbers of alveoli and capillary beds, presents as severe respiratory distress. Small lungs and a small thoracic cage are seen on x-ray. A major cause of this syndrome is diminished amniotic fluid volume (oligohydramnios), which can result from early rupture of fetal membranes or lack of fetal urine formation because of nonfunctioning kidneys or urinary tract obstruction. Diaphragmatic hernia or other intrathoracic space-occupying lesions may also result in pulmonary hypoplasia. When oligohydramnios is the cause, the infant may have the characteristic facies of **Potter's syndrome.**

In the premature infant in particular, one must look beyond cyanosis for clues to differentiate congenital heart disease from respiratory distress syndrome, which occurs in about 20% of infants born between 28 and 32 weeks of gestation. Shortly after birth, these infants develop nasal flaring, grunting, tachypnea, chest wall retraction during inspiration, and cyanosis. During the next 12 to 24 hours, these symptoms worsen and respiratory acidosis develops. X-rays of the lungs show diffuse ground-glass opacification of the lung fields.

Therapy includes assisted ventilation, often with continuous positive airway pressure. Oxygen delivery is monitored and acid-base disturbances corrected. More recently, surfactant preparations have been blown into the airway of such infants, and these early trials are encouraging. Bronchopulmonary dysplasia with eventual pulmonary fibrosis may develop in some infants who have required prolonged assisted ventilation and oxygen therapy. Another complication in these premature infants who have required high concentrations of oxygen is **retrolental fibroplasia**, a major cause of blindness in childhood.

NEONATAL SEPSIS

Neonatal sepsis can in large measure be attributed to a poorly developed immune defense system in the newborn infant. These developmental deficiencies include defects in leukocyte function as well as the fact that only IgG and not IgM antibodies cross the placenta. The incidence of neonatal sepsis varies but can be up to 9 or 10 per 1,000 in some nurseries. Scrupulous hand washing by personnel as well as meticulous care with even minor invasive procedures can contribute to reduction in nursery infection rates. Bacterial sepsis can be due to almost any organism, and the major cause varies from nursery to nursery as well as with time. In the past, group A beta-hemolytic streptococci and *Staphylococcus aureus* were major threats. In recent years, group B beta-hemolytic streptococci have been a major etiologic agent. Other organisms colonizing the maternal vagina or GI tract may cause sepsis in the newborn without adversely affecting the mother.

The signs of neonatal sepsis are subtle at first, but progression may be rapidly overwhelming. Initial lethargy and poor feeding, hypotonia, or rapid respirations may be the initial signs, with rapid development of septic shock. Fever is not a common sign, and the normal leukocytosis of the neonate gives way frequently to leukopenia and even agranulocytosis (i.e., less than 500 absolute neutrophil count) early in the course of sepsis.

Evaluation and initiation of therapy should be done rapidly. A spinal tap is indicated to detect meningitis. Broad antibiotic coverage, directed at both gram-negative and gram-positive organisms, should be initiated immediately without waiting for identification of the causative agent; it can be changed or curtailed if necessary after identification and knowledge of antibiotic sensitivity are obtained. Attempts to augment therapy of this catastrophic event through the administration of granulocytes and/or intravenous gamma-globulin are being studied.

Not only are newborns uniquely susceptible to bacterial infections, but they are also subject to **congenital infection** acquired in utero. These infections may be viral, protozoal, spirochetal, or bacterial; the degree and nature of the effect on the fetus depend not only on the dose of the infecting agent but also on the time in gestation when the infection occurs. Congenital defects of the heart, eyes, and liver occur as a result of maternal infections such as rubella during morphogenesis of the embryo.

Maternal varicella in early pregnancy can lead to an infant who is small for gestational age (SGA), with chorioretintis, mental retardation, seizures, muscle atrophy, scarring of the skin, and an increased susceptibility to infection. If the maternal infection occurs later in pregnancy, it may lead to subclinical infection in the infant and an increased likelihood of herpes zoster infection later in childhood. Maternal varicella at the time of delivery can result in severe disease in the infant.

A newborn infant who has hepatosplenomegaly, anemia, thrombocytopenia, frequently with petechiae or purpura and jaundice, often with evidence of CNS involvement, and signs characteristic of multisystem congenital infection is said to have **TORCH syndrome,** and a search is made for the causative agent. These causative agents have been grouped under the acronym TORCH, which stands for **T**oxoplasmosis, **R**ubella, **C**ytomegalovirus, and **H**erpes simplex virus.

An increasing number of infants are born infected with the acquired immunodeficiency syndrome (AIDS) virus, or human immunodeficiency virus (HIV), formerly called HTLV-III. These infants are not usually recognized until they show signs of failure to thrive or develop secondary infections, usually pneumonia. Most of these infants are born to mothers who have acquired the virus through intravenous drug abuse or from infected partners. The mothers need not have overt signs of disease at the time of delivery. Some infants have acquired the virus from blood products administered in the nursery. There is growing awareness of the need for screening for viruses and special treatment of blood products to make them safer, especially for this very susceptible newborn population.

AIDS is becoming a leading cause of death in infants and children beyond the neonatal period.

JAUNDICE IN THE NEWBORN

Newborn infants are born with an umbilical cord bilirubin level of 1.8 to 2.8 mg/100 ml, a value that is elevated by adult standards. After birth, the level usually rises, and in full-term infants the mean peak value of 4.5 to 5.0 mg/100 ml is reached between the second and third day of life. By the end of the first week of life, the serum bilirubin level has fallen to 1 to 2 mg/100 ml in normal full-term infants.

Many factors can alter this pattern of physiological jaundice. The primary factor is the degree of prematurity or immaturity. This phenomenon can be best understood by appreciating that the fetal metabolism of bilirubin is different from that required in extrauterine life, and the more immature the infant the more fetus-like will be his or her system for clearing this lipid-soluble tetrapyrrole that is the end product of heme metabolism. In intrauterine life, unconjugated bilirubin formed from the degradation of heme is cleared from the fetal circulation via the placenta. Only unconjugated bilirubin and not conjugated bilirubin crosses the placenta. Several steps in the clearance of bilirubin are not needed and in fact would be disadvantageous for the fetal clearance of bilirubin, since it reaches the maternal circulation if it remains in the unconjugated form. Therefore, it is not surprising that the fetus does not develop the glucuronide-conjugating system until late in gestation.

It is interesting that the fetus also has an increased amount of intestinal beta-glucuronidase, which can degrade any conjugated bilirubin glucuronide back to the unconjugated form. Further, the fetus has an enhanced capacity for the intestinal reabsorption of unconjugated bilirubin. These fetal characteristics promote the clearance of unconjugated bilirubin via the placenta even during late gestation, when systems that will be required after birth are in the process of developing.

The more immature the infant, the more likely it is that he or she will, like the fetus, tend to keep the bilirubin in the unconjugated form. The glucuronyl transferase system will be limited, intestinal beta-glucuronidase will be increased, and the capacity to reabsorb bilirubin from the intestine will be high. In extrauterine life, these fetal characteristics are disadvantageous, since the infant can no longer clear this potentially toxic substance via the placenta. In the infant as in the adult, clearance of bilirubin is accomplished by hepatic conjugation of bilirubin and subsequent excretion of the bilirubin-diglucuronide into the intestine, where it is reduced to form urobilinogen and stercobilinogen through the action of bacteria. In a sense, the intestine completes the process of clearance initiated by the liver. Conjugation by the liver not only renders the pigment water soluble, but, in that form, the pigment, once excreted into the bile, is not reabsorbed across the intestinal mucosa.

From this description, it is evident that the more premature the infant the greater the likelihood that he or she will have a high level of unconjugated bilirubin (hyperbilirubinemia). The mean peak bilirubin in prematures is 9 to 10 mg/100 ml, and this peak occurs later than in term infants, at about the seventh day of life or later, depending on the degree of prematurity.

Hyperbilirubinemia in an infant is described as bilirubin level above the physiological range. Although definitions vary, there are pragmatic reasons for considering a level of 10 to 12 mg/100 ml as deserving special attention in either full-term or premature infants, and such infants should carry the diagnosis of hyperbilirubinemia rather then physiological jaundice. This is done to alert those caring for the infant to examine the infant closely, seeking factors that might account for this exaggerated finding: Hemolysis is the leading cause of rapid rise in bilirubin and jaundice *in the first day of life.* Other pathology is often characterized by jaundice, such as sepsis, maternal diabetes, and galactosemia. In term breast-fed infants, the level of bilirubin is often exaggerated, particularly if feeding is not kept up during the night.

It is equally important to assess the infant for factors that might render bilirubin toxic to the infant regardless of the cause of the elevated bilirubin. These factors include hypoxia, acidosis, extreme prematurity, hemolysis, and drugs that displace bilirubin from albumin.

Unconjugated bilirubin can cause **kernicterus** (bilirubin encephalopathy). It is generally thought that unconjugated bilirubin that is dissociated from albumin (i.e., free bilirubin) is the toxic form. Sulfisoxazole (Gantrisin) causes kernicterus in infants by displacing bilirubin from albumin. The serum bilirubin is deceptively low in such infants, since the dissociated bilirubin moves into the tissues including the brain. Osmotic opening of the blood-brain barrier to bilirubin has recently been proposed as a major factor in the production of kernicterus or bilirubin encephalopathy.

Hyperbilirubinemia can be prevented in very small infants by the early institution of **phototherapy**.

Exchange transfusion is still the only means of rapidly removing bilirubin that has risen to levels above about 15 mg/100 ml, but phototherapy instituted when bilirubin is 10 mg/100 ml or less can usually curtail the rise.

Levels of **direct-reacting (conjugated) bilirubin** in normal infants are less than 1 mg/100 ml; levels above that may mean poor laboratory technique or a type of pathology that leads to biliary tract obstruction. An increased level of conjugated bilirubin is never physiological; it occurs commonly in association with sepsis, congenital systemic infections, galactosemia, or alpha$_1$-antitrypsin deficiency, as well as in neonatal hepatitis and biliary atresia. Urinary tract infections are often associated with a cholangitis, which leads to direct bilirubinemia.

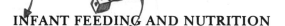

INFANT FEEDING AND NUTRITION

Most term infants gain weight satisfactorily during the first 6 months of life if their calorie and water requirements are met by the consumption of 90 to 120 calories/kg and 150 to 200 ml/kg/day. Although this can be accomplished with either breast milk or formula feeding, human milk is the ideal food for these infants. **Breast-feeding** has many advantages, including the high biologic value of the protein in human milk, the presence of antibodies, low electrolyte content, and a calcium-to-phosphorus ratio favorable for high calcium absorption. In addition, breast-fed infants have a low incidence of allergy and a lower rate of infection. In recent years, there has been increasing effort to develop formulas that more closely simulate human milk by lowering the saturated fat content, increasing the unsaturated fat, lowering the protein and salt content, adjusting the calcium-to-phosphorus ratio, and using lactose almost exclusively as the source of carbohydrate.

Breast-fed infants of mothers who are well nourished do not require vitamin supplements, unless the mother is not exposed to sunlight. Infants of such mothers should be given 400 IU of vitamin D. If water in the area is not fluoridated, 0.25 mg of fluoride should be given daily.

ARTIFICIAL MILK FORMULAS

Artificial formulas that simulate human milk are diluted to contain 67 calories/100 ml and are fed to provide 150 to 200 ml/kg/day in infants less than 1 year of age. These formulas contain sufficient vitamins so that no supplementation is necessary. In areas in which water is not fluoridated, fluoride drops should be given daily.

Although solid foods may be introduced at 4 to 6 months, the potential for obesity is increased because of the high caloric density.

At 1 year of age, the calorie requirement decreases to 80 to 100 calories/kg; after that, most children adjust calorie requirements to need. A general estimate is 1,000 calories + (age in years × 100 calories).

FAILURE TO THRIVE

Calorie deficiency is the leading cause of failure to thrive and in severe form it is known as marasmus. In developed countries, maternal ignorance, neglect, or emotional disturbance is usually responsible. Other causes include failure to compensate for increased calorie requirements or losses.

Since children should be gaining weight, the diagnosis of failure to thrive applies not only to children with obvious weight loss, but also to children who fail to gain. As the calorie deficiency progresses, there is not only weight loss but failure of head and chest circumference to increase, and wasting of cheeks, buttocks, and fat pads.

Disorders in which calorie requirements are increased include hypermetabolic states such as fever, infection, heart disease, hyperthyroidism, and anemia.

Calories are lost or wasted in renal disease, diabetes, diarrheal disorders, regional enteritis, ulcerative colitis, celiac disease, and cystic fibrosis. Calorie intake in excess of calorie expenditure leads to obesity; the exact role of genetics and

---

family patterns is unknown. Hypothyroidism, hypothalamic lesions, and emotional disturbances can lead to obesity.

PROTEIN MALNUTRITION

There are several grades of protein malnutrition, and when calorie intake is adequate, weight loss may not occur. When protein malnutrition is severe, **kwashiorkor** develops. In this disorder, serum proteins are low and there is anemia. The striking characteristic physical findings include a change in hair color to a reddish blond, abdominal distension, edema, and rash. There is usually lethargy and diarrhea, and infections are frequent.

HEALTH SUPERVISION

Guidelines for health supervision of children and adolescents have been developed for children receiving competent parenting and in whom there are no manifestations of serious health problems and no problems in growth and development. Health supervision, beginning with the care of the newborn in the hospital as well as continuity of care, comprehensive in nature, is strongly advocated for the health maintenance of children.

A major feature of the health supervision visits is the recording of objective measurements of height and weight throughout childhood, and additionally measurement of head circumference in the first year of life. Developmental and behavioral assessment are also important features of the regular comprehensive care offered to infants and children.

Another major feature of preventive pediatric care is the regular schedule for active immunization. Table 4-1 represents the presently recommended schedule for immunization in normal infants and children. Other schedules have been developed for immunization of those who missed being immunized in the first year of life.

Table 4-1. Recommended Immunizations of Normal Infants

Age	Immunization
2 months	DPT and trivalent oral polio vaccine (TOPV)
4 months	DPT and TOPV
6 months	DPT (TOPV optional)
1 year	Tuberculin test (should be done at the time of or preceding administration of measles vaccine; repeat annually or biannually
15 months	Measles, rubella, and mumps
18 months	DPT and TOPV
4–6 years	DPT and TOPV
14–16 years	Tetanus and diphtheria toxoids

OBJECTIVE MEASUREMENTS OF PHYSICAL GROWTH

The average full-term male infant weighs 3.27 kg at birth; the female infant averages 3.23 kg. The range is from 2.5 kg to 4.6 kg. Infants weighing less than 2.5 kg are considered low birth weight and may be term or preterm (see the section on the newborn).

Approximately 10% of initial weight may be lost in the first 3 to 4 days of life and represents loss of extracellular fluid and meconium as well as relatively limited intake. Most infants regain their birth weight by 10 days of age. Weight gain in the first 6 months of life averages 20 g/24 hours, decreasing to 15 g/24 hours during the second 6 months of life. In term infants of average weight, the weight usually doubles by 4 to 6 months and triples by 1 year of life. In the second year, the average weight gain is 2.5 kg, and then 2.0 kg/year for the next 3 years. From age 5 years until the adolescent growth spurt, there is steady gain of about 3 kg each year. Table 4-2 lists useful formulas for determining normal height and weight.

At birth, the term male infant's median length is 50.5 cm, (49.9 cm for females). In the first year of life, length increases by about 50%. In the second year, the child grows about 12 cm, and between the third and fifth year, the child grows at a rate of about 7 cm/year. From 5 years of age until the adolescent growth spurt, height increases by about 6 cm/year.

Head circumference during infancy is an index of brain growth. The DNA content of the brain increases during the first 6 months of life and then plateaus; head circumference follows the same pattern. Head circumference at birth is 34 to 35 cm; it increases by 10 cm in the first year. After that, the rate of increase diminishes, and from 5 years of age until maturity, it averages 1.25 cm/year. Small head size is commonly encountered with congenital infections. In addition, in severe prenatal as well as in severe postnatal malnutrition, growth failure can include failure of the brain and head to grow, even though there is a tendency to spare the brain in comparison with other parts of the body.

BONE AGE

Ossification centers form at different ages, and therefore analysis of x-rays of the hands and feet provides a basis for estimating bone age. At birth, about 90% of full-term infants have five ossification centers: the calcaneus, the cuboid, the talus, and the ends of the distal femur and proximal tibia.

Until the age of 6 years, an estimate of bone age is roughly as follows: age in years + 1 = the number of ossification centers in the wrist.

Table 4-2. Useful Formulas for Height and Weight

3 to 12 months of age: weight in pounds = age in months + 11

2 to 12 years: (age in years × 5) + 18

Between 2 and 12 years, a child's height can be estimated as: height in inches = (age in years × 2) + 32

MOTOR DEVELOPMENT

As indicated above, preventive pediatric management requires assessment of development throughout the formative years of childhood. There is orderly progression in the child's capacity to function; the sequence is dependent in large measure on the gradual maturation and myelination of the nervous system.

Assessment of development includes evaluation of gross and fine motor skills as well as language and social development. Major developmental milestones are outlined in Table 4-3.

Milestones in language and social skills are outlined in Tables 4-4 and 4-5.

Evaluation of these developmental sequences is important in order to recognize signs of either delayed development or regression. The precise timing of the deviation from the

Table 4-3. Milestones in Motor Development

Motor function	Approximate age
Grasp reflex	At birth
Sits with support	3 to 4 months
Intentional reaching	4 to 5 months
Palmar grasp	6 to 8 months
Sits unaided	7 to 8 months
Pincer grasp	9 to 10 months
Stands alone briefly	12 to 13 months
Walks unaided	12 to 15 months
Builds a 6-block tower	24 months
Climbs onto furniture	24 months
Walks up stairs (one step at a time)	24 months
Rides tricycle	36 months
Reproduces a cross with crayon	36 months

Table 4-4. Milestones in Language Development

Language skill	Approximate age
Indistinct noises	3 to 5 weeks
Cooing	10 to 12 weeks
Syllables	6 to 8 months
Three-word sentences	36 months
Six- to seven-word sentences	48 months

Table 4-5. Milestones in Social Development

Social skill	Approximate age
Responsive smile	4 to 6 weeks
Smiles at self in mirror	6 months
Responds to "no"	8 months
Frightened by strangers	8 to 10 months
Knows own gender	24 to 30 months
Plays in parallel with another child	24 to 36 months

normal sequence is invaluable in identifying the cause of poor development or regression.

ADOLESCENT DEVELOPMENT

The average age of onset and duration of the stages of pubertal development in the female and the male are outlined in Table 4-6.

Most pubertal physical changes occur during early adolescence, usually through age 14. During this period, adolescents need reassurance that their bodies are developing normally. These physical changes are accompanied in many adolescents by mood swings and problems related to peer pressure, the need for privacy, and the development of adult identity. These problems may become quite stressful. These stresses may lead to depression and attempted suicide.

Special health problems emerge in adolescents, such as disorders of menarche as well as sexually transmitted diseases like *Chlamydia*, gonorrhea, *Gardnerella*, syphilis, and trichomonas vaginitis. Eating disorders including anorexia nervosa and bulimia are common. Bulimia is binge eating followed by purging through vomiting and/or the use of laxatives or diuretics.

Substance abuse with cigarettes, alcohol, and drugs is a common problem. Cocaine use, particularly in the form of "crack," has been increasing. All these abuses compromise health, and chronic substance abuse leads to disordered psychosocial development.

CHILDHOOD INJURY AND POISONING

During the past 4 years, injuries (accidents) have become the leading cause of death in childhood. Each year 20,000 children (to age 19) die from injuries.

In childhood, the death rate of 30.3 per 100,000 from injury is four times greater than from any disease. Each year, about 20% of all children receive injuries severe enough to require an emergency visit; 17% of hospitalizations of children are related to injuries.

Obviously, the types of injuries that children experience relate chiefly to their stage of development, their degree of

Table 4-6. Stages of Pubertal Development

Male genital development

Stage I   Preadolescent; testes, scrotum, and penis are the same as in childhood.

Stage II   Testes and scrotum enlarge, skin over the scrotum becomes red and altered in texture; penis enlarges slightly.

Stage III Testes and scrotum continue to grow; penis enlarges.

Stage IV   Testes and scrotum continue to grow; scrotal skin darkens; penis grows in width and glans penis develops.

Stage V   Mature; penis, testes, and scrotum are adult size and shape.

Female breast development

Stage I   Preadolescent; juvenile breast has elevated papilla and small, flat areola.

Stage II   Breast bud forms, papilla and areola elevate as a small mound, and diameter of areola enlarges.

Stage III Breast increases in size, elevating papilla; areola continues to enlarge.

Stage IV   Areola and papilla separate from the contour of the breast to form a secondary mound.

Stage V   Mature; the areolar mound recedes into the general contour of the breast; papilla continues to project.

Pubic hair development

Stage I   Preadolescent; fine vellus hair covers the genital area.

Stage II   Sparse distribution of long, slightly pigmented hair at base of penis in males, bilaterally along medial border of labia majora in females.

Stage III Pigmentation increases; hair begins to curl and spread laterally but in scant amount. Spreads over mons pubis in females.

Stage IV   Hair continues to curl and becomes coarse in texture. Adult distribution is attained, but amount remains sparse.

Stage V   Mature. Hair has adult distribution with spread to surface of medial thigh; forms triangular pattern in females; pubic hair grows along the linea alba in 80% of males.

mobility, and their sense of danger. For example, in the second 6 months of life, infants can reach and grasp and put objects in their mouths. As a result, mechanical suffocation becomes a leading cause of death.

Among adolescents, peer pressure may lead to dangerous activities including injuries related to substance and alcohol abuse. Adolescence is also a period when a sense of peer or family rejection may lead to suicide attempts. A stressful or disorganized home environment is thought to be a major factor accounting for increased risk of injury or "accident."

CHILD ABUSE

Child abuse can present as an acute injury or the history of recurrent injury. The circumstances surrounding any injury must be sought in detail to screen for abuse or neglect. Suspicion of child abuse is raised when there are recurrent injuries, marks of inflicted injury, injuries atypical for the child's developmental stage, or a history of events inconsistent with the nature or degree of the injury.

Particular injuries known to be associated with child abuse include scald burns of the buttocks, burns from cigarettes, subdural hematoma, retinal hemorrhage, rib fractures from the "shaken baby syndrome," and spiral fractures of the femur.

SUICIDE

Both suicide attempts (a serious effort) as well as gestures that represent cries for help occur primarily among adolescents. Injuries from gunshot wounds, single-passenger automobile accidents, or poisonings must not only be managed acutely but the underlying motive or problem must be explored in order to prevent repeat attempts.

Suicide is the third leading cause of death among adolescent males and the fourth leading cause among female adolescents.

MOTOR VEHICLE ACCIDENTS

The leading cause of death between the ages of 6 months and 19 years is trauma from motor vehicle accidents in which the injured child is a passenger; 9,000 such deaths occur each year. The peak ages are infancy, 2 months, and adolescence.

Drivers 16 to 18 years of age have a fatality rate that is 8 to 10 times higher than that of 30-year-old drivers, and adolescent drivers are also more likely to kill others in a collision. Alcohol abuse is a major factor in adolescent motor vehicle-related death.

Use of infant car seats, as well as the use of seat belts in older passengers, is the most useful means of preventing injury or death among passengers in automobile accidents. Such use potentially promises to reduce fatality rates by 90% and morbidity by 50%. Falls are the most common cause of injury in the home and rank as the fourth leading cause of death from injuries.

DROWNING

Drowning is the third most common cause of accidental death in children and the second most common cause of accidental death among adolescents. The peak incidence for both sexes is between the ages of 1 and 5 years. There is a second peak for males 10 to 15 years of age.

CHOKING

The most common cause of injury-related death in children under 1 year of age is foreign body aspiration. The younger the child, the higher the involved site; the larynx is the common site in children younger than 1 year. In children 1 to 4 years old, the trachea and bronchi are most commonly involved. Upper airway obstruction, which is manifested by gagging, choking, wheezing, aphonia, or dysphonia, may cause asphyxiation and is an immediate threat to life.

Wheezing and asymmetric or absent breath sounds signal lower tract obstruction. The more distal the site of obstruction, the longer it may be tolerated.

ACCIDENTAL POISONING

Each year, poisoning occurs in 2,000,000 children younger than 5 years. A second peak occurs among adolescents, most often as a suicide gesture or attempt. Over-the-counter and prescription medications account for 45% of all childhood poisonings; aspirin and acetaminophen (Tylenol) are commonly used drugs. Fifty percent of ingestions involve cleaning agents, insecticides, toiletries, paints, and paint solvents. Parental consultation with poison control centers is helpful both in management of potentially serious ingestions and in providing reassurance in cases of ingestion of benign substances.

In one survery of poison control centers, 75% of calls were related to poisons of low toxicity; 20% of cases required rapid removal of the poison, and fewer than 5% required intensive emergency medical management. Removal of gastric contents as soon after ingestion as possible is the first line of defense. Among children, emesis is more effective and less traumatic than gastric lavage; administration of syrup of ipecac (10 ml in children younger than 1 year; 15 ml in those over 1 year) is followed by emesis in about 20 minutes. Its use is contraindicated in infants younger than 6 months of age, in children with a decreased level of consciousness, or when volatile hydrocarbons or corrosive substances have been ingested.

Emetics are not effective in cases of ingestion of antiemetics or the chlorpromazine group of tranquilizers.

Activated charcoal quickly absorbs a wide spectrum of material. Some agents that are not absorbed include iron, boric acid, cyanide, mineral acids, caustics, and lithium. Since the activated charcoal renders ipecac ineffective, it should not be administered until vomiting induced by ipecac is over.

After the gastric emptying and charcoal absorption, administration of a cathartic reduces transit time and moves toxins through the GI tract.

LEAD POISONING

Five to 15% of children in the United States have absorbed abnormally high amounts of lead. Plumbism is a chronic disorder in which acute episodes occur. Some sources of the lead include paint in old buildings, household dust in old houses, exposure to lead smelting or to contaminated work clothes, food from lead-glazed ceramic pots, burning of battery cases, and sniffing leaded gasoline.

Symptoms include pica, apathy, clumsiness, and intermittent vomiting. Lethargy, stupor, ataxia, vomiting, and eventually coma and seizures are symptoms of acute encephalopathy. Chronic lead poisoning may manifest as behavioral or attention disorder, developmental delay, seizures, and peripheral neuropathy, particularly in children with sickle cell anemia. Biochemical evidence for plumbism includes elevated blood lead level, increased free erythrocyte protoporphyrin (FEP), as well as increased urinary excretion of lead following calcium EDTA.

The most important aspect in the management of childhood lead poisoning is the interruption of the child's intake of lead, usually by separating the child from home until the home environment is lead free.

Children with systemic lead poisoning should receive a chelating agent. Following this, oral D-penicillamine can be given for 2 to 6 months to prevent rebound increases in the blood lead level. Although treatment of asymptomatic children is controversial, chelation is also suggested for children with both an elevated blood lead level and biochemical evidence of adverse effects of the lead such as an elevated FEP.

GENETIC DISORDERS AND BIRTH DEFECTS

The background risk for medically significant birth defects is of the order of 3 to 5% of live-born infants. Not all of these defects are detected at birth. Some are diagnosed later in life, such as forms of kidney disorders, congenital heart disease, and mental retardation. Congenital anomalies cause about 10% of all neonatal deaths. Birth defects are caused by environmental factors as well as genetic disorders. Environmental factors cause about 10% of all birth defects. Teratogens from the environment include infection, chemicals, and radiation, as well as physical or structural forces that cause congenital anomalies by interfering with fetal organogenesis or cellular physiology. The cause of some birth defects is of course unknown, and such defects are termed sporadic. Some may be due to new autosomal dominant mutations; these are difficult to distinguish from sporadic birth defects.

Dysmorphism is an abnormality in form; there are many causes of dysmorphic features. For example, inadequate amniotic fluid (oligohydramnios) results in severe fetal constraint and may be associated with hypoplasia of the lung. External mechanical forces can lead to disruption of fetal blood supply. Among such forces is the formation of bands of tissue from the amniotic sac, which can cause hypoplasia of the limbs or transverse amputations.

An important example of a teratogenic disorder is the fetal alcohol syndrome (FAS). Alcohol is the most common known teratogen to which the fetus may be exposed. FAS occurs in 1 to 2 per 1,000 in most populations, and it is estimated that 10 to 20% of mild to moderate mental retardation may be due to the effects of alcohol in utero.

Fetal alcohol syndrome manifests as a growth deficiency with facial dysmorphism and other anomalies, as well as CNS dysfunctions. The average IQ of the affected child is about 63. There is poor fine motor coordination, tremulousness, and irritability in infancy. Brain disorganization, or scrambled brain, due to aberrant nerve cell migration may occur. There may also be microcephaly. Birth weight and length may be below the third percentile. The facies show a characteristic dysmorphism, including a small midface area; a long, smooth philtrum; and a smooth, thin upper lip with poor definition. There may be decreased joint mobility, clinodactyly, rib abnormalities, renal structural malformations, and cervical vertebral fusion (Klippel–Feil anomaly). There are no data to support a safe amount of alcohol use during pregnancy, but the syndrome usually occurs in offspring of pregnant women who drink more than 4 to 6 alcoholic drinks a day. The effect of small amounts of alcohol or even occasional binge drinking are really not known, and women are advised to avoid alcohol entirely during pregnancy.

GENETIC DISORDERS

Genetic disorders are classified as single-gene disorders, chromosomal disorders, or multifactorial disorders. Individuals have between 30,000 and 50,000 genes. There have been 3,000 disorders already described due to alterations of single genes. Single-gene disorders may be inherited as autosomal dominant, autosomal recessive, or X-linked.

CHROMOSOMAL DISORDERS

Human individuals have 46 chromosomes, 22 pairs as autosomes and one pair of sex chromosomes. Females have two X chromosomes and males one X chromosome and one Y chromosome. One member of each pair of chromosomes comes from each parent; alterations in the amount of chromosomal material are usually associated with birth defects.

Autosomal dominant disorders

Genes on chromosomes numbers 1 to 22 are autosomal genes, and autosomal dominant conditions become manifest when one gene of a gene pair is altered. An individual who has an autosomal dominant condition has a 50% chance of passing the mutant gene to each offspring and thus a 50% chance that each child will be affected.

An example of a common autosomal dominant disorder is **Marfan's syndrome**. This disorder of connective tissue occurs with an incidence of 1 in 20,000. A syndrome believed to be due to an abnormal cross-linking of collagen results in structural abnormalities in four major systems. In the skeletal system, the characteristic body habitus includes unusually long, thin limbs; scoliosis, a spine deformity; pectus excavatum; long spider-like fingers and toes; hypermobile joints and a long thin face with a high, narrow palate. The eyes are usually affected; severe myopia is common, and lens subluxation may occur. The most serious medical complication occurs because of the effect on the cardiovascular system. There is dilatation of the aortic root due to abnormal connective tissue in the vessel wall, leading to aortic insufficiency; dissection and rupture of the aorta can occur. Frequently there is mitral valve prolapse. In childhood, there is a high incidence of spontaneous pneumothorax due to rupture of pulmonary blebs and emphysema because of abnormal connective tissue in the bronchial tree. Since there is a high incidence of new mutations in this disorder, only 70 to 85% of affected individuals have an affected parent. Therefore, in addition to taking a family history, it is necessary to examine parents and siblings of a patient suspected of having this disorder. There is marked variability of expression of Marfan's syndrome. Preventive surgery to replace the proximal aorta after aortic enlargement has occurred can significantly decrease the mortality rate.

Autosomal recessive disorders

Autosomal recessive disorders occur when both genes of a gene pair are mutant. When both members of a gene pair are mutant, the individual is said to be homozygous for that specific gene or disorder. If an individual carries only one mutant and one normal gene for a gene pair, the individual is said to be heterozygous for that gene pair and usually displays no clinical effect from the single mutant gene. Parents of a child who has an autosomal recessive disorder and who are clinically well are heterozygous for that gene. With each pregnancy, there is a 25% risk of having another child with the same disorder.

Many autosomal recessive disorders are due to mutations in genes that code for enzymes. The amount of normal enzyme activity found in the heterozygote, although only half that of normals, is adequate under most circumstances.

Inborn errors of metabolism are usually due to autosomal recessive disorders, although a few may be X-linked. Clinical features that are helpful in detecting inborn errors include vomiting, acidosis, or hyperammonemia; in disorders of amino acid metabolism or carbohydrate metabolism, the unusual odor of urine or sweat occurs, as in maple syrup urine disease. Hepatosplenomegaly can occur as a result of accumulation of metabolites within the liver or spleen. Other common symptoms include growth retardation and seizures. Mental retardation occurs with the accumulation of metabolites in disorders such as **phenylketonuria** (PKU). A family history of early infant death should alert one to the possibility of an inborn metabolic error. Certain ethnic groups have an increased risk of specific metabolic errors; **Tay-Sachs disease** is seen most frequently among Ashkenazi Jewish as well as French Canadian populations.

Perhaps the best-studied and most common of amino disorders is **PKU**, an autosomal recessive disorder occurring in 1 in 12,000 live births. The defect is in the enzyme phenylalanine hydroxylase. The deficiency prevents the conversion of phenylalanine to tyrosine, and there is buildup of toxic metabolites. Although the damage is done very early, PKU may not be symptomatic in early infancy; the most significant manifestation is moderate to severe mental retardation. Since there is a block in the conversion of phenylalanine to tyrosine, hypopigmentation is a common sign since tyrosine is necessary for the production of melanin. Dietary restrictions of phenylalanine must start very early in infancy, before the age of 1 month, and lifelong restriction is recommended. Most states in the United States have mandatory newborn screening programs to identify infants with this disorder so that proper dietary restriction may begin early to prevent mental retardation. Women who have PKU and who have discontinued dietary restrictions are at increased risk of having children with birth defects including microcephaly, congenital heart disease, and mental retardation.

Galactosemia is an example of a serious inborn error of carbohydrate metabolism. In this autosomal recessive disorder, there is a deficiency of the enzyme galactose-1-phosphate uridyl transferase resulting in impaired conversion of galactose-1-phosphate to glucose-1-phosphate. Symptoms are noted within a few days to weeks of initiation of milk feedings; initial symptoms include hepatomegaly, vomiting, amino aciduria, and grwoth failure. One can detect nonglucose reducing substances in the urine, including galactose and galactose-1-phosphate. Confirmation of the diagnosis is made by demonstrating the absence of galactose-1-uridyl transferase in erythrocytes. Therapy for galactosemia is the elimination of all formulas and foods containing galactose. If the diagnosis is made and treatment is initiated early, most treated individuals have normal intelligence. Untreated infants often die from inanition or *Escherichia coli* sepsis; untreated survivors suffer from birth retardation, mental retardation, and cataracts.

X-linked disorders occur when a male inherits a mutant gene on the X chromosome that he has received from his mother. His mother is usually hereterozygous for that gene, since she usually has one normal and one mutant gene. She may demonstrate partial manifestation of the disorder, since only one of the two X chromosomes in any cell is transcriptionally active, according to the Lyon hypothesis. Common X-linked disorders include **hemophilia A, color blindness, Duchenne's muscular dystrophy, and glucose-6-phosphate dehydrogenase deficiency,** as well as **ornithine transcarbamylase deficiency.** In this latter disorder, the male infant usually dies from severe hyperammonemia.

Chromosome disorders occur in 5 of 1,000 live births (0.5%). Among chromosomal disorders are autosomal trisomies, the word *trisomies* referring to the fact that three rather than two copies of specific chromosomes are present in the cell. The most common autosomal trisomy is **trisomy 21, Down's syndrome,** which occurs in 1 of 700 live births. Ninety-five percent of children with Down's syndrome have 47 chromosomes, since there are 3 number 21 chromosomes. The risk of having a child with Down's syndrome increases with maternal age; this risk increases dramatically after maternal age of 35 years. (Nevertheless, most children with trisomy 21 are born to women younger than 35, since most women bear children before age 35.) Four percent of children with Down's syndrome have 46 chromosomes, with translocation of a third chromosome 21 to another chromosome, usually in a D group or G group.

Children with Down's syndrome have a characteristic appearance due to dysmorphic features: a flat facial profile; a short, upslanting palpebral fissure; Brushfield's spots; a flat nasal bridge with epicanthal folds; and a small mouth with a protruding tongue. The ears are short, and the earlobes are folded down. Other dysmorphic features include microcephaly, flat occiput, excess posterior neck skin, short stature, and short hands. There is an incurved fifth finger with a hypoplastic middle phalanx and a single palmar crease. There is a gap between the first and second toe.

Hypotonia is most apparent in the newborn. Cardiac defects are a major cause of death. Fifty percent of these children have endocardial cushion defects and/or septal defects; about half of these are fatal. GI abnormalities, chiefly duodenal atresia and Hirschprung's disease, are the second most common abnormalities of the intestinal organs.

Developmental delay is seen early; mental retardation is later evident in most individuals. The mean IQ is 50. As more children survive into adulthood, it has become apparent that a pattern of dementia that resembles Alzheimer's disease develops in the third or fourth decade.

Another common trisomy is trisomy 13, occurring in 1 in 4,000 to 1 in 10,000 live births. Characteristically there is microcephaly, with open skin lesions of the scalp, cleft lip and often cleft palate, severe CNS malformation, eye malformations, polydactyly, omphalocoele, genital malformations including ambiguous genitalia in males, congenital heart disease, and severe mental retardation.

Sex chromosome disorders affect the number or actual structure of the X or Y chromosomes. Included in this group is **Turner's syndrome,** which affects 1 in 2,500 newborn girls. More than half of those with the Turner's phenotype have a 45,X karyotype. Others (about 10%) have an alteration in the structure of one of the X chromosomes. About 15% of the Turner's phenotype are mosaic for two or more cell lines; usually one is 45,X and the other 46,XX or 46,XY. If a girl with Turner's syndrome has a cell line with Y chromosome, bilateral gonadectomy is indicated because of the risk of a gonadoblastoma.

The dysmorphic features of Turner's syndrome include lymphedema of hands and feet at birth, webbed neck, shield-shaped chest, short stature, increased carrying angle of the forearm, and multiple pigmented nevi. Malformations that occur include gonadal dysgenesis and congenital heart disease (aortic stenosis, bicuspid aortic valve, or coarctation of the aorta). Renal anomalies such as horseshoe kidney or reduplication of the collecting system occur in about 40% of the cases. Autoimmune thyroiditis is common, as are learning disorders.

Klinefelter's syndrome is a sex chromosome disorder that occurs in 1 in 1,000 live-born boys. Most patients have a 47,XXY karyotype. Clinical features in Klinefelter's syndrome vary. The affected male is taller than others in the family; arm span is greater than height. After puberty, there is incomplete masculinization and a female body habitus. The testes are small and spermatozoa production low, leading to infertility; the latter may be a feature that leads to a diagnosis missed in childhood. There is slight increased frequency of mental retardation; the mean IQ is 90. There may be behavioral problems.

SOME MARKERS OF GENETIC DISORDERS

Mental retardation is frequently an indicator of a genetic disorder. Autosomal dominant disorders that cause mental retardation include **tuberous sclerosis and mytonic dystrophy;** autosomal recessive disorders include **PKU** and **mucopolysaccharidoses.** An example of an X-linked cause of mental retardation is the **fragile X syndrome. Prader-Willi syndrome** and **Down's syndrome** are also examples of chromosomal disorders associated with mental retardation.

Pubertal disorders can in some cases be linked to sex chromosome abnormalities, such as Turner's, Klinefelter's, or Prader-Willi syndrome.

Predisposition to cancer is evidenced by cancers occurring at an earlier age than expected, which may be related to single-gene disorders including those leading to breast cancer and colon cancer (e.g., **Peutz-Jegher's syndrome, familial polyposis**).

Autosomal dominant seizure disorders may present in adolescence or adulthood.

INFECTIOUS DISEASES

STREPTOCOCCAL AND NONSTREPTOCOCCAL PHARYNGITIS

One of the most common problems in pediatric practice is the management of the child with pharyngitis. The main concern relates to group A streptococci (GAS), which are recovered from 20 to 40% of cases. There are many nonstreptococcal causes of pharyngitis, including *Mycoplasma pneumoniae*, adenoviruses, influenza and parainfluenza viruses, and enteroviruses. The most common cause among young children is adenovirus; in older children it is Epstein-Barr virus. Diphtheria is rare, and usually a membrane is present. Pharyngitis due to *Neisseria gonorroheae* also should be considered in adolescents as well as in abused children; a special medium is required for culture of these organisms.

Since studies have clearly demonstrated that penicillin therapy of GAS can prevent acute rheumatic fever, the management of children with pharyngitis includes throat cultures and the administration of penicillin for 10 days to those children with cultures positive for GAS. This is still the recommended practice even though there has been a marked decline in the incidence of rheumatic fever in the United States in recent decades. There is, however, an ongoing reevaluation of this practice, including more rigorous attempts to identify the factors that characterize the manifestations of GAS pharyngitis in children in an effort to exempt some children from this approach while still assuring appropriate therapy to those with GAS.

The clinical manifestations of GAS pharyngitis classically include fever, chills, severe sore throat, headache, and abdominal pain in a child with a beefy red pharynx, petechiae on the soft palate, pharyngeal exudate, and tender anterior cervical adenitis. However, this picture is only found in about 20% of children with this infection. Age is one of the determinants of a variant pattern. Children less than 3 years of age, for example, usually have moderate fever, cough, coryza, vomiting, anorexia, pharyngeal injection without exudate, and moderate cervical adenitis. In this age-group, suppurative complications including otitis media are common.

SEPSIS AND BACTEREMIA

Both sepsis and septicemia are severe and overwhelming infections with bacteria in the bloodstream. Bacteremia is a laboratory diagnosis referring to a positive blood culture. The clinical features usually include fever and the appearance of being seriously ill, though in septic neonates these symptoms may be lacking. There may be septic shock and disseminated intravascular coagulopathy (DIC). The history and physical examination should address the possibility of an obvious source of infection such as a site of infection elsewhere or previous instrumentation such as cannulas or contaminated infusions; possible host defense defects should be sought.

Meningitis

Bacterial meningitis is an emergency; early, intensive appropriate therapy is essential for the prevention of brain damage and death. Purulent meningitis is predominantly a disease of childhood; more than 65% of cases occur in children younger than 5 years. *Hemophilus influenzae* meningitis accounts for more than half the cases between 1 month and 5 years of age. Between 5 years and 30 years of age, more than half the cases of bacterial meningitis are due to meningococci; after the age of 30, pneumococci are the predominant cause.

As mentioned in the section on the neonate, the most common causes of meningitis in the first 30 days of life are enteric bacteria, chiefly *E. coli* and group B streptococci. Other organisms that cause meningitis in the newborn but only rarely later on include other enteric gram-negative rods, as well as *S. aureus* and *Listeria monocytogenes*.

Meningococcemia

Meningococcemia is the prototype of fulminating bacteremia in a previously normal child. There is usually high fever and a petechial rash. Progression is rapid; myocarditis, shock, and DIC with purpura may occur early and are the common mechanisms of death. Securing an intravenous route for fluid therapy takes precedence over a lumbar tap in children who present in septic shock. In meningitis, CSF pleocytosis is variable and is usually not among the early fulminant manifestations. Early diagnosis and prompt appropriate management offer the only hope.

Fulminant pneumococcemia

The clinical picture and typical course of this disease are similar to that described above for meningococcemia. However, fulminant pneumococcemia usually occurs in individuals with impaired host defense, notably in those with absent or nonfunctioning spleens as in sickle cell disease. These children also have an increased susceptibility to fulminant septicemia from another encapsulated bacterium, *H. influenzae*. Vaccines are available for both of these organisms, but unfortunately they are not very effective in infants less than 2 years of age because they lack the capacity to respond optimally to polysaccharide capsular antigens. Antibiotic prophylaxis against pneumococci is employed prior to the age of 2 years. It should be noted that *H. influenzae*, *Streptococcus pneumoniae*, and *S. aureus* are the most frequent causes of positive blood cultures in children.

Staphylococcal sepsis

Acute disseminated staphylococcal septicemia can occur with or without a preceding focus of infection in previously healthy children, especially in older children and adolescents. The patient appears very ill and toxic. DIC with petechiae and purpura can occur. As part of the process of dissemination, bone and joint pain, rashes, lung nodules, hematuria, jaundice, and seizures can occur. Focal microabscesses may occur anywhere. The CSF and urine may show a minimal number of leukocytes.

Group A streptococcal sepsis

Typically, bacteremia due to GAS occurs as a complication of cellulitis or bone or joint infection, with wound infections, or with the skin lesions of chicken pox. Less frequently, a primary bacteremia without an obvious focus can occur and can be followed by overwhelming sepsis, often with embolization and secondary foci in the lungs, meninges, and skin.

Antibiotic treatment of presumed septicemia

When children present with presumed septicemia, antibiotics should be begun immediately even though information concerning bacterial susceptibility is not yet available. The selection is based on clinical assessment and opinion concerning the likely organism; therapy should be optimal for all likely possibilities.

Throughout infancy and childhood, infections are the most common causes of diarrhea; these include both infectious diarrheas as well as infections outside the GI tract that are frequently associated with diarrhea in infants. In contrast to infants with diarrhea from improper feeding, infants with infectious causes of diarrhea appear ill. They may have fever, and some may have CNS signs, depending on the causative agent.

Enteropathogenic *E. coli* as well as the enterotoxigenic and enteroinvasive *E. coli, Shigella, Salmonella,* and reovirus-like organisms are common causes of infectious diarrhea. Diarrhea associated with non-GI infections and diarrhea due to anti-biotics are more common in children than in adults.

Chronic diarrhea in children has a host of causes, extending from minor disorders or even misinterpretation of physiological responses to those that are severe and life threatening. These problems are discussed in the section on gastrointestinal disorders.

SPECIAL CONSIDERATION CONCERNING FLUID THERAPY IN INFANTS AND CHILDREN

The pathophysiological effects of reduction of fluid intake or increase in fluid losses occur more rapidly in infants than in adults. As a result, infants and young children are particularly at risk from illnesses that lead to vomiting and/or diarrhea, which seriously affect fluid balance.

Fluid therapy for children with dehydration should be considered in three phases: **deficit therapy** to replace losses of fluid and electrolytes that occurred prior to institution of medical care, **maintenance therapy** to make up for ongoing normal and abnormal losses, and **supplemental therapy** to provide specific fluids that may be required in certain diseases.

Basal amounts of fluid and electrolytes are lost in urine, sweat, and feces. In addition, water is lost from the lungs as evaporation in exhaled air. The amount and type of these losses vary with disease states.

Maintenance fluid and electrolyte requirements are related to metabolic rate and can be determined if the patient's caloric expenditure can be estimated.

A relatively simple method for calculating caloric expenditure from body weight is outlined in Table 4-7. These values are for the average hospitalized patient with normal activity in bed.

For every 100 kcal expended, 100 ml of fluid should be

Table 4-7. Simplified Method for Calculating Caloric Expenditure From Body Weight

Body weight (kg)	Caloric expenditure per day
Up to 10	100 kcal/kg
11–20	1,000 kcal + 50 kcal/kg for each kg above 10
>20	1,500 kcal + 20 kcal/kg for each kg above 20

administered; this solution should contain 25 mEq of sodium and 20 mEq of potassium per liter and 5% dextrose. If there is physical activity, these caloric expenditure estimates should increase by 20%. Reduced intake with normal losses and excessive losses with or without usual intake lead to deficits in body water and electrolytes. Deficits in water and electrolytes are relatively similar irrespective of the precipitating cause. Therefore, management is dictated chiefly by the severity and type of deficit rather than the underlying cause.

The type of deficit depends on the relative magnitudes of loss of water and of electrolytes, chiefly sodium. In dehydrated patients, serum sodium may be normal, low, or high depending on the relative loss of fluid and electrolyte. When serum sodium is 130 to 150 mEq/L, dehydration is termed isonatremic; if the level is less than 130 mEq/L, dehydration is hyponatremic. When serum sodium is above 150 mEq/L, dehydration is hypernatremic.

In **isonatremic dehydration**, the major fluid loss is from the extracellular compartment. In **hyponatremic dehydration**, there is movement of fluid from the extracellular compartment into cells, leading to further depletion of extracellular fluid and some increase in intracellular fluid. In **hypernatremic dehydration**, fluid moves out of the cells, depleting the intracellular volume; depletion of extracellular fluid is less than expected. These three types of dehydration lead to differing physical findings, as outlined in Table 4-8.

In addition to the relative loss of sodium, dehydration is classified according to the extent of fluid loss; on this basis, the degree of dehydration may be mild, moderate, or severe. Table 4-9 outlines the major signs of these three degrees of dehydration.

The **principles of therapy** of dehydration are essentially the same for widely different etiologies. Though management of a dehydrated patient in shock is a medical emergency, it should be remembered that most errors in fluid management occur in the initial stages of rehydration. Every effort must be made to assess the patient's state of hydration and the magnitude of electrolytes required for patients with severe dehydration. *Oral rehydration is usually appropriate for those with mild or moderate dehydration.*

Parenteral rehydration is accomplished in three phases: first, the emergency phase; second, the phase of repletion; and third, the phase of early recovery.

The goal of the **initial or emergency phase** is rapid reexpansion of extracellular fluid volume to improve circulatory dynamics and renal function. If there are no manifestations of circulatory deficit (no tachycardia), the emergency phase may merely consist of a more rapid rate of infusion during the subsequent or repletion phase of therapy.

If emergency-phase treatment is required, it may be implemented by administration of 20 ml/kg of single-donor plasma or 5% albumin. This is followed by administration of 20 ml/kg of a solution of 10% glucose in water. These infusions are given rapidly. The total volume for the emergency phase is 40 ml/kg to be administered over a 1-hour interval. (An alternate approach to this phase involves the use of an aqueous solution. Initially a 10% glucose solution to which 75 mEq/L of sodium, 55 mEq/L of chloride, and 20 mEq/L of bicarbonate is added, for a total volume of 40 ml/kg in the first hour.)

Over the next 7 hours, the **repletion phase** should be accomplished to restore the interstitial fluid. *In the first 8 hours of*

Table 4-8. Physical Signs in Various Types of Dehydration

	Isonatremic dehydration	Hyponatremic dehydration	Hypernatremic dehydration
ECF volume*	Markedly decreased	Severely decreased	Decreased
ICF volume*	Maintained	Increased	Decreased
Physical signs			
Skin turgor	Poor	Very poor	Fair
Mucous membrane	Dry	Slightly moist	Dry
Eyeball	Sunken and soft	Sunken and soft	Sunken
Fontanel	Sunken	Sunken	Sunken
Mentation	Lethargic	Coma	Hyperirritable
Pulse†	Rapid	Rapid	Moderately rapid
Blood pressure†	Low	Very low	Moderately low

*ECF = extracellular fluid; ICF = intracellular fluid.
†Signs of shock rather than of dehydration itself.

Table 4-9. Clinical Aspects of Various Degrees of Dehydration

Signs and symptoms	Mild dehydration	Moderate dehydration	Severe dehydration
General appearance and condition:			
Infants and young children	Thirsty; alert; restless	Thirsty; restless or lethargic but irritable to touch or drowsy	Drowsy; limp, cold, sweaty, cyanotic extremities; may be comatose
Older children and adults	Thirsty; alert; restless	Thirsty; alert; postural hypotension	Usually conscious; apprehensive; cold, sweaty, cyanotic extremities; wrinkled skin of fingers and toes; muscle cramps
Radial pulse	Normal rate and strength	Rapid and weak	Rapid, feeble, sometimes impalpable
Respiration	Normal	Deep, maybe rapid	Deep and rapid
Anterior fontanel	Normal	Sunken	Very sunken
Systolic blood pressure	Normal	Normal or low	Less than 90 mm; may be unrecordable
Skin elasticity	Pinch retracts immediately	Pinch retracts slowly	Pinch retracts very slowly (>2 seconds)
Eyes	Normal	Sunken (detectable)	Grossly sunken
Tears	Present	Absent	Absent
Mucous membranes	Moist	Dry	Very dry
Urine flow	Normal	Reduced amount and dark	None passed for several hours; empty bladder
% body weight loss	4–5%	6–9%	10% or more
Estimated fluid deficit	40–50 ml/kg	60–90 ml/kg	100–110 ml/kg

Modified from World Health Organization guide.

therapy *(in the first two phases of emergency, 1 hour + 7 hour repletion)* *50% of the planned first day's fluid volume should have been administered.* Five percent glucose rather than 10% is used after the first hour. The sodium content of the fluid is adjusted according to need, ranging from 40 to 80 mEq/L. After the patient voids, parenteral potassium, 20 mEq/L, may be added.

The **early recovery phase** takes place over the remaining two-thirds of the day. The rate of fluid administered during this period is slower than in the first 8 hours. For example, in a patient with 10% deficit (100 ml/kg), 60 ml/kg is given over a period of 16 hours. If tolerated, an oral glucose and electrolyte solution may be substituted for intravenous fluids.

A special approach must be used in **hypernatremic dehydration.** The therapy must take into account its distinct pathophysiology and potential complications. In 20% of such patients, hypocalcemia may occur, and in about one-third there is hyperglycemia.

Rapid infusion of 5% glucose must be avoided since it causes a rise in CSF pressure from swelling of brain cells (not edema) and may lead to convulsions.

A solution that has a low glucose as well as a high potassium content to offset cerebral swelling should be administered at a slow, even rate. One ampule of 10% calcium gluconate should be given for every 500 ml of infusion. In infants with hypernatremic dehydration, the rate of infusion of fluid should be relatively slow, about 6 to 7 ml/kg/hour.

DISEASES OF THE KIDNEYS

This section addresses the common disorders of the kidney in childhood and includes a discussion of the differential diagnosis of the symptoms of edema, hypertension, and/or hematuria of renal and nonrenal origin. Renal tumors are discussed in the section on tumors of childhood.

CONGENITAL RENAL DEFECTS

As with other organ systems, congenital defects of the kidneys should be given strong consideration when confronting a child with renal disease. Congenital hydronephrosis and congenital hydroureter are relatively common disorders in infants and may even be detected by sonography before birth. They are often associated with anomalies of the lower GI tract. Posterior urethral valves are a significant cause of hydronephrosis in boys, and such infants may present because of failure to thrive.

NEPHROTIC SYNDROME

Idiopathic nephrotic syndrome of childhood is a disorder of unknown etiology characterized by proteinuria, hypoproteinemia, edema, and hyperlipidemia. About 60% of the children between the ages of 1 and 6 years with nephrotic syndrome have minimal change (nil) disease. This term refers to the "nil lesion" of the kidney on light microscopy, consisting of effacement of epithelial foot processes.

Renal biopsy is no longer recommended in nephrotic syndrome in children between 1 and 6 years of age unless unusual features are present, such as findings suggestive of a nephritic component such as hematuria, severe hypertension,

depressed C3, or symptoms of arthralgia, rash, and abdominal pain. These findings suggest **Henoch-Schönlein purpura nephritis** (now considered to be an IgA-related small artery vasculitis), **systemic lupus,** or **membranoproliferative or focal segmental glomerulonephritis,** all of which may present as nephrotic syndrome. A failure to respond to steroid therapy also suggests that one is not dealing with classic idiopathic nephrotic syndrome of childhood. Furthermore, if the child is older than 6 years, minimal change disease is unlikely and renal biopsy may be required in order to make the diagnosis. Adolescent girls with nephrotic syndrome are likely to have systemic lupus. Nephrotic teenagers with long-standing diabetes mellitus can be assumed to have **Kimmelstiel-Wilson syndrome.**

Renal biopsy may also be needed to make a diagnosis in infants under the age of 1 year, because they may have causes of the syndrome unique to this age-group in addition to those mentioned above. In these young infants, one should consider hereditary congenital nephrosis of the Finnish type or nephrotic syndrome from congenital infections such as syphilis or the agents of the TORCH syndrome (i.e., Toxoplasmosis, Rubella, Cytomegalovirus, and Herpes).

It should be remembered that generalized edema may be due to disorders other than renal disease, including liver disease, particularly cirrhosis, or to heart disease, as well as to poor diet and other disorders that lead to low serum protein, especially serum albumin.

HYPERTENSION AND ACUTE NEPHRITIS

In contrast to adults, an organic cause for hypertension in childhood is usually found; most often it is due to renal disease.

The most common cause of hypertension of acute onset is acute glomerulonephritis. Hematuria and headache occurring 7 to 14 days following a streptococcal infection of the throat or skin is the characteristic onset. Oliguria and renal failure may occur. Antistreptococcal enzymes are elevated, as are the BUN, creatinine, and erythrocyte sedimentation rate (ESR), while the C3 complement component is decreased. Early complications include hyperkalemia and hypertension following acute fluid overload, usually requiring salt and fluid restriction and the use of antihypertensives. Penicillin should be administered to eliminate any persisting source of streptococcal antigen. Most of these children recover; however, if the child does not improve in 10 to 14 days after onset or if anuria or severe renal insufficiency develops, another diagnosis should be sought and renal biopsy may be necessary.

OTHER RENAL DISORDERS

Hereditary nephritis, usually in the form of **Alport's syndrome,** is an autosomal dominant disorder with preferential segregation with the X chromosome. It usually presents in males in the second decade of life. There is hematuria and frequently hypertension. There is a history of deafness in the patient and in male relatives. While males progress to renal failure and need dialysis, females are less severely affected even though they have the disease more often.

Hemolytic uremic syndrome presents in children 1 to 4 years of age, a day or two following gastroenteritis, with hematuria, oliguria, pallor, edema, and usually hypertension. Fibrin deposition in the renal vascular bed is thought to be responsible for both the renal insufficiency and the microangiopathic hemolytic anemia, as is seen in DIC. The peripheral blood shows characteristic fragmented cells, and there is thrombocytopenia. Peritoneal dialysis is the treatment for the many complications. There is a recurrent form of the disorder in older children; low-dose aspirin therapy is used in these children to prevent recurrence. In a familial form of hemolytic uremic syndrome, the disease occurs in siblings with the onset months or years apart.

Nonrenal causes of hematuria in children include coliform and viral cystitis, pinworms, bubble baths causing vaginitis and/or cystitis, and urethral foreign bodies. Trauma to any part of the GU tract must always be considered in the differential diagnosis of hematuria, and, in this regard a careful history is taken to rule out **battered child syndrome,** which is prevalent in all levels of society. *Hematuria is commonly found in sickle cell anemia as well as in sickle cell trait.*

Nonrenal causes of hypertension in children include labile hypertension, which may not be related to true hypertension; excess ingestion of licorice, which contains an aldosterone-like compound; heavy metal exposure; coarctation of the aorta (upper extremities are hypertensive, lower extremities are not); hyperthyroidism; increased intracranial pressure; catecholamine-producing lesions such as neuroblastoma; carcinoid; and pheochromocytoma, as well as familial dysautonomia (Riley-Day syndrome). While obese children may be hypertensive, *it is important to use the proper size blood pressure cuff in all children.*

KEY THERAPEUTIC DECISIONS

Hypertensive emergencies, such as a confirmed diastolic blood pressure reading above 120 and hypertensive encephalopathy, require immediate treatment with intravenous hydralazine or diazoxide. For children with mild hypertension, dietary sodium should be reduced and weight controlled. Children with blood pressure determinations consistently in the 95th percentile for age or 140/90 mm Hg despite dietary measures should be given pharmacologic agents to control hypertension.

METABOLIC DISORDERS OF CHILDHOOD

RICKETS

In children, deficiency of vitamin D results in rickets, a disorder of *growing* bone; therefore, the bones affected in any given patient are those that are growing at the time. For example, if rickets occurs in the first year of life, the skull is principally involved since it is growing fastest. Excess osteoid and noncalcified cartilage pile up and produce characteristic frontal bossing. In the second year of life, when long bones are growing fast, widening of the epiphyses at the wrists and ankles is seen. Wrist deformities are increased by crawling, and bowing of the legs develops as the child begins to support weight and walk. In this disorder, the cartilage cells in the growing end of bone fail to arrange themselves in orderly columns and the cartilage cells in the zone of provisional clacification fail to degenerate as they should; the matrix is not impregnated with

calcium salts. These abnormalities result in the formation of a wide, irregular zone of noncalcified cartilage and osteoid much less rigid than normal bone. Osteoid rather than bone surrounds the length of the shaft. These pathological findings account for the characteristic x-ray findings in children with this disorder.

Deficiency of vitamin D causes the blood phosphorus level to fall. Though the absorption of calcium is affected, the calcium level is maintained in the early stages of the disorder through increased parathyroid activity. Osteoporosis develops as calcium is withdrawn from bone; if this fails to maintain the serum calcium level, tetany may result. Usually, however, the serum calcium is normal, the phosphorus level is low, and the alkaline phosphatase level is markedly elevated.

Rickets can develop in children with epilepsy receiving phenobarbital or phenytoin. These drugs enhance hepatic hydroxylase activity, which inactivates vitamin D metabolites.

Infants require 400 IU of vitamin D daily to prevent rickets. Treatment of rickets requires 10,000 units of vitamin D daily.

VITAMIN C DEFICIENCY

Vitamin C deficiency leads to disordered collagen formation, which manifests as the clinical entity of scurvy. The major manifestations of scurvy are spongy gums, hemorrhage, pseudoparalysis due to pain on motion, and marked irritability. There is easy bruising and a positive tourniquet test. Radiographic findings as well as a low blood level of vitamin C are diagnostic. Infants and children require 35 to 50 mg of vitamin C daily, depending on their age.

JUVENILE DIABETES

Juvenile or insulin-dependent diabetes is the most common endocrine disorder of childhood. Its prevalence in children less than 15 years of age is estimated to be between 1 in 600 to 1 in 1,200. The onset in children is accompanied by polydipsia and polyuria. If untreated, there is progression to weight loss, ketoacidosis, dehydration, coma, peripheral circulatory collapse, and death. These manifestations result from almost complete lack of insulin production by the pancreas. The onset in children may be abrupt, and the initial presentation may be ketoacidosis. This type of onset often occurs in infants who are not toilet trained or who are nonverbal, whose initial symptoms of polydipsia and polyuria may go undetected. Several features distinguish juvenile diabetes from the adult-onset type; these are outlined in Table 4-10.

Although predisposition to diabetes appears to be genetically determined, there is strong evidence for an immunologic element. Antibodies against pancreatic islets have been found, and they are thought to develop following a viral infection. Antibodies against thyroid, adrenal, or gastric antigens are also found more frequently in diabetic children than in normal children.

A diagnosis of diabetes mellitus in children is made in the presence of classic symptoms of polydipsia, polyuria, ketonuria, rapid weight loss, and a random plasma glucose > 200 mg/100 ml. In asymptomatic patients, the diagnosis depends on finding both an elevated fasting glucose concentration and a sustained elevated glucose concentration during the oral glucose tolerance test on more than one occasion. Symptomatic

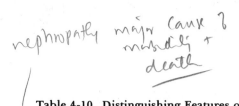
nephropathy major cause of
morbidity +
death

**Table 4-10. Distinguishing Features of
Juvenile- and Adult-Onset Diabetes**

	Juvenile type	Adult type
Insulin response to glucose	Decreased or absent	Dealyed, may be increased
Need for exogenous insulin	Required, long-term	Rarely required
Quality of control	Labile	Stable
Ketosis	Prone	Resistant
Oral hypoglycemic agents	Partial effect	Effective
Major complications	Microangiopathy	Atherosclerosis
Reduced life expectancy	Approximately 30%	Less, especially with older onset
Obesity	Unusual	About 80%
Calorie restriction	Poor response; leads to cachexia	Can restore glucose tolerance

diabetes mellitus in children always requires insulin therapy.

Vascular injury is the most important complication of juvenile-onset diabetes. Retinopathy is the earliest microangiopathic lesion. Large-vessel calcification occurs in 6.5% of diabetic children ages 10 to 19 years. Nephropathy is the major cause of morbidity and early death.

HEMATOLOGIC PROBLEMS IN PEDIATRICS

PHYSIOLOGICAL ANEMIA OF THE PREMATURE AND NEWBORN

Erythropoiesis is erythropoietin mediated even in fetal life. During gestation, the intrauterine environment is relatively hypoxic and erythropoietin levels are high. There is a progressive increase in red cell mass and at term the infant is born with a relative polycythemia, with the mean hemoglobin level about 18 g/100 ml.

Preterm infants have somewhat lower hemoglobin levels at birth than do those born at term since they have not completed the progressive increase in red cell mass.

After birth, the arterial oxygen saturation rises from about 45% to 95% and the level of erythropoietin falls to barely detectable levels by the end of the first week of life. Both the hemoglobin concentration and the hemoglobin mass begin to decrease by the end of the second week of life and reach their nadir at approximately 6 to 8 weeks in the premature infant and by 2 to 3 months in the full-term infant. This phenomenon is known as physiological anemia of the newborn. A more pronounced anemia is seen in the premature infant than in the full-term infant, but both are due to the same process (i.e., marrow depression due to increased oxygenation of the blood and consequent decrease in erythropoietin). The hallmark of this anemia is a reticulocyte count less than 1% during the period of marrow depression (1 to 6 weeks of age). The nadir in

hemoglobin concentration during the period is dependent on the hemoglobin at birth, as well as the length of the period of postnatal marrow depression. The hemoglobin concentration will of course be influenced by any superimposed events such as hemolysis, bleeding, or transfusion, but in otherwise normal infants the time course as well as the degree of anemia is predictable. Recovery is heralded by a rise in the reticulocyte count to about 3%, with subsequent gradual increase in the concentration of hemoglobin to about 11 g/100 ml.

ANEMIAS IN INFANCY AND CHILDHOOD

Diagnostic decisions concerning the causes of anemias in children must begin with a consideration of the age of the patient at the time of onset of the anemia. Not only do the causes of anemia vary with age, but normal hematologic values also vary with age. Other useful diagnostic considerations include the red cell indices, whether or not there is involvement of white cells and platelets, and whether or not there is marrow hypoplasia or evidence of response with reticulocytosis.

Anemia in the newborn

Anemia at birth is usually related to hemorrhage or to hemolysis. It should be remembered that hemoglobin values from capillary specimens from neonates are about 1.5 to 2 g/100 ml higher than those from venous samples. Since normal full-term infants have a *capillary* hemoglobin concentration of 18.5 g/100 ml, anemia should be considered when the value is 16 g/100 ml or less on the first 3 days of life. The anemia may be due to events that are ongoing or to events such as hemorrhage that occurred in utero or at the time of delivery. In these instances, although the degree of anemia varies widely depending on the time and degree of the hemorrhage, there may be profound anemia and shock. The abdomen is scaphoid, and hepatosplenomegaly and jaundice are not present. An important diagnostic stratagem, in addition to a thorough prenatal and obstetric history, is to get a sample of blood from the mother and look for fetal cells in it using the acid elution test of Betke and Kleihauer. The number of cells containing fetal hemoglobin in the maternal circulation can be used to quantitate fetal maternal hemorrhage that might have occurred during gestation. Such bleeding can lead to varying degrees of anemia in the newborn, and therapy ranges from none to the use of a simple transfusion.

In twin pregnancies, **fetal-fetal transfusion** can occur, rendering one infant pale, anemic, and often smaller than the other twin with the higher hemoglobin. This latter twin may have polycythemia and jaundice and symptoms related to hyperviscosity.

Both hemolysis and hemorrhage that have begun more than 24 to 48 hours before birth are usually associated with a reticulocyte count that is elevated above the expected count of up to 5% in the first day of life; this is a useful means of determining whether the cause of the anemia is related to prenatal events. Obviously, if the test is delayed for 24 or 48 hours, an elevated reticulocyte count only indicates a response to anemia but gives no clue to the pre- or postnatal timing of the event producing the anemia.

Hemolysis secondary to maternal-fetal blood group incompatibility and isoimmunization in the Rh or in the ABO blood groups is the major cause of hemolytic anemia in the neonate. Such phenomena should be looked for immediately in any anemic newborn, as well as in any that have jaundice in the first 24 hours of life, by performing blood typing and a direct Coombs' test. Such early jaundice can only be explained by increased production of bilirubin either from hemolysis or internal (i.e., enclosed) hemorrhage. If heterospecificity of blood types exists between mother and child and the direct Coombs' test is negative, an indirect Coombs' test or an elution of antibody from the infant's cells should be performed to determine whether isoimmunization is the cause of the hemolysis.

Hereditary defects in red cell enzymes can present in the newborn, usually giving rise to anemia and jaundice. The most common of these is glucose-6-phosphate dehydrogenase deficiency, an X-linked disorder that occurs in 10 to 14% of black males and about 2% of black females in the United States and Africa. This defect is also widespread among Mediterranean, Chinese, Malaysian, and Sephardic Jewish populations. Pyruvate kinase deficiency in which the red cells are markedly distorted in shape may also present with anemia and jaundice early in the newborn period. Hemolytic anemia secondary to inherited disorders of the red cell membrane such as hereditary spherocytosis, elliptocytosis, and stomatocytosis often have their initial presentation as neonatal hyperbilirubinemia because of the increased bilirubin load from red cell destruction. Later in life when there is adequate development of the mechanisms for clearance of bilirubin, jaundice is a much less prominent feature, though the red cell defects and hemolysis persist.

Another common cause of anemia in the neonate is that frequently seen with infection, whether bacterial, viral, or protozoal. It is a very common feature of *E. coli* infections as well as of congenital infections such as syphilis or the agents of the TORCH syndrome. The anemia is due to hemolysis; in some cases, particularly in gram-negative septicemia, it may be accentuated by the red cell fragmentation that occurs in DIC, a frequent complication of neonatal sepsis.

Hemoglobinopathies are only rarely the cause of anemia in the first weeks of life, since the preponderant hemoglobin at this age is fetal hemoglobin with little expression of the abnormal hemoglobin. However, when the abnormality is in one of the chains of fetal hemoglobin (i.e., alpha or gamma chains), decreased synthesis results in alpha-thalassemia trait or gamma-thalassemia, which can be manifest in the newborn period.

Anemia due to failure of production of red cells can be manifest in the first week of life and is characterized by a reticulocytopenia. The rare disorders responsible for such bone marrow failure include Diamond-Blackfan syndrome, congenital leukemia, and osteopetrosis, disorders that require bone marrow aspiration for confirmation. The causes of anemia of infancy and childhood change with the age of the child, and so do the normal hematologic values. Table 4-11 outlines the major causes of anemia in relation to age. Table 4-12 outlines some of the important changes in hematologic values in relation to age.

Between 2 and 3 months of age, the anemias of the hemoglobinopathies become evident as the relative concentration of fetal hemoglobin declines and that of the abnormal hemoglobin increases. While normal infants at this age are in the period of physiological anemia, infants with sickle cell anemia have a more rapid and greater drop in hemoglobin and, in contrast to normal infants, have a reticulocytosis. Sickle cell anemia is an autosomal recessive disorder that occurs in 1 in 500 black infants. The hemoglobinopathy can be diagnosed in newborn infants even though the anemia is not usually apparent until 6 to 12 weeks of life.

Infants who have had blood loss may show evidence of iron deficiency, although nutritional iron deficiency does not make its appearance until infants have more than doubled their birth weight, usually after 6 months of age.

Iron deficiency anemia

Although iron deficiency anemia is statistically the most common anemia of childhood, it must be stated that it is common only at specific ages—that is, *in infants 6 months to 2 years and in adolescents*. These are both periods of rapid growth with increased demand for iron intake. Between these periods, one must be very cautious in making the assumption that anemia is due to iron deficiency. Blood volume and body iron are related to body weight; 35 to 45 mg of iron are needed for each kilogram increase in body weight. Rapid growth with the concomitant increase in blood volume leads to dilution of the hemoglobin mass. The rapid growth during the first year results in a need for 200 mg of iron, or 0.6 mg/day, to maintain adequate stores. From *2 years until puberty*, the weight gain is steady at about 2.5 kg/year, with an attendant reduction in iron requirement to 0.3 mg/day.

Nutritional iron deficiency in infants and toddlers is related to inadequate dietary intake of iron during a period of rapid growth. The incidence, based on the criterion of a hemoglobin concentration of 10 g/100 ml, ranges from 17 to 44% and varies in different population groups. Though iron deficiency anemia

Table 4-11. Major Causes of Anemia in Relation to Age

Age	Causes
At birth	Hemorrhage (obstetric accidents, fetomaternal, twin-twin)
	Internal hemorrhage
	Hemolytic disorders
	Isoimmunization as a result of antibody from mother to fetal Rh or ABO red cell antigens
	Inherited red cell abnormality (e.g., hereditary spherocytosis or enzyme deficiency)
	Acquired red cell abnormality (e.g., in association with congenital or neonatal infection, or acidosis)
	Rare disorders (e.g., Blackfan-Diamond syndrome, congenital leukemia, osteopetrosis)
2–6 months	Late manifestation of isoimmunization
	Hereditary red cell defects
	Thalassemia major
	Sickle cell anemia
	Vitamin E deficiency
	Iron deficiency as consequence of neonatal hemorrhage
	Folate deficiency
	Persistent infection
	Renal disease; acidosis
> 6 months	Iron deficiency
	Hemorrhage
	Hemoglobinopathies
	Hereditary red cell enzymatic or membrane defects
	Chronic infection
	Renal disease
	Leukemia

can occur by 6 months, the peak incidence occurs between 10 and 15 months of age. By this age, infants have outgrown their iron endowment, which at birth amounts to about 75 mg/kg, most of which is in the red cell hemoglobin. Under normal circumstances, there is minimal iron loss from the body and it is not until the infant's weight has more than doubled that the iron endowment becomes inadequate. Preterm infants who receive less iron during their limited period of gestation may become iron deficient earlier, because they rapidly outgrow their endowment of iron.

Though cow's milk and human milk each contain less than 1.5 mg iron per 1,000 calories, breast-fed infants absorb 49% of the extrinsic iron as compared with 10% absorption from cow's milk. Because of the greater bioavailability of iron to breast-fed infants, these infants have higher iron stores during the first year of life than do those fed cow's milk formulas.

Iron deficiency anemia is characterized by hypochromasia and microcytosis; the mean corpuscular volume (MCV) in these infants is <70 μm^3 and the serum ferritin is <10 ng/ml.

The deficiency of iron is not limited to the red cell hemoglobin. The normal body iron content of 3.4 to 4.5 g is distributed in three compartments:

1. Oxygen transport and storage: Hemoglobin, 65% (of body iron); myoglobin, 5%
2. Iron storage and transport: Ferritin and hemosiderin, 29%; transferrin, 0.2%
3. Iron-containing enzymes, 0.2%, in iron porphyrin proteins (e.g., cytochromes, catalase, etc.)

In addition, several enzyme systems are iron responsive or iron dependent, and therefore during iron deficiency their function is impaired. For example, mitochondrial monamine oxidase (MAO) is sensitive to the state of the body's iron stores, and it has been postulated that some of the behavioral abnormalities noted with iron deficiency may be caused by impaired MAO function and consequent excess of catechols. These latter nonhematologic points are still controversial.

Not all microcytic hypochromic anemias are due to iron deficiency. Alpha- and beta-thalassemia syndromes, lead

Table 4-12. Major Hematologic Values in Relation to Age
(Mean values)

Age	Hemoglobin g/100 ml	Hct %	Retics %	WBC/mm³ (× 10³)
Birth (cord blood)	16.8	55	5.0	18
2 weeks	16.5	50	1.0	12
3 months	12.0	36	1.0	12
6 months–6 years	12.0	37	1.0	12
7–12 years	13.0	38	1.0	10
Adult (female)	14.0	42	1.6	8
Adult (male)	16.0	47	1.6	7.5

poisoning, chronic infection, and sideroblastic (pyridoxine-responsive) anemias also have these characteristics.

Anemias occurring after the age of 3 years require careful scrutiny and should never be assumed to be due to iron deficiency. This is an age of high frequency for leukemia, and a normocytic anemia may be the presenting sign. There is a low reticulocyte count and usually an associated leukopenia and thrombocytopenia early in the course of childhood leukemia; these findings are also characteristic of aplastic anemias. Bone marrow examination is essential. Chronic renal disease as well as chronic infection, hypersplenism, and the effect of drugs can produce similar peripheral blood findings and should be considered in the differential diagnosis if no abnormal cells are found.

Reticulocytosis with normal neutrophil and platelet counts usually indicates hemorrhage or a hemolytic disorder. In such anemias, examination of the peripheral blood usually gives a major clue to the diagnosis through identification of red cell morphological changes characteristic of inherited or acquired red cell disorders, including spherocytes, elliptocytes, stomatocytes, fragmented cells, burr cells, and sickle cells. Polychromasia and often nucleated red cells in the peripheral smear are indicative of marrow response to the anemia and are evidence for a hemolytic process if hemorrhage has been ruled out. A Coombs' test is done at this age to diagnose autoimmune hemolytic disease.

Anemias with low reticulocyte counts represent bone marrow failure. These anemias may be due to a pure red cell aplasia or in other instances may be associated with neutropenia or thrombocytopenia. Pure red cell aplasias may be congenital or acquired. **Diamond-Blackfan anemia** is an autosomal recessive anemia that becomes evident within the first few months of life. Macrocytosis and a high fetal hemoglobin are characteristic. About half of these patients respond to corticosteroids, and red cell production can often be maintained by the stimulatory effect of very low doses of prednisone.

Transient erythroblastopenia of childhood is an acquired, normochromic, normocytic anemia of short duration and of unknown etiology; it may result from prolonged renal suppression of erythropoiesis. The hemoglobin F level is normal. Most patients recover in 2 to 4 weeks without therapy.

Parvovirus infection is often associated with a hypoproliferative anemia. When the patient has an underlying hemolytic disease (such as sickle cell anemia), an aplastic crisis may develop with parvovirus infection since the marrow becomes unable to meet the demands of rapid red cell turnover.

WHITE BLOOD CELL DISORDERS

Inherited disorders of leukocyte morphology include **Chédiak-Higashi syndrome**, the **May-Hegglin anomaly**, and the **Pelger-Huët anomaly**.

Chédiak-Higashi syndrome is an autosomal recessive disorder characterized by giant cytoplasmic granular inclusions; patients have severe pyogenic infections, photophobia, lymphadenopathy, and hepatosplenomegaly. Lymphoreticular malignancies may develop.

In the May-Hegglin anomaly, a rare autosomal dominant disorder, large blue inclusions (Döhle bodies) are found in the cytoplasm of neutrophils, as well as in eosinophiles, basophils, and monocytes. There are also large granules in oversized platelets, together with thrombocytopenia.

The Pelger-Huët anomaly is a common autosomal dominant trait characterized by decreased nuclear segmentation of neutrophils; however, neutrophil function is intact.

Neutropenia

When the **absolute neutrophil count** (ANC) is below 1,500/mm³, **neutropenia** exists. When the ANC is less than 500/mm³, the condition is termed **agranulocytosis**.

Patients can be at increased risk of infection when the neutrophil count is between 500 and 1,000/mm³, and mouth ulcers and gingivitis usually appear. At levels of neutrophils less than 500/mm³, the risk of overwhelming septicemia is great.

Neutropenia may occur as a result of failure in production or through the mechanism of increased destruction. Failures in production of neutrophils occur in **congenital neutropenia** and in **cyclic benign neutropenia**. Severe congenital neutropenia or **Kostmann's disease** leads to severe or lethal infections of the skin or respiratory tract. These infections develop in the first month of life in this autosomal recessive genetic disorder.

Metabolic disorders such as methylmalonic acidemia and idiopathic hyperglycinemia are associated with neutropenia beginning in the neonatal period. **Schwachman-Diamond syndrome** is a disorder in which neutropenia occurs in association with pancreatic exocrine insufficiency, metaphyseal chondrodysplasia, and dwarfism. Infants present with diarrhea, recurrent sinopulmonary infections, and failure to thrive. There is no known therapy for the neutropenia or dwarfism in this syndrome.

Neutropenia secondary to infections

Many bacterial and viral infections in children are associated with neutropenia. Among the viral agents causing neutropenia are varicella, rubella, respiratory synctyial virus (RSV), influenza A and B, hepatitis A and B, and the Epstein-Barr virus.

Among bacterial infections associated with neutropenia are typhoid and paratyphoid fevers, as well as brucellosis and tularemia.

It should be noted that in the neonate, neutropenia is a common accompaniment of neonatal sepsis, notably with *E. coli*, *Pseudomonas*, and group B streptococcal infections.

Neutropenia associated with drugs

Drugs and toxic substances may produce neutropenia. Some such as the cytotoxic agents (e.g., methotrexate) do this by dose-dependent marrow suppression of all elements. Others, such as the phenothiazines, sulfonamides, and synthetic penicillins, may cause idiosyncratic suppression of neutrophil production. Neutropenia is also produced by toxic agents such as heavy metals and benzene.

Neutropenia can result not only from marrow suppression but also from increased destruction through autoimmune processes. In the fetus, isoimmune neutropenia can result from transfer of antineutrophil antibodies from the mother. Drugs may induce neutropenia not only through marrow suppression, but also by acting as haptens in immune neutropenia.

Neutrophils as well as red cells and platelets may be sequestered in the spleen in illnesses in which there is splenomegaly.

Handwritten annotations (top margin):
- Hemophilia (B) / Christmas dise — IX
- PTT Prolong
- Rx FFP
- def g Cofactor / VIII:C
- prolonged PTT / Rx Cryoprecip
- Hemophilia A / X-linked
- VIII
- VIII:R
- von willebrand (involve different part of factor VIII molecule
- von willebrand (incl) PTT/Bleeding time
- only PTT is abn. other coag OK

PLATELET DISORDERS AND THROMBOCYTOPENIA

The platelet count is normally between 150,000 and 300,000/mm³; even premature infants have platelet counts above 100,000/mm³. A decrease in platelet number is the most common cause of abnormal bleeding. Decreased platelet production (usually evaluated by assessing the adequacy of megakaryocytes in the marrow) or increased destruction of platelets can cause thrombocytopenia. *Bleeding from thrombocytopenia alone does not usually occur unless the platelet count is less than 50,000 mm³.*

Thrombocytopenia due to decreased production of platelets occurs in bone marrow failure, usually with pancytopenia. It also occurs in amegakaryotic thrombocytopenia, including **thrombocytopenia-absent radius syndrome**, which is an autosomal recessive disorder, and **Wiskott-Aldrich syndrome**, an X-linked recessive disorder with eczema, recurrent infections due to deficient T- and B-cell function, and **thrombocytopenia with characteristically small platelets.**

Thrombocytopenia due to increased destruction of platelets is characteristic of **childhood immune thrombocytopenia**, frequently termed **idiopathic thrombocytopenic purpura (ITP)**. Most childhood ITP is different from adult ITP; it characteristically follows a viral infection or active immunization; it is usually self-limited, 80 to 90% of children recovering within 1 to 6 months, the majority within 1 month. It is an immune process, and antibodies to platelets can be demonstrated. Severe hemorrhage is rare despite very low platelet counts (10,000 to 30,000/mm³). Intracranial hemorrhage, which occurs in less than 1% of the cases, has not been associated with platelet counts above 20,000/mm³ in this disorder. Although recovery may be speeded up with the use of prednisone or intravenous gamma-globulin, the condition usually resolves spontaneously.

Splenectomy is to be avoided in children because of the lifelong threat of overwhelming sepsis due to loss of important splenic function. In the 10 to 15% of ITP patients who develop chronic ITP, splenectomy can be postponed and perhaps avoided altogether through the judicious use of intravenous gamma-globulin. This is important, since some of the children who develop a chronic form of thrombocytopenia may recover after 1 or even 2 years of the disease.

Thrombocytopenia in the newborn has many causes. The most common is infection, whether congenital infection, such as those of the TORCH syndrome, or bacterial sepsis. The latter may be associated with DIC in which there is consumption of platelets during the coagulopathy. DIC is best treated by treating the underlying sepsis.

Immune thrombocytopenia may be due to maternal autoimmune antibodies, which affect the infant's platelets as well as the mother's. This phenomenon occurs in maternal ITP and systemic lupus erythematosus (SLE), or it may be drug induced. Thrombocytopenia in the infant can result from maternal isoimmune antibodies directed at the fetus's platelet antigens, which differ from her own.

Qualitative platelet disorders or thrombocytopathies result in bleeding because of dysfunction of the platelet rather than a reduced number of platelets. In the **Bernard-Soulier syndrome**, in which there is an absence of platelet glycoprotein Ib, there is also a mild thrombocytopenia and giant platelets visible on blood smears. In **Glanzmann's thrombasthenia**, there is a deficiency of platelet membrane glycoprotein IIb-IIIa complex, and tests of platelet aggregation are abnormal. In **storage pool** disease, there is a deficient release of ADP by stimulated platelets, but the platelets aggregate normally when stimulated by exogenous ADP.

Aspirin-induced thrombocytopathy is common. Aspirin inhibits platelet release of ADP, and the second wave of aggregation is deficient.

DISORDERS OF HEMOSTASIS

In addition to platelets, normal hemostasis requires integrity of blood vessels and soluble clotting factors. The nature of the problem is often suggested by the type of bleeding that is described in the history or is evident on physical examination. Petechiae and purpura suggest a quantitative or qualitative platelet defect. Severe recurrent epistaxis or menorrhagia suggests a disorder such as **von Willebrand's** disease. Recurrent hemarthrosis suggests a form of **hemophilia.**

The tests of the integrity of the hemostatic system include examination of blood smear, platelet counts, bleeding time (which tests both vascular integrity and platelet function), partial thromboplastin time (PTT) (which tests the intrinsic pathway), and prothrombin time (PT) (which tests both the extrinsic pathway and the common pathway).

Vascular abnormalities affecting coagulation occur in **Ehlers-Danlos syndrome**, which is an inherited disorder of collagen synthesis, and in scurvy. Deficiency of vitamin C leads to an acquired impairment of collagen synthesis and also to qualitative platelet defects. **Hereditary hemorrhagic telangiectasia**, an autosomal dominant disorder characterized by vascular abnormalities on mucosal surfaces throughout the body, may lead to severe GI bleeding.

The most common inherited coagulation diseases are disorders involving Factor VIII, including hemophilia A and von Willebrand's disease. These disorders involve different parts of the Factor VIII molecule. **Hemophilia A** results from a deficiency of the Factor VIII procoagulant protein, known as antihemophiliac factor or VIII:C, which is a cofactor in the intrinsic pathway. **Von Willebrand's disease** results from a deficiency of VIII:R, the von Willebrand factor, which is important in platelet adhesion. There is also a deficiency of VIII:C.

Hemophilia A is a sex-linked inherited disorder. The severity of the disease relates to the degree of deficiency of VIII:C. Severely affected boys with less than 1% of VIII:C bruise easily and develop hemarthrosis readily, usually after the age of 1 year when they begin to walk; infants may bleed at circumcision. Trauma may lead to life-threatening internal hemorrhage. The PTT is prolonged as a result of the defect in the intrinsic pathway. Other coagulation tests are normal. Replacement therapy is accomplished through the use of cryoprecipitate or Factor VIII concentrates. Before replacements were screened for the AIDS virus, more than 90% of hemophiliacs became HIV positive; however, only about 5% of those who became positive have manifested AIDS or AIDS-related complex (ARC). Now all products are processed to eliminate the virus.

The inheritance pattern of von Willebrand's disease is variable. As with hemophilia A, the severity of the disorder varies with the degree of deficiency of Factor VIII. Bleeding is usually mild, and as in platelet disorders, mucosal and cutaneous bleeding is most common. Epistaxis and menorrhagia are common. Trauma may result in more severe hemorrhage. In von Willebrand's disease, both the PTT and the bleeding time are prolonged. Characteristically, ristocetin-induced platelet aggregation is abnormal and there is a deficiency of VIII:R antigen. Cryoprecipitate rather than Factor VIII concentrates is the preferred replacement treatment.

Hemophilia B (Factor IX deficiency or Christmas disease) is an X-linked recessive disorder with bleeding similar to that in hemophilia A. PTT is prolonged, and Factor IX activity is decreased. Fresh-frozen plasma or prothrombin complex concentrate (a mixture of Factors II, VII, IX, and X) may be used as replacement therapy.

Vitamin K-dependent coagulation factors are Factors II, VII, IX, and X; they are synthesized in the liver. Warfarin interferes with vitamin K activity and is therefore an anti-coagulant.

Vitamin K must be given to affected newborn infants in order to prevent **hemorrhagic disease of the newborn.** Since all coagulation factors other than Factor VIII are synthesized in the liver, severe liver disease is associated with prolonged PT as well as PTT. In addition, there may be impairment in clearance of activated clotting factors. Fresh-frozen plasma rather than prothrombin complex is the preferred mode of treatment, since activated factors may lead to DIC.

In the newborn infant, in whom DIC is common, one should distinguish DIC from vitamin K deficiency and from liver disease. Specific determination of Factors V and VIII distinguishes hepatic disease from DIC, since in DIC both factors are decreased but in hepatic disease Factor VIII is normal since it is not made in the liver.

TUMORS AND NEOPLASMS IN CHILDHOOD

Brain

Brain tumors are the most common solid tumors of childhood; among childhood malignancies, they are exceeded in frequency only by leukemia. About 75% of brain tumors in children arise from glial cells; among the most common tumors are astrocytomas (including brain stem gliomas) and medulloblastomas. Brain stem gliomas though histologically benign are inoperable because of their location. Optic gliomas (which are often associated with neurofibromatosis) are curable by surgical resection if they do not involve the chiasm.

Medulloblastomas are of embryonal origin, and the period of high risk following surgical resection and neuraxis radiation is like that of other congenital tumors (e.g., age at presentation plus 9 months—Collin's law).

Brain tumors may become symptomatic at any time in childhood; the peak incidence is from 5 to 10 years of age. Symptoms are related to the location and rate of growth of the tumor rather than to its histological characteristics. Focal neurological deficits and increased intracranial pressure are the characteristic presentations. Early morning headache produced by increased intracranial pressure is caused by expansion of the lateral ventricles and cerebral hemispheres. This stretches the pain-sensitive dura. Since these structures are innervated by the trigeminal nerve, pain is referred to the bifrontotemporal areas. Headache is dull and steady and occurs in the morning.

In the upright position, venous drainage from the head is facilitated and the symptoms gradually subside after the child is up and active. Other symptoms related to increased intracranial pressure include personality changes such as apathy, somnolence, or irritability. Rapid head enlargement secondary to hydrocephalus is produced by obstruction of the CSF. Normally, the posterior fontanel is closed by age 4 months and the anterior by 2 years; closure of the fontanels may be delayed in the presence of increased intracranial pressure. Papilledema is usually not found until the child is older than 2 years and the fontanels and sutures are closed. Focal neurological symptoms due to CNS tumors are related to their location in the following areas: cerebral hemisphere, parasellar-optic chiasm, quadrigeminal region, posterior fossa, or spinal column.

In the child presenting with signs and symptoms of brain tumor, including focal seizures or a focal abnormality on EEG, investigation is usually begun with a CT scan. Conditions with symptoms like those of a brain tumor include brain abscess, lead encephalopathy, subdural hematoma, hydrocephalus, pseudotumor cerebri, tuberculoma, and encephalitis. In herpes simplex encephalitis, in which there may be memory loss, olfactory hallucinations, seizures, stupor, and hemiplegia, a CT scan shows a frontal or temporal lobe mass as well as other encephalitides.

Wilms
↙ neuroblastoma

ABDOMINAL TUMORS

The most common abdominal tumors of childhood are Wilms' tumor and neuroblastoma. *Neuroblastoma* About 50% of neuroblastomas manifest in infants less than 2 years of age. These tumors arise most often in the abdomen (50%). About one-third arise from the adrenal and about 15% occur in nonadrenal sites in the abdomen. Although the common presentation is that of an abdominal mass, the majority of children have metastatic lesions at the time of initial diagnosis. In contrast to Wilms' tumor, metastases to bone are common in neuroblastoma, whereas those to lung are rare. Proptosis of the eye, with attendant periorbital swelling and ecchymosis secondary to retrobulbar soft-tissue involvement, should alert one to the possible presentation of neuroblastoma. Symptoms related to catecholamine production in the tumor include diarrhea, flushing, perspiration, tachycardia, hypertension, and paroxysmal headaches.

In recent years, it has become evident that not all children are at equal risk for the development of cancer. There are some children at higher risk than others, and some of the risk factors including associated conditions have recently been identified. For example, neuroblastoma has been found to occur in children with aganglionic megacolon as well as in association with neurofibromatosis and with the fetal hydantoin syndrome. The underlying factor apparently is an error in development related to the neural crest. The degree of malignancy in neuroblastoma appears to be related to the number of copies in the tumor tissue of a DNA sequence related to v-myc and c-nyc oncogenes, designated N-myc in neuroblastoma. The less-malignant stage I and IV-S have only one copy of this gene; more malignant cell lines have an increased number.

Although the prognosis is generally poor for neuroblastoma patients, it is more favorable for infants less than 1 or 2 years of age and for those patients with well-encapsulated tumors.

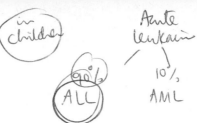

WILMS' TUMOR

Almost all children with Wilms' tumor present before the age of 5 years. The initial finding is a palpable abdominal mass or abdominal enlargement. The mass is usually large, firm, and nontender. Abdominal x-ray findings reveal a soft-tissue mass displacing the intestine to the opposite side. Intravenous pyelography (IVP), sonography, or CT scan reveals an intrarenal mass. In contrast to neuroblastoma, calcification in the mass is unusual. The tumor spreads locally but also to the lungs, liver, and brain. In contrast to neuroblastoma, spread to bone is rare.

As with neuroblastoma, there are children at increased risk for the development of Wilms' tumor. This tumor is found in association with congenital aniridia, which is due to a partial deletion of the short arm of chromosome 11. The chromosomal abnormality leads to a dysfunction in the regulation of growth of renal tissue; this dysplasia predisposes to neoplasia. Wilms' tumor also occurs with excessive frequency in children with Beckwith-Wiedemann syndrome, characterized by visceral cytomegaly, omphalocele, macroglossia, and hemihypertrophy. In this syndrome, cancer occurs in organs with cytomegaly: the kidneys, the adrenal cortex, and the liver.

Early cancer detection and the potential for cure can be augmented by the recognition of the factors that identify children at high risk for the development of this and other childhood cancers. The prognosis for children with Wilms' tumor is now very good; with appropriate surgery, radiation, and chemotherapy almost 90% of children can now be cured.

Although several other tumors, including teratoma, ovarian neoplasms, hepatic tumors, etc., may present as intra-abdominal masses, not all masses in the abdomen represent tumors. Renal enlargement results from renal malformations, multicystic or polycystic kidneys, multilocular cysts, or hydronephrosis. Abdominal enlargement as well as masses can result from liver masses including hemangiomas, hepatomas, cystic disease, or hepatic abscesses. Volvulus of the gut as well as intussusception must also be considered when one finds an abdominal mass. Intussusception produces a sausage-shaped mass usually palpable on the right side. Dance's sign occurs when the mass moves into the right upper quadrant, leaving an empty right lower quadrant with no bowel palpable there.

As in almost all disorders of childhood, the age of the patient is a major factor to be considered in approaching the differential diagnosis of masses in the abdomen as well as tumors at any site.

LEUKEMIA IN CHILDHOOD

Acute leukemia can occur at any age in childhood, but the peak incidence is between 2 and 5 years. About 2,500 new cases occur each year in the United States. The risk for white children to develop leukemia is higher than that for blacks and is 1 in 2,880 for the first 10 years of life. The risk is higher for siblings of leukemic patients (1:1,000), and 20% of monozygotic twins of children with leukemia develop the disease within weeks or months of the co-twin. Other genetic factors that are associated with leukemia include chromosome anomalies (e.g., trisomy 21 or Down's syndrome, trisomy G), Fanconi's anemia, Bloom's syndrome, and Klinefelter's syndrome.

Approximately 90% of childhood acute leukemia is of the acute lymphoblastic (ALL) or acute undifferentiated (stem cell) type. The remaining 10% is chiefly acute myeloblastic (AML) or acute monocytic leukemia. Chronic lymphocytic leukemia does not occur in childhood; chronic myelocytic leukemia accounts for about 2% of leukemia in childhood.

Lymphosarcoma arising outside of the marrow can enter a leukemic phase indistinguishable clinically from ALL.

The presenting symptoms of leukemia vary; low-grade fever, lassitude, and pallor with varying degrees of anemia are common initial findings. Bone marrow involvement affects all cell lines; a decrease in normal granulopoiesis often leads to infection and ulceration of the buccal mucosa. At the outset there is often a low total white cell count with few if any blast forms noted in the peripheral smear, though the bone marrow shows clear evidence of infiltration with the abnormal cell population. The marrow involvement not only leads to anemia and granulocytopenia, but to thrombocytopenia. This is associated with petechiae, purpura, and commonly with bleeding from the gums. Fatal intracranial hemorrhage, although not uncommon early in the course of AML, is rare in ALL. Lymphadenopathy and hepatosplenomegaly resulting from infiltration of these tissues are common features of ALL but are less common in AML.

In childhood leukemia, the CNS is the most common site of extramedullary involvement. Over 50% of children who do not receive prophylactic CNS therapy at the time of induction develop this complication, compared with only 10% of those who do receive that therapy. CNS involvement may be manifest with diffuse or focal symptoms. Most commonly it presents as a meningeal syndrome with morning headache, vomiting, papilledema, and often bilateral sixth nerve palsy. Parenchymal involvement results in focal neurological signs. In unusual cases, CNS leukemia may present as the hypothalamic syndrome, with polyphagia, weight gain, behavior disturbance, and hirsutism.

The diagnosis of CNS leukemia is based primarily on CSF findings of elevated pressure, increased protein, normal or decreased glucose, and pleocytosis. While cells can be found in the CSF as a reaction to intrathecal chemotherapy, as well as to CNS infection such as with Cryptococcus, leukemic blast cells can be distinguished by cyto centrifugation of the CSF and subsequent staining of the cells with Wright's-Giemsa stain.

Testicular enlargement as a result of leukemic infiltration occurs in 10 to 23% of boys in the course of their disease. Both CNS and testicular involvement represent metastases to "sanctuary" areas in which leukemic cells are less accessible to chemotherapeutic agents. The clinical presentation is painless enlargement of one or both testicles, which on palpation are rock hard. This complication can occur even when there is bone marrow remission; however, hematologic relapse usually follows within 6 months.

Bone pain is one of the initial symptoms of acute childhood leukemia, occurring in about 25% of patients. This has frequently been misdiagnosed as rheumatoid arthritis or rheumatic fever, since there may be migratory joint pain with swelling and tenderness. There may be direct infiltration of the periosteum, bone infarction, or expansion of the marrow cavity with leukemic cells. Patients may have bone pain without characteristic radiological changes.

Bone marrow aspiration and examination are required to establish the diagnosis. Normal marrow contains less than 5% blasts. At initial diagnosis, the leukemic marrow usually has more than 50% blast cells. In the marrow, there is a reduction of erythroid and granulocytic precursors. Megakaryocytes are decreased or absent. These normal elements are in large measure replaced by the leukemic cells.

In some cases, there may be hypocellularity of the marrow that is difficult to distinguish from aplastic anemia, and a bone marrow **biopsy** or biopsy of other tissue such as a lymph node may be required in order to make the diagnosis.

ALL is a heterogeneous disease and has been classified by immunologic techniques into three major groups: T-cell ALL; B-cell ALL, and non-T/non-B cell ALL. Each of these classes has been subdivided depending on the presence or absence of various immunologic (surface) markers. The three morphological types of lymphoblasts that have been designated L1, L2, and L3 do not correspond to immunologic type except for the L3 cell, which is associated with B-cell ALL. L3 cells are large cells with a round nucleus, one or more vesicular nucleoli, deep blue cytoplasm, and prominent cytoplasmic vacuolation. These cells are found in Burkitt's lymphoma.

Eighty percent of children with ALL have the non-B/non-T cell type; this type is further subdivided into three groups, depending on the presence of specific surface markers. Subgroup III is the most common subgroup; almost all children with non-B/non-T cell leukemia have this cell type, which is devoid of classical T and B markers but has Ia-like and ALL antigens and has a relatively favorable prognosis.

The T-cell group and most of its subgroups have a less favorable prognosis. The clinical picture has identifiable features. It occurs in an older age-group (median 12 years) and has a male:female ratio of 4:1, high initial white count (often >100,000), poorer response to treatment, and median disease-free survival of only 12 months. The relapse pattern is different in that a significant number of relapses occur in extramedullary sites, principally CNS and often testes, whereas in non-T disease relapse occurs in marrow.

These considerations are important to keep in mind when discussing the prognosis with parents, for much progress has been made toward cure of the more favorable types of childhood leukemia. Every effort is being made today to design treatment regimens based on the specific cell types and their prognosis. In general, poorer prognosis is associated with factors of age, race, sex, and white blood cell count. Children less than 2 or more than 10 years of age have a poor prognosis; this is also true for black children as well as those with high white cell counts. Boys have a shorter remission than do girls. This may relate to the fact that the testes may serve as an occult sanctuary of disease and that males are more likely than females to have the lymphoma-leukemia syndrome.

Treatment today consists of specifically designed regimens of combined chemotherapeutic agents. The role and efficacy of bone marrow transplantation are under intense investigation.

GASTROINTESTINAL DISORDERS

The nature of disorders of the GI tract of infants and children is greatly influenced by the age and developmental status of the host and therefore differs from that of adults. For example, in children under the age of 6 years, gastric ulcers are as common as duodenal ulcers. In children over the age of 6, duodenal ulcers are more common than gastric and are more frequently found in boys than girls. Gastroesophageal reflux is very common in young infants and can be expected to resolve as development progresses and the lower esophageal sphincter matures. Structural abnormalities due to congenital malformation of the GI tract can lead to life-threatening events, as in congenital tracheoesophageal fistula, which may present with recurrent pneumonia due to aspiration.

Pyloric stenosis occurs in about 1 in 150 male and 1 in 750 female infants. Familial occurrence is noted in about 15% of cases. Hypertrophy of the smooth muscle of the gastric antrum causes the gastric outlet obstruction. The onset of vomiting is usually manifest between 2 and 4 weeks of age. Nonbilious vomiting is the main feature, but, when the diagnosis is delayed, constipation and poor weight gain become evident. Dehydration may occur, and hypochloremic alkalosis is common as a result of persistent vomiting. Peristaltic waves proceeding from the left upper quadrant toward the pylorus in the right upper quadrant may be seen after feeding. A mass like an olive can be felt in the epigastrium, confirming the diagnosis, and immediate surgery is indicated.

Intussusception, the invagination of a proximal part of the intestine into a distal area, is one of the most common causes of intestinal obstruction in infancy. Neonates as well as children over 5 years of age with intussusception may have a specific pathology serving as the lead point, such as a Meckel's diverticulum, lymphoma, a foreign body, or a polyp; in infants between 1 month and 2 years of age, usually no lead point is found. There may be a sudden onset of colicky pain; vomiting is common. Currant jelly stools that contain red blood and mucus may occur. Therapy is surgical.

Cystic fibrosis is discussed in the section on pulmonary disease.

DIARRHEAL DISORDERS

Improper feeding is the most common cause of acute diarrhea in early infancy. There is wide variation in tolerance among infants to both the quality and quantity of food. There is also wide variation in both the amount and type of protein, fat, and carbohydrate in the commonly used formulas. Stool water and volume vary with the fat and sugar content of the formula. Infants fed formulas with high polyunsaturated fat content have looser stools than those fed formulas containing more saturated fat. If the formula has a high sugar content, stools may also become watery. As the GI tract matures, this intolerance decreases.

Throughout infancy and childhood, infections are the most common causes of diarrhea. These include both infectious diarrheas as well as certain infections outside the GI tract that are frequently associated with diarrhea in infants. In contrast to infants with diarrhea from improper feeding, infants with infectious causes of diarrhea appear ill; there may be fever and, in some, CNS signs, depending on the causative agent. Although in 20 to 30% of the cases of infectious diarrhea no specific infectious agent is identified, in temperate climates human rotavirus is responsible for 50% of all diarrheal illness and up to 80% of cases of severe diarrhea in infants in winter. Parvovirus-like agents have been associated with major outbreaks of acute diarrhea in Norwalk, Connecticut, Hawaii, and Montgomery County, Maryland. Bacterial pathogens probably cause 10 to 15% of acute diarrheal disease in children. The most commonly identified pathogens in children in North America are *Campylobacter jejuni*, strains of *Salmonella* and *Shigella*, and *Yersinia enterocolitica*. Although *E. coli* is a normal inhabitant of the distal bowel, some strains have been found to be pathogenic and enteroadherent strains have been found to produce severe diarrhea in children. Parasitic agents, including *Entamoeba histolytica* and *Giardia lamblia*, produce diarrhea; toddlers, particularly those in day-care centers, commonly acquire giardiasis.

Diarrheas associated with non-GI infections as well as with the use of antibiotics are more common in children than in adults. Chronic diarrhea in children has a host of causes extending from minor disorders or even misinterpretation of physiological responses to those that are severe and life threatening. The diagnostic challenge is further accentuated by the extreme diversity in the nature of the etiology, including such diverse causes as cow's milk protein intolerance, inborn errors of metabolism, and tumors such as neuroblastoma that produce catecholamines. The etiology of diarrhea has a definite relationship to age. For example, Hirschsprung's disease, cystic fibrosis, antibody deficiency syndromes, and neurogenic tumors usually manifest in infancy and early childhood, whereas regional enteritis, chronic ulcerative colitis, and hyperthyroidism more commonly present after 8 years of age.

Of greatest importance in the approach to diagnosis is taking a thorough history with emphasis on feeding history, growth and development, general health, and the stool description. Examination of the stool can give a major clue to the nature of the problem. For example, purulent mucus suggests infection; bloody mucus suggests mucosal ulceration. Dissacharidase deficiency is unlikely if free water is absent from the stool, for in such patients nonhydrolyzed sugar acts osmotically to increase stool water. The unabsorbed sugar is found in the stool; some is metabolized by enteric flora to lactic acid, lowering the pH of the stool.

Chronic nonspecific diarrhea in children less than 5 years of age is not associated with a failure to thrive and is usually associated with diets low in fat content (less than 27% of total calories); caloric content may be normal or low normal. The stool contains mucus but no blood. These children respond to an increase in fat content in the diet of 4 g/kg body weight.

General therapeutic considerations for children with diarrhea

1. Assess for shock, which requires immediate administration of appropriate fluids and electrolytes.
2. The less severely affected should have their state of hydration evaluated as mild, moderate, or severe. Moderate implies some dehydration, which is usually absent in mild diarrhea.
3. Severity also should be assessed based on weight loss per 24 hours. Acute diarrhea is usually considered as mild if weight loss is less than 3%, moderate if 3 to 6%, and

severe if over 6%. Severe diarrhea merits hospitalization for fluid replacement and treatment of the specific cause.

LIVER DISEASES

Bilirubin metabolism and the pathogenesis of various types of jaundice are discussed in the section on the newborn, where the primary problem of jaundice in the pediatric age-group is reviewed.

Neonatal hepatitis implies that there is intrahepatic cholestasis. The syndrome manifests as idiopathic neonatal hepatitis of unknown etiology, as neonatal infectious hepatitis, or as intrahepatic bile duct hypoplasia.

Neonatal infectious hepatitis is often shown to be due to a specific agent; a variety of viruses have been identified as causes of neonatal hepatitis, including hepatitis B, cytomegalovirus (CMV), herpes simplex, rubella, and coxsackievirus infections. Pregnant women who are carriers of hepatitis B surface antigen (HBsAg) are of little risk to the fetus, but there is a high incidence of neonatal infection among women who develop evidence of acute infectious hepatitis during the third trimester of pregnancy or within 2 months postpartum. In infants with intrauterine rubella, neonatal hepatitis and in some cases biliary atresia occur, and it is now thought that biliary atresia is the consequence of intrauterine viral infection. The 17-18 trisomy syndrome, consisting of neonatal hepatitis and biliary atresia, may also be of viral etiology.

The neonatal cholestasis syndrome can result from other causes:

1. Toxoplasmosis can occur in the newborn infant, with hepatomegaly, jaundice, and evidence of a generalized infection with CNS, eye, and cardiac involvement.
2. Bacterial infections that produce septicemia, pyelonephritis, and pneumonia also are associated with neonatal hepatitis; in addition, syphilis must always be considered.
3. Alpha$_1$-antitrypsin deficiency is also a major cause of the syndrome of intrahepatic cholestasis.

Intrahepatic cholestasis may result from hypoplasia or paucity of the intrahepatic ducts. These disorders, often referred to as **intrahepatic biliary atresia**, may result from a derangement in development or from a segmental destructive process within the liver. Distinctive syndromes associated with a paucity of intrahepatic bile ducts and an intact extrahepatic biliary tree have recently been identified. These include arteriohepatic dysplasia (Alagille syndrome); cerebrohepatorenal syndrome (Zellweger syndrome), in which there is absence of peroxisomal function; glutaric aciduria; and the rare, familial, fatal disorder of bile canalicular membranes known as Byler disease.

Extrahepatic biliary atresia is a term that refers to a group of anatomic abnormalities of the extrahepatic bile ducts, which lead to complete obstruction and cholestasis. It is thought to be developmental, but some cases may be the result of viral infection. Persistent and progressively increasing jaundice with acholic stools, impaired growth, malabsorption, development of cirrhosis with portal hypertension, hypoproteinemia, and bleeding problems occur. Afflicted children usually develop rickets. Stools are pale, urine dark, and serum bilirubin very high and mostly conjugated; serum transaminase levels are usually below 400 units, and alkaline phosphatase is moderately elevated.

Clinically, neonatal hepatitis usually begins in the second or third week of life; children show persistent jaundice with elevated levels of conjugated bilirubin and often develop acholic stools, suggesting complete absence of bile flow. It is difficult to differentiate neonatal hepatitis from cholestasis due to extrahepatic biliary atresia. In all cases of complete biliary obstruction, it is important to differentiate extrahepatic biliary atresia from neonatal hepatitis since an attempt at surgical correction of the former is mandatory, although successful in only 10 to 15% of cases. In the majority of cases, it is necessary to attempt to provide bile drainage by experimental procedures such as hepatoportoenterostomy (the Kasai operation) or even by liver transplantation.

Although hepatobiliary scintigraphy using labeled imidodiacetic acid analogues may be of some use in differentiating neonatal hepatitis from biliary atresia, liver biopsy provides the most definitive means of diagnosis. In biliary atresia there is bile ductular proliferation but the basic hepatic lobular architecture is intact. In neonatal hepatitis there is disturbed architecture, diffuse hepatocellular disease, and marked infiltration of inflammatory cells.

The relative incidence of the various cholestatic syndromes should also be considered in the differential diagnosis. Idiopathic neonatal hepatitis occurs in 1 in 5,000 to 10,000 births; biliary atresia is less common, occurring in 1 in 10,000 to 15,000 births. Intrahepatic bile duct atresia or hypoplasia is still less common, occurring in 1 in 50,000 to 75,000 births.

Intrahepatic biliary atresia is associated with more prolonged survival than is extrahepatic obstruction; children usually live for a decade and characteristically develop cutaneous xanthomas. Severe itching is a problem because of bile salt retention. Treatment with cholestyramine increases extrahepatic elimination of bile salts and is helpful.

There are many complications of chronic cholestasis:

1. Retention of substances such as cholesterol, bilirubin, bile acids, and trace elements (e.g., copper) normally excreted into the bile.
2. Decreased intraluminal bile acid concentration, which results in malabsorption of long-chain triglycerides and fat-soluble vitamins (A, D, E, and K) with steatorrhea.
3. Growth is retarded.
4. Rickets is common.
5. Vitamin E deficiency, which leads to muscle degeneration.
6. Progressive fibrosis in the liver leads to biliary cirrhosis.

Hepatitis in older infants and children

The mode of transmission, clinical manifestations, and laboratory findings in hepatitis A, hepatitis B, and non-A/non-B hepatitis are very similar to those found in adults (see Chapter 1).

Therapy may require 4 to 6 weeks of corticosteroid administration if jaundice does not improve after a few weeks of observation. Isolation precautions are indicated for these patients while hospitalized, and parents should be advised on precautions to take at home.

Severe hepatitis. Although mild, anicteric cases of hepatitis are more common in children than in adults, prolonged or persistent hepatitis occasionally occurs, with continued hepatomegaly and laboratory abnormalities for several months. With severe hepatitis, fluid retention and ascites may occur, in part as a result of increased sodium retention by renal tubules; restriction of sodium intake and diuretics are necessary in these instances. Encephalopathy occurs in part as a result of shunting of portal venous blood around the liver and may be aggravated by diuretic therapy. Protein should be eliminated from the diet. GI bleeding is common, adding to the protein load causing the encephalopathy. Adequate carbohydrate intake is important to minimize protein breakdown, and unabsorbable antibiotics (e.g., neomycin) can decrease bacterial ammonia formation in the gut; lactulose helps convert some of the ammonia in the gut to ammonium ion, which is less absorbed.

Fulminant hepatitis can occur, with acute massive hepatic necrosis and death within a few weeks. Mental changes (lethargy, confusion, EEG changes) develop, the liver size decreases rapidly, and widespread bleeding associated with prolonged prothrombin time not corrected by vitamin K are characteristic. Other serum proteins, as well as hepatic enzyme levels, may fall in these patients as a result of failure of synthesis by liver cells.

Chronic hepatitis and cirrhosis. Chronic liver disease with cirrhosis most commonly results from biliary atresia or cystic fibrosis; occasionally it is the result of undiagnosed Wilson's disease, alpha$_1$-antitrypsin deficiency, or neonatal hepatitis. Most cases of cirrhosis in the pediatric population occur between the ages of 10 and 20, with a female preponderance. Portal hypertension with bleeding esophageal varices and ascites occurs late. Multisystem disease is present in many cases, including nephritis, thyroiditis, myositis, arthralgia, colitis, and acquired hemolytic anemia, suggesting an autoimmune mechanism. A positive test for antinuclear antibody is common, and the term "lupoid hepatitis" is used, but the disease process appears to be distinct from true SLE, and liver involvement is extremely rate in SLE. Liver biopsy shows piecemeal necrosis, with areas of regeneration, lymphoid and plasma cell accumulation, and erosion of the limiting plate separating the portal tract and the lobule, as well as fibrosis. Therapy usually includes corticosteroids, but more than 80% of patients with chronic liver disease die within 5 years.

A number of developmental congenital metabolic abnormalities lead to cirrhosis of the liver (Table 4-13).

Other causes of portal hypertension. Portal vein thrombosis is usually secondary to neonatal omphalitis or trauma to the umbilical vein during cannulation. Anomalies of the portal circulation occur but are rare. Portal hypertension is more often due to postnecrotic cirrhosis or extrahepatic biliary obstruction. Collateral circulation is prominent, with a caput medusae apparent on the abdominal wall. Hematemesis occurs frequently, and the overall prognosis is very poor. Radiological esophagography or careful esophagoscopy usually establishes the presence of varices and confirms the diagnosis; celiac arteriography is also useful. Surgical relief of the portal hypertension is helpful but should be delayed until age 4 to 6 if possible.

Table 4-13. Examples of Congenital Metabolic Abnormalities Leading to Cirrhosis of the Liver

Syndrome	Autosomal dominant (D) or recessive (R)	Associated findings
Polycystic liver disease	D or R	Usually associated with polycystic kidneys
Congenital hepatic fibrosis	R	
Hereditary-hemorrhagic telangiectasia	D	Muscosal hemangiomas
Wilson's disease	R	Increased hepatic copper, decreased ceruloplasmin, Kayser-Fleischer rings. Effective control with penicillamine
Galactosemia	R	Nonglucose-reducing substance in urine; cataracts; treatment with galactose-free diet
Cystic fibrosis	R	Increased sweat chloride, pulmonary infections
Fructose intolerance	R	Hypoglycemia
Thalassemia major	R	Repeated transfusions lead to secondary hemochromatosis
Glycogen storage disease, Type IV	R	
Tyrosinosis	R	Rickets; renal tubular disorders; may present as neonatal hepatitis
Cystinosis	R	Rickets; renal tubular disorders
Alpha$_1$-antitrypsin deficiency	R	May present as neonatal hepatitis; decreased levels of inhibitor in serum; cytoplasmic inclusions in liver

REYE'S SYNDROME

Reye's syndrome, an acute process involving the liver and CNS, is frequently fatal. It usually follows a mild viral infection; influenza B, herpes simplex, and varicella viruses have been implicated. *Other agents, particularly salicylates, may be precipitating factors and should be avoided in children with viral infections.*

Patients begin vomiting, rapidly followed by delerium, which progresses to stupor and coma. There is moderate hepatomegaly, signs of brain stem involvement such as altered pupillary reflexes, and evidence of increased intracranial pressure. Laboratory findings include increased serum transaminases but little or no increase in serum bilirubin; coagulation factors synthesized in the liver are decreased, and bleeding may become a problem.

Liver biopsy reveals pale tissue, with fatty vacuoles in hepatocytes; lipid stains are positive, showing evidence of increased triglycerides and fatty acids. Electron microscopic examination reveals mitochondrial swelling and pleomorphism. Fatty infiltration in other organs, including the myocardium, renal tubules and pancreas, has been reported. These abnormalities may account for the arrhythmias, aminoaciduria, and hypoglycemia that occur in some of these patients. Reduction in urea cycle enzymes, including carbamyl phosphate synthetase and ornithine transcarbamylase, have been reported and may acount for the inability of the liver to convert ammonia to urea.

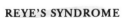

There is no specific therapy yet. Treatment of hypoglycemia with IV glucose, correction of acidosis, and infusion of mannitol and dexamethasone to control cerebral edema are tried. Exchange transfusion has been reported to reduce neurological changes and improve survival.

PEDIATRIC CARDIOLOGY

The major cause of heart disease in children is congenital heart disease; approximately 5 to 7 per 1,000 newborn infants have a cardiovascular anomaly. Among the most common anomalies are **ventricular septal defects, patent ductus arteriosus,** and **atrial septal defects.** Although rheumatic heart disease is the second most common cause of heart disease in childhood worldwide, in the United States the incidence of this disorder has declined radically over the past 25 years. Recent sporadic reports of outbreaks of rheumatic fever have led to renewed concern, however. Since congenital heart disease is highly lethal in early childhood, the proportion of heart disease due to the effects of rheumatic fever and other causes makes up about 30% of the total in children of highschool age.

Chest pain is rarely the initial presentation of hert disease in childhood, in contrast to that in adults. Ninety-five percent of children present with a cardiac murmur. The time when murmurs first appear is helpful in suggesting the diagnosis. Murmurs from obstructive lesions are usually heard in the immediate neonatal period; those murmurs related to pressure differences between the right and left chambers of the heart may not appear for weeks or months. Other murmurs whose intensity is dependent on large stroke volume may not be appreciated for years. Since 50% of all children may have functional murmurs that disappear over time, it is important to recognize their distinguishing characteristics. **Functional murmurs** are of short duration and occur in midsystole, never in diastole. They are usually soft and low pitched. These soft murmurs are best heard at the upper left sternal border. A second type is a loud, low-pitched murmur heard best to the right of the apex, sometimes transmitted to the left of the sternum.

Infants with congenital heart disease may present initially with cyanosis and symptoms of hypoxia. It has been shown that only at arterial oxygen saturations below 75% is clinical cyanosis apparent to all observers in all patients. Three of the most common congenital anomalies producing cyanosis are **tetralogy of Fallot, transposition of the great vessels,** and **pulmonary stenosis with atrial or ventricular septal defects.** When the right-to-left shunt leads to a concentration of reduced hemoglobin of 5 g/100 ml or greater in capillary blood, cyanosis becomes apparent.

In some children with congenital cardiac defects, congestive heart failure precipitated by a respiratory tract infection may be the first sign of the disorder. The finding of an abnormal cardiac silhouette on x-ray may also be the initial clue to heart disease in children.

The evaluation of the cardiovascular system in infants and children must include three important measurements: (1) blood pressure, (2) cardiac rate as well as peripheral arterial pulse rate and character, and (3) respiratory rate and pattern.

Blood pressure should be measured in both upper extremities and in at least one lower extremity. The contrast of high blood pressure in the upper extremities and low or undectectable pressure in the lower extremities points to the diagnosis of **coarctation of the aorta.** The blood pressure of a child increases steadily with age and correlates with height and weight. Ranges of blood pressure in normal children have been published and serve as the standards for comparison and evaluation.

Cardiac rate varies with development from fetal life through adolescence. The normal fetal heart rate varies between 120 and 160/minute. A slow heart rate may indicate fetal distress or may signal congenital heart block. Average rates for a full-term infant during the first week of life are 120 to 140/minute. The heart rate slows as the infant ages, and by 2 years the resting rate is 110/minute. By 10 years, the rate is about 90/minute, and by adolescence the values are 60 to 80/minute.

Anemia, shock, and fever are associated with rapid heart rates. Slower rates may be normal with physical training, but pathological states such as increased intracranial pressure, hypothyroidism, or increased serum potassium levels are also associated with slow cardiac rates.

The normal rate of respiration ranges from 30 to 50/minute at birth and decreases to 16 to 20 by age 6 years. At adolescence, the respiratory rate is 14 to 16/minute. Rapid or slow rates of respiration as well as depth of respiration and use of accessory muscles are important signs of pathological processes.

PULMONARY DISEASES

Special features of pulmonary disease occurring in infants and children will be covered in this section.

Respiratory tract infections are common in childhood, but many respiratory tract symptoms are produced by noninfectious diseases as well. The nature of the accompanying symptoms is very helpful in the differential diagnosis. The presence of stridor is an especially serious finding, warranting immediate attention and often emergency therapy.

Stridor is a harsh sound caused by obstruction in the larynx or trachea during breathing; it usually is caused by a serious problem and should never be ignored. Stridor can resemble a wheeze and may be minimal at rest. Inspiratory stridor is usually due to obstruction at or above the larynx, whereas subglottic or tracheal lesions usually cause expiratory stridor. The soft, easily collapsible nature of the trachea and larynx makes children more susceptible to narrowing of the airway during expiration.

Stridor present since birth suggests a developmental abnormality or birth trauma. Difficulty in breathing in the newborn is usually accompanied by difficulty in feeding, and there may be regurgitation with aspiration, leading to episodes of pneumonia.

In young children, stridor is usually due to inhaled foreign bodies, and the history of what the child was doing when the stridor first appeared is important; if he was playing with a toy that is missing, or if she was eating easily aspirated foods (e.g., peanuts, popcorn, food such as watermelon with seeds, etc.), x-ray and endoscopy (laryngoscopy and bronchoscopy) for foreign body should be performed immediately. Examination may reveal unilateral or localized noise during inspiration, helping to point to the location of the obstruction; muscles of respiration show retraction during inspiration.

Acute infectious croup is a major cause of stridor in young children; it is usually of viral origin today, particularly due to parainfluenza viruses.

Acute epiglottitis, usually caused by *H. influenzae*, can result in a life-threatening laryngeal obstruction; emergency restoration of the airway by intubation or tracheotomy may be necessary. Infectious mononucleosis can also cause sufficient swelling of tonsillar and adenoidal lymphatic tissue to produce airway obstruction, as can a retropharyngeal abscess.

Angioneurotic edema due to allergic reaction and laryngospasm due to an irritant gas can also cause severe, life-threatening stridor.

Paralysis of the vocal cords due to a congenital anomaly can cause stridor in early infancy, with difficulty feeding. Other congenital or recurrent lesions that can cause respiratory obstruction include nasal polyps or foreign bodies, laryngeal webs or cysts, thryoglossal cysts, congenital goiter, mediastinal masses, double aortic arch, anomalous innominate or left carotid artery, and anomalous pulmonary artery.

Wheezing is usually due to narrowing of medium or small airways. Table 4-14 lists the common causes of wheezing in childhood.

Acute viral bronchiolitis is usually due to respiratory syncytial virus (RSV) in children and is accompanied by marked tachypnea and dyspnea; cyanosis may be present. The differentiation from asthma may be difficult (see below).

Cough can be a feature of many types of pulmonary disease, including infections in the bronchi or pulmonary parenchyma, allergies, pulmonary edema, aspiration of foreign material, extrinsic irritation of the tracheobronchial tree by tumors or infection, etc. Psychogenic cough or a habit-spasm tic can also cause a chronic cough. Some diagnostic features of coughs worth keeping in mind include the following:

1. Sinusitis causes a cough because of postnasal drip entering the trachea; it is usually worst at night or shortly after arising in the morning.
2. Bronchitis can cause a deep, productive cough that can persist 4 to 6 weeks after other signs of the upper respiratory tract infection have disappeared.
3. Pertussis cause paroxysms of harsh, repetitive coughs followed by an abrupt, deep, noisy inspiration (the whoop).
4. *Chlamydia* causes a cough in infants, usually 2 to 6 weeks of age, with a distinctive series of harsh, staccato coughs separated by a brief inspiration; there is no posttussic whoop. An inclusion conjunctivitis is present in about half the cases.
5. Bronchiectasis produces paroxysms of coughing productive of purulent sputum, sometimes with blood, often induced by changes of posture.
6. Coughing occurring with feeding of an infant suggests a bronchopleural fistula.
7. A harsh, repetitive, brassy cough often results from compression or infiltration of the bronchial wall by mediastinal adenopathy or tumor.
8. An associated stridor suggests larygneal or tracheal obstruction.
9. A chronic cough in an adolescent suggests smoking.
10. Cough due to habit spasm is usually short, dry, absent during sleep, and worse when attention is directed to it. It often begins with a respiratory infection but persists and is magnified by parental concern.

BRONCHIOLITIS AND RESPIRATORY SYNCYTIAL VIRUS

RSV is the major cause of bronchiolitis and pneumonia in infants under 1 year of age and is considered the most important respiratory tract pathogen of early childhood. It accounts for 45 to 75% of bronchiolitis, 15 to 25% of childhood pneumonia, and 6 to 8% of croup.

Epidemics of RSV occur in temperate climates each winter and last 4 to 5 months. In urban settings, it is estimated that half the susceptible infants develop a primary infection in each epidemic. In day-care centers, the attack rate approaches 100% in young infants.

Bronchiolitis is common after the first year of life. After that age, acute infective wheezing is called asthmatoid bronchitis or asthma attacks. Many children with asthma give a history of bronchiolitis in infancy.

In infants 1 to 4 years of age, *Chlamydia trachomatis* may cause interstitial pneumonia. There may be conjunctivitis. Although coughing is prominent, wheezing is not.

Although coryza, pharyngitis, and fever are the common symptoms produced by this infection, lower respiratory tract infections, including bronchitis, bronchopneumonia, and/or bronchiolitis, occur in 10 to 40% of infants. Bronchiolitis is the

Table 4-14. Causes of Wheezing in Children

Acute bronchiolitis:
  Viral (especially respiratory syncytial virus)
  Aspiration of toxins (especially hydrocarbons such as gasoline, turpentine, lighter fluid)

Recurrent wheezing:
  Bronchial asthma
  Hypersensitivity pneumonitis (pigeon-breeder's lung, farmer's lung, etc.)
  Aspiration bronchitis
  H-type bronchoesophageal fistula (which can be a subtle lesion, causing repeated aspiration)

Infectious bronchitis:
  Cystic fibrosis
  Immune deficiency disorders
  Nonspecific infections

Alpha$_1$-antitrypsin deficiency (not usually evident until third decade of life)

Obliterative bronchiolitis (usually an end-stage result of viral infection)

Congenital heart disease with hyperperfusion, or other congenital vascular anomalies (as listed above)

most common clinical diagnosis established in infants hospitalized with RSV infection; it is most common in the second month of life. Reinfections occur. Recurrent wheezing occurs in 33 to 50% of infants who have had bronchiolitis; humidified oxygen therapy is often needed in these cases. Ribavirin therapy has been found to be useful in very sick or high-risk cases.

BRONCHIAL ASTHMA

Asthma is a common problem in childhood. Attacks may be infrequent or almost constant. The symptom complex may due to extrinsic factors (allergic asthma, usually due to pollens or dusts, immunologically mediated with release of mediators from mast cells, especially histamine) or intrinsic, due to nonallergic factors. Exercise-induced and aspirin-induced asthma also occur.

Narrowing of bronchi due to smooth muscle spasm, mucosal edema, and accumulation of thick mucus produces the wheezing typical of asthma. Children with asthma have recurrent attacks of wheezing and usually have airways that are hyperreactive to various stimuli, an important diagnostic point helping to differentiate asthma from other causes of wheezing.

Childhood asthma usually begins by age 5 and is twice as common in boys as in girls and is more common in black than in white children. Asthma seems to decrease in early adolescence and recur in late teen years. The prevalence of asthma increased 58% (from 4.8% to 7.6%) among 6- to 11-year-old black as well as white children of both sexes during the decade of the 1970s. During the same period, there was an increase in both severity of and mortality due to asthma. Death from asthma occurs more frequently in childhood than in adult asthmatics.

There is a greater prevalence of asthma in the South than in the North, both in the United States and in Europe.

Smoking is especially harmful for asthmatics.

Pathophysiology

In asthma, narrowing of airways occurs because of bronchospasm, edema of the mucosa, and increased amounts of secretions. Since the resistance to flow of a fluid in a tube is inversely proportional to the fourth power of the radius of the tube, this effect increases resistance to expiration more than inspiration. Asthmatics use accessory muscles of respiration to augment the pressure on expiration, and there is prolongation of the expiratory phase and wheezes, especially during expiration. The high intrathoracic pressure can exceed the intraluminal pressure in the bronchi, at least in some areas, and bronchial collapse can occur. Air trapping results. The patients have hyperpnea and dyspnea, and the air trapping results in hyperinflation of the thorax. The asthmatic lung becomes stiffer (decreased compliance). The work of breathing is greatly increased, and fatigue can result.

Irregular ventilation of areas of the lung that remain well perfused (ventilation-perfusion mismatch) results in some blood moving through the lung without being fully oxygenated; anoxemia results, and cyanosis may become detectable. The greater diffusibility of carbon dioxide than oxygen allows the adequately ventilated areas to compensate in this regard, and

patients with mild to moderate asthma show normal or even decreased $PaCO_2$ because of the hyperpnea and overcompensation of well-ventilated areas of lung. When the asthma is severe, however, the ability of the relatively well-ventilated areas to compensate is lost and carbon dioxide retention develops.

Clinical features

Extrinsic asthma is allergic and mediated primarily by IgE; it is often seasonal, such as when ragweed pollen is airborne. Dust, feathers, mold, and animal dander are other common causes. Allergic rhinitis and conjunctivitis may accompany the asthma. Positive skin tests are usually detectable. Avoidance of the allergen, specific anti-immune therapy, and bronchodilators are usually adequate therapy.

Intrinsic asthma results from highly irritable bronchi that react on exposure to a variety of stimuli, including air pollutants, weather changes, respiratory tract infections, exposure to cold air, and emotional stress. Immune mechanisms are not involved, and skin tests for allergies are negative. Symptoms may occur in any season but tend to be more frequent in winter because of the greater frequency of respiratory tract infections. Mixed-type cases occur, and asthma may relate to strenuous exertion (exercise-induced asthma, usually subsiding within 1 to 2 hours) or may be induced by aspirin or other prostaglandin inhibitors (i.e., the nonsteroidal anti-inflammatory agents).

Clinically, in very severe cases of asthma, wheezing may not be heard because of almost total airway obstruction. Patients will show a hyperinflated thorax, with raised shoulders and hyperresonance on percussion. They may be cyanotic, and the anoxia produces anxiety, restlessness, irritability, or confusion. Carbon dioxide retention causes headache, muscle twitching, somnolence, and even coma. These patients will show a greatly exaggerated pulsus parodoxus, and this is a useful finding.

Examination of the sputum in patients with allergic asthma usually reveals eosinophils, Charcot-Leyden crystals (probably the result of breakdown products of eosinophils), and Curschmann's spirals (mucoid casts of the bronchioles). Neutrophils and bacteria will be present if there is infection. Asthmatic children usually have elevated white blood cells and eosinophils during attacks, whether or not the asthma is allergic, but secondary polycythemia is rare. X-rays show evidence of hyperinflation, but evidence of pneumonia, atelectatic areas, and pneumothorax may be present.

Status asthmaticus is defined as a persistent attack of asthma not responding to treatment with the usual measures; asphyxia and death can occur, and a true medical emergency exists. Such episodes are often precipitated by abuse of sympathomimetic nebulizers and by complicating respiratory tract infections. Assessment includes examination for cyanosis, intensity of wheezing, evidence of fatigue of accessory muscles of respiration, dehydration, cerebral function, existence of underlying disease, severity of pulsus paradoxus, chest x-ray, white blood cells, throat culture, sputum examination and culture, serum electrolytes, and arterial blood gases (ABGs). Patients not responding to oxygen, fluid, and electrolyte therapy require intravenous aminophylline and corticosteroid therapy.

Diagnostic decisions

Evaluation of patients with severe asthma includes chest x-ray and ABG determination. During mild attacks, the child usually hyperventilates; the Pa_{O_2} is slightly decreased, and excessive removal of carbon dioxide gives a low Pa_{CO_2}. With increased severity of the attack and loss of the compensatory removal of carbon dioxide, the Pa_{CO_2} decreases to a level that appears normal, but the Pa_{O_2} decreases further. With maximal bronchial destruction and fatigue of respiratory muscle, the Pa_{CO_2} increases; levels above 55 mm Hg indicate impending respiratory failure, and above 65, frank respiratory failure.

Pulmonary function tests are usually normal between attacks of asthma; during attacks, the peak expiratory flow rate (PEFR), vital capacity (VC), and forced expiratory flow rate in 1 second (FEV_1) become abnormal. Although the FEV_1 (normally >86% of VC) is a good indicator of airway obstruction, the value obtained depends on the effort expended. A good measure of small-airway resistance is the maximal mid-expiratory flow rate (MMEFR), the mean flow rate in the middle of the FEV. Measured on a spirogram, it is usually the earliest sign of airway obstruction and the last finding to return to normal.

Before and after the use of an inhaled bronchodilator (e.g., isoproterenol), asthmatics usually show an increase in PEFR and FEV_1 of over 15 to 20%, whereas patients with chronic bronchitis, emphysema, and other forms of chronic obstructive lung disease show a lesser degree of improvement.

Children with allergic asthma usually have elevated IgE levels, and radioallergoabsorbent skin tests (RAST) can identify specific allergens.

Therapeutic decisions

Removal of antigens from the environment of children with allergic asthma, as much as possible, is of paramount importance. Hyposensitization measures are also useful, although it is doubtful if bacterial vaccines are of value. Food allergies rarely cause asthma; milk and eggs are the most frequent offenders.

Pharmacologic measures.   Modification of intracellular levels of cyclic AMP (cAMP) and cyclic GMP (cGMP) forms the basis of drug therapy for asthma. An increase in intracellular cAMP inhibits release of mast cell mediators and promotes dilatation of bronchial smooth muscle; increase in intracellular cGMP has the opposite effects. The level of cAMP is increased by stimulation of bronchial cell receptors by catecholamines (e.g., isoproterenol or epinephrine), while stimulation of the alpha receptors in these cells by phenylephrine decreases cAMP. Cellular cGMP is increased by stimulation of cholinergic receptors (e.g., by acetylcholine) and is decreased by anti-cholinergic agents (e.g., atropine). Prostaglandin E increases cAMP, but prostaglandin $F_{2\alpha}$ increases cGMP. Theophylline inhibits the enzyme that breaks down these cyclic nucleotides (phosphodiesterase), resulting in higher levels of cAMP. Corticosteroids enhance catecholamine effects on beta receptors in asthmatics; prostaglandins have different receptors.

Theophylline, which depresses phosphodiesterase activity, is the most useful drug; therapeutic levels, 10 to 20 μg/ml, are usually obtained with 5-mg/kg doses 3 to 4 times a day. If an adequate response is not obtained, measurement of blood levels and appropriate adjustment of dosage regimen is worthwhile. Toxicity, usually at blood levels greater than 20 μg/ml, includes nausea, vomiting, hypotension, arrhythmias, hematemesis, and convulsive seizures.

Sympathomimetics produce bronchodilatation by increasing cAMP. Some are inactivated by intestinal enzymes (epinephrine, isoproterenol) and are only effective parenterally or by inhalation. Terbutaline and metaproterenol are more specific for the $beta_2$ receptors and produce better bronchial smooth muscle relaxation without the $beta_1$ effects on the heart. Epinephrine is very effective subcutaneously or by inhalation but has a short duration of action and causes CNS and cardiac stimulation. Ephedrine is cheap and effective orally and has a longer duration of action, requiring administration 3 to 4 times a day, but it is less effective and produces headache and insomnia in some children. Isoproterenol (Isuprel) is effective by inhalation, but a metabolite has some bronchoconstrictor effect. Newer $beta_2$ agonists, such as metaproterenol (Alupent), have longer action with a lower incidence of $beta_1$ effects. It can be administered orally or by inhalation, as can terbutaline sulfate and salbutamol, which are more potent $beta_2$ stimulators and can also be given subcutaneously.

Expectorants are thought to increase the flow of mucus and thus decrease its viscosity; iodides and glyceryl guaiacolate are used.

Cromolyn sodium apparently works by stabilizing mast cell membranes, preventing release of bronchoconstrictive mediators, and is most effective as preventive therapy in maintenance doses.

Corticosteroids affect a variety of mechanisms and are the most effective therapy for intractable cases of asthma. Maintenance doses of prednisone given every other day do not affect the hypothalamico-pituitary-adrenal axis (HPA) and therefore do not prevent growth; more frequent administration, even as low as 2.5 mg every day, does suppress the HPA. An inhaled steroid, beclomethasone, is effective topically without suppressing the HPA.

Therapy of severe attacks in a hospital emergency room usually begins with oxygen by nasal cannula and subcutaneous epinephrine every 15 to 20 minutes. If response is adequate, a long-acting form (Sus-Phrine) can be injected, oral theophylline given, and the child sent home. If response is not adequate, hydration and IV theophylline are given. If there is still not adequate response, the child should be considered in status asthmaticus and admitted. Complications should be sought (evidence of infection, including white blood cell count, sputum examination, and chest x-ray, which also will detect pneumothorax). Intravenous corticosteroids are usually needed. If clinical findings and ABG determinations reveal that respiratory failure is developing, IV isoproterenol and artificial mechanical ventilation are added.

Maintenance therapy for chronic asthma includes oral theophylline, sometimes other oral sympathomimetic agents (e.g., metaproterenol) and cromolyn sodium. Short-term steroid therapy may be needed, but long-term steroids, often needed in adults, can depress growth and also have many other adverse side effects. Beclomethasone (Vanceril) inhaled up to 4 times a day is preferable.

It is impossible to give an accurate prognosis, because childhood asthma is extremely variable. Between one-half and two-thirds of affected children outgrow the problem and are free of asthma as adults.

CYSTIC FIBROSIS

Cystic fibrosis, the most common life-threatening genetic trait among Caucasians, is due to an autosomal recessive gene located on chromosome 7. It is estimated to occur in 1 in 2,000 live births among whites and 1 in 17,000 live births in blacks. There are abnormalities of the exocrine glands, affecting primarily the lungs, pancreas, and GI tract, varying greatly in severity.

Cystic fibrosis is the major cause of severe chronic obstructive lung disease in childhood. Thickened secretions in the bronchi lead to dyspnea and cough. Secondary infections, bronchiectasis, and fibrosis are common sequelae in severe cases. Malabsorption can result from the thickened secretions in the GI tract, causing pancreatic exocrine insufficiency, fatty stools, deficiencies of fat-soluble vitamins, failure to gain weight, and retarded growth.

In almost 10% of newborn infants with cystic fibrosis, the thick intestinal secretions can cause obstruction of the distal small bowel (meconium ileus) within the first 24 to 48 hours of life. Ileal obstruction with fecal matter occurs occasionally in older children as well. Fibrosis of the pancreas can result in abnormal glucose tolerance; insulin-dependent hyperglycemia develops in 1 to 2%.

Nasal polyposis, pansinusitis, and rectal prolapse are also encountered in this disorder. Virtually all men with cystic fibrosis are sterile because of obstructive lesions in the vas deferens.

Hepatic lesions occur; 25% of the patients develop a focal biliary cirrhosis, occasionally diffuse enough to produce portal hypertension and esophageal varices.

Clinical manifestations of the pulmonary involvement can include hemoptysis (due to pulmonary infections leading to bronchiectasis) and pneumothorax; cor pulmonale can develop as result of severe obstructive pulmonary disease. Hypertrophic pulmonary osteoarthropathy can develop.

The wide spectrum of system involvement may lead to difficulty in differential diagnosis. The diagnosis is suggested by failure of a newborn infant to pass a stool in the first 24 hours. The presence of small bowel obstruction (usually at the ileocecal valve) and evidence of an underdeveloped colon (microcolon) are diagnostic of meconium ileus. Even before birth, meconium peritonitis may occur and peritoneal calcification can be seen. In milder cases, development of respiratory symptoms in early childhood (cough, recurrent pneumonia, persistent lung crackles) and repeated finding of *Pseudomonas, Staphylococcus,* or in infants, *Klebsiella* or *E. coli* in the sputum is very suggestive. Failure to thrive and gain weight, steatorrhea, evidence of biliary cirhosis, malnutrition, edema, nasal polyposis, hypochloremic hyponatremic metabolic acidosis, and a positive family history are also suggestive.

Electrolyte concentrations in the sweat are abnormally high in these patients, leading to heat intolerance. The quantitative sweat test is diagnostically useful; after pilocarpine iontophoresis, sweat is collected, and a chloride concentration above 60 mEq/L is abnormal (normal children have chloride levels below 50). False-positive test results can occur in myxedema, nephrogenic diabetes insipidus, untreated adrenal insufficiency mucopolysaccharidoses, severe malnutrition, and ectodermal dysplasia.

The diagnosis depends on a positive sweat test plus a family history, documented exocrine pancreatic insufficiency, or typical chronic obstructive pulmonary disease.

Therapy consists of antibiotics to combat the repeated infections, bronchodilators, and the mucolytic agent acetylcysteine (Mucomyst) by inhalation. Chest physiotherapy including postural drainage is very important. Administration of pancreatic enzymes orally can help the problem of malabsorption; vitamin supplementation and stool softeners help. Surgery is usually needed for meconium ileus.

The prognosis has improved with intensive medical therapy, and the mean duration of life is about 20 years; most patients die of the pulmonary disease.

BIBLIOGRAPHY

Behrman RE, Vaughan VC III: Nelson Textbook of Pediatrics, 13th ed. WB Saunders, Philadelphia, 1987.

Dworkin PH: National Medical Series for Independent Study. Pediatrics. John Wiley and Sons, New York, 1987.

Finberg L: Treatment of diarrhea in infancy. Pediatr Rev 3:113, 1981.

Gergen PJ, Mullally DI, Evans RE III: National survey of prevalence of asthma in the United States, 1976 to 1980. Pediatrics 81:1, 1988.

Haggerty RJ (ed): Symposium on chronic disease in children. Pediatr Clin North Am 1984.

Kaye R, Oski F, Barness L: Core Textbook of Pediatrics, 2nd ed. JB Lippincott, Philadelphia, 1982.

Krugman RD: Review of Pediatrics. WB Saunders, Philadelphia, 1983.

Nathan D, Oski F: Hematology of Infancy and Childhood, 3rd ed. WB Saunders, Philadelphia, 1987.

Rudolph A, Hoffman J: Textbook of Pediatrics, 18th ed. Appleton & Lang, East Norwalk.

SAMPLE QUESTIONS

DIRECTIONS: Each question below contains four suggested answers of which **one** or **more** is correct. Choose the answer:

A if **1, 2, and 3** are correct
B if **1 and 3** are correct
C if **2 and 4** are correct
D if **4** is correct
E if **1, 2, 3, and 4** are correct

1. Indications of sepsis usually observed in a neonate include

   1. leukopenia
   2. rapid respirations
   3. poor feeding
   4. fever

2. Which of the following statements about neonatal jaundice are true?

   1. The normal bilirubin level in cord blood is over 3 mg/100 ml
   2. The peak bilirubin level expected in normal infants is over 6 mg/100 ml
   3. Both conjugated and unconjugated bilirubin cross the placenta
   4. In normal infants, virtually all the bilirubin in cord blood is unconjugated

3. Which of the following statements about bilirubin in the newborn are true?

   1. Hemolysis is the main cause of rapid rise in bilirubin in the first day of life
   2. Drugs such as sulfisoxazole (Gantrisin) can increase the toxicity of unconjugated bilirubin by dissociating it from albumin
   3. Elevated conjugated bilirubin levels in newborn infants can indicate sepsis, neonatal hepatitis, or biliary atresia
   4. Phototherapy is useful in lowering levels of unconjugated bilirubin

4. Breast-feeding has which of the following advantages over milk formulas?

   1. Breast-fed infants have a lower incidence of allergies
   2. The protein of human breast milk is of higher biologic value
   3. Antibodies present in human breast milk are of clinical value
   4. Breast-fed infants do not require supplemental vitamins

5. Normal growth and development include which of the following parameters?

   1. Weight gain in the first 6 months of life averages 20 g per day
   2. Normal infants are expected to double their birth weight by 4 to 6 months
   3. Normal infants are expected to triple their birth weight by 1 year
   4. After 2 years of age, normal weight gain is about 2 kg/year

6. U.S. mortality statistics during childhood reveal which of the following statements to be true?

   1. The leading cause of death between the ages of 6 months and 19 years is motor vehicle accidents
   2. Suicide is the third leading cause of death among male adolescents
   3. The death rate from trauma in childhood is about four times higher than that due to disease
   4. Mechanical suffocation due to inhalation of objects put into the mouth is rare before the age of 1 year

7. Which of the following statements about Marfan's syndrome, a common genetic disorder, are true?

   1. In Marfan's syndrome, a family history is absent in a considerable proportion of the cases because of the high frequency of spontaneous mutations
   2. Aortic root dilatation can become a serious problem leading to aortic valvular insufficiency
   3. The weakened collagenous structure usually results in larger than normal eyeballs, associated with severe myopia
   4. Marfan's syndrome is an autosomal recessive disorder

8. Which of the following statements about inherited disorders are true?

   1. If a given set of parents have a child with an autosomal recessive disorder, the chances of the next child having the same disorder are still 25%
   2. More cases of Down's syndrome occur in children born to women under the age of 35 than to older women
   3. Mental deficiency seen in untreated galactosemia is preventable
   4. Hemophilia A and Duchenne's muscular dystrophy are sex-linked disorders

9. Organisms that are common causes of pharyngitis, other than group A hemolytic streptococci, include which of the following?

   1. *Mycoplasma pneumoniae*
   2. Adenoviruses
   3. Enteroviruses
   4. Epstein-Barr virus

10. In the syndrome of meningococcemia,

　　1. a fulminating syndrome that is rapidly fatal can occur
　　2. an IV line should be established immediately, before performance of a spinal tap
　　3. spinal fluid can have normal cellularity
　　4. a rash is not a usual finding

11. Which of the following statements about infections are true?

　　1. *Hemophilus influenzae, Streptococcus pneumoniae,* and *Staphylococcus aureus* are the most common causes of positive blood cultures in children
　　2. Overwhelming pneumococcal infection occurs most frequently in patients with absent spleens, such as those with sickle cell anemia
　　3. Acute disseminated staphylococcal infection can occur without predisposing cause, in previously healthy children
　　4. Acute meningococcemia can occur without predisposing cause, in previously healthy children

12. Which of the following statements are true about the treatment of severe dehydration?

　　1. The goal of the initial or emergency phase of treatment of severe dehydration is rapid reexpansion of extracellular fluid volume to improve circulatory dynamics
　　2. The goal of the second or repletion phase is complete restoration of lost volume within 8 hours
　　3. Oral fluids and glucose should be substituted for IV fluids as soon as possible
　　4. The correct procedure for replacement of fluid varies with the cause of the dehydration, not its severity

13. Which of the following statements about nephrotic syndrome are true?

　　1. Nephrotic syndrome can result from infection with a TORCH virus
　　2. Generalized edema can result from nephrotic syndrome, liver disease, or nutritional hypoalbuminemia
　　3. Idiopathic nephrotic syndrome of childhood would not be expected to respond to steroid therapy
　　4. Nephrotic syndrome can be due to systemic lupus erythematosus, IgA nephropathy, membranous glomerulonephritis, or diabetic nephropathy

14. Which of the following statements about hematuria are true?

　　1. Hematuria can be caused by pinworms
　　2. Foreign bodies in the urethra can be a cause of hematuria in childhood
　　3. Sickle cell trait is associated with hematuria
　　4. Hematuria would not be expected to occur in cystitis due to a virus

15. Which of the following statements about diabetes in childhood are true?

　　1. Genetic predisposition is not thought to be a significant factor since only 50% of monozygotic twins both get the disease
　　2. Environmental factors, such as viral infections, play no role in the etiology of childhood diabetes
　　3. Symptomatic diabetes in childhood can usually be treated without insulin
　　4. Antibodies against pancreatic islet cells have been demonstrated in children who develop diabetes

16. Which of the following statements about anemias in childhood are true?

　　1. A hemoglobin of 15 g/100 ml on the first day of life indicates a significant anemia
　　2. Hemorrhage by the newborn may not be apparent, since it could be bleeding in the placenta directly into the maternal circulation
　　3. Iron deficiency without hemorrhage is rare in the first 3 months of life
　　4. Isoimmunization due to ABO incompatibility can cause a hemolytic anemia presenting at 3 months of age

17. Which of the following statements about clotting disorders are true?

　　1. Idiopathic thrombocytopenic purpura in childhood usually requires splenectomy
　　2. Both von Willebrand's disease and hemophilia A result from deficiencies of components of Factor VIII
　　3. Both von Willebrand's disease and hemophilia A are sex-linked disorders
　　4. Coagulation Factors II, VII, IX, and X all are synthesized in the liver and are vitamin K dependent

18. Pyloric stenosis

　　1. rarely causes vomiting before 1 month of age
　　2. is usually familial
　　3. can usually be treated without surgery
　　4. can result in peristaltic waves that are visible across the surface of the abdomen

19. Which of the following statements about Reye's syndrome are true?

　　1. It usually follows a viral infection such as herpes simplex
　　2. Abnormal CNS function rapidly progresses to stupor and coma
　　3. It can apparently be precipitated by aspirin
　　4. It causes abnormal hepatic function with jaundice

20. Which of the following statements about murmurs in childhood are true?

1. Functional murmurs can extend into diastole
2. Murmurs due to septal defects may not be evident in the first few months of life because of the lack of a pressure difference between right- and left-sided circulations
3. Murmurs due to obstructive lesions are usually not heard in the neonatal period because of the rapid heart rate and low pressures in the newborn circulation
4. Murmurs are the most common presenting manifestation of cardiac disease in children

21. Evidence for an inhaled foreign body in a child can include which of the following?

1. A missing small toy
2. A localized wheeze
3. Retraction of muscles of respiration during inspiration
4. History of eating popcorn

22. Which of the following statements about childhood asthma are true?

1. Asthma is twice as frequent in boys as in girls
2. The prevalence of childhood asthma has increased in recent years
3. Death from asthma occurs more frequently in children than in adults
4. Exercise-induced asthma is usually relieved by aspirin

23. Which of the following statements about cystic fibrosis are true?

1. Pancreatic exocrine insufficiency can occur with malnutrition due to malabsorption
2. Repeated pulmonary infections with bronchitis and bronchiectasis are common
3. Heat intolerance is common as a result of increased electrolyte loss in sweat
4. Chronic obstructive pulmonary disease is not a usual clinical problem

DIRECTIONS: The group of questions below consists of lettered choices followed by several numbered items. For each numbered item, select the **one** lettered choice with which it is **most** closely associated. Each lettered choice may be used once, more than once, or not at all.

Questions 24–27. For each of the following descriptions of cough, choose the most likely cause.

A. Sinusitis
B. Pertussis
C. Bronchiectasis
D. Bronchoesophageal fistula
E. Habit spasm fistula in infant

24. Aggravated by changes in posture

25. Worst on arising in morning

26. Appears during feeding

27. Paroxysmal, followed by noisy inspiration

ANSWERS

1. A (1, 2, 3)	15. D (4)
2. D (2, 4)	16. A (1, 2, 3)
3. E (all)	17. C (2, 4)
4. A (1, 2, 3)	18. C (2, 4)
5. E (all)	19. A (1, 2, 3)
6. A (1, 2, 3)	20. C (2, 4)
7. A (1, 2, 3)	21. E (all)
8. E (all)	22. A (1, 2, 3)
9. E (all)	23. A (1, 2, 3)
10. A (1, 2, 3)	24. C
11. E (all)	25. A
12. B (1, 3)	26. D
13. C (2, 4)	27. B
14. A (1, 2, 3)	

5

PSYCHIATRY

Martin S. Kesselman

Symptoms causing mental distress are widely prevalent, and their recognition and treatment are an inextricable part of patient care no matter what the presenting problem. For example, the Midtown Manhattan study, which surveyed the prevalence of psychological symptoms in residents between the ages of 20 and 59 living in a circumscribed urban area, found that about 80% of subjects interviewed described psychological symptoms severe enough to cause significant distress. Surveys in rural settings have indicated lower but still significant prevalence rates.

Not all patients with such distress will present themselves to mental health workers. In general, only about 15% do so. Primary care physicians see by far the largest number of such patients, and many of these come with physical rather than psychological complaints. The relationship between physical illness and psychological distress is a complicated one. Psychological symptoms often appear as part of the clinical picture, not only because many medical illnesses directly affect cerebral function but because the patient must bring his or her personality with its strengths and weaknesses to bear on the threats that such illnesses present. Patients' capacity to respond to their symptoms, to seek medical care in an appropriate manner, and to comply with treatment are all affected by their mental state. Psychiatric illness often presents with physical symptoms. Patients with depression, for example may minimize their mood state and present with fatigue, insomnia, or weight loss instead. Finally, the incidence of medical illness is increased in patients with psychiatric disorders. There is some evidence that psychological stress may influence the immune system directly and make patients more vulnerable to physical illness.

Pilot programs in which psychiatrists or other mental health workers are integrated into the primary care health team have proved quite effective in identifying concomitant psychiatric disorder and in enhancing treatment. This system has not been widely adopted, most often on grounds of lack of feasibility or cost-effectiveness. Much of the primary care of psychiatric disorders remains in the hands of nonpsychiatric physicians. Therefore it is important to learn to assess and refer such patients as needed. In order to do so, one must be familiar with the major psychiatric disorders and know something about their treatment.

In accomplishing this goal, the third *Diagnostic and Statistical Manual* (*DSM-III*) is an invaluable guide. This manual was developed by the American Psychiatric Association in an attempt to respond to criticisms of previous diagnostic schemes. The authors of *DSM-III* were concerned that psychiatric diagnosis be **reliable**—that is, that well-trained psychiatrists would generally agree on the diagnosis no matter where the patient was seen. In order to assure this, diagnosis was based as much as possible on **objectifiable** signs and symptoms rather than on inference. Often, *DSM-III* indicates not only what symptoms must be present but how severe they must be and how long they must have persisted in order to be significant. Diagnoses often are **hierarchically arranged**; one must diagnose the most severe disorder possible even if the patient's presenting complaint might otherwise fit a less severe diagnosis. (For example, patients with schizophrenia might initially present with depressive symptoms and the more severe signs of symptoms of schizophrenia may be discovered only after more detailed scrutiny.) To the extent it is possible at our current state of knowledge, *DSM-III* tries to make diagnoses **valid**. A specific diagnosis should imply a course and treatment plan. Finally, to make the complex interaction between psychiatric, medical, and psychosocial aspects of the patient's condition explicit, *DSM-III* uses a **multiaxial scheme**. Axis I encodes the patient's clinical syndrome, Axis II the more long-standing personality disorder (and developmental disabilities) that might underlie the Axis I diagnosis. Axis III is used to encode the patient's physical disorders and conditions. Axes IV and V are used less commonly. Axis IV is used to encode the severity of the psychosocial stressors that the clinician believes may have contributed to the development of the psychiatric disorder. For example, illnesses that follow a severe stress may be more likely to resolve when the stressor is no longer present. In Axis V, the physician is asked to assess the highest adaptive level of functioning in the patient's social life, at work, and in leisure time activity in the year prior to the illness. This assessment allows the physician to determine whether treatment has at least returned the patient to baseline. It also has considerable prognostic import. The use of a multiaxial system allows the clinician to attempt to disentangle factors that might otherwise confound the diagnostic picture.

The following survey of clinical psychiatry is based on the major *DSM-III* disorders in adult psychiatry. Since there is considerable overlap in the application of therapies to various diagnostic categories, these are treated in a separate section at the end of the chapter.

ORGANIC MENTAL DISORDERS

Compromised brain function can be manifested in behaviors that are referred to the psychiatrist for diagnosis or management. Indeed, these changes may be the first manifestation of an otherwise silent disease process. Fortunately, despite the complexity of brain function and the many different disease processes that may impinge on them, there are a relatively few organic mental *syndromes* that are characteristic of underlying organic dysfunction. One may not know the etiology of an organic mental syndrome at the time of diagnosing it. That is the basis for the workups we will describe. Often, the etiologic diagnosis is apparent from the clinical context.

Two common types of specific organic mental disorders are diagnosed on Axis I. They are disorders arising in the presenium or senium and those that arise from substance abuse. If the medical cause of an organic mental syndrome is diagnosed, it will usually arise from a disease that is coded outside *DSM-III*, and this should be indicated on Axis III. In these cases, and when the etiology is unknown, the Axis I diagnosis should reflect the nature of the presenting organic mental syndrome.

DELIRIUM

Deliria are caused by conditions that compromise brain metabolism, such as hypoxia, hypoglycemia, electrolyte imbalance, or toxic states. Neoplasms, trauma, or hematomas may affect intracranial dynamics sufficiently to produce a delirium. Many commonly used drugs such as digitalis, sedatives, and tranquilizers produce direct toxic effects on the brain. If brain function is already compromised through loss of neural function (as in dementias), the patient will be more susceptible to these effects. Reduced alcohol tolerance, for example, may be an early sign of dementias.

In view of the manifold causes of delirium, it is not surprising that several studies have found that as many as a third of patients on a general medical ward will have more or less subtle signs of delirium, and in some settings where elderly patients predominate the incidence will be far higher.

Despite this, physicians are often insensitive to the signs of delirium or misdiagnose it as stemming from functional causes.

The cardinal manifestation of delirium is a reduced state (or clouding) of consciousness, which in turn affects attention, orientation, memory, sleep patterns, and motor behaviors. Consider these one at a time: Patients with delirium are distractible. It is difficult to gain and hold their attention, and their affect is relatively shallow even when one attempts to engage them on serious topics. They may be disoriented to time, place, or person, but this is not reliably present in early deliria and is not necessary for the diagnosis if other signs are present. Orientation for "time, place, and person" is lost in that order as the delirium progresses. Patients who are disoriented for person (particularly for personal identity) are apt to be severely ill. If they are not, one should consider a functional dissociative state. As the patient improves, orientation is recovered in reverse order. Disturbances of memory result from the patient's inability to attend to and register the requisite information. Frequently, delirious patients will mis-

identify stimuli in the environment because they can only grasp at partial cues and are restricted to superficial similarities. They may state that they are in a butcher shop, for instance, because the white coats of the staff recall that setting. Speech is often incoherent but not because, as in the functional psychosis, the patient is distracted by idiosyncratic or bizarre associations so much as because of the vacillating state of alertness and disattentiveness. Since the diffusely represented small-celled reticular activating system is particularly disrupted by metabolic insults, the patient's state of alertness will wax and wane (this instability is particularly characteristic of organic states) and the patient's sleep patterns may be disrupted or even reversed. Hallucinations may occur. They are often visual (in contrast to the idea-like auditory hallucinations of schizophrenia). In some cases, microptic hallucinations are present. Tactile or olfactory hallucinations also occur but do not present so clear a diagnostic indicator. Finally, the patient may show either psychomotor retardation or agitation. Agitation is perhaps more common in drug withdrawal states. Because of the possibility of injury from either of these conditions, patients are usually kept under close observation and in loose restraints.

Since any factor that interferes with the metabolism of brain cells can cause a delirium, the differential diagnosis is extensive. Common causes of delirium in the general hospital are as follows:

Hypoxia
Hypoglycemia
Electrolyte imbalance
Infection
Fever
Medication (e.g., digitalis)
Drug withdrawal states
Hepatic or renal failure

The diagnostic workup for delirium is intended to adduce evidence for both intra- and extracranial metabolic disturbances. A complete history and physical examination will provide the surest basis for an informed guess as to etiology. Withdrawal syndromes and specific intoxications can be deduced from the relevant historical data or from the patient's social and psychiatric background. Endocrine, cardiovascular, and neurological causes usually manifest themselves in physical findings. Infections are accompanied by fever, x-ray findings, or immunologic studies. A complete blood count, urinalysis, ECG, and automated blood tests for electrolytes, blood urea, glucose, and liver enzymes will allow assessment of the patient's metabolic status. In delirium, the EEG is slowed, with beta and even delta activity predominating.

One must recall that compromise of brain functioning, whether because of dementia or from more transient causes such as operative stress, may lower the patient's resilience to any of these factors. Some patients will show findings of delirium when, in a compromised state, they are exposed to reduced or exaggerated levels of environmental stimulation. Patients in an ICU, who are both overstimulated by the constant ambient activity and who are often deprived of social supports, are particularly susceptible to deliria. Elderly organic patients may show signs of confusion in the evening or nighttime when stimulus levels are low. Patients who are receiving low doses of sedative-hypnotic drugs may show "sundowning," confusional states during periods of inadequate ambient stimulation. The appearance of a delirium should always suggest the possibility of an underlying dementing process.

Obviously, the treatment of a delirium is the treatment of the underlying pathogenic process. Certain general measures are usually of help, however. Patients should be loosely restrained to avoid harming themselves. Delirious patients should be housed in well-lit areas and, if possible, constantly attended. It must be recalled that sedation is often the cause of the problem. If feasible, sedatives should be lowered or withdrawn. If this is impossible, adequate doses of a non-sedative tranquilizer (e.g., a butyrophenone) should be employed.

DEMENTIA

Deliria are disorders characterized by **disorganization** of mental functioning, whereas dementias are characterized by **loss of mental abilities** sufficient to interfere with normal social and vocational functioning. Although dementias are often irreversible or progressive, if the loss of function is related to metabolic or nutritional factors (e.g., hypoglycemia, endocrine disturbances, thiamine deficiency), cognitive deficits may be at least partially reversible. Therefore, the equation of dementias with nonreversible organic mental disease has been discarded in *DSM-III*. A particularly dramatic instance of this is so-called pseudodementia, a syndrome sometimes indistinguishable from other dementing syndromes but due to psychiatric causes. In the elderly, almost all such cases are due to underlying depression; these patients respond well to antidepressants. In younger patients, schizophrenia, hysteria, and mania must be included in the differential diagnosis as well. Pseudodementias account for about 10% of cases evaluated for intellectual deterioration. When anatomic findings are present in dementia, they are usually in the form of thinning of the cortical mantle or enlargement of the ventricles. In other instances, normal brain tissue may be replaced by tumor or gliosis. Since nerve tissue does not regenerate, organic mental syndromes that evince the presence of a dementing process are characteristically irreversible and often progressive. The changes in the EEG are usually in the form of slowing; however, the EEG may remain normal well after symptoms appear.

The clinical presentation of a dementia depends on many factors. The neurological function of the part of the brain affected is certainly a major determinant. Thus it is important to understand the neuropsychological function of the major areas of the cortex. However, early in the course of a dementing illness, it is not these *direct* effects that are most prominent but the adaptive changes in the patient's personality by which he or she attempts to compensate for or conceal the progressive loss of function. We are all highly invested in maintaining our sense of mental competence and mastery. Even minor changes in our mental capacity are apt to evoke those mechanisms we use to deal with frustrations and obstacles in our daily lives. Thus, paradoxically, the earliest sign of a dementing process may be an **exaggeration of the patient's premorbid personality**—that is, a heightening of the patient's usual defensive operations. Thus, scrupulous and overorganized patients may become even more exact as they attempt to overcome an encroaching handicap. A patient who uses denial or "giving up" as a coping style may appear hypomanic or depressed. In other patients, normal defense mechanisms break down and patients become sufficiently unlike their "usual self" to draw attention. For example, an ordinarily repressed and straitlaced person may become talkative and sexually preoccupied. Thus patients who present with changes in psychiatric symptoms incongruous with their premorbid status should be examined closely for dementia.

As a corollary, the clinical presentation of dementia will depend to some extent on the rate at which the dementing process progresses. Slowly developing processes allow the patient to adapt and may be manifested—in the early phases at least—by psychological symptoms. Fulminant processes may be manifested by anxiety and confusion. In the latter case, the patient is less able to deny the underlying process. Similarly, dementias often come to light when patients are forced to change their external circumstances drastically, since this sort of change stresses their adaptive capacity. So long as patients can coast along on habit, those around them may see little change. For this reason, elderly patients may show what appears to be a drastic deterioration of function when they are widowed or are forced to move to new surroundings.

Finally, patients with impaired cortical functioning will be more apt to develop superimposed delirious states when brain metabolism is compromised.

Common symptoms of dementia include the following:

1. **Personality changes** (as noted above). Demented patients may present with a variety of organic personality disturbances. They may seem shallow or silly (*witzelsucht*). They may display behavioral inertia, trouble starting on a task, and trouble stopping once started. For example, the demented patient may be unable to name 10 states. Social judgment may be sufficiently impaired as to affect personal hygiene or appearance. Impulses may be disinhibited; the patient may manifest uncharacteristic and inappropriate sexual tendencies. Patients with frontal lobe disease may become bland and apathetic.

2. **Disturbances in memory.** Characteristically, recent memories are difficult to retrieve while, initially at least, long-term memory is preserved (Ribot's law). For example, older people may dwell with precision on episodes in their youth but forget events of the day before. With progression of the disorder, even these memories may be lost or confused and patients may have difficulty responding to persons and situations with which they have been long familiar.

3. **Loss of abstract attitude.** This refers to the capacity to see relationships between objects that are quite unlike (e.g., to see that both an orange and a banana are examples of a fruit), to flexibly deploy attention to the significant (as opposed to the salient) features of a situation, and to respond to the symbolic rather than the "signal" aspect of a stimulus. Demented patients will stop at a red light and proceed on a green one; they will not know what to do when the light is stuck on red. During the mental status examination, abstraction is usually tested with similarities or proverb interpretation. (The demented patient will not see that "You can't tell a book by its cover" is intended to apply to people, not books.)

4. **Impaired judgment.** To some extent, judgment is a faculty that depends on abstract attitude. Inappropriate

behavior in social situations or at work may be in the initial presentation of dementia. It is difficult to capture this quality by formal testing. Patients may have difficulty responding to such questions as "What would you do if fire broke out in a crowded theater?"

If the underlying illness affects specific brain areas, the patient may demonstrate aphasic, apraxic, or agnostic signs or show disturbances in the sensory or motor spheres. In these cases, the diagnosis is easily made by the neurological consultant. Cases of dementia referred to psychiatrists usually show these signs relatively late in their course.

Finally, patients with dementia may complain of hallucinations or exhibit delusional thinking. As in deliria, hallucinations are more apt to be visual and less bizarre or difficult to understand than in the functional psychoses. Depression is a common and understandable concomitant of dementias and may present diagnostic difficulties.

As defined above, dementia is an organic mental *syndrome*. Investigating the etiology of such syndromes involves consideration of infectious, metabolic, toxic, neoplastic, traumatic, cerebrovascular, and genetic factors. Entities that can produce dementia are listed in Table 5-1.

Aside from the routine laboratory investigations, therefore, patients with dementia should receive a CT scan, EEG, and metabolic studies including studies of thyroid, adrenal, and pituitary function, serum B_{12} and folate levels, serum ammonia levels, and a full range of liver and renal function tests. Depending on history, toxicological and drug studies may be indicated as well.

DSM-III defines two major dementing disorders, **primary degenerative dementia** and **multi-infarct dementias**. The former are further categorized as senile or presenile in onset but otherwise differ little in their symptoms or course.

Alzheimer's disease is the most common cause of primary degenerative dementia, occurring in about 6% of the population. Pathological changes in the brain include neurofibrillary tangles, senile plaques, and granulovacuolar bodies. Although the cause is at present unknown, recent interest has focused on decrease in brain cholinergic function. Decreases in both choline acetyltransferase and acetylcholinesterase levels have been demonstrated in the brains of affected individuals. Administration of choline or physostigmine (an acetylcholinesterase inhibitor) has produced brief improvements in memory function. Hence it is likely that this aspect of the illness may be related to neurotransmitter disturbances. Genetic factors have been implicated as well. In some families, Alzheimer's disease is passed on as a mendelian dominant. Patients with Down's syndrome develop primary degenerative dementia if they survive sufficiently long, an indication that the genetic defect (trisomy 21) from which they suffer may influence the appearance of the illness. Chromosomal anomalies on this same chromosome have recently been described in affected individuals. Other suggested causes include a hypothesized slow virus, aluminum toxicity, and autoimmune mechanisms.

Earlier workers made a distinction between primary dementias occurring in the senium and those occurring in the presenium (i.e., ages 50 to 65). The neuropathological changes in both these groups of illnesses are similar, and there is no reason to limit the designation of Alzheimer's disease to the presenium as was previously done.

The course of Alzheimer's disease is usually divided into three stages. In the first, characteristic changes involve frontal lobe functions and memory. The patient's personality may become less spontaneous and lively, small lapses in social appropriateness may become evident, and changes in emotionality including uncharacteristic irritability or depression may be noted. Memory impairment affects new or recent learning particularly. Frequent episodes of forgetfulness may be noted. Visuomotor skills are lost, and the patient gets "lost" even in familiar surroundings. Word-finding skills are affected; the patient is often at a "loss for words." Often, patients themselves are unaware of these changes and those around them dismiss them as symptoms of "getting older." In the first phase, EEG and CT scans are usually normal. In the second phase, as abstract attitude is affected, patients become less flexible in their planning in the face of change. They may exhibit periods of frank confusion, particularly when confronted with novel situations. Memory is more severely impaired, and aphasic signs and apraxias are elicited on formal examination. The patient shows difficulty with calculations and performs poorly on visuomotor tests. Affect is usually bland and apathetic. In this phase, the EEG shows some slowing and the CT scan shows beginning signs of cortical atrophy or ventricular dilatation. Finally, as the disease progresses to the third and final phase, clear evidence of intellectual deterioration becomes inescapable. The patient has difficulty with calculations, memory loss, and language impairment. The rate of progression is variable but progressive; there are no evidences of remission.

Multi-infarct dementia, as its name implies, is the result of a series of strokes that cumulatively impair cognitive functioning.

Table 5-1. Causes of Dementia

Infectious
Encephalitides (including herpes B encephalitis and acquired immuno-deficiency syndrome [AIDS] encephalitis)
Meningitis
Cerebral toxoplasmosis
CNS syphilis

Metabolic
Hypoglycemia
Liver failure
Hypothyroidism
Hyperthyroidism
Cushing's disease
Hypopituitarism
Hypercalcemia
B_{12} and folate deficiency
Chronic thiamine deficiency
Pellagra (niacin deficiency)
Chronic uremia

Toxic
Heavy metal intoxication (e.g., lead, manganese, mercury)
Chronic alcoholism
Carbon monoxide poisoning

Neoplastic
Brain tumors
Remote effects of neoplasm
Metastatic brain disease

Traumatic
Posttraumatic
Postanoxic

Cerebrovascular
Stroke

Genetic
Huntington's chorea
Machiafava-Bignami syndrome
Wilson's disease
Leukodystrophies

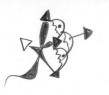

In contrast to Alzheimer's disease, it characteristically follows a stepwise course, with some return of functioning between episodes. Unlike Alzheimer's disease, in which the frontal lobes are affected early, the disturbances of judgment and planning that are early symptoms of that disorder are less consistently found in multi-infarct dementia and the patient's premorbid personality is less affected.

Other dementias should be coded as organic mental syndromes with the etiologic basis (if known) indicated on Axis II.

ORGANIC AMNESTIC SYNDROME

Although memory disturbances are common in both deliria and dementias, in the organic amnestic syndrome they are present without the clouding of consciousness characteristic of deliria or the intellectual deterioration typical of dementias. Patients may be unable to learn new information (commonly tested by asking them to recall three objects some 3 minutes later) or older, well-learned information (for example, the events preceding an auto accident). A common concomitant is **confabulation:** The patient "fills in" a memory gap by making up a story that may be more or less persuasive. Although the underlying pathophysiology of memory is imperfectly understood, the structures that subserve it are widely distributed and include the mesencephalic reticular activating system, the mammillary bodies, the medial forebrain bundle, the dorso-lateral thalamus, the cingulate gyrus, and the hippocampus. **Bilateral hippocampectomy,** sometimes used for the control of intractable epilepsy, produces a relatively pure deficit of short-term memory; patients are incapable of new learning. However, in most instances the mental status will consist of a more mixed picture of memory disturbances. In chronic alcoholics, an organic amnestic syndrome, **Korsakoff's syndrome,** is often accompanied by peripheral neuropathies. In this latter disorder, pathological findings often include hemorrhage into the mammillary bodies. **Head trauma** or electroconvulsive therapy (ECT) can also affect memory. Amnesia for events that preceded the incident are spoken of as retrograde amnesia; amnesia for events that follow are antero-grade. While anterograde amnesia persists—presumably because of continuation of the inciting causes—the patient may be confused, agitated, or impulsive. In closed head trauma, the persistence of the anterograde phase is an indicator of prognosis.

OTHER ORGANIC MENTAL SYNDROMES

At times an organic cause may give rise to syndromes characterized by hallucinations, delusions, or personality changes not accounted for by the release of an underlying functional disorder. For example, cocaine abuse may give rise to a short-lived depression indistinguishable from a major affective disorder. Chronic alcoholics may present with hallucinations, often in the auditory sphere, in a clear sensorium (**alcoholic hallucinosis**). Patients with frontal lobe tumors may present with personality changes. In the presence of a confirmatory history or of appropriate physical or laboratory findings, an organic hallucinosis, organic delusional syndrome, organic hallucinosis, or organic personality syndrome is diagnosed.

Intoxication and withdrawal from substances of abuse produce a range of complex syndromes that do not fall into one of the organic mental syndromes already delineated. In many instances, they will fall into the specific organic mental disorders discussed below.

ALCOHOL ORGANIC MENTAL DISORDERS

Alcoholism is a major public health issue afflicting approximately 10,000,000 Americans. Its etiology appears to be complex. In about 15% of cases, a familial—possibly genetic—factor appears to be implicated. Genetic factors appear particularly to be implicated in severe cases. Characteristic neurophysiological changes have been identified in the children of alcoholic parents. In the remainder, social and psychological factors are likely to play a role. However, alcoholism is distributed among all social classes; the concept of an "alcoholic personality" has generally been discarded. A small minority of patients suffer from a concurrent Axis I disorder and self-medicate to reduce their symptoms. A group of alcoholic bipolar patients whose drinking responds to lithium treatment has been described. There are differences in the behavioral effects of similar alcohol blood levels in alcoholics and nonalcoholics. Normal subjects will manifest characteristic behaviors of intoxication at blood levels of approximately 100 mg/100 ml. Heavy drinkers may tolerate much higher blood levels without these manifestations. For these individuals, symptoms of withdrawal may appear in the face of high blood levels (which are relatively depressed for that patient).

Although some attempts have been made to teach alcoholics controlled drinking, there is general agreement that abstinence is the most effective course. Subtle psychological and physiological disturbances appear in abstinent patients for 6 months to a year after cessation of drinking, the so-called "prolonged abstinence syndrome"; these effects serve to undermine the patient's resolve. Patients will frequently require several attempts before they remain "on the wagon." Programs such as that provided by Alcoholics Anonymous are effective in supporting the patient through this period and, although they are in many ways antithetical to a medical approach, have generally been accepted as part of rehabilitation regimens. Patients who have continued difficulty with compliance may benefit from disulfiram (Antabuse) administration. Disulfiram is a drug that inhibits the breakdown of acetaldehyde by its dehydrogenase. If patients on disulfiram drink, they experience nausea, vomiting, and flushing. Severe alcoholics may choose to drink despite these aversive effects.

Of particular importance is the occurrence of multiple medical problems in the alcoholic population. Malnutrition is common, even in the face of apparently adequate intake. Concurrent infections are common. Alcohol has direct and invidious effects on many organ systems, such as the cardiovascular (cardiomyopathies and hypertension), GI (peptic ulcer, pancreatitis, hepatic cirrhosis), and nervous system (cerebral atrophy, Korsakoff's and Wernicke's syndromes, cerebellar degeneration, and peripheral neuropathies), compromising the functioning of those organs. Alcoholics are more prone to develop certain cancers such as those of the upper GI tract.

Alcoholism is a disease with a significant psychosocial morbidity and mortality. Direct and indirect effects produce an increase in death rate from natural causes and accidents. There is a significantly elevated suicide rate among alcoholics.

ALCOHOLIC INTOXICATION

Patients are commonly brought to emergency rooms because of maladaptive behaviors (including drunk driving and assaultiveness) and a history of drinking or of alcohol on the breath. Screening may be done with a Breathalyzer, but blood levels are more accurate. Physical signs include slurred speech, incoordination, ataxia, nystagmus, and flushed facies. Behavioral signs include signs of disinhibition such as labile mood, irritability, talkativeness, and impaired attention or concentration. A common treatment strategy is to allow the patient to metabolize the alcohol off safely by administering a single dose of 50 mg of Librium PO.

ALCOHOL IDIOSYNCRATIC INTOXICATION

Some patients become assaultive or frankly paranoid on the ingestion of even small amounts of alcohol. In extreme instances, these patients are quite dangerous. At times, a temporal lobe focus may be identified, but positive findings are uncommon.

ALCOHOL WITHDRAWAL

Alcohol withdrawal syndromes occur only after protracted abuse, commonly 5 to 15 years. Patients who concomitantly are taking other drugs, particularly methadone, may display it after a shorter interval. Manifestations commonly appear 48 to 72 hours after cessation or reduction of the level of alcohol intake or after an infection or unusual physical stress. Symptoms include tremulousness, nausea, elevated temperature, heightened blood pressure and pulse rate, and anxious mood.

Untreated, alcohol withdrawal may proceed to frank delirium (delirium tremens [DT]), usually within a week. DT has an appreciable mortality. Formerly, as many as 15% of patients died, often from high-output cardiac failure. Current treatment methods using drugs cross-tolerant to alcohol that may be gradually withdrawn has improved treatment outcome. The patient is medicated with a dose high enough to suppress symptoms, generally about 200 mg/day of Librium. This is decreased over a period of about 5 days. Thiamine, folic acid, and multivitamins are also administered. Since magnesium levels are often depleted, it is the practice in some centers to give the patient supplements of this mineral.

Some patients will manifest a hallucinosis (alcohol hallucinosis) as a dramatic early sign of withdrawal, generally within the first 48 hours after the cessation of drinking. Hallucinations may be in the auditory or visual sphere, the former being more typical. Hallucinations may be threatening, and patients' fearfulness can pose a significant danger to themselves or others as they try to avoid their persecutors. These patients are sometimes misdiagnosed as paranoid schizophrenics. Specific medication (like that used for DT) is necessary to avoid progression to more severe withdrawal syndromes.

Fulminant withdrawal may result in Wernicke's syndrome, a severe reduction in the state of consciousness, ataxia, and ophthalmoplegia, which may progress into coma and death if untreated. Patients who are subjected to this sort of severe withdrawal state may be left with a characteristic memory disturbance, the alcohol amnestic disorder (a form of Korsakoff's syndrome), characterized by disturbances in short-term memory and often complicated by peripheral neuropathies. Amnestic syndromes with a more insidious onset and course have also been described. The provision of vitamin replacement therapy (particularly the B complex vitamins) appears to ameliorate the course of this illness, although memory dysfunction may persist despite treatment efforts.

Finally, some patients who have a history of protracted heavy alcohol abuse may show signs of dementia that persist more than 3 weeks after the remission of other withdrawal effects. Although there is some controversy about its direct relationship to alcohol abuse, this concatenation of circumstances is sufficiently common as to justify as separate coding in DSM-III.

SUBSTANCE-INDUCED ORGANIC MENTAL DISORDERS

BARBITURATE/SEDATIVE/HYPNOTIC DISORDERS

Sedatives, hypnotics, and minor tranquilizers—particularly the latter—are widely prescribed for insomnia and the control of anxiety. About 16% of the general population received benzodiazepines in any given year; 30% of drug-related deaths are due to benzodiazepines or barbiturates. Clearly, the potential for abuse and for medically serious complications is high.

INTOXICATION

Barbiturates are obtainable by prescription or, more commonly in cases of abuse, as street drugs or "downers." In the latter case, they may be adulterated with other drugs or taken separately to bring the patient down after stimulant ingestion. Since these are cerebral depressants, the symptoms of intoxication are most commonly those of disinhibition: euphoria, loquacity, restlessness, and irritability. Users may become belligerent or exhibit inappropriate sexual activity. At higher doses, sedative effects may predominate. The patient may evince ataxia, slurred speech, and incoordination. Memory and concentration may be adversely affected. At high doses, the patient may become comatose. Death from respiratory arrest presents a significant danger.

WITHDRAWAL

Prolonged use of barbiturates (generally for a period of 1 to 3 months) can result in addiction. Barbiturate withdrawal represents a true medical emergency. Symptoms include nausea and vomiting, tachycardia, hypertension (or orthostatic hypotension), tremor, anxiety, and depression. Seizures may occur—generally within the first 2 to 5 days of withdrawal.

When addicted patients are to be withdrawn from barbiturates in the hospital, the pentobarbital test is often a helpful guide: 200 mg of pentobarbital is administered PO. If patients fall asleep, they have little tolerance and do not need a withdrawal regimen. If they show signs of intoxication, the 24-

hour requirement is in the range of 400 to 600 mg of pentobarbital. If they show only lateral nystagmus, the daily requirement may be set at 600 mg to 1 g. If there are no signs of intoxication and patients appear comfortable, they have probably been using more than a gram a day. The patient's estimated requirement is provided in divided doses as pentobarbital or as phenobarbital (100 mg of pentobarbital being equivalent to 30 mg of phenobarbital). After a few days, the dose may be reduced by about 10% a day.

Signs and symptoms of minor tranquilizer and sedative-hypnotic withdrawal are similar. Controlled withdrawal may be effected by gradual reduction of the drug involved or of a drug cross-tolerant with it.

OPIOID DISORDERS

Intoxication

The use of opioids as drugs of abuse has remained relatively constant over the past decade. About half a million individuals are said to be opiate abusers nationwide. Because of the relation between hard drug abuse and criminality, the problem has attracted national concern, and treatment centers using drug-free or methadone-maintenance modalities have been widely established. More recently, the IV drug-abusing population has also been identified as a high-risk group for AIDS and a source of infection to the general population.

Besides AIDS, IV drug addicts are subject to a variety of other medical conditions including hepatitis, bacterial endocarditis, pneumonia, thrombophlebitis, and tetanus.

It is clear that not all individuals who try opiates become long-term addicts. Factors such as social and family disorganization play a major role.

Patients receiving opiates such as Dilaudid, Demerol, Percodan, and Talwin as pain killers may become addicted. Physicians and nurses are particularly vulnerable to this form of addiction.

Opioid intoxication is manifest by pupillary constriction, drowsiness, slurred speech, and impaired attention and memory. Psychological effects of the drug range from euphoria to apathy, dysphoria, and psychomotor retardation. Obviously, repeated episodes of intoxication interfere with the patient's capacity to maintain a job or to conduct social relationships.

In cases of profound stupor when the possibility of an opiate overdose is a diagnostic consideration, naloxone—an opiate antagonist—may be administered. In addicted patients, this drug may produce a fulminant withdrawal syndrome.

Withdrawal

Signs of opiate withdrawal include piloerection (hence the phrase "cold turkey"), tearing, runny nose, pupillary dilatation, sweating, and diarrhea. Blood pressure may be mildly elevated and heart rate increased. The patient may run a low-grade fever.

Hospital detoxification is usually done with methadone. If the extent of the patient's habit cannot be accurately ascertained, 20 mg of methadone can be safely given on a b.i.d. basis. Dosage is then reduced by 10% daily. Recent reports indicate that clonidine may reduce the most troublesome autonomic symptoms of opiate withdrawal.

AMPHETAMINE AND COCAINE ORGANIC MENTAL DISORDERS

Cocaine and amphetamine intoxication

In the past decade, the use of cocaine—once thought to be nonaddicting— has become a major public health problem, particularly when it is used in the inexpensive and rapidly absorbed form called "crack." Crack is a relatively impure form of cocaine that can be smoked and hence absorbed almost immediately through the respiratory tract.

Cocaine and the amphetamines, which share similar pharmacologic actions, are stimulants or "uppers." Intoxication produces a sense of euphoria and is behaviorally manifest by agitation, loquacity, and a hypervigilance that easily shades into paranoia. These drugs are sympathomimetics. They increase heart rate and blood pressure, cause sweating, and produce pupillary dilatation. Once on his "high," the patient will attempt to avoid the profound drop in mood or "crash" that follows it. Drugs such as crack that have brief, intense effects may be repeated several times an hour. Amphetamine highs are more sustained. Characteristically, patients attempt to continue their high until they run out of drugs, attract the attention of police, or exhaust themselves.

High doses of these substances may produce a delirium.

Of considerable theoretic interest is the fact that after sustained use, amphetamines produce a paranoid psychosis sometimes indistinguishable from paranoid schizophrenia. Presumably, cocaine and amphetamines produce their effects through activation of dopaminergic pathways similar to those involved in the pathogenesis of the latter syndrome.

In a similar vein, patients "coming off" crack or amphetamines may experience a profound depression quite similar to an endogenous depressive disorder. This state is characterized by psychomotor retardation, suicidal ideation, and ideas of hopelessness and worthlessness. In some patients, delusional thoughts occur. Characteristically, patients experience either insomnia or hypersomnia during this phase. Increased dreaming—presumably due to rapid eye movement (REM) rebound— is frequently reported.

PCP or similarly acting arylcyclohexylamine organic mental disorder

Phencyclidine (PCP) was originally developed as an anesthetic agent but withdrawn after reports that it produced an agitated delirium. It is widely available as a street drug, "angel dust," and is often a contaminant in drugs sold under other names. It is commonly smoked, although it is active by other routes.

Although a euphoriant at low doses, PCP is capable of producing psychotic states with a wide range of manifestations. Without an adequate history, the diagnosis may be unclear. Patients show severe emotional lability. Periods of calm may vacillate with dangerous excitement. Many of these patients appear profoundly anxious; it is this fearfulness and unpredictability that make them dangerous in emergency rooms. Physiological effects of the drug include hypertension, nystagmus, ataxia, and a characteristic muscle rigidity, particularly of the face and neck. Patients may show any of the manifestations of an agitated acute schizophrenic disorder.

Treatment is symptomatic. Both diazepam and haloperidol have been reported as useful. In most cases, the patient recovers within 48 hours.

HALLUCINOGEN ORGANIC MENTAL DISORDER

Hallucinogenic halucinosis is caused by a heterogeneous group of drugs including mescaline (from the peyote cactus), LSD (lysergic acid diethylamide, a synthetic substance related to compounds naturally occurring in morning glory seeds), psilocybin, and dimethyltryptamine. As a group, they produce an altered state of consciousness marked by perceptual distortions, alterations in the sense of time, changes in the flow and content of thought, emotional lability, and at times hallucinations and delusion-like thinking. They do not produce disorientation or other symptoms of delirium. They have been used in religious rituals and in psychotherapy to disinhibit rational, goal-directed thinking.

Hallucinogenic hallucinoses, or "bad trips," occur in a small percentage of cases. Individuals so affected are in a panic state; paranoid thinking is prominent, sometimes accompanied by referential thinking and delusional percepts. There is a pervasive sense of being out of control. It is likely that the occurrence of such hallucinoses is related to the circumstances under which the drug is taken ("bad vibes"), the patient's predominant state of mind, and the premorbid psychiatric status. A small number of individuals remain psychotic after the drug is metabolized. In these cases, it is likely that the drug experience has triggered off a preexisting psychosis.

Some individuals will report the spontaneous, usually transient recurrence of drug experiences ("flashbacks") subsequent to recovery. Flashbacks tend to be precipitated by stress or by subsequent drug use.

In general, patients with hallucinogenic hallucinosis will respond to a quiet, reassuring atmosphere and a calming attitude. Minor tranquilizers or sedatives may be used. Since some street hallucinogens contain potent anticholinergics, the use of major tranquilizers with similar effects may produce an anticholinergic crisis and is generally to be avoided.

Cases in which delusional thinking or affective elements are prominent are classified as hallucinogenic delusional or affective disorders.

CANNABIS ORGANIC MENTAL DISORDER (CANNABIS INTOXICATION)

Marijuana use has increased dramatically in the past 30 years. Well over half of all high school students have tried it, although for most, use is only occasional or for social purposes. Use is almost entirely by smoking. Signs of intoxication include a mild euphoria ("high"), slowing of time sense, sharpening of perception, preoccupation with visual imagery, and inappropriate laughter. In adverse reactions, individuals may become paranoid, depersonalized, and panicky. The active ingredient of marijuana is tetrahydrocannabinol (THC).

Prolonged daily use of marijuana has been reported to produce an apathetic, amotivational state.

As with all psychedelic agents, the reactions to marijuana are dependent on the patient's mood, setting, and premorbid psychiatric history. Adverse reactions usually respond to reassurance and mild sedation, but the possibility of an underlying psychiatric disorder must be borne in mind.

CAFFEINE ORGANIC MENTAL DISORDER (CAFFEINE INTOXICATION)

Heavy doses of caffeine have been reported to produce prolonged episodes of sympathetic activation that resemble generalized anxiety but that respond to cessation of intake.

SUBSTANCE USE DISORDERS

When use of a psychoactive agent is daily or frequent, when the altered state of consciousness is prolonged, when use interferes with social or occupational functioning, and when the disturbance has lasted for a protracted period (usually 1 month), the patient is said to suffer from a substance use disorder.

AFFECTIVE DISORDERS

Affective disorders have as their cardinal sign disturbances of the quality, intensity, or appropriateness of mood. **Depression** is by far the most common presenting symptom, but patients may present with elevated mood (mania), irritability, and anger or less easily definable dysphorias as well. Although other psychiatric disorders may (and generally do) include mood disturbances, the latter will, in general, be clearly subordinate to or follow the appearance of more the characteristic signs and symptoms of the primary disorder. In practice, however, "borderline" states are quite common and clinicians often resort to hybrid diagnostic terms (e.g., schizoaffective states, anxious depressions, etc.). Despite this, diagnosis is usually straightforward since, especially in the depressions, insight is commonly preserved and patients can describe the history of their painful state quite accurately. Because of the grave risk of suicide as a complication of this disease, all physicians should know how to recognize depression, even in its less typical presentations (as for example, when somatic symptoms predominate). The student should also be aware of the subtypes of depression recognized by *DSM-III* and the general indications for treatment in uncomplicated cases.

Depressions are *common* in the general population. Recent epidemiologic studies based on interview samples of large populations indicate a prevalence rate of 9 to 11% for depressions of moderate intensity and 3 to 5% for severe depressions. Hospitalized patients show a far higher incidence: About a quarter of medical inpatients are clinically depressed. Indeed, the loss of physical well-being and vigor undermines resistance to depression. The disorder is more common in the elderly, in whom differential diagnosis from organic mental disorders may be difficult. Finally, for most types of depression (*excluding* bipolar disorder) women are more apt to be affected than men.

Everyday clinical observation would suggest that environmental stressors and biologic diathesis would play complementary roles in the susceptibility to depression. Older terminologies attempted to distinguish between "endogenous" and "exogenous" (or reactive) symptom pictures. In fact, it is impossible to make this distinction on the basis of the clinical appearance of the patient, and *DSM-III* has discarded the distinction in favor of separating off the major affective disorders (which have severe disruptive effects on the patient's functioning) and other specific symptom complexes.

ETIOLOGIC THEORIES OF DEPRESSION

Psychological theories

Although depression appears to represent the "final common pathway" on which a number of etiologic pathways converge, depressed patients express a surprisingly similar set of concerns: helplessness, worthlessness, guilt, and lack of pleasure (anhedonia). Psychological formulations are useful because they help to explain these particular manifestations of depression. They have *therapeutic* utility because they guide clinicians in helping their patients to cope effectively with stresses that might precipitate acute episodes. Many clinicians believe that they also provide useful clues as to the origins of depression in particular patients. Many psychological theories are difficult to formulate in a manner that is rigorously testable. Despite this, research has provided a modest amount of support for the importance of psychological antecedents of depression.

Freud's paper "Mourning and Melancholia" was an important early formulation. Freud noted that many depressive patients torment themselves with feelings of worthlessness and blame, often in the face of strong contrary evidence. He postulated that the delusional accusations were best understood as being unconsciously intended for an object of the patient's love whom the patient had lost or by whom he or she felt abandoned. Underlying patients' dilemma was their strong ambivalence toward their love object. Unable to express their anger directly, they turned it inward toward themselves (or toward that part of themselves that identified with—or had introjected—the lost object). In fact, in a small number of cases where there is a clear precipitating loss, one can recognize the patient's guilty ruminations as being more easily understandable in this manner. More importantly, Freud's theory pointed to the association between difficulties with feelings of anger and loss. The role of unresolved ambivalent feelings in retarding the "work of mourning" has found application in helping patients suffering from unresolved grief reactions.

Depressives are often consumed with feelings of lowered self-worth and shame. The American psychoanalyst Bibring has suggested that depressives set unrealistic expectations of themselves, expectations that they are often unable to attain. The patient experiences these failures as disastrous drops in self-esteem, and, if no restitutive mechanisms are available, a painful depression ensues. Bibring's formulation certainly describes a premorbid personality that is common in many people who are prone to depression: They are perfectionistic and demanding—of others as well as themselves. They have difficulty in maintaining a continuing sense of their own worth and depend unduly on the opinions and attitudes of others for recognition and praise. Many patients who are now considered as suffering from a narcissistic personality disorder meet this criterion. Not all such individuals suffer from clinical depression, however, and Bibring's formulation must be considered as only a partial explanation of depression. Recently, there has been considerable interest in the cognitive therapy of depres-

sion. Using behavioral techniques, clinicians attempt to identify and help patients to overcome unrealistic and self-defeating attitudes that they have learned to hold concerning their self-worth.

Another group of theoreticians have called attention to the relation between depression and loss. John Bowlby, an English ethologist and psychiatrist, has called attention to the resemblance between the reactions to separation and loss in young mammals (including humans) and the manifestations of depression. Research studies have indicated that patients with early experiences of parental loss are more apt to become depressed later in life than a comparable group without such experiences. Research in this area is fraught with difficulties. For many people, even the disastrous experience of losing a parent is compensated for by the presence of alternate caregivers. Similarly, parental abuse and rejection may occur in subtle forms for which our present research methodology is too insensitive. Recent workers have demonstrated the importance of the amount and quality of the patient's social support network in the course of depression.

Not all psychological theories stress unconscious motivation or past experiences. Behavioral theories have postulated that depressed patients have learned to use their depressive symptoms as gestures of helplessness which influence others to fulfill their needs. Clinicians who are guided by this formulation attempt to substitute more assertive and direct responses for the old unsatisfying and self-defeating ones.

Finally, work on "learned helplessness"—a construct originally developed in experimental psychology—has been influential in writings on depression. Animals subjected to a painful and inescapable experimental situation develop behavioral signs that resemble some signs of clinical depression (and that may be reversed by antidepressants)! Certainly, depression often appears to be a form of frustration behavior. Patients cannot escape from a web of circumstances in which there is no winning solution. Since escape is impossible, they "learn helplessness." Forms of brief psychotherapy that help to clarify patients' interpersonal dilemmas and support them to find solutions that they had previously been unable to supply or to carry through solutions that they had not been able to pursue have proved effective for some depressive patients.

Biologic theories

Biogenic amines.   When the antihypertensive drug reserpine was introduced, physicians discovered that its use was associated with the precipitation of a depressive episode in a number of cases. Since reserpine depletes stores of biogenic amines—particularly noradrenaline and serotonin (or 5-hydroxytryptophan [5-HT]) in the hypothalamus—investigators in the biochemistry of affective disorders have vigorously pursued the role of these transmitters in depression. Indeed, several lines of investigation have converged to support their role:

1. A number of other pharmacologic agents that affect the synthesis or release of biogenic amines also act to induce depressions. Among these are several antihypertensive agents including alpha-methyldopa, guanethidine, and propranolol.

2. Antidepressant agents act to increase the availability of these transmitters either by inhibiting reuptake (tricyclic anti-

depressants [TCAs]) or intracellular catabolism (monoamine oxidase [MAO] inhibitors). Lithium, whose therapeutic action is less well understood, appears to decrease sodium reuptake.

3. Metabolic products of both epinephrine (3-methoxy-4-hydroxyl-phenylglycol) and serotonin (5-hydroxyindoleacetic acid [5-HIAA]) are decreased in the urine in patients with severe depression. Unfortunately, the largest part of these metabolites is derived from *peripheral* rather than central biogenic amine catabolism, so such studies provide only inferential evidence.

4. There is evidence that depressed urinary 5-HIAA may be a predictor of **suicide potential**.

5. Psychological stress can affect the levels of brain amines. When it is possible to study brain sodium levels in animals, such as by separating infant monkeys from their mothers or exposing dogs to a learned helplessness paradigm, depressed brain sodium levels have been demonstrated.

Although observations like these do implicate the role of sodium and 5-HT, we are still far from clear about the exact role that they play in depression. For example, although antidepressants have the effect indicated on brain transmitters (in animal studies), the *clinical* effect appears delayed by up to 2 weeks, suggesting that the symptoms of affective disorder involve a more complex chain of events than simply increasing or decreasing the availability of biogenic amines.

Acetylcholine. Although less studied, the cholinergic system appears to be implicated in the pathophysiology of depression and mania. Some patients will show a brief improvement when given small doses of physostigmine (a cholinesterase inhibitor). The same drug will produce a period of depression in some subjects.

The endocrine system. Depressive symptoms have been reported in hypothyroidism, in hyperparathyroid disorders, in hypopituitarism, and in adrenal insufficiency. Manic symptoms have been reported in Cushing's disease. Endocrine studies are therefore appropriate in cases of secondary affective disorders. In the majority of cases, however, endocrine function will be normal.

Researchers have demonstrated reduced responsiveness of the pituitary hormone thyroid-stimulating hormone (TSH) after administration of thyrotropin releasing hormone (TRH), a hypothalamic hormone that ordinarily controls its secretion. Clinical utility of this finding is restricted to a few academic settings.

In severe depressions, the normal feedback loop by which rising blood corticosteroid levels dampen pituitary adrenocorticotrophic hormone (ACTH) output appears to become less sensitive and blood cortisol levels remain high. This has become the basis of the dexamethasone suppression test (DST):

A blood sample for blood cortisol is drawn, and the patient is given 1 mg of dexamethasone by injection at 11 P.M. Subsequent blood samples are drawn at 8 A.M. the following day and again at 4 P.M. The 8 A.M. sample should show a return to normal, preinjection blood levels. Failure to suppress is regarded as positive.

About half of patients with a clinically significant depression will have a positive DST. However, the effect is influenced by the patient's age and by associated organic illness. Hence, the DST has proved too undiscriminating to be a primary diagnostic instrument and is best used as a supplementary investigation.

CNS effects of depression. Major affective disorders are associated with other changes in brain functioning that are currently chiefly of research interest but of which the student should be aware. These include the following: (1) decreased latency of the first REM episode, (2) reduced stage 4 sleep time, (3) disruption of the ordinary diurnal periodicity of peripheral cortisol secretion, and (4) reduced sensitivity to hypothalamic tropic hormones.

MAJOR DEPRESSIVE DISORDER

Diagnosis

The criteria for the diagnosis of major depressive disorder are as follows:

1. Dysphoric mood is "prominent and persistent" although not necessarily the most dominant symptom. Some patients are inattentive to their emotional state or quick to repress uncomfortable perceptions by dint of their personality or because sociocultural influences render these unacceptable. These patients may minimize changes in mood. However, sustained and severe depression will inevitably result in objectifiable changes in physiological activity or in behavioral patterns that can be elicited in the interview. These patients often present with apparently nonpsychological problems, and the practitioner must maintain a high index of suspicion.

2. Among these symptoms will be changes in appetite and sleep habits, easy fatigability, difficulty in concentration, and feelings of helplessness and hopelessness. The latter may lead patients to complain (often with some truth) that they are no longer able to function at home or at work with their usual degree of effectiveness. Close inquiry may reveal that reduced feelings of interest or pleasure or lowered self-esteem are the cause rather than the result of the impairment. Close inquiry about suicidal feelings—either suicidal preoccupations or actual attempts—is an essential part of the history in these cases.

This cluster of findings is almost always accessible on interview once a trusting relationship has been established. If a sufficient number of such symptoms are present and they are sustained over a significant period of time (*DSM-III* requires four to have been present at least daily over a 2-week period), then the degree of depression justifies considering the diagnosis.

Depressive symptoms commonly occur in other psychiatric disorders, however. In many (e.g., organic affective disorders related to drug use), they are seldom sustained for an extended period. In more chronic and severe cases such as schizophrenia or dementia, however, the patient may appear chiefly depressed for long periods in the course of illness. The clinician must be careful not to miss the underlying diagnosis. Delusions and hallucinations not easily understood as deriving from the primary mood disturbance (so-called mood-incongruent psychotic features). Bizarre behaviors are not typical of depressions and, although they are not in themselves diagnostic, should raise the question of schizophrenia or some other psychotic disorder.

Finally, uncomplicated bereavement may present a picture that is typical in almost every respect of major depressive disorder. In these cases, the patient's circumstances will usually make the diagnosis clear.

Two **subcategories** must be considered when the diagnosis of major depressive disorder is made.

The easier one to understand relates to the presence of psychotic features, chiefly **delusions or hallucinations**. These features are present in about 10% of patients with major depressive disorders. There are convincing data to suggest that the presence of these symptoms will affect response to treatment. *DSM-III* distinguishes between delusions and hallucinations that are mood congruent—that is, understandable in the context of the primary mood disturbance—and those that are mood incongruent. For example, it is easy to understand why a depressed woman might hear voices speaking of her (fantasied) promiscuity, but it is not immediately understandable if she feels that her body is being tampered with by incubi. It is unclear at present whether the distinction between mood-congruent and mood-incongruent psychotic features is related to treatment response, however.

The criteria for the other category, **melancholia,** include the following: (1) a "distinct quality of depressed mood" that the patient can readily distinguish from feelings of sadness or grief; (2) diurnal mood variation; depressed feelings are worse in the morning and lighten toward evening; (3) early morning awakening; (4) psychomotor agitation or retardation; (5) anorexia or weight loss, and (6) feelings of excessive or inappropriate guilt.

At least three are required to justify the diagnosis. The features of melancholia correspond to those clinical features that have been shown to predict a good response to antidepressants and ECT. In the past, clinicians have tended to identify this syndrome with an endogenous depression, one in which biologic factors played a predominant role. In fact, research data have failed to support this assumption. In many cases, it is possible to point to a situational precipitant in patients with this symptom complex. Despite this, many patients insist that there is a characteristic difference in the "feel" of this sort of depression from their ordinary periods of sadness or discouragement. Furthermore, there is no question that physiological signs are quite distinct in this disorder. Although all patients with major depressive disorder may demonstrate **diurnal mood variation,** patients with melancholia characteristically feel worse on wakening. Patients with other forms of depression may feel worse at the end of the day. Similarly, although appetite disturbances are common in all depressed patients, melancholic patients tend to have *diminished* appetite. They *lose* weight, characteristically 10 to 20 pounds, instead of gaining it. Melancholic patients are more apt to show disruption of their capacity for day-to-day activities. They are immobilized by psychomotor retardation or they are too agitated to attend to anything but their distress. They are frequently plagued by guilty ruminations. This symptom picture was at one time thought to be most characteristic of patients who fell ill in the **involutional period** (45 to 55 in women; 50 to 60 in men). Recent research has failed to substantiate this association.

Clinical course

Older clinical studies antedate the new *DSM-III* classification. In light of the availability of effective treatment measures for major depressive disorder, it is unlikely that naturalistic studies of the course of untreated illness will be justifiable or feasible. It is therefore necessary to extrapolate between the less rigorous diagnostic standards they used and our current nomenclature.

Major depressive disorder is *more common among women than men by a ratio of 2:1*. It is not clear to what extent this represents a biologic or a social phenomenon. Social circumstances certainly influence the occurrence and course of depressions and probably reflect the extent to which major social roles are supportive and free of conflict. Depression is more common among **married women** (compared with married men) and more common among unmarried men than unmarried women. Depressed women with several children, few confidantes, and distant or absent husbands are apt to have difficulty in recovering from depression. Psychotherapeutic interventions make use of these findings.

The **occurrence of the first episode** tends to be in the third and fourth decade of life. Childhood depressions have been increasingly recognized but are relatively rare. Onset after age 40 is considerably more common. Careful history will often elicit a history of a prior untreated depressive episode in these cases.

Major depressive disorder follows an **episodic** course. Untreated, an episode lasts from 6 to 9 months, and early studies have indicated that recovery occurs in approximately 85 to 90% of cases. However, recent work has suggested that these studies may have underestimated the incidence of a more prolonged low-grade depressive disorder on which subsequent episodes may be superimposed—so-called double depressions.

About 50% of patients will have one or more subsequent depressions. Each episode of recurrence appears to increase the patient's vulnerability to a further episode.

Over 15% of patients will attempt suicide.

There is a strong clinical impression that obsessional character traits are overrepresented in the premorbid personalities of patients with major depressive disorder.

Pathogenesis

We do not know the cause of major depressive disorder, and the speculations about why patients become depressed in general apply equally to this subgroup.

Patients will describe a positive family history to varying degrees. There are some patients who present a strong family history of similarly afflicted relatives. In others, the patient represents what appears to be the sporadic occurrence of major depression. In an interesting subgroup, depression occurs in the proband but the male family members present with a higher than expected incidence of alcoholism and sociopathy. It has been suggested that this grouping corresponds to valid subgroups, but most clinicians have resisted adapting them as the basis of subcategorization.

BIPOLAR AFFECTIVE DISORDER

In some patients, depressed episodes are interspersed with relatively sustained periods of elevated mood. At times, the two mood states may alternate within a single episode so rapidly that they appear admixed. Although this set of circumstances is relatively rare—it appears in about 3% of depressed patients—it is striking and has captured the public imagination. In the lay mind, *all* major depressions and many minor mood swings are referred to as "manic-depressive." What is less self-evident is

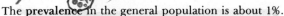

that the presence of such symptoms is not just a reflection of how particular patients will show affective pathology but that it marks a group of patients who appear to be suffering from a different disease than those whose symptoms are consistently drawn from the depressive pole alone. Although bipolar patients resemble patients with unipolar disease when they are depressed, they differ from that group in family history, clinical course, and response to treatment. Somewhat less well-established differences exist in premorbid personality and in the patient's functioning between episodes. Thus the distinction between unipolar and bipolar disease is the basis of a major diagnostic distinction in *DSM-III*.

Even in this group, manic episodes are relatively rare. The initial episode is most likely to be one of depression. The diagnosis may be based on the occurrence of bipolar symptoms in the patient's family, or it may have to await the occurrence of manic features in a subsequent episode. Some clinicians have proposed that if one includes episodes of hypomania (a less intense form of mania) that were insufficiently severe to warrant hospitalization, one may broaden the category. These workers call this latter form of illness bipolar disease II—a form of nomenclature that has not come into general use.

The existence of "pure" unipolar manic disorder is controversial. Certainly, if it exists, it is quite uncommon. The student will be interested in the diagnostic criteria for mania because of the importance of distinguishing between unipolar and bipolar disorders.

Like depression, mania may occur as a primary disease or may be secondary to some other psychiatric, medical, or substance abuse disorder. Because it is an uncommon symptom, it is essential to keep in mind that *every case of mania must be viewed as a secondary mania until proved otherwise.*

Salient points in the *DSM-III* criteria for mania include the following:

1. Compared with depression, symptoms must be sustained for only *1 week*.

2. Manic symptoms may be interspersed with depressive symptoms during the interval of observation. Mixed manic and depressive symptoms (easier to recognize than to try to imagine) are allowable toward meeting this requirement.

3. One cannot make this diagnosis in the presence of symptoms suggesting a schizophrenic, paranoid, or organic disorder.

Course of bipolar illness

Bipolar affective disorders tend to present themselves in the third and fourth decades of life. Classic cases beginning in childhood or in later life have been well documented but are infrequent. Earlier presentations are said to carry more ominous prognostic significance. Such cases *must* be worked up as secondary manic or depressive disorders.

In the past, American psychiatrists have tended to underapply this diagnosis, particularly in severely psychotic patients or in patients from the lower socioeconomic classes. It has been claimed that the disorder is rare in blacks, for example. Recent evidence has failed to support this contention.

Untreated manic episodes are said to last 4 to 6 months, untreated depressive episodes 6 to 9 months. However, since the adoption of effective treatment methods, both the course and frequency of episodes of decompensation have decreased.

The **prevalence** in the general population is about 1%.

The long-term course of the illness is highly variable. The potential for recurrence after a single episode is somewhat higher than for unipolar disease. Cases of strict alternation between manic and depressive episodes occur but are rare and chiefly of theoretic interest. **Rapidly cycling manics** have been closely studied; they are poor treatment responders and have a correspondingly poorer prognosis. Most patients will have an inter-illness period of months to years. About 5% of bipolar patients may become increasingly psychotic and be reclassified as schizophrenic. The unpredictable clinical course presents practical problems for prophylactic treatment. Occurrence of acute episodes is unreliably associated with clear precipitating factors.

The **premorbid personality** of bipolar patients is said to be characterized by mood swings (**cyclothymic personality disorder**). Many patients show a high degree of social adaptation when well. It is likely that this stereotyped view admits many exceptions. Bipolar illness places severe demands on the patient's family and disrupts work functioning, and adverse changes in social role functioning across episodes are common.

Pathogenesis

In contrast to unipolar affective disorder, in which several subgroups appear to exist, there is strong evidence for a genetic contribution to the pathogenesis of bipolar disorder. From 10 to 25% of first-degree relatives will be similarly afflicted. Concordance rates for monozygotic twins is about 68% and for same-sexed dizygotic twins about 23%.

Although the prevailing assumption is that the illness is transmitted as a dominant gene, controversy exists as to details of its inheritance. Some researchers have used sex-linked markers (among them genes for color blindness, human leukocyte antigen [HLA], and the XG_a blood group) as markers in the study of family pedigrees. The hypothesis that bipolar illness is inherited in a sex-linked manner in *some* patients remains controversial.

TREATMENT OF MAJOR AFFECTIVE DISORDERS

Mania

Lithium, prescribed as the carbonate or citrate salts, is a specific antimanic agent. Administered in the course of an acute manic or hypomanic episode, it will normalize mood in about 70% of patients. Patients on chronic lithium maintenance show a dramatic decrease in the frequency of subsequent manic and depressive episodes. Because its antimanic effects are seldom apparent for the first 10 to 14 days, however, it is general practice to begin treatment of an acutely disturbed patient with a neuroleptic. Haloperidol (Haldol) seems to have some specificity in mania. Lithium is begun either concurrently or as the manic episode remits. As the therapeutic effect of the lithium becomes apparent, the required dose of neuroleptic decreases, and it will usually be possible to withdraw it entirely. It should be noted that the combination of haloperidol and lithium has been implicated in a rare but sometimes fatal neurotoxic syndrome characterized by confusion, fever, and seizures. Patients on this regimen must be observed closely.

Not all manic patients will benefit from lithium. Some will

fail to respond to adequate doses; others will find it difficult to tolerate side effects. For others, compliance may become an issue. Many manic patients value at least mild highs because of the degree of creativity they allow and because of the apparent release from daily frustrations and cares.

Several as yet unproven antimanic agents, generally drugs with other applications in neurology or medicine, have been the object of investigational studies. Among these are carbamazepine, clonazepam, and verapamil. It is likely that these and other new drugs will extend our capacity to treat lithium-resistant manic patients.

Depression

The treatment of depression is somewhat more complex. Nonpsychotic depressives are generally treated with TCAs in the initial phase. If the patient fails to respond to an adequate dose over an adequate trial period (generally 5 to 6 weeks), an MAO inhibitor is begun. A 10-day interval should intervene between the two regimens to minimize the possibility of a toxic interaction.

Patients with psychotic symptoms do not respond as reliably to TCAs. Treatment is initiated with a major tranquilizer (to which a TCA *may* be added). Remission is usually apparent within a few days. If the patient fails to respond adequately, ECT may be considered.

Bipolar patients in the depressed phase may respond to antidepressant medication or ECT by "overshooting" into a manic phase. For this reason, as well as to provide adequate prophylaxis, lithium should be initiated along with the antidepressant medication.

ECT is used in some centers for patients in whom the degree of suicide potential or agitation presents an acute danger. It has been cogently argued, however, that the duration of such treatments (generally eight treatments over a period of 3 weeks) is no briefer than a pure psychopharmacological regimen. In any case, relapses are frequent unless ECT is supplemented with antidepressants or lithium.

Because of the recurrent nature of affective disorders, medication should not be withdrawn when the patient's acute symptoms are under control. In general, antidepressants are continued for a period of 6 to 9 months after the onset of the acute episode. Patients with bipolar disorder may not require as lengthy a period of maintenance if lithium prophylaxis is initiated.

Finally, one must consider prophylaxis. Patients with frequent episodes of unipolar depression may benefit from a long-term antidepressant regimen. The use of lithium in these patients is a less reliable measure but may be better tolerated. For patients with bipolar disease, long-term lithium prophylaxis is indicated. There are bipolar patients whose episodes are sufficiently infrequent that they will resist this recommendation. Counterpoised against this cause is the drastic impact of even a single episode on the patient's social functioning and the high degree of suicidal risk.

SCHIZOPHRENIA

Although a relatively rare disorder, its prevalence in the general population generally estimated as about 1%, schizophrenia takes a tragic toll because of its chronicity and the severe disability it entails in personal, vocational, and social functioning. It is a disease of young people; the age of onset is commonly between 18 and 35. Many of its victims are unable to establish independent lives, and responsibility for their care commonly falls to public and community institutions, which are increasingly unable to provide adequate resources for their care. In the past, when it was the custom to care for chronic schizophrenic patients in large state hospitals, they accounted for almost half of the patient in these settings. The introduction of neuroleptics and the development of methods to treat them in the community lead to largely unrealized hopes that they might be reintegrated into community life. In recent years, however, because of the nationwide policy of deinstitutionalization from state inpatient facilities, many of these chronic patients have become a prominent part of the homeless population.

Despite these failings, the past decade has seen progress in our understanding of the illness. The reliability and validity of diagnosis has been enhanced, research on treatment methodology has guided the development of more rational regimens, and continuing investigation of the biologic bases of the illness has provided a clearer picture of the nature of the illness.

Historical background

Partly because of the elusive nature of the pathophysiology of the disorder, observations made early in this century continue to exert a strong influence on our current views. Emil Kraeplin described **dementia praecox** as an illness of young people that leads—in most cases—to deterioration in intellectual and social function. He regarded this as a pleomorphic disorder and included several previously described syndromes such as catatonia and hebephrenia within this category. Bleuler's monograph *The Group of Schizophrenias* provided an extensive description of these patients and incidentally suggested the name for the disorder that is more commonly used today. As indicated in his title, Bleuler was careful to emphasize that the term *schizophrenia* included not one but several illness. Under the influence of early psychoanalytic theories, he described how the content of the patients' symptoms reflected psychological concerns. His description emphasizes the possibility of remission or even recovery in some patients. His description of a supportive and encouraging hospital environment still applies to inpatient work today. Bleuler thought that schizophrenic psychopathology reflected weakening of associational bonds and that loosening of associations could be detected in patients if one looked hard enough. He theorized that the other symptoms could be understood in terms of this primary defect. American psychiatry in particular has been strongly influenced by Bleuler, and medical students are still taught the "four A's" (associational loosening, affective flattening, ambivalence, and autism) that he emphasized. However, these criteria cannot be observed reliably, nor are they always unique to schizophrenia.

Two American psychiatrists made important contributions to our understanding of schizophrenia early in this century. Adolf Meyer stressed the importance of understanding the patient's life circumstances in the development of the illness. Harry Stack Sullivan viewed schizophrenia as deriving from severely disordered *interpersonal* relations, especially a fear of intimacy that led patients to isolate themselves from close

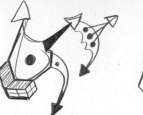
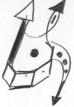

relationships at important points in their development. German psychiatrist Kurt Schneider described particular symptoms that he felt were of diagnostic importance in schizophrenia when they occurred in sufficient number. Among these symptoms were delusions of influence and particular hallucinatory experiences such as hearing voices arguing or commenting on the patient. When these symptoms are elicited from patients, it is easy for examiners to agree on their presence (that is, they are reliable) and they have formed part of the basis of some *DSM-III* criteria.

In the second half of this century, thinking about schizophrenia has derived less from broad clinical theories and more from the work of individual researchers. After World War II, social scientists began to study the social settings in which patients became sick and in which they were treated. Ferris and Dunham published their classic studies of urban setting and psychopathology, and Hollingshead and Redlich studied the relation between social class and mental disorder. Goffman studied the mental hospital as a total institution, and Stanton and Schwartz described its dynamics. In Scotland, Maxwell Jones's work on the open community began the movement toward less institutionalized settings, which strongly influenced the development of the community psychiatry movement in this country in the 1960s. Investigations of the role of the family in the genesis of schizophrenia dominated the 1950s and 1960s. More recently, the impact of the family environment on maintaining patients in the community has led to the development of the so-called psychoeducational approach.

Meanwhile, the adventitious discovery of an effective class of psychotropic agents, the phenothiazines, renewed the search for biologic factors in schizophrenia. Genetic studies begun in the 1960s established the importance of genetic factors in some patients but just as clearly underscored the importance of environmental factors. Biochemical studies centered largely around the dopamine hypothesis, which related psychotic symptoms to excess dopaminergic activity in some brain centers, probably the mesolimbic system. Finally, the introduction of new brain-imaging techniques allowed investigation of brain functioning in living patients.

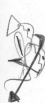

Signs and symptoms

There are no pathognomonic signs or symptoms of schizophrenia. Neither laboratory studies nor imaging procedures can establish the diagnosis. At different times in its course, especially at the outset, its symptoms may mimic almost any other psychiatric illness including drug-induced psychoses. Few other disorders, however, exhibit the characteristic longitudinal history of schizophrenia including onset relatively early in life, a tendency toward deteriorating course punctuated by episodes of psychosis, and, in many of its victims, the increasing dominance of negative symptoms. The symptoms of schizophrenia therefore consist of a varying admixture of two symptom clusters, one related to the occurrence of episodic psychoses and the other to a deterioration in the patient's psychosocial functioning. The manifestations of the disorder may vary widely; as Bleuler demonstrated, many of the patient's symptoms may even be psychologically understandable. Only if the patient shows *both* sorts of symptoms and one can rule out other causes for the distress should one diagnose a schizophrenic disorder.

As in most chronic illnesses, patients may look quite different depending on just when in their course they are examined. A patient who is brought to the emergency room in an agitated and psychotic state will look very different from a well-compensated outpatient or a chronically hospitalized "back ward" patient. Yet they all suffer from the same disorder. In an attempt to capture this heterogeneity, the authors of *DSM-III* have resorted to a somewhat labyrinthine set of criteria. If one appreciates their task, to assure that the patient exhibits those traits that are most characteristic at each point in what may be a complicated course, one can understand more easily how to apply these criteria.

Patients who present their first symptoms after the age of 45 cannot be diagnosed as suffering from a schizophrenic disorder by *DSM-III* criteria, since other disorders such as presenile dementias and affective disorders are more likely to present this way at that age. In fact, late onset *does* occur with some frequency and, if all other causes may be ruled out, should be diagnosed as an atypical psychosis.

Transient and remitting psychoses may arise from a large number of sources (including, for instance, complications of substance abuse, reactions to stress in patients with borderline disorders, and ICU psychoses) and may resemble a true schizophrenic psychotic episode rather closely. However, in these instances, symptoms are rarely sustained for 6 months, the *duration* criterion for schizophrenic disorder. Past diagnostic criteria were not so insistent on this feature. As a consequence, patients who displayed a prolonged psychotic episode without psychosocial deterioration (e.g., major affective disorders) or a brief but severe psychotic episode (e.g., a drug-induced psychosis) were falsely diagnosed as schizophrenic. Prematurely labeling patients discouraged further critical review of the diagnosis on subsequent episodes, led to inappropriate treatment regimens, and saddled the patient with a lifelong expectation of vulnerability to further episodes. Confronted with a heterogeneous group of patients so labeled forced researchers into developing a more stringent diagnostic set, which was at variance with that used by clinicians in their day-to-day work.

In the **active phase** of the psychosis, the schizophrenic patient usually complains of hallucinations or exhibits delusions. (In some cases—when the patient is incoherent or displays disorganized or stuporous behavior—it may be difficult to elicit these symptoms.) Since paranoid psychoses are considered separately, delusions of persecution or jealousy *unaccompanied* by hallucinations are insufficient by themselves to justify the diagnosis of schizophrenia. Certain types of hallucinations, those that are bizarre or that consist of isolated words unrelated to affective content, are considered more specific for schizophrenia. Hallucinations in which the "voices" comment on the patient's behavior or argue with each other also fall into the latter category. These are useful clinical guidelines, but the clinician should never be tempted to make the diagnosis on the basis of the *content* of hallucinations or delusions alone. What is important is that they occur as part of an illness that is *sustained for at period of at least 6 months*. Rarely, the active phase will last this long, but in treated patients, at least several months of this requisite 6-month period will consist of a prodromal or residual phase.

Not all cases of schizophrenia announce themselves with

the onset of an acute hallucinatory or delusional episode. More commonly, there is a **prodromal period** during which the patient or patient's family will give a history of withdrawal from social life, preoccupation with fantasy over reality (autism), impairment in "role" performance (at school or at work), and neglect of self-care. Sometimes patients' idiosyncratic preoccupations affect their way of speaking or thinking, which may become less realistic and more "magical" (dereism). They may, for example, become preoccupied by ideas such as clairvoyance or telepathy. Their speech may become vague or disorganized and hard to follow. Metaphorical expressions may be taken literally or become the object of obsessive ruminations. These changes may be accompanied by blunted or inappropriate affect. Often the patients or their families have rationalized these changes as related to a disappointment in love or an adjustment to a new social demand such as marriage or parenthood.

Similar changes may occur not before but *after* an active psychosis, when they are called **residual symptoms.** A diagnosis of schizophrenia requires that for a continuous period of 6 months the patient display some combination of prodromal, active, or residual symptoms.

Several **subtypes** of schizophrenia are recognized. The **disorganized** type is distinguished by frequent episodes of incoherence and blunted, inappropriate, or silly affect; the **catatonic** type by inhibited, stuporous, or excited motor behavior; the **paranoid** type by persecutory, grandiose, jealous delusions (or hallucinations with a similar content); the **undifferentiated** type—the most commonly diagnosed—by a mixture of these features. **Residual** schizophrenia is diagnosed when the patient has a history of schizophrenia but chiefly shows symptoms of the residual phase.

Patients whose illness has lasted 6 months to 2 years are called **subchronic;** longer than 2 years, **chronic.**

Etiology

Researchers attempting to elucidate the pathogenesis of schizophrenia have pursued a wide variety of approaches. It is hard to think of a discipline that has not been brought to bear in schizophrenia research. Much has been learned about the nature of the disorder, but to date both the cause and the mechanism of the disease remain obscure. We know a good deal about those factors that are likely to increase the possibility of a schizophrenic outcome (genetic, familial, psychological, and social), but their influence varies from cohort to cohort and no one factor has proved to be either sufficient or necessary. Many psychiatrists agree with Bleuler that schizophrenia is not one disease but many and that what we observe in the clinic is the result of one or more invidious circumstances on a complex and vulnerable developmental process. Given the rapid development of the neuroscience in the past two decades, it is possible that newer techniques will allow us to clarify the mechanism by which all these factors finally come to exert their effect on the behaviors we study. Whatever the outcome, we now know that the causes of schizophrenia are complex and that biologic mechanisms play an important role. Therapeutic approaches are more apt to combine both pharmacologic and psychotherapeutic modalities. Patients and their families have learned to think of schizophrenia as an illness with a course that may be ameliorated or worsened by compliance with treatment

and modification of the social milieu. The search for a single causative agent (such as the influence of a "schizophrenogenic mother"), which characterized treatment in the past, is no longer a part of our theoretic armamentarium.

Research on genetics

Clinicians have known for a long time that the incidence of schizophrenia in the families of many of their patients is higher than in the population at large, and indeed in recent **family studies** the risk of relatives of a diagnosed proband suffering from the disorder is 5 to 15 times higher than in the general population. Families are similar in more respects than in sharing a common genetic pool, however (for example, they may share a predisposing psychological environment). **Twin studies** are, in theory, more specific. Genetic similarities between monozygotic (identical) twins are greater than between dizygotic (fraternal) twins. Differences between the concordance rates of the two kinds of twins should generally reflect genetic influences. To the extent this is so, research has supported a genetic role. Concordance rate in identical twins is about 40% as compared with about 15% for dizygotes. Although these differences are large enough to establish the major contributions of genetic factors in liability to schizophrenia, one should also note that some 60% of even identical twins are **discordant** for schizophrenia. Clearly other factors come into play. Twin studies do not entirely rule out environmental influences. Twins—but particularly identical twins—are apt to be reared more similarly than nonidentical twins and are more apt to be exposed to familial and social risk factors in a similar fashion. **Adoption studies** of the offspring of schizophrenic mothers who have been adopted away early in life shed some light on the influence of genetic as opposed to environmental factors. Despite the fact that these children are raised by mostly nonschizophrenic families, the incidence of schizophrenia among them is considerably higher than among adopted away children of nonschizophrenic mothers. Similarly, if one identifies a cohort of schizophrenic adoptees, the incidence of schizophrenia among their biologic relatives is significantly higher than among their adoptive relatives. In summary, it is clear that genetic influences affect the risk for a schizophrenic outcome, but neither the mode of transmission nor their mechanism is yet clear.

Research on families of schizophrenics

Familial influences on schizophrenics are complex. It is in the family that the tasks of early development are first undertaken: the development of a feelings of safety and trust, the beginnings of a sense of autonomy and initiative, and the taming of paralyzing guilt. Social and sexual roles are tested and internalized. The developing child acquires language and, equally important, learns to use it in a logical and communicative manner. The admixture of fantasy and reality so characteristic of very young children is refined so that the two separate modes of thought are maintained as separate. All these processes would appear to be relevant to the failures in ego functioning that are characteristic of schizophrenia (as well as other disorders). It is not surprising that family process in schizophrenia has been the object of psychological research for some time.

Psychoanalytic theories have emphasized the preemptive

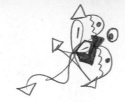

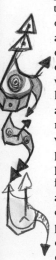

influence of early experience on later functioning. Psychoanalytic clinicians noted the **disturbed ego boundaries** in schizophrenic patients. Such patients have difficulty in maintaining clear boundaries between themselves and others (as in the common delusional conviction that their thoughts are being influenced or broadcast). Accordingly, it was postulated that these patients had failed to successfully resolve the symbiotic relationship with their primary object (usually their mother). Later observers noted that the mothers of schizophrenics were often anxious or depressed women who more or less subtly discouraged attempts at separation by their offspring. The schizophrenic-to-be was often "selected" by a covert agenda that involved the other family members, who thus avoided the fate of this crippling attachment. The patient's covert struggle for autonomy engendered unconscious feelings of aggression and guilt, which further crippled normal development. Although such family patterns are commonly observed, there is no evidence that they are specific for a schizophrenic outcome. Furthermore, the emphasis such theories place on the mother's responsibility for the patient's outcome (however much she may herself have been under the sway of her own unconscious needs) introduces an element of blame that may have an invidious effect on attempts at therapeutic intervention.

Other authors have focused their observations on **family process.** Lidz and colleagues have described two patterns that they feel are commonly found in the families of schizophrenic offspring. In schismatic families, the parents' role functioning and values are both contradictory and vested with sufficient emotional force that the children cannot safely internalize either without guilt. If a child attempts to placate both parents' values, there is a serious weakening in the coherence of his or her personality. Skewed families are dominated by the personality of one or the other parent. Since normal development requires some degree of identification and separation from the values of *both* parents, children from this family constellation—particularly those of the opposite sex from the dominant parent—are at a severe disadvantage. Unlike unconscious fantasies, family process admits to observation and research, although instruments that are both reliable and valid may be difficult to develop. Important questions remain as to the prevalence and specificity of the patterns that Lidz has described. Brown and Brierly have developed an **expressed emotion scale.** Families high in expressed emotion are hostile, critical, and intrusive toward their sick member. The offspring of such families are less apt to do well at home after hospitalization. Interestingly, high expressed emotion behavior is subject to modification. Although less ambitious that other descriptions of family process—it makes claims neither to explaining etiology nor to specificity for schizophrenia—therapeutic approaches based on this concept appear to be effective in modifying the course of schizophrenia.

The occurrence of bizarre, eccentric, or deviant modes of communication not only in patients but in their families has attracted the attention of other workers. Bateson described the phenomenon of the "double bind"; patients are presented with a double and contradictory message and are placed under strong emotional pressure to avoid pointing out the contradiction. Wynn and colleagues developed an instrument for measuring communication deviance, the extent to which communication within a family is fragmented, contradictory, or illogical. Families who rate high on both communicative deviance and expressed emotion appear to predispose toward schizophrenic members.

Biologic factors

Neurotransmitters. The antipsychotic effect of neuroleptics correlates with these agents' ability to block postsynaptic dopamine receptors. Inevitably, biologic research has focused on the possible role of an increase in dopaminergic activity in the etiology of schizophrenic symptomatology. Little direct evidence has been elicited. Most schizophrenics who come to autopsy have been exposed to neuroleptics (which are likely to have increased the number of postsynaptic dopamine receptors indirectly). Furthermore, some of the *negative* symptoms of schizophrenia (i.e., blunted or flat affect, impoverishment of speech and thought, and a decrease in volitional behavior) appear to be related to a *reduction* in dopaminergic activity, perhaps in other pathways.

Since some hallucinogens (e.g., PCP) can produce a schizophrenia-like syndrome, attempts have been made to identify endogenous hallucinogens that might simulate their action in schizophrenics. Since methyl donors (like methionine) exacerbate symptoms in some patients, it has been suggested that biogenic amines may be subject to methylation along abnormal pathways. However, it is questionable whether such abnormal metabolites are found in differentially greater concentrations in schizophrenics.

Both elevated levels of creatinine phosphokinase (CPK) and decreased levels of platelet MAO have been reported in patients with schizophrenic psychoses but are probably nonspecific.

In summary, although there is much indirect evidence that neurotransmitter abnormalities play an important role in the mechanism of schizophrenic psychoses, their role is highly complex and may be more nonspecifically related to psychotogenesis than to schizophrenia as such.

Anatomic and functional brain studies. The development of techniques for in vivo brain imaging has offered neuroscientists an opportunity to investigate brain structure and function in schizophrenic patients. On CT scans, groups of schizophrenics show significantly more lateral and third ventricle enlargement than a group of matched controls. Another common finding is cerebral atrophy. These findings do not appear to be an effect of neuroleptic treatment and, in some studies, correlate with the prevalence of negative symptoms. Although substantiating the view that, for some patients at least, schizophrenia represents a neurological illness, they are not universally present and their implications for our understanding of the pathogenesis of the illness remains unclear.

Several recent studies have attempted to study regional cortical functioning by means of blood flow (using xenon-133, a radioactive tracer) or by means of positron emission tomography (PET scanning). Although results have not always been consistent, both techniques demonstrate a tendency toward reduced activity in the dorsolateral prefrontal cortex, a finding that may relate to negative symptoms.

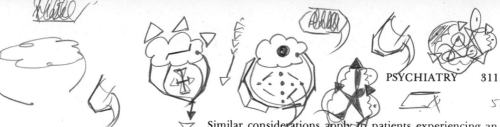

Psychological functioning

It has been known for some time that schizophrenics are not able to maintain an appropriate state of readiness (mental set) in learning tasks and that they are more easily distracted by irrelevant stimuli than normal persons. On timed tests (e.g., reaction time procedures) they are slower than normals, particularly in the presence of distractors. They are less apt to use efficient organizational strategies in recall. They cope poorly with high-intensity stimulus demands and do better on self-paced task in which they can control task demands than on other-paced tasks. Attention is a difficult concept to operationally measure, but many workers believe that schizophrenics' inability to focus and deploy attention appropriately is an important cognitive deficit in these patients.

Sociological factors

Schizophrenic patients are more apt to come from the lower socioeconomic strata. In large cities, patients are more apt to live in the more crowded, inner city areas than in the more affluent, less densely populated suburbs. Certainly, economic stress is a major component of hospitalization rates, which are better predicted by economic measures than by purely psychiatric ones. It has been proposed that the disabling effects of the illness lead to a **downward drift** in the social status of patients and their families. Alternatively, it has been proposed that the "culture of poverty" inhibits the development of specific ego strengths, leaving the patient more vulnerable to the effects of the illness.

Economic status also affects the pattern and quality of care provided to patients. Patients from developing third world countries are less apt to require frequent rehospitalization, probably because their families are more apt to attempt to care for them at home.

Treatment

Treatment of the active phase.   Although many "first-break" patients will present themselves during the prodromal period, during which withdrawal, eccentricity, and deterioration in self-care are common symptoms, the appearance of symptoms of incoherence, hallucinations, and delusions represents a psychiatric emergency. The experience is frightening to both patients and to their families, and the disinhibition of behavior and intrusion of dereistic thinking may put patients and those around them at serious risk. In most instances, hospitalization will be indicated to confirm the diagnosis, to stabilize the patient's medical regimen, and to establish a relationship with the family in regard to posthospital course. The patient's family is bewildered, frightened, and angry at the patient for "doing this to them." A period of surcease may be necessary for them to gain perspective on what has been happening. Patients are commonly terrified; their subjective experience is often one of fragmentation and unstable perceptions. They are particularly dependent on cues from those around them but at this stage are particularly apt to misinterpret or exaggerate the intentions of others. They are prone to relate in a helpless and regressed fashion. The hospital milieu has been developed to minimize the cognitive stress on patients and to reduce the behavioral regression attendant upon the disease.

Similar considerations apply to patients experiencing an acute exacerbation of a subchronic or chronic disorder. If the patient has been noncompliant with medication, a common reason for such deterioration, the reasons for noncompliance should be explored. Subtle side effects may have made the patient uncomfortable. Or family or occupational stress may have lead the patient to "give up" efforts to remain well and to comply. In the presence of a supportive family and when the patient's illness follows a familiar and predictable course, hospitalization may be avoided or partial hospitalization (e.g., a day hospital setting) may be used instead.

Medication.   Most patients will require a neuroleptic. Initially, the therapeutic effects of major tranquilizers are nonspecific, and for very agitated patients, more sedative, low-potency tranquilizers may be helpful. Paranoid and hyperalert patients may become more fearful when partially sedated; for this group, less-sedating medication is indicated. Although clinicians have turned to rapid tranquilization regimens for acutely disturbed patients, neither rapid tranquilization nor megadose regimens have proved superior to more moderate dose regimens on controlled study. Since the extrapyramidal side effects (EPS) are a major source of agitation and noncompliance, it is generally helpful to add an anticholinergic agent to the initial regimen. Specific antipsychotic effects of medication will usually become manifest in a week to 10 days; however, in some patients adequate neuroleptization may require 4 to 6 weeks of treatment for optimal effect. About 30% of patients will fail to show an adequate response even after an extended trial. For these patients, a trial of another class of neuroleptic might prove helpful.

A number of patients will demonstrate depressive symptoms after recovery from their acute psychotic episode. There is some controversy as to whether this represents a true depressive sequel or the reemergence of negative symptoms after neuroleptic medication. The addition of an antidepressant to the patient's neuroleptic regimen is of some value in the management of this complication.

Supportive psychotherapy.   Interpretive psychotherapy is contraindicated. Patients will need assurances about their present safety and the likelihood that their frightening psychotic experiences will come under control. The therapist must provide a measure of reality testing. Since patients' feelings about themselves and the world about them are primitive and ambivalent, they require assurances that they are not in immediate danger from malevolent outside forces or from their frightening sense of grandiosity or of distancing from what is familiar and comforting. Communications should be simple and direct since patients may misinterpret what they hear. The regularity and accessibility of meetings with the therapist are in themselves reassuring. Sessions may be brief and take into account the patient's limited capacity to maintain attention and to ward off fears of closeness and engulfment.

Milieu therapy.   Wards that treat schizophrenic patients are organized to take into account the patient's ego impairment. The mutual obligations of staff and patients are clearly delineated. Ward activities proceed along rules that are made explicit. Every effort is made to reduce regression to a passive or infantile role. Patients are expected to take an active role in

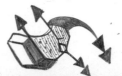

their self-care and in activities of daily living on the ward. Decision making is shared with the patients in community meeting. On some wards, a patient government takes responsibility for ward regulations and privilege levels. To minimize passivity, hierarchical role structure is kept to a minimum; staff eschews uniforms and other accoutrements of rank. In some units, staff and patients eat together. Patients are encouraged to express their feelings, but the difference between thought and action is emphasized. Because of the cognitive limitations of psychotic patients, nonverbal activities are a prominent part of the patient's day. Violation of ward rules leads to explicitly delineated loss of privileges. Some wards are organized along specifically behavioral principles and maintain a token economy in which patients gain or lose "points" depending on their behaviors. Perhaps most important, the ward atmosphere is a predictable and benign one, well insulated from the pressures and inconsistency that the patient may have experienced outside the hospital setting. At the same time, expectations are clear and regression is not reinforced.

Family therapy. The patient's family plays an important role in allaying the need for rehospitalization. **Psychoeducational programs** work with the family to help them cope with the manifold problems of a schizophrenic offspring or relative. As the term indicates, such programs rely on an educational rather than a therapeutic model. The family is taught about schizophrenia and what we know about the factors that lead to compensation. Schizophrenia is presented as a brain disease. Usually a "stress-diathesis" model emphasizes the relationship between specific stressors to which patients are vulnerable and their characteristic ways of responding to them. Commonly, families feel they are responsible for having made their relatives sick, and an illness model relieves them of a sense of blame. At the same time, the family learns to modify their expectations that the patient will be cured or resume his or her previous level of achievement. Both the frustrations they experience with these patients and the demands they place on them are ameliorated. More traditionally oriented **family therapy** also has a place in the treatment of schizophrenia. Role relationships in skewed or schismatic families can be clarified, and the family may be helped to express difficult or shameful issues clearly and without the obfuscation characteristic of such families. The therapist must listen for communication deviance and help the family to maintain an effective and consistent focus on issues at hand.

Treatment of the maintenance phase. The goals of this phase are assuring continued compliance with medication, evaluating and minimizing side effects, assisting patients to improve their psychosocial competence through vocational training, and attempting to reduce the morbidity caused by negative symptoms. After the acute phase, a day hospital or a residential treatment facility may provide the optimal setting for structuring a long-term program. In some cases, the family may have sufficient strength to serve as cotherapists in this effort.

Medication. As in any chronic illness, patients are apt to become noncompliant with medication when they are under stress. At times, they consciously wish to return to the regressive environment of the hospital. At other times, the patient may be "getting back" at the family or the therapist by becoming noncompliant. In contrast, for a few patients in

whom decompensation follows a predictable and more gradual course, the patient may be kept on a medication-free regimen until prodromal signs appear. This course must be followed with caution, however. Finally, some have advocated a very low-dose IM fluphenazine (Prolixin) regimen (0.1 mg every 2 weeks). Although patients are more apt to decompensate on this schedule, such episodes are usually manageable without hospitalization by increasing the dose of medication. However, it is claimed that the incidence of long-term side effects is decreased.

Tardive dyskinesia. Medicolegal considerations require that the clinician inform patients and their families of the risk of tardive dyskinesia (TD) as a side effect of chronic neuroleptic maintenance therapy. The patient should be examined carefully for early signs of this complication, and, if they appear, neuroleptics should be discontinued. Unfortunately, since there is no consistently effective treatment for TD, there will be instances in which the clinician must weigh the potentially disabling effect with the effects of the primary disorder.

Social and vocational rehabilitation. Because schizophrenia is a disease of young people and interferes with development, many patients will have lacked the experience of independent socialization and of time in the work world. Even when they had such experience, the disorder itself will have had a psychological effect on their capacity for attention and concentration. The experience of psychosis itself has corrosive effects on self-esteem that will in themselves impair learning. Socialization and vocational rehabilitation programs attempt to teach patients such skills in settings that are sensitive to the cognitive impairments imposed by the illness. Patients often begin in a prevocational setting where basic skills can be assessed and corrected. They may move on to a full vocational skills training program or may be assigned to a real workplace that has agreed to integrate a number of patients with their work staff. Such work-related programs have proved quite effective in maintaining patients in the community.

Prevention of negative symptoms. During the first flush of enthusiasm for outpatient treatment for schizophrenia, the prevalence of negative symptoms was often ascribed to the effects of chronic hospitalization in settings that isolated patients from the demands of ordinary adult life and kept them in a passive and powerless role. Although one cannot deny the reality of the phenomenon of "hospitalism," negative symptoms are currently viewed as a component of the schizophrenic symptom complex. When active social and rehabilitation programs are attempted, it is partly in hopes of counteracting or retarding the development of such symptoms as social withdrawal, lack of motivation, and flattening of affect. Precisely because they display these symptoms, however, some patients may be unable to participate fully in such programs. The precise therapeutic effectiveness of such interventions is difficult to assess. Because negative symptoms resemble those of parkinsonism, levodopa or similar drugs have been used to counteract them. Such treatments remain experimental, however.

Prognosis and course

In spite of our best efforts, as many as 40% of patients who are fully compliant with medication will require rehospitalization within 2 years of their first episode. About 80% of patients who *fail* to take medication will be rehospitalized in this period. The posthospital setting strongly affects these expectations.

In general, early symptoms consists of symptoms drawn from both positive and negative clusters. Positive symptoms— which are the components of the active psychotic episode— become somewhat less prominent after the disease has been present for about 5 years. Individual symptoms of the psychotic episode have little prognostic value. In general, adjustment after 5 years is best predicted from the patient's premorbid level of social and vocational functioning. Paranoid schizo- phrenics, who generally fall ill late and in whom ego functioning may be relatively well preserved, have a somewhat better prognosis than other subtypes.

In long-term follow-up studies, about 30% of patients function in the community with mild to moderate impairment and another 30% will require institutional or extensive out- patient or institutional support. The remainder will fall between these two extremes.

ANXIETY DISORDERS

Although almost everyone has experienced transient anxiety on occasion, about 5 to 7% of the population will suffer from relatively prolonged and incapacitating episodes of a sufficient intensity to warrant the diagnosis of an anxiety disorder. Such manifest symptoms must be differentiated from latent or unconscious anxiety, which most psychodynamic theories postulate as underlying the deployment of defense mechanisms and the determination of neurotic behaviors. Over the past several years, clinicians have begun to distinguish among these disorders more carefully, and specific pharmacological and behavioral therapies have been demonstrated to be of great utility.

Signs and symptoms of anxiety will vary from person to person, although any one individual will demonstrate a characteristic cluster of symptoms (response stereotypy) from episode to episode. Anxious patients experience a sensation of apprehension or dread, usually manifest by hypervigilance. In extreme cases, they fear they will lose consciousness or die, although unlike delusional patients, anxious patients usually have only a vague sense of the source or content of the danger. Symptoms are usually "ego-alien"—that is, the patient recog- nizes them as being of psychological origin and out of proportion to the stimulus. Somatic sensations include rapid pulse, palpitations, dry mouth, rapid and shallow respiration, muscle tension or tremor, abdominal discomfort or cramps, diarrhea, and urinary frequency.

In the context of a dangerous or life-threatening situation, these symptoms would be easily recognized as intense fear or panic, but in the anxiety disorders the reaction is out of proportion to the stimulus (which may not be evident at all), and, in a surprisingly high proportion of cases, neither the patient nor the physician correctly diagnoses the disorder. Patients are often worked up for somatic conditions related to one or another of their complaints; patients may fasten on this medical workup as a more concrete object of their fears.

Neither the psychophysiology of fear reactions nor, by extension, of the anxiety disorders is well understood. When subjects are confronted with stressful or dangerous circum-

stances, catecholamine (that is, epinephrine and norepine- phrine) secretion and turnover increase. Corticosteroid levels in the blood rise, as do blood glucose, free fatty acids, and several endocrine measures including blood testosterone. Urinary MHPG increases. The EEG becomes desynchronized; activity in the beta and theta ranges increases. However, the pattern and extent of these changes vary with individuals and with the situation. Benzodiazepines, which are in effect antianxiety agents, bind to sites in the cortex, limbic system, cerebellum, and spinal cord. It is possible that the experience of anxiety is mediated at these sites, but no endogenous receptor has been discovered.

Given our limited understanding of pathogenesis, the etiology of anxiety disorder has provoked numerous theories. Both generalized anxiety disorder and panic disorder appear to run in families, and a positive family history may be a diagnostic aid. Panic disorders have been linked to both a disrupted family environment and to a family history of depressive illness. Psychoanalytic clinicians have sought to demonstrate a link between precipitating events and sensitizing trauma in the patient's past. Certainly, severe traumatic events can lead to the characteristic symptoms of posttraumatic stress disorder. Since only a small proportion of patients exposed to trauma will develop sustained symptoms, it is likely that personality and constitutional factors play a role in this disorder as well. Learned fears may be demonstrable in simple phobias, and behavioral techniques may be quite effective in resolving them quickly.

Since anxiety will occur in the context of other psychiatric and medical disorders, careful diagnostic investigation is necessary. Anxiety disorder often coexists with drug and alcohol abuse, either because patients are self-medicating an underlying disorder or because of the disruptive effects of the medication on their mood. Anxiety symptoms occur very commonly in depressions, and the clinician may be taxed to determine the primary diagnosis.

ANXIETY STATES

Panic disorder

The distinct quality of panic attacks arises not so much from the component symptoms that they share with other anxiety disorders so much as from the fact that they are circumscribed and intense and that they arise independent of any apparent phobic stimulus, external stress, or period of physical exertion. Patients' subjective state of distress is intense, and no matter how often they may have this experience, each episode may be accompanied by the conviction they are about to die. It is usual to diagnose panic disorder in patients with agoraphobia. Other medical disorders such as pheochromocytoma and hyperthy- roidism may mimic this disorder, but they are relatively rare causes. Withdrawal from drugs or alcohol may produce panics, but the underlying cause is generally self-evident. Caffeine intoxication is a more commonly overlooked differential diagnosis.

Panic disorder has been reported as occurring in about 1% of the population and is more common among women than men.

In order to justify the diagnosis, *DSM-III* requires that the patient report three episodes in a period of as many weeks. In fact, the condition is so distressing and evident that the diagnosis will present few difficulties if the examiner is aware of the entity. A surprising number of patients will go from physician to physician without the condition being recognized, and the average period from onset to diagnosis has been reported to be about a year.

Panic disorder has been demonstrated to respond to treatment with TCAs or to MAO inhibitors such as phenelzine. Alprazolam, a triazolobenzodiazepine, also has demonstrated efficacy in this condition. Treatment must be maintained for several weeks prior to a response. If treatment is successful, the regimen is maintained for 9 to 12 months before the drug is gradually withdrawn. Recurrence is common.

Generalized anxiety disorder

When symptoms of anxiety are sustained for a month or more in the absence of panic attacks or when phobic or obsessive-compulsive symptoms and no underlying psychiatric or medical disorder can be diagnosed, the patient is considered to be suffering from a generalized anxiety disorder. Its prevalence is said to be from 2 to 6% and, like panic disorder, it occurs more commonly in women.

An association between generalized anxiety disorder and mitral valve prolapse has been suggested. The specificity of this relationship has not been definitively established, however.

Minor tranquilizers have proved effective in symptom amelioration, but because of their addictive potential, can play only a limited role in treatment. Patients who fail to respond to psychotherapy may benefit from antidepressants.

Obsessive-compulsive disorder

Obsessions are **forced ideas or images** that intrude themselves repetitively in an uncomfortable manner in spite of one's efforts to avoid them. They commonly deal with dirt or germs, with sexuality, or with profane religious conceits. **Compulsions are forced impulses.** In some patients, they may have a direct and disquieting impact (e.g., the new mother who is afraid she will stick her baby with pins), and in other cases they appear to be less threatening defenses against other ideas or impulses (compulsive hand washing, cleaning, "checking"). An uncommon form of compulsive disorder is compulsive slowness. Patients with obsessive-compulsive disorder feel their symptoms as ego alien. Symptoms characteristically wax and wane over the duration of the illness, and the patient may experience considerable social impairment. The disorder occurs with a prevalence rate of about 4%, and the sex ratio, although slightly favoring women, is considerably closer to 1:1 than for other forms of anxiety disorders. No definitive treatment exists, although antidepressants (particularly clomimipramine, a drug not available in the United States) have been reported as showing promising results when used over a sustained period of time.

Posttraumatic stress disorder

After the Vietnam War, public interest fastened on a group of returning veterans who displayed a characteristic set of symptoms including recurrent dreams of combat, "flashbacks" (i.e., imagery of wartime experiences evoked by stimuli reminiscent of Vietnam and sometimes so vivid as to transiently cause the veteran to act as though he were back there), emotional numbing with constriction of affect, sleep disturbances, and general symptoms of anxiety. Such syndromes have been recognized after other episodes of trauma, individual or collective, and have been designated in *DSM-III* as the posttraumatic stress disorder. Stress in this context is difficult to define precisely; *DSM-III* defines it as an experience that "would evoke significant symptoms of distress in anyone." Initially, it was assumed that a latent period intervened between the experience of stress, but there is some evidence that early symptoms may occur almost immediately. Acute and chronic forms have been recognized. No one treatment has been found effective, and it is likely that a multimodal treatment plan including supportive psychotherapy and medication is indicated. Support groups of victims who have undergone similar trauma may have great utility, particularly when issues concerning survivor guilt or self-blame are prominent. When phobic anxiety is prominent, behavioral treatments have been reported to be effective.

Agoraphobia

Although agoraphobia is often defined as fear of open spaces, it is the unavailability of help or assistance that patients fear. Thus some patients with agoraphobia will be frightened of public places because they may be trapped in crowds; others may specifically fear crowded, closed spaces such as elevators because they cannot escape quickly if they are in distress. In extreme instances, patients will not leave their homes or will only go out in the presence of a trusted friend or family member ("phobic companion"). The prevalence of agoraphobia is generally estimated to be about 4%, and women are affected more frequently than men. When severe, it is a disabling condition.

Many patients with agoraphobia will give a history of antecedent panic attacks, and many clinicians have argued that the phobic symptoms are based on the patient's apprehension about developing such attacks away from sources of succor or safety. This supposition is supported by the finding that agoraphobia without a history of panic attacks is quite infrequent.

Although it may appear as a separate condition, agoraphobia can also occur in the context of other psychiatric disorders such as severe personality disorders and schizophrenia.

Although agoraphobia may be ameliorated somewhat by minor tranquilizers, these agents are not effective in controlling the syndrome. Behavioral techniques such as systematic desensitization have proved effective. Alprazolam, TCAs (imipramine), and MAO inhibitors have also been reported to be effective. Most clinicians combine these latter two modalities and use minor tranquilizers to help control apprehension about recurrence.

Other phobias

Many people have "irrational" fears that do not fall into the category of agoraphobia. Individuals with **social phobias** will avoid public situations in which they feel they may be scrutinized and subject to embarrassment or humiliation. For example, a patient may refuse restaurant invitations for fear she will not know how to act or that her eating habits will embarrass her. Many individuals fear public speaking.

Phobias that fall neither under the rubric of agoraphobia nor social phobias are called **simple phobias.** This is a diverse category and includes fear of animals (e.g., snakes), fear of heights, etc.

Although social and simple phobias may be limiting in particular occupations, they are seldom as incapacitating as other anxiety disorders. Behavioral treatments have been of great help in alleviating these disorders. **Stage fright** has been treated with propranolol, a beta-adrenergic blocker, with some success.

PERSONALITY DISORDERS

Most people have a clear intuitive notion of what is meant by **personality,** the habitual style of behaving and responding that we and others recognize as being peculiarly our own. It is frequently difficult to characterize this style because it must be abstracted from many different circumstances over a lengthy period of time and because real life requires that responses be sufficiently flexible and adaptive to a variety of different situations.

Patients with personality disorders have a response repertoire that is limited, rigid, and maladaptive. It is easier to characterize them because they tend to react to stress the same way over a range of instances even when others consider it inappropriate. The patient with a paranoid personality disorder, for example, is distrustful even in instances when this is inappropriate. Frequently, patients are unaware of this inflexibility; they are often referred by significant others or outside agencies who can no longer tolerate their behavior. Since these individuals have a limited number of coping mechanisms, questioning the ones they habitually use may evoke anxiety or depression, and they understandably resist efforts at therapy without sufficient incentive for change. Although patients may feel comfortable, their behavior interferes with their work, their attempts at intimacy, and their sense of psychological comfort. That is why these conditions represent psychiatric disorders.

Little is known about the etiology of these disorders. Some appear related to more easily definable syndromes such as paranoid disorders, schizophrenia, and affective disorders and may represent *formes frustes* or partial manifestations. Others seem to represent an interaction of genetic, familial, and experiential influences. By providing clear, objectifiable diagnostic criteria, *DSM-III* has fostered research in this area.

Paranoid personality disorder

These patients are chronically suspicious, distrustful, and hypervigilant to threat. They consistently "overread" others' intentions. Pathological jealousy is a special and particularly virulent form of the disorder. Cold and remote to others, persons with paranoid personality disorder respond to the merest intimation of slight by "going on the attack"; yet they seldom court the sort of relationships that would support their needs for confirmation and love.

Some patients who present with paranoid personality disorder will, on closer examination, have signs of paranoid

disorder or schizophrenia. The great majority will present a developmental history of great stress or deprivation to which they have responded by maintaining a safe distance from others while subordinating their desires for intimacy and love. In these latter instances, psychotherapy—the indicated treatment—may be difficult since it represents just the sort of threat the patient fears.

Schizoid personality disorder

These people are, in lay terms, "introverts" or "loners." They eschew social interactions, have few friends, and appear remote and indifferent to the opinions of others. They are often unmarried and may prefer solitary occupations (e.g., night watchman). They appear to have difficulty understanding social rules; at best this makes them appear awkward, at worst it leads to difficulties with employers and with the law. Psychotherapy is often an educative and supportive process in which therapists lend their "social self" to allow patients to ford more difficult transitions.

Schizotypal personality disorder

Although included among the personality disorders, many of these patients appear to have "just missed" qualifying for the diagnosis of schizophrenia. Like patients in the previous categories of personality disorder, they are often socially isolated and inappropriately distrustful and suspicious. Where they differ is that their sense of reality appears impaired. Although they are seldom frankly delusional, they hold magical or illogical ideas. Neutral or insignificant stimuli may be experienced as referring to patients themselves. Hallucinations are absent, but patients may report extraordinary or quasi-religious experiences such as "visions" or out-of-body experiences. Speech may be digressive or difficult to follow without a formal thought disorder. In general, these patients are able to recoup their sense of reality. Some of these patients will have grown up in a household where a dominating figure was in fact mentally ill. In other cases, the clinician may come to the conclusion that the patient is in fact a relatively well-compensated schizophrenic.

Histrionic personality disorder

The lay term *hysterical* applies to these patients. They are volatile, self-dramatizing, egocentric, and prone to tantrums. Generally seeking to surround themselves with excitement and stimulation, they are often described by others as colorful, but on closer contact their emotions are often superficial or false. They are adept at manipulating others through their emotional display; in some patients this manifests itself in repeated suicide attempts. Beneath the surface, they are often dependent and in need of constant reassurance.

Histrionic behavior patterns are often socially learned. They are more characteristic of women but far from infrequent in men. Some patients appear to suffer from an underlying affective disorder. In others, more careful examination may reveal characteristics of a borderline personality disorder. Assorted psychopharmacological interventions such as neuroleptics or antidepressants have been proposed but are inconsistently helpful. In general, these patients will benefit best from supportive psychotherapy.

Narcissistic personality disorder

Like patients with histrionic personality disorders, these patients are egocentric, attention seeking, and exploitative in their interpersonal relationships. Their inner life is fueled by feelings of specialness, and they remain aloof and distant even from their intimates. If they are subjected to criticism, they may respond with exaggerated feelings of humiliation and rage. Despite this, they have little capacity to empathize with the vulnerability or needs of others. A common feature is their feeling of "entitlement," which causes them to take from others with little sense of reciprocal obligation. In their close relationships, they alternate between idealization and derogation.

The same difficulties that cause problems in ordinary relationships interfere with psychotherapy. Narcissistic patients are distrustful and difficult to engage; attempts to induce them to distance themselves from and examine their behavior are apt to be met with feelings of rage and shame.

Antisocial personality disorder

Although the term appears to allude to persons given to criminal acts, most lawbreakers do not suffer from antisocial personality disorder, nor do afflicted persons always run afoul of the law. Patients with this disorder appear to have difficulty in making stable, meaningful, affectional attachments to family, friends, and lovers. They also suffer with impulsiveness that prevents them from sustaining adequate work and love relationships and that may be manifest in difficulties with authorities in school or on the job, in drug or alcohol abuse, and in promiscuous or polymorphous perverse sexual behaviors.

The etiology is unclear. A significant number of patients have signs of neurological dysfunction on examination or in their EEGs. Some patients have a history of maternal neglect or abandonment. Others come from families in which antisocial disorder has been manifest in other members, particularly among males. It has been well established that the history of antisocial behaviors tends to establish itself early. *DSM-III* requires confirmatory history before the age of 15, but signs are often apparent by an earlier history of lying, truancy, and other delinquent acts. In antisocial patients, this history is continuous over many years. It must be emphasized that episodic delinquent or irresponsible behaviors occur during periods of stress (in adolescence, for example) or as features of other psychiatric illnesses including schizophrenia and major affective disorders.

The treatment of these patients is difficult. Substance abuse problems may require attention. Psychotherapeutic interventions are difficult, because these patients form tenuous therapeutic alliances (often motivated by fear of more stringent punishment) and may be untrustworthy. Behavioral techniques have been used but are most effective in institutional settings.

Borderline personality disorder

These patients maintain a "stably unstable," sometimes chaotic life-style that is difficult to capture in a fixed set of criteria. Outwardly, their lives may be replete with incident, characterized by emotional storms, impulsivity, and emotional storms. Inwardly, they complain of a sense of "empty" depression or chronic rage. They are "object hungry" and sensitive to withdrawal or abandonment by others, but they are equally threatened by a sense of engulfment in close relation-

ships. They have little sense of identity, and in fact it is often difficult to describe them in consistent terms (something that is not true of patients with histrionic personality disorder, whom they may superficially resemble). In extreme cases, patients may resort to suicidal attempts or to self-mutilation just to convince themselves that they "really exist." In therapy, their emotional distance from the therapist may swing from closeness to distance with dizzying speed, and their attitude may shift as readily from tender idealization to a devaluating rage. Brief psychotic episodes (usually with a paranoid flavor) lasting hours to days may occur in periods of stress and cause them to be labeled schizophrenic (one source of the "borderline" description). Nevertheless, under more neutral circumstances, these patients may perform well, and the history may show a dissociation between their functioning in relatively well-structured settings and in intense interpersonal relationships. In a parallel fashion, structured psychological tests (such as the Wechsler Adult Intelligence Scale [WAIS]) may indicate less psychopathology than unstructured projective tasks (like the Rorschach), where they may produce regressed and near-psychotic responses.

It is likely that this is a heterogeneous group of disorders, and inevitably, many different treatment approaches have been proffered. At present, long-term psychotherapy appears to offer the most effective approach, although there is a high dropout rate and the treatment process may be eventful and arduous.

Avoidant personality disorder

Like schizoid patients, patients with avoidant personality disorder have adopted social withdrawal to escape the threat of humiliation or rejection at the hands of others. Unlike schizoid patients, they are usually conscious of their wish for closeness and affection; they are less likely to substitute an internal fantasy life for reality. Patients may harbor a profound contempt for themselves and their social deficit. They may appear awkward and distant at first but can give a painful history of life at the fringes of groups and relationships. Such patients often have difficulty in interpreting the social signals of others and in engaging in the social give-and-take necessary to learn them. In psychotherapy, therapists may have to "lend" the patient their social skills. Even then, patients may find little pleasure in their successes.

Dependent personality disorder

This is an essentially descriptive category. Dependent patients submit readily to others and fail to assert their own needs or wishes. They perceive themselves as having little ability to control or determine their own lives. Lacking a sense of self-confidence, they allow others to make major decisions in their lives. An extreme example is the wife who habitually submits to verbal and physical abuse.

Psychologically, dependence and anger are mirror images of each other; the opposite of each is healthy assertiveness. In general, dependency is viewed as a learned behavior; it is a way (albeit self-harmful) of control. These patients are denying their own aggressiveness and allowing others to express it against them. Effective assertiveness training techniques have been developed. However, the change in the patient's personality is apt to disrupt existing relationships and threaten the patient's security.

Compulsive personality disorder

So-called compulsive traits such as orderliness, parsimony, goal-directedness, and cleanliness are highly adaptational in our society. Patients with compulsive personality disorder exhibit maladaptive traits that are almost parodies of these. They are overorganized, inflexible, and perfectionistic. They are apt to become so concerned with the task at hand that they lose sight of why they are engaged in it in the first place. They tend to be workaholics. To others they seem overly cold and distant. Emotional relationships appear to be subordinated to the goals they are seeking. They substitute willfulness and stubbornness for real interpersonal engagement. Some patients become so concerned with detail that they paradoxically appear indecisive and unable to complete the task at hand.

By missing the larger picture, patients with compulsive personality disorder retain a sense of order and control and defend themselves against the emotions that they might otherwise find overwhelming. Since psychotherapy may evoke similar conflicts, these patients may bring their compulsive traits into therapy. The defense mechanisms of intellectualization, isolation (of thought from affect), and doing and undoing (indecisiveness) will be prominent. Because of this, these patients may be difficult to work with. However, psychotherapy remains the therapy of choice. Patients with this disorder may be particularly prone to episodes of depression, which are then treated as indicated.

Passive-aggressive personality disorder

Like those with dependent personality, these patients have difficulty in expressing healthy self-assertion and instead substitute such traits as stubbornness, procrastination, and repeated forgetfulness as indirect expressions of their anger. Although these mechanisms may be displayed from time to time in everyone, the patient with passive-aggressive personality disorder exhibits them in a consistent manner over a protracted period. Patients come into therapy as others become alienated from them and they experience repeated failures in their social or work spheres.

Psychotherapy is directed at helping these patients to accept responsibility for their seemingly inadvertent behavior and substituting more adaptive forms of assertiveness.

PSYCHIATRIC DISORDERS MANIFESTED BY PHYSICAL SYMPTOMS

The general physician is frequently confronted with symptoms that appear to be related to the patient's psychological state either because emotional factors appear to play a predominant role in provoking or maintaining such symptoms or because they cannot be adequately accounted for on the basis of known physiological mechanisms. In these instances, the physician must be guided by two apparently contradictory principles. On one hand, psychological states *do* manifest themselves somatically and it does the patient no good to "fix" such symptoms by focusing concern on somatic manifestations through a fruitless series of diagnostic tests. On the other, some

illnesses (e.g., collagen diseases, some endocrinopathies, and neurological illnesses such as multiple sclerosis) may present in an obscure and atypical fashion. Thus, a high index of suspicion is indicated even when a psychological diagnosis appears most certain. In a high proportion of cases, psychological and organic symptoms may be admixed. Even the most apparently hypochondriacal patient may fall physically ill.

Somatization disorder

In a small proportion of the population, about 1 or 2%, stress will be manifested by multiple somatic complaints, often of a vague but disabling nature. Most, but not all, of these patients are women whose pattern of response has begun in late adolescence, and the patient usually reports she has been "sickly" most of her life. The patient's life-style is frequently organized around this perception; she may ingest large amounts of different medications and take to bed frequently. *DSM-III* has attempted to quantify the disorder. Patients are required to report 12 out of 37 such symptoms if they are men, 14 out of 37 if they are women. Not surprisingly, pseudoneurological or conversion symptoms (see below) are common, as are GI, menstrual, psychosexual, and cardiopulmonary complaints, many of them reminiscent of symptoms of anxiety. Psychogenic pain is frequently reported by these patients, although it is more commonly encountered as an isolated complaint. Although the level of the patient's complaints may vary with stress, the symptom picture is a relatively stable one and there is no specific treatment beyond supportive psychotherapy. The etiology is obscure. Social factors are probably of some importance, since the sick role has been institutionalized in some places and during certain historical periods. However, why only a small proportion of individuals at risk adapt this posture remains unexplained and may point to some underlying physiological mechanism that has yet to be delineated. Somatization disorder is said to run in families; the patient's male relatives are said to show a higher than expected incidence of alcoholism and sociopathy.

Conversion disorder (hysterical neurosis, conversion type)

Conversion symptoms involve the somatosensory or motor systems or the special senses (in contrast to pschophysiological disorder, which involve autonomic nervous system functioning) in a manner that is inexplicable by ordinary pathophysiological mechanisms. For example, hysterical anesthesia or pain syndromes often fail to follow anatomic pathways. The psychodynamic origins of these symptoms are often surprisingly easy to deduce. They frequently arise in response to a psychological conflict (unconscious in that the patient is unaware of it) and often may be interpreted as expressing a symbolic communication. For example, patients with hysterical blindness may not "want to see," and patients with hysterical aphonia may not "want to speak" about what is troubling them. Instead, the focus of concern is shifted to the dramatic and disabling symptoms. The consequent attention and concern that the patient's illness arouses and the degree of support that it elicits are often spoken of as **secondary gain. Primary gain** is derived from the patient's success in continuing to repress the unacceptable part of the conflict that initiated the complaint. The onset or exacerbation of symptoms is temporally relatable to the psychological stimulus. Patients with conversion disorders sometimes act relatively unconcerned about the seriousness of their illness; they exhibit so-called **belle indifference.**

Although conversion disorders may be multiform, frequently encountered examples include difficulty in swallowing (**globus hystericus**), dizziness, blindness, aphonia, dizziness, amnesias, seizure, failure in balance, paralyses, convulsions, paresthesia, and loss of sensation. Despite the apparently non-atomic and dramatic nature of the symptom, patients cannot appreciate its psychological etiology *nor can they control it*.

When seen as an isolated symptom, pain is diagnosed as psychogenic pain disorder and psychosexual symptoms as psychosexual dysfunctions.

As many as a third of patients with conversion disorders will have some other major psychiatric diagnosis. Another third will have some associated *physical* disorder including neurological illness. Hence, the diagnosis should not preclude the search for other serious illness.

Many conversion symptoms remit spontaneously or when environmental attention and support are withdrawn. In these cases, supportive therapy is all that is indicated.

Psychogenic pain disorder

Patients with this disorder complain of pain that is unrelatable to an anatomically founded ailment or that is out of proportion to what can be explained by objective findings. Careful history will often reveal that pain is exacerbated when the patient is under stress. In some instances, particularly when compensation elements are involved, patients' symptoms allow them to escape from an intolerable work situation or to receive support from those around them in a manner that would otherwise be impossible.

In general, these are difficult ailments to treat. Since anxiety or depression decreases pain tolerance, these elements should be sought. Even when frank depressive symptoms are absent, antidepressants may be of value. Behavioral techniques aimed at modifying the pain behavior and helping the patient to develop more effective interpersonal skills are sometimes useful but are best implemented in specialized settings. Psychotherapy is often of little use; these patients tend to have limited introspective skills and to express their feelings somatically.

Hypochondriasis

Hypochondriacal patients are preoccupied with the conviction that they have a serious illness, a fear that is not assuaged by a thorough physical examination and objective tests. In severe cases, the patient's life is limited by his or her need to seek further reassurances. Although the cause of this disorder is unknown, the patient's continual struggle with skeptical physicians for attention and belief is thought to sustain it. Many patients have severe personality disorders and an impaired body image that allows them to express unacceptable feelings through their symptoms.

Factitious disorder with physical symptoms

Unlike other patients in this group, these patients appear to be driven to seek a "patient status" by consciously inventing or exaggerating symptoms requiring extensive workup or multiple hospitalizations. Some patients are adept at inducing skin lesions or fever. They may evade even subtle efforts of hospital staff to discover the source of their symptoms. Patients with **Munchausen's syndrome** amass voluminous hospital charts (usually at many different institutions); their complaints often center on symptoms suggestive of polysystem disease (such as collagen diseases, porphyria, and multiple sclerosis). They are frequently the victims of polysurgery, polypharmacy, and long and fruitless laboratory investigations. These patients are frequently expert in avoiding identification. Psychiatrically they often resemble imposters and patients with antisocial personality disorder. The etiology and treatment are obscure.

DISSOCIATIVE DISORDERS

Dissociative disorders are relatively uncommon conditions in which patients attempt to escape from conflict-laden or unsolvable situations by consigning them to an inaccessible part of their personality. Whole areas of experience that would ordinarily cohere to provide a continuous sense of identity are repressed or are only intermittently available to the patient. The most dramatic instances occur in **multiple personality,** in which patients may experience (and present) themselves as different people, often with contrasting personalities that act out conflicting aspects of themselves such as a "good" or "bad" self. In complex cases, many such personalities coexist and each may have a differing awareness of the others.

Less dramatic are **fugue states,** in which patients unexpectedly travel from their usual habitation and assume a new identity without awareness of their old one. In **psychogenic amnesia,** patients have extensive memory loss for personal details (sometimes including their own identity). In **depersonalization disorder,** patients feel sufficiently separated from or apart from a normal sense of self to be distracted from their ordinary functioning.

Although the dynamics of these patients' illness may be clear to outsiders—they are attempting to escape from an intolerable inner or outer reality—they are usually unaware of these factors and may show a rather bland affect about their disability. Dissociative disorders are commonly found in patients with neurological impairment (including chronic alcoholism), and organic disorders should be included in the differential. They also occur during the course of psychotic disorders such as schizophrenia. Psychogenic amnesia and fugue states often remit spontaneously; the patient should be observed in a safe setting. Depersonalization disorder may occur in the presence of an underlying depression, and antidepressants may be helpful. Patients with multiple personalities usually require extensive psychotherapy.

Dissociative disorders sometimes occur in the context of forensic cases (e.g., the patient may be unable to remember an act committed in a state of "temporary insanity"). In these instances, differentiation from malingering may be difficult.

Repressed material may be made accessible by giving the patient sufficient IV amytal to produce light sedation ("truth serum"), as well as through hypnosis. In most instances, patients will forget what has been recovered once they are alert. In general, it is best to allow the patient to reintegrate the repressed material in a more gradual manner and in a fully conscious state.

ADJUSTMENT DISORDERS

In some instances, the onset of symptoms appears to be temporally associated with the onset of an identifiable psychosocial stressor and the patient's reaction does not appear to be only the latest in a pattern of maladaptive responses. These adjustment disorders may present with anxiety, depression, conduct disturbances, withdrawal, or work inhibition (e.g., writer's block). There may be a mixture of symptoms. In general, the patient will respond to supportive psychotherapy, but, where they are intense, presenting symptoms may require psychopharmacological treatment.

PSYCHIATRIC THERAPIES

PSYCHOPHARMACOLOGY

Until the early 1950s, the only behaviorally active drugs available to psychiatrists were sedatives and hypnotics. The introduction of lithium carbonate and of chlorpromazine and related phenothiazides in the 1940s and 50s provided the first *specific* antipsychotic agents. The TCAs are structurally derived from the phenothiazines. MAO inhibitors were serendipitously discovered when physicians using related antitubercular drugs noted mood-elevating side effects. Antianxiety drugs appeared in the 1950s; since then, the benzodiazepines have become the predominant group of such agents. Compounds from more diverse structural groups have been developed, but the four major categories—antipsychotics, antimanics, antidepressants, and anxiolytics—still represent the major available classes.

It is important to appreciate the fact that even with optimal management a considerable number of patients will fail to respond adequately to drug treatment. From 20 to 30% of patients with schizophrenia or major affective disorder will prove to be medication resistant. In some cases, age or concurrent medical disorders will limit their usefulness. All psychotropic drugs have side effects that may affect the patient's willingness to comply with the prescribed regimen; Tardive dyskinesia (TD), a long-term effect of antipsychotics, may affect the patient's and physician's willingness to continue these drugs. Finally, although useful in a single episode, none of these agents are curative. Patients may relapse or deteriorate despite continued treatment. Combinations of medications may be necessary to control symptoms fully. On the other hand, many psychiatric disorders, including the major psychoses, have a tendency toward remission. For this reason, clinical investigators of a new agent have the difficult task of ascertaining whether the drug is more effective than placebo or than a proven and standard treatment.

Drugs treat the patient, not the disease. Although some patients may respond to a simple course of medication, most patients will need psychological support, behavioral prescriptions, or psychotherapy for maximum benefit. In this regimen, drugs are only a single, although frequently a necessary, component. Finally, although it is simple to group medications

in the categories outlined above, one must remember that the indications for a particular drug may be more extensive than the category indicates. For example, some antidepressants are effective in phobic disorders and some anxiolytics appear to have antidepressant effects. As research continues, we may expect that the indications for drugs in our armamentarium will become broader and more specific.

The antipsychotic drugs

Antipsychotic agents are particularly effective in reducing the "positive" symptoms of psychosis, including hallucinations, delusions, agitation, and attention deficits. They are less effective in treating "negative" symptoms such as attenuated effective expression, retardation of speech, and thought and avolitional behaviors. Thus, except in acute and circumscribed psychoses, they must be supplemented with psychological support and social rehabilitation programs.

The phenothiazines and butyrophenones (chiefly haloperidol) are the most commonly used "front line" antipsychotics.

The antipsychotics can be categorized according to their chemical structures:

Aliphatic phenothiazides. The best-known example is chlorpromazine (Thorazine). These are low-potency drugs. They tend to be sedating and to produce orthostatic hypotension. They produce prominent anticholinergic side effects. Extrapyramidal symptoms (EPS) occur with moderate frequency.

Piperazine phenothiazines. Examples are trifluoperazine (Stelazine), fluphenazine (Prolixin), and perphenazine (Trilafon). They are high-potency medications, and their use is attended by a high incidence of EPS. They are nonsedating, and some clinicians believe they "activate" withdrawn patients. Fluphenazine is available in IM depot preparations and is particularly helpful in the treatment of poorly compliant patients.

Piperidine phenothiazines. Examples are thioridazine (Mellaril) and mesoridazine (Serentil). These molecules appear to have strong intrinsic anticholinergic properties. Some clinicians prefer them because they produce fewer manifest EPS. However, they are apt to produce male sexual disturbances (retarded ejaculation and anorgasmia). In high doses, thioridazine has been reported to produce retinopathies and cardiomyopathies; thus its dose is generally limited to no more than 800 mg/day.

Butyrophenones. Haloperidol is the best-known example. These drugs are high potency and moderate in their tendency to produce EPS. Haloperidol is generally well tolerated in liquid form because it is tasteless. A depot preparation for IM administration has recently been introduced.

Thioxanthines. Thiothixene (Navane) is the most widely used drug of this class, which resembles the piperazine phenothiazines in their pharmacological profiles.

Indoles. Molindone (Moban) is a less frequently used antipsychotic. It is said to produce less weight gain than other antipsychotics.

Dibenzapines. Loxapine is the most widely used drug in this class.

Choice and regulation of medication are determined by clinical response (including tolerance to side effects). There is no evidence for a systematic difference in overall clinical efficacy among antipsychotics, nor are any of them highly specific against particular symptoms.

There is a wide variation in dose range: For psychotic patients, a minimal dose of about 400 mg of chlorpromazine or its equivalent is necessary. In general, antipsychotic effects are not clearly manifest for the first week, although patients may show side effects early and a 4- to 6-week trial is necessary to evaluate the full therapeutic effect. Clinicians have attempted to produce more rapid response by "rapid neuroleptization" (or digitalization) of the initial dose regimen, but there is no firm evidence that this improved response rate. If patients fail to respond to an adequate trial of 2 g of chlorpromazine equivalent, further increases in dose are unlikely to appear and consideration should be given to another agent.

Both fluphenazine and haloperidol are available in depot preparations, which are given IM every 2 to 4 weeks and which may be helpful in the management of noncompliant patients.

The neuroleptics commonly produce side effects that limit the acceptability and safety of their use. Common side effects include the following:

1. **Sedation,** particularly with low-potency medications. This symptom often disappears after a week.

2. As described above, **orthostatic hypotension** is a particular side effect of low-potency compounds.

3. **Anticholinergic** side effects (particularly notable in the piperidines including thioridazine and mesoridazine) include dry mouth, orthostatic hypotension, constipation, retrograde ejaculation, urinary retention, blurred vision (due to interference with accommodation), and exacerbation of narrow-angle glaucoma.

4. EPS include the following:
   a. **Parkinsonism** including bradykinesia, tremor, and mask-like facies. Antiparkinson medication will relieve these symptoms.
   b. **Dystonias** of the muscles of the tongue, jaw, and neck. Since patients are often alarmed by these reactions, the use of parenteral antiparkinsonian drugs (e.g., diphenhydramine) is indicated.
   c. **Akathisia and akinesia.** These are disturbances of voluntary motor activity, the first marked by an uncontrollable restlessness, often confined to the lower extremity, the latter by severe inhibition of movement.

5. **Neuroleptic malignant syndrome** (NMS). This idiosyncratic but serious complication of neuroleptic administration has come to be increasingly recognized. It may affect as many as 1 to 4% of patients at risk. NMS is characterized by muscle rigidity, fever, and change in state of consciousness. Transient elevations of blood pressure and pulse may also be noted. The illness is progressive, especially if medication is not withdrawn. Treatment consists of the withdrawal of medication and symptomatic measures. Calcium channel blocking agents (e.g., dantrolene) or bromocriptine may be of some help.

6. **TD** is generally encountered in patients who have been receiving neuroleptics for a protracted period. It is manifest by abnormal motor movements, often of a choreiform or athetoid quality and generally involving the tongue, lips, mouth, or upper extremities. Older patients, particularly women and those with a marked affective component, are thought to be more vulnerable. As many as a fifth of patients exposed to protracted administration of these drugs are thought to be affected in varying degrees, and since it may progress to the point of severe disability, early detection is necessary. Common early signs involve overactivity or fasciculations of the tongue and lips, but tic-like movements of facial muscles or of the upper extremity may also be noted. In fact, the illness, particularly in its more severe manifestations, may present as a variable syndrome. Many patients will show only mild symptoms that are nonprogressive. The possibility of progression is a serious one that must be discussed with the patient and family. If it is possible to safely withdraw the neuroleptic, this should be done since in many patients symptoms will remit over time. However, in some patients, lowering medication will *worsen* symptoms. No standard and effective treatment exists for TD. It is generally believed to be related to dopamine hypersensitivity attendant on proliferation of postsynaptic dopaminergic receptors (a secondary effect of the neuroleptic's dopamine blocking action), but this understanding has not lead to a corresponding rational treatment regimen.

Less common or minor side effects of neuroleptics include the following: (1) agranulocytosis, which is rare and unpredictable but serious; patients on neuroleptics should have a blood count when any sign of infection appears; (2) allergic skin rashes; (3) dermatologic photosensitivity; and (4) gynecomastia and galactorrhea. Cholestatic jaundice was noted by early investigators but is now an uncommon side effect.

The antipsychotic activity of neuroleptics correlates well with their capacity to block postsynaptic dopamine receptors.

Antidepressant drugs

Antidepressants fall into two major classes: the TCAs and the MAO inhibitors. In addition, a benzodiazepine, alprazolam (Xanax), possesses significant antidepressant properties.

Tricyclic antidepressants and related compounds. A broad range of TCAs are on the market. A few compounds with a different molecular structure but similar clinical indications are also available. These include tetracyclic compounds such as amoxapine (Asendin), which is related to the antipsychotic dibenzapine loxapine, and maprotiline (Ludiomil). It should be noted that these drugs may also be useful in the treatment of disorders other than mood disorders, notably in some anxiety disorders and in the schizoaffective disorders. These drugs appear to have a similar degree of clinical efficacy; about 75 to 80% of appropriately selected patients will show symptom remission. (It should be noted that depressions are commonly remitting conditions and about a third of patients will show spontaneous remission). The choice of drug is determined by the patients' drug history, by their susceptibility to or tolerance of side effects, and by the presenting clinical picture.

Patients will generally respond well to a medication to which they have responded in the past. This forms a reliable guide to drug choice. If a member of the patient's *family* has demonstrated a good response, it is likely that this will be predictive of a good response in the proband.

Antidepressants of this group have a wide range of side effects. The most troublesome common side effects include sedation, tremor, orthostatic hypotension, and a variety of anticholinergic symptoms (e.g., dry mouth, constipation, urinary retention, and exacerbation of angle-closure glaucoma). Many of these drugs affect cardiac conduction, and all patients over age 40 should have an ECG prior to institution of therapy.

Anticholinergic side effects may be particularly troublesome. Desipramine and nortriptyline have a lesser degree of anticholinergic action and may be useful when these effects are to be avoided. In patients with cardiac disease, doxepin is said to be less apt to produce conduction abnormalities. There are claims that the tetracyclic maprotiline has a somewhat more rapid onset.

The mode of action of these drugs is not commonly understood. As a group, they tend to inhibit reuptake of biogenic amines, increasing their availability at the synapse. This mechanism does not adequately explain the common observed delay of 10 days to 2 weeks in onset of therapeutic action, however.

Accurate blood level testing is now widely available. Since a therapeutic response is poorly predictable from the oral dose, this procedure will assure that patients are attaining adequate therapeutic levels (perhaps the single most important determinant of efficacy). A few of these drugs display therapeutic windows—that is, they produce less effect when the dose level is either too low *or* too high. Blood levels may be used to monitor the oral regimen more accurately.

Once the patient is receiving an adequate therapeutic dose, the antidepressant effects are usually delayed for a period of 10 days to 2 weeks. To maintain a good response, the drug should be maintained for a period of 6 months to prevent relapse. It should then be withdrawn gradually. Rapid withdrawal may lead to a flu-like syndrome.

MAO inhibitors.   In the United States, these are used as second-line drugs. Many clinicians use them only when a trial of the first group has failed. As their name indicates, they act by inhibiting the enzyme MAO, which is responsible for the intracellular metabolism of biogenic amines. Patients on these drugs may become sensitized to "false" sympathetic transmitters such as tyramine. Foods rich in these substances may produce crises manifested by hypertension and fever. Deaths from stroke have been reported. Hence patients on MAO inhibitors must observe dietary precautions and must exclude such foods as "stinky" cheeses, yogurt, pickles, pickled meats, beer, and flat beans from their diets.

Common side effects include sedation, hypotension, and malignant interaction with other drugs (e.g., meperidine).

Despite the precautions one must observe, these are effective agents. They are said to be particularly useful in the treatment of atypical depressions (where characterological or hysterical features are admixed with the depressive ones).

Alprazolam.   This benzodiazepine has demonstrated antidepressant features in moderately severe depressions. It has a rather high addictive potential and should be used with caution. Other side effects include sedation and motor incoordination.

Lithium

Lithium salts (carbonate and citrate) are effective antimanic agents in about 70% of affected patients. Lithium maintenance reduces the frequency of *both* manic and depressive episodes in bipolar patients. In some patients, lithium may also have antidepressant effects, but this is less reliable.

The therapeutic range of lithium is rather narrow (blood lithium levels of about 0.8 to 1.5 mEq/L, the upper end of that range being necessary for the control of acute mania). Even in well-tolerated doses, lithium can effect such physiological parameters as the kidney's concentrating ability and thyroid functioning. Long-term loss of renal concentration has been reported, although its clinical significance is unclear. Acute toxic effects may become apparent if this range is exceeded. Hence the drug must be used with caution, especially under circumstances that impair electrolyte imbalance such as supervening infections and fever, vomiting or diarrhea, concomitant diuretic therapy, or circumstances that promote excessive heat loss or sweating. Toxic effects include tremor, muscle weakness, vomiting, diarrhea, and in severe cases confusion and impairment of consciousness.

Therapeutic effects may not be evident for 10 days to 2 weeks, and in severely manic patients it is common to "cover" the patient with a neuroleptic in this interval. In rare cases, however, the combination may lead to a malignant syndrome characterized by fever, confusion, and collapse.

Because of this potential toxicity, patients should receive careful medical evaluation before therapy is initiated. Commonly, this workup includes a complete blood count, ECG, urinalysis, serum creatinine level, BUN, and thyroid function studies. These tests should be repeated at intervals during the course of lithium maintenance.

Lithium levels are generally obtained three times a week or even more frequently during initial dose adjustment. Once stable and effective blood levels are attained, the frequency may be reduced to weekly, monthly, and even less-frequent intervals.

Anxiolytic agents

Anxiolytic agents reduce anxiety but with little of the sedative effects of older agents such as barbiturates. Although a number of categories of antianxiety drugs (minor tranquilizers) have been marketed, the benzodiazepines have in effect dominated the market in this category. They are not the only effective agents, however. Antidepressants (both TCAs and MAO inhibitors) are highly effective in panic disorder, and propranolol, a noradrenergic blocking agent, has found some usefulness in patients in whom *peripheral* manifestations of anxiety are most bothersome. Because of the ubiquity of anxiety as a symptom, these drugs are among the most widely prescribed in the pharmacopoeia.

Benzodiazepines have a number of therapeutic actions. They are muscle relaxants and anticonvulsants; because of their cross-tolerance with alcohol, they are useful in the treatment of withdrawal states. In relatively low doses, they are effective anxiolytics. In somewhat higher doses, they are useful soporifics. (Flurazepam and temazepam are more apt to produce sedation and are marketed as sleep medications.) These drugs have a large therapeutic margin, and death is rare even from massive overdoses so long as the drug is not mixed with other medications.

Specific benzodiazepine-binding sites have been discovered in the CNS. These receptors appear to be functionally linked to gamma-aminobutyric acid (GABA) receptors, whose activity may account for the therapeutic effects of these drugs.

The two most widely prescribed benzodiazepines chlordiazepoxide and diazepam (Valium) are examples of the 2-

ketobenzodiazepine group. Metabolized in the liver, often to derivatives that are themselves active (e.g., desmethyldiazepam), these drugs have a relatively long half-life. Oxazepam (Serax) and lorazepam (Ativan) have shorter half-lives and do not have active metabolites and are often used in the elderly when the clinician is concerned about the accumulation of obtunding medications. Recently, several reports on the adjuvant use of lorazepam (along with major tranquilizers) in calming agitated psychotic patients have appeared.

Chlordiazepoxide is available in an IM form, but absorption is unreliable and should be avoided.

Benzodiazepines are addicting on prolonged use, and withdrawal symptoms may occur, although these are usually mild and limited to tremulousness, feelings of anxiety, and nausea. Rarely, patients will develop withdrawal seizures. Patients on alprazolam seem particularly prone to withdrawal symptoms, and the dosage must be reduced slowly to avoid discomfort.

Alprazolam is an example of the triazolobenzodiazepines. Along with its antianxiety properties, it is an effective anti-depressant, presumably because of direct effects on central noradrenergic systems. Probably for the same reason, it is a useful agent in treating panic disorders.

ELECTROCONVULSIVE THERAPY

ECT can be a highly effective form of treatment. The major indication for its use is in major depression, particularly when signs of melancholia are present. It is also indicated in delusional depressions, in which antidepressant medication is often less effective. Its use in schizophrenia is more controversial. It has proved helpful in cases of schizophrenia, especially when the patient demonstrates catatonic or affective features. In other cases of schizophrenia, occasional good results have been reported but with far less frequency. It may be tried in patients who fail to respond to drug treatments.

The major advantages of ECT are its rapid therapeutic action and its relative safety. The mortality rate is about the same as for that of short-term general anesthesia. Thus, in cases in which the patient's suicidal inclinations or life circumstances dictate rapid intervention, ECT presents an alternative to drug therapies, which may be slower acting. Ambulatory ECT is feasible, but treatments are now chiefly given in an inpatient setting.

Pretreatment workup includes, besides the routine labora-tory studies and chest film, ECG and skull and spine films. If feasible, an EEG may be obtained. Antidepressant medication and lithium should be lowered or withdrawn during the course of treatment.

In general, treatments are given 3 days a week; a course of eight treatments is considered minimal, but treatment may be extended based on the patient's response.

The patient is premedicated with a muscle relaxant (succinylcholine) to "soften" the seizure and prevent fractures and with a short-acting barbiturate (usually Brevital). In *unilateral* treatment, electrodes are placed on the nondominant hemisphere. Unilateral treatment results in a lesser degree of amnesia and confusion. Many clinicians believe that bilateral treatment, in which the electrodes are placed bitemporally, is more effective, however.

Depressed patients often show therapeutic effects after the first three treatments. Some patients may demonstrate a manic rebound. All patients should, however, have a complete course of treatment. Follow-up treatment with antidepressants, lithium, or neuroleptics is generally necessary to avoid relapse.

Although there are no absolute contraindications to ECT, it should be administered with great caution to those for whom an increase in intracranial pressure presents a high risk (i.e., those with intracranial masses or strokes) and to those with heart disease.

The use of ECT has proved an object of controversy. Most states have enacted restrictive legislation governing proper procedures for informed consent, and these must be strictly adhered to. The degree to which a long-standing memory deficit persists after ECT is controversial. Most patients will report lacunar deficits around the period of treatment. Patients who have repeated or lengthy courses of ECT may have more persistent problems with memory. As with all forms of therapy, the clinician must be careful to balance the risk-benefit ratio.

PSYCHOTHERAPY

This broad group of therapeutic interventions includes approaches other than the use of medication or other somatic therapies such as ECT. Behavior therapy, in which an attempt is made to correct maladaptive learned responses, is sometimes discussed apart from other psychotherapies. However, approaches that integrate behavioral and more traditional approaches have become common.

In the 1960s, several highly influential critiques of psycho-therapy brought into question its specificity and effectiveness. Better-designed research followed, and there is now a general consensus that psychotherapy can be highly effective if patients are appropriate selected and treatment goals are clearly and effectively defined. New techniques of brief psychotherapy have been developed. The use of adjunctive psychotherapy in medical and surgical patients has been demonstrated as shortening hospital stay and reducing the number of post-hospital complications.

Most forms of traditional psychotherapy are based on classic psychoanalysis. The patient's presenting symptoms are considered to be related to unconscious wishes or impulses that the patient has failed to successfully integrate at an appropriate earlier phase of development. Freud placed a strong emphasis on innate sexual drives (the term *sexual* being more broadly defined as related to need-gratifying behaviors). He grouped such drives into oral, anal, and phallic clusters based on the parts of the body around which they were organized at successive stages of development. If the environment provided excessive stimulation or frustration of these drives, successful integration into behavior was impeded and they (or their psychic representations) were repressed. The patient then became vulnerable to the development of neurotic symptoms when confronted with related issues in later life. For example, the anal period is one in which drive expression often comes in conflict with parental attempts to control the child's toilet habits. If the child fails to find a successful solution to the problem of balancing self-assertion with the demands of authority, neurotic symptoms may reemerge in struggles with authority figures later in life. Symptoms are unlikely to directly reflect the earlier conflict but are relatable to it by symbolic means (e.g., a person may make a mess of things, hold back on requests, or may evince such personality characteristics as stubbornness and severe parsimony, which lead to difficulties with others).

In psychoanalysis, the therapist is usually most silent and affectively neutral. The patient is often asked to lie on a couch and to free associate. Thus, the situation is removed as far as possible from normal social situations, and the power of repression is weakened. In this setting, patients are more apt to project onto the therapist their feelings about past figures and to reveal less-disguised thoughts about their basic conflicts. This **transference** of attitudes toward past figures onto the therapist is considered a key element, and its interpretation to the patient so it becomes accessible to awareness and to adult coping mechanisms is considered a critical therapeutic element. Psychoanalysis is an **uncovering psychotherapy**. It involves a detailed reconstruction of the past, which allows patients to see they are fighting "old battles" in a new setting. Thus, it is a reeducational procedure. It is often quite lengthy and expensive. It requires a fair degree of psychological insight and at least average intelligence. It is not suitable for patients with limited capacity to stand apart from themselves and subject themselves to the often painful experience of redefining themselves so drastically.

In **psychoanalytic psychotherapy,** the therapist's attitude is less neutral. He or she actively attempts to focus the patient on specific issues in the current life situation. Transference (to the therapist at least) is less likely to be interpreted, but, as in classic psychoanalysis, a major goal is to help patients understand the basis of their distress. The patient usually sits facing the therapist. Free association is discouraged.

In **supportive psychotherapy,** therapists intervene more actively as benign and mature participants in the patient's life. They may do this by actively clarifying patients' life situation and presenting them with alternatives, or they may actually advise patients as to a course of action. Clearly, supportive therapy is helpful for patients who lack the capacity to tolerate frustration and its attendant anxiety or who lack the capacity to distance themselves from their life problems and to think fruitfully about themselves. This includes patients with borderline personality disorders or major psychoses whose sense of self is so disorganized that they may need to "borrow" the therapist's ego when they are under stress.

The same range of techniques is used in **group therapy** and in **family therapy.** In both these modalities, the therapist may adopt a neutral or actively intervening attitude toward the participants. Some therapists believe that if one treats the family or therapy group as a **system** that itself can function adaptively or maladaptively in relation to its goals, one can promote the health of its individual members. Family therapy, in particular, has proved helpful to the families of patients with major psychiatric disorders. In the **psychoeducational** approach to working with families of schizophrenics, the therapist uses formal educational and casework techniques to teach families to accept their relatives' psychopathology without inappropriate feelings of guilt or excessive emotionality and shares techniques that other, better-adjusted families have found useful.

Although all forms of psychotherapy can be thought of as educational, **behavior therapy** explicitly uses **learning theory** to modify behaviors that the patient finds distressing. Behavioral therapists are interested in **objective** behaviors; they are interested in identifying those contingencies that enforce or inhibit desired behaviors or promote the undesirable ones. **Positive reinforcers** increase the likelihood of a behavior being emitted; **negative reinforcers** do the reverse. Anxiety generally disrupts behaviors and prevents the patient from engaging in adaptive, desirable behaviors. For example, a patient with an elevator phobia is too anxious to use elevators when she wishes to. A major set of techniques available to behavioral therapists are those that help the patient to relax and hence to counteract the development of anxiety. Once the patient masters a relaxation technique, he or she is presented with a **hierarchy** of stimuli ranging from those that elicit minimal anxiety to those that elicit intense anxiety. (A patient may be asked to imagine waiting by an elevator, taking a short ride on an elevator, getting stuck in a crowded elevator, etc.). In one procedure, the patient is asked to image the hierarchy along with the relaxation technique. He or she gradually is able to image even intensely fearful scenes with little manifest anxiety. The effect is then generalized to real-life situations by requiring the patient (often accompanied by the therapist or a companion) to actually enter into the feared situation. In **flooding,** the patient is actually exposed to the most anxiety-provoking situation at once; imagery or in vivo exposure may be used. Patients will experience intense anxiety, but, if they are forced to remain in the feared situation, their anxiety will subside. In effect, they will have learned that there is nothing to be afraid of. A variety of specialized techniques for providing behavioral contingencies that increase adaptive behaviors have been developed. Anxiety and phobia clinics based on these principles have become commonplace and, using behavioral techniques with or without medication, have proved to be clinically efficacious and cost-effective. However, many patients with apparently circumscribed phobic and anxiety symptoms will also have other psychiatric diagnoses for which other forms of therapy are indicated.

BIBLIOGRAPHY

American Psychiatric Association. Diagnostic and Statistical Manual of Mental Disorders, 3rd ed. Washington, DC, American Psychiatric Association, 1980.

Bassuk EB, Schoonover SC, Gelenberg AJ: The Practitioner's Guide to Psychoactive Drugs, 2nd ed. Plenum Press, New York, 1983.

Frances A, Clarkin JF, Perry S: Differential Therapeutics in Psychiatry: The Art and Science of Treatment Selection. Brunner/Mazel, New York, 1984.

Glickman LS: Psychiatric Consultation in the General Hospital. Marcel Dekker, New York, 1980.

Kaplan HI, Sadock BJ (eds): Comprehensive Textbook of Psychiatry IV. Williams and Wilkins, Baltimore, 1985.

Karasu T (ed): American Psychiatric Association Commission on Psychiatric Therapies: The Psychiatric Therapies. American Psychiatric Association, Washington, DC, 1984.

Lazare A (ed): Outpatient Psychiatry: Diagnosis and Treatment. Guilford Press, Baltimore, 1979.

Millman R (ed): Drug Abuse and Drug Dependence. In Frances AJ, Hales RE: Psychiatric Update, Vol. 5., American Psychiatric Association, Washington, DC, 1986.

Pasnau RO (ed): Diagnosis and Treatment of Anxiety Disorders. American Psychiatric Association, Washington, DC, 1984.

Paykel ES (ed): Handbook of Affective Disorders. Guilford Press, New York, 1982.

Sederer LI (ed): Inpatient Psychiatry: Diagnosis and Treatment. Williams and Wilkins, Baltimore, 1983.

Strauss JS, Carpenter WT: Schizophrenia. Plenum Press, New York, 1981.

SAMPLE QUESTIONS

DIRECTIONS: Each of the following questions contains four suggested answers. Choose the one best response to each question.

1. In general, signs of delirium will be found in what proportion of patients on a general medical ward?

A. 10%
B. 30%
C. 50%
D. 90%

2. In deleria, the EEG characteristically shows

A. alpha blocking
B. spikes and waves
C. slow beta and delta activity
D. K-complexes

3. When an elderly patient displays evening disorientation ("sundowning") one should consider

A. increasing the dose of minor tranquilizer or hypnotic
B. decreasing the dose of minor tranquilizer of hypnotic
C. adding a major tranquilizer to the evening medication
D. adding a stimulant to the patient's evening medication

4. The best treatment for pseudodementia in an elderly patient is usually

A. antidepressants
B. multivitamin therapy
C. thyroid replacement therapy
D. brief supportive psychotherapy

5. All of the following are characteristic of dementias EXCEPT

A. disorientation
B. loss of abstracting ability
C. impaired judgment
D. impared recent memory

6. The neurotransmitter system most directly implicated in the memory deficit of Alzheimer's Disease is:

A. adrenergic
B. serotonergic
C. cholinergic
D. gabanergic

7. Which of the following entities may serve as the basis for Korsakoff's psychosis?

A. Diabetes
B. Alcoholism
C. Head trauma
D. Any of these

8. The prevalence rate of depressions of moderate intensity in the general population is

A. 1%
B. 5%
C. 10%
D. 20%

9. Sleep disturbances in depressives include all of the following EXCEPT

A. decreased REM latency
B. decreased time in Stage 4 sleep
C. reduction in REM time
D. disruption of the ordinary diurnal periodicity of peripheral cortisol secretion

10. Delusional depressive disorders are most apt to respond to

A. tricyclic antidepressants
B. MAO inhibitors
C. a combination of major tranquilizers and antidepressants
D. no treatment

11. In order to qualify for a diagnosis of an acute schizophrenic disorder, symptoms (including pre- and postpsychotic symptoms) must persist for

A. 1 week
B. 2 weeks
C. 6 months
D. 1 year

12. The antipsychotic effects of a phenothiazine appear to be correlated with the molecule's

A. ability to block dopamine
B. anticholinergic activity
C. ability to produce EPS
D. molecular weight

13. A persistent and sometimes disabling effect of long-term phenothiazine administration is

A. dystonia
B. neuroleptic malignant syndrome
C. tardive dyskinesia
D. dementia

14. All of the following are characteristic of the psychophysiological response to anxiety EXCEPT

    A. increased urinary MHPG
    B. desynchronized EEG
    C. increased blood fatty acids
    D. increased galvanic skin resistance

15. Mrs. X is a shy, sensitive woman who pursues her occupation as a librarian with competence. She has few friends of either sex, indeed she seems unconcerned about social relationships and appears to have little understanding of why they are important to most people. She has never required psychiatric treatment and, except for some blunting of affect, her mental status examination is unremarkable. The most likely diagnosis is

    A. schizotypal personality disorder
    B. schizoid personality disorder
    C. latent schizophrenia
    D. chronic schizophrenia

16. Which of the following is NOT true of patients with antisocial personality disorders?

    A. Onset of their symptoms begins in late adolescence
    B. The clinical picture is continuous rather than intermittent
    C. Drug and alcohol problems are common
    D. All of the above

17. The LOWEST incidence of extrapyramidal side effects is produced by

    A. aliphatic phenothiazines
    B. piperazine phenothiazines
    C. piperidine phenothiazines
    D. thioxanthines

18. Which of the following is NOT likely to be a side effect of a tricyclic antidepressant?

    A. Dry mouth
    B. Extrapyramidal side effects
    C. Tremor
    D. Constipation

19. The earliest sign of lithium toxicity is apt to be

    A. gastrointestinal distress
    B. failure to concentrate urine
    C. extrapyramidal side effects
    D. depression

20. A medication that has both anxiolytic and antidepressant therapeutic effects is

    A. lithium carbonate
    B. alprazolam
    C. amitryptiline
    D. chlorpromazine

21. Which of the following is NOT true of classical psychoanalytic treatment?

    A. Use of free associations
    B. Interpretation of the transference
    C. The analyst presents himself as a "real" person to the patient
    D. The patient must have at least normal intelligence

22. The treatment of delirium tremens generally includes all of the following EXCEPT

    A. hydration
    B. multivitamins
    C. a minor tranquilizer
    D. a sedative

23. Behavior therapy of phobic disorders may include all of the following EXCEPT

    A. relaxation training
    B. interpretation of the unconscious meaning of the phobia
    C. flooding
    D. in vivo exposure to the feared stimulus

24. Characteristic symptoms of posttraumatic stress disorder include of the following EXCEPT

    A. emotional numbing
    B. hallucinations
    C. flashbacks
    D. insomnia

25. The percentage of medication-compliant patients who return to the hospital within 2 years after their first schizophrenic episode is

    A. 10%
    B. 20%
    C. 30%
    D. 40%

ANSWERS

1. B	14. D
2. C	15. B
3. B	16. A
4. A	17. C
5. A	18. B
6. C	19. A
7. D	20. B
8. B	21. C
9. C	22. D
10. C	23. B
11. C	24. B
12. A	25. D
13. C	

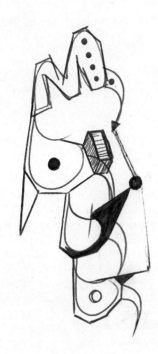

6

PUBLIC HEALTH AND COMMUNITY MEDICINE

Robin J. O. Catlin

BIOSTATISTICS AND METHODS OF EPIDEMIOLOGY

CONCEPTS OF MEASUREMENT

Of the many aspects of medical practice in this age, a thorough understanding of **probability** may be one of the most perplexing. Most physicians do not regard themselves as mathematicians, nor as biostatisticians. Yet patients are continually posing questions about the possibilities of the outcome of their disease. They are entitled to answers that are both accurate and intelligible. This section is intended to assist the student in formulating such advice. It will not be a full treatise on biostatistics. For that, the student must search elsewhere. Some of the most important points about concepts of measurement in relation to the practice of medicine will first be considered.

Perhaps the first important point is a consideration of what is "normal." This question has to be addressed in relation to the "usual" outcome of a particular disease. It is also essential to have a concept of what is appropriate in this regard in relation to the interpretation of a test. What is an acceptable normal range? If the readings are one or two units of measurement outside the given range of a test, does this indicate that further investigation or treatment has to be undertaken?

The first principle to be understood relates to **measures of central tendency**. When is it appropriate to consider a mean reading? Would a median reading or a modal reading be more appropriate?

The **mean** is the sum of all the readings in a particular series of measurements divided by the number of measurements. This is commonly understood to be the average. Suppose we have a series of nine systolic blood pressure readings: 132, 163, 150, 150, 170, 120, 120, 131, 165. The mean is

$$\frac{132+163+150+150+170+120+120+131+165}{9} = \frac{1301}{9} = 144.6$$

Since it is not possible to measure blood pressure below 1 mm Hg by an office sphygmomanometer, a mean using a decimal fraction is inappropriate. The mean should be rounded to the nearest whole number, or 145 for the example given above.

A better approach might be to consider the **median** reading. This is the value of the "middle" reading or observation when these have been ranked according to size. Thus, we could first rank the above nine systolic blood pressure readings with the largest first to read 170, 165, 163, 150, 150, 132, 131, 120, 120. For an odd number of readings, we find the middle reading by first adding 1 to the number of readings and dividing by 2. This gives the fifth reading (i.e., 150) as the median. For an even number of readings, the median is the average of the two middle readings after ranking by size. The first of the two readings is located simply by dividing the number of readings by two.

In other circumstances, the consideration of the most commonly occurring reading may be more useful. This reading is known as the **mode**. In the series of systolic blood pressure readings given above, two readings occur twice: 150 and 120. Thus, this series of readings does not have a single mode. In fact, one of the more commonly occurring readings is at the lower end of the series. This can therefore be described as bimodal. In larger series, the modal (or bimodal) pattern can best be recognized diagrammatically. A histogram (bar graph) or a simple graph of readings and their frequency of occurrence may be drawn, leading to instant recognition of the modal peaks. Histograms may also be superimposed on one another in order to facilitate comparisons of modal readings from another parameter. For example, from Figure 6-1 it becomes immediately apparent that in spite of efforts to increase public awareness and therefore to increase the percentage of the population of childbearing age who are protected against rubella infection by immunization, there is still a second modal peak in these years. The incidence declined over the years under review, indicating that the program has had some success.

The next principle to be understood relates to **measures of variation**. If we are considering a mean reading from a series, may we assume that it is a reliable estimate? There are two factors that we might feel intuitively would be important in answering this question, assuming always that there was lack of bias in measuring the sample. The first is the size of the sample. Testing a sample of 500 persons in a larger community will obviously give a better picture than testing only 5. This will be true whether the characteristics being measured are social, biologic, or medical. The second is the variation or scatter or spread of the observations. The wider the range of readings, the less likely it is that the mean—or the median—will be representative of the series. The **range** is the difference between

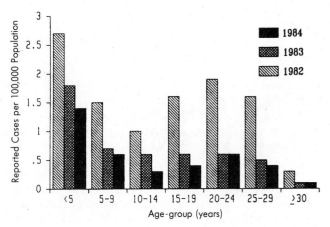

Figure 6-1. Rubella (German measles). Estimated rates by age-group in the United States, 1982–1984. Rates were calculated by multiplying the percentage of cases with known age-group by total reported cases and dividing by the population in that age-group. (Centers for Disease Control: Annual summary 1984: Reported morbidity and mortality in the United States. MMWR 33(54):52, 1986.)

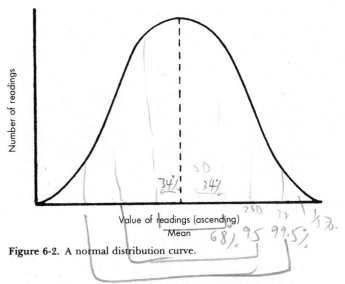

Figure 6-2. A normal distribution curve.

the minimum and maximum readings of a particular series. The usual method of measuring the variation or spread of data is to study the dispersion of the observations about the mean.

Two series of figures may have the same mean reading, but the range of one series may be greater than that of the other series. In order to assess this, the term **variance** is used. This measures the average amount by which readings in either series differ from the mean. These differences may be above or below the mean: In other words, they may have negative (−) or positive (+) values. If they were simply summed (added), the result would be zero. If they are squared, both differences from the mean have positive values. This makes mathematical calculations possible, giving numerical definition to the concept. However, the variance thus produced is geometrically related to the actual differences rather than arithmetically related. For this reason, the measurement is converted back to its original units by calculating the square root of the variance. This is known as the **standard deviation**.

Some people puzzle over this question: Why, when calculating the average differences from the mean to arrive at variance or at standard deviation, is the divisor not the total number of readings (n), but the total number of readings less 1 ($n - 1$)? This makes allowance for the fact that a sample rather than the whole population is being studied.

If a whole normal population is studied, it may be expected that there will be an equal number of readings falling above and below the mean. If drawn as a graph or as a histogram, the mean will demonstrate the highest number of readings, with a symmetrical distribution of readings higher and lower than the mean (Fig. 6-2). Both mathematically and graphically it may be demonstrated that in a **normal (Gaussian) distribution curve** a range of 1.96 standard deviations on either side of the mean will cover 95% of the area under the curve. Only 2.5% of each sample will lie in each "tail." Similarly, a range of 3.09 standard deviations from the mean will cover 99.8% of readings. These two important statistical statements are often simplified for ease of calculation to 2 and 3 standard deviations covering 95% and 99.5% of readings, respectively.

The variance or its square root, the standard deviation, is the measure of spread that is used in statistical tests of significance. A large spread will be associated with large deviations from the mean, and this in turn with a large variance. Other things being equal, statistical tests are less likely to show that two samples are significantly different if their variances are large.

In medicine, a sample from which it is intended to extrapolate to describe a population is frequently taken. How close the sample mean is to the population mean is a very relevant question. When the sample is small, there is a high probability that the distribution of the members does not approximate to the distribution of the members of the whole population. If it is possible to take several samples, the average of the sample means is more likely to approach the true population mean. The sample means are themselves normally distributed around the population mean and have a deviation from it which may be calculated. To avoid confusion, this deviation from the estimated population mean is known as the **standard error of the mean**.

Earlier it was seen that, in normal distribution, a range of ±1.96 standard deviations about the mean will cover 95% of the area under the curve. In large samples of more than 30 readings ($n > 30$), 95% confidence limits may be calculated using the mean and its associated standard error. These are the mean value ±1.96 times the standard error.

To this point, normal distribution has been considered. In practice, biologic and other medical data often have a skewed distribution. When this is so, it is inappropriate to calculate the mean or the variance. Appropriate descriptive statistics are the mode and the median. Another way of dealing with skewed data is to transform it. Probably the most common way of doing so is to convert the data to logarithmic values, generally using the base 10. This may normalize the distribution of the data.

A binomial distribution occurs whenever the possession of a particular character or attribute or the lack of it is under consideration. For example, if it is known that of a randomly selected population of individuals only 40% are smokers, it may be inferred that 60% are nonsmokers. Individuals in such a sample possess the attribute with a probability P or fail to possess it with a probability of $1 - P$.

CONCEPTS OF STATISTICAL INFERENCE

One of the first problems to be faced is whether a particular sample is representative of the whole population being studied. Another version of the same problem may seek to assess whether the characteristics of the sample group are chance findings that may be discovered in a section of the whole population or whether the sample group differs in a significant way from the whole population. This can be useful, for example, in determining whether freedom from disease in the sample population may be due to a particular mode of therapy that is being received by the sample group but not by the whole population.

The principles on which these inferences are made are important and have wide application. As sample size increases, most observers become more confident in their estimations of the population means. The standard error of the mean quantifies the uncertainty of the estimate of the true population mean based on the sample. As the sample size increases, the standard error of the mean decreases. This logic can be expressed in the following ratio:

$$t = \frac{\text{difference in sample means}}{\text{standard error of difference of sample means}}$$

To calculate the t ratio, the most difficult part is the calculation of the standard error of the difference of the sample means. The extreme values of t that would lead to the rejection of the hypothesis that there is no difference between the groups lie in both tails of the distribution. This leads to the definition of the test being employed as the **two-tailed t-test**. Occasionally a single-tailed t-test is used, but this is *only* correctly used when values at both ends of the range of readings are impossible or inappropriate for consideration. The t-test or **Student's t-test** is the most common statistical procedure in the medical literature, but it is frequently misused or misapplied. A frequent misuse is its application to compare multiple groups. The significance of different calculations of t in relation to the size of the variance may be calculated by comparison with tables. When the experimental design involves multiple groups, analysis of variance should be used.

The X^2 or **chi-square test** allows the assessment of whether the observed frequency (O) of an event departs significantly from the expected frequency (E) on the basis of a null hypothesis. First calculate by how much the observed frequencies (O) differ from the expected (E). This can be expressed as (O−E). Because some of the differences will be negative, this difference is squared, removing the negative sign. Each difference is then divided by the expected number to allow for group size, giving an average difference per unit group. These averages are then added together. This summation is known as the "chi-square."

$$\chi^2 = \text{sum of } \frac{(\text{observed} - \text{expected number of individuals in cell})^2}{\text{expected number of individuals in cell}}$$

$$\chi^2 = \Sigma \frac{(O - E)^2}{E}$$

When the chi-square has been calculated for a number of groups (g), there are g − 1 degrees of freedom. This application of the test to goodness of fit to any predicted pattern is only one use of the chi-square test. It is important to remember that for the test to be applied correctly, the expected number in any group should not be less than five. If it is, two groups may frequently be combined. Also, the total number of observations should not be less than 20. Finally, chi-square tests must be carried out on actual numbers and *not* on percentages or ratios. The assessment of significance of a chi-square test must be read from a table of chi-square distribution.

All significance tests are designed to assess the probability of the observed result arising if the null hypothesis is valid. By convention, if the result is likely to arise less than 1 in 20 times, the result is statistically significant, $P < 0.05$, and the null hypothesis is rejected. Whenever the effect of the intervention or treatment can be summarized on a better/worse or more/less (±) scale, a sign test may be used to assess significance. In such situations, if there are "uncertain" (don't know) or unchanged readings, such data should not be included in the calculations. The chi-square test may also be applied to data of this kind. However, if the sample size is small, a correction for continuity, such as Yates's correction, should be applied. Contingency tables may be prepared using this modified test to assess whether two or more factors are exerting a significant effect on two or more groups.

The question of **probability** must now be considered further. In statistics, the probability of an event or outcome that is certain to occur is 1. The probability that a patient will survive or die is 1. An example with more than two mutually exclusive events is provided by an illness in which the outcome may be death, survival with one or more permanently handicapping sequelae, or survival unscathed. Consider rheumatic fever, the study of which in a large series of cases reveals the probability of death (P_1), the probability of persistent valvular disease of the heart (P_2), and the probability of full recovery (P_3). The probability of surviving with or without sequelae would be $P_2 + P_3$. The probability of these two would not be 1 or certainty, since it does not cover all possible outcomes. The probability of either one of two or more mutually exclusive events occurring is the sum of their separate probabilities. But the probability of two or more independent events occurring is the product of their separate probabilities.

In health care, most events are not mutually exclusive and are also not independent. It is still possible to calculate the probability of two events happening by using the same multiplication rule as for independent events, if the probability of one event occurring given that the other event has occurred is known. This is called conditional probability since the occurrence of the second event is dependent or "conditional" on the first event. The probability of X happening on condition that Y has occurred is called the conditional probability of X on Y. It is expressed mathematically as P (X/Y).

Following this concept further, it is now necessary to discuss the degree of association or correlation between two variables. A common use is for testing for any relationship between the administered dose of a substance and the evoked response. The expectation is that by altering one variable, the other will be changed. It is a study of cause and effect. However, it is important to remember that the existence of a statistically significant correlation may not necessarily be taken as evidence of causality. All that may be inferred from nonexperimental data is that there is a possibility of association, which may be worth testing experimentally.

Once again, a chi-square test may be adapted to test such an association. Alternatively a Pearson correlation coefficient or a Spearman's rank correlation coefficient may be employed. A full description of these tests must be sought elsewhere. Linear regression analysis is yet another possibility. Leading statistics textbooks present varying views on the question of when correlation should be used and when regression should be used. In some journals and articles, these methods are frequently and inaccurately interchanged. Although these points may be subtle and beyond the scope of the present text, there are some things that are important to remember. One is that when drawing a regression line, it is not correct to extrapolate the line beyond the known data points. In other circumstances, there may be more than two dependent variables; in this situation, multiple linear regression may be used.

TYPES OF STUDY DESIGN

Epidemiology is the study of the distribution and determinants of health-related states and events in populations and the application of this study to the control of health problems. This definition was recently agreed on by an international panel. Distribution may refer to different "areas," which may be geographic, cultural, age, sex, or time related. Determinants may be either causal or accessory factors. Even if a disease is recognized to have a single and specific cause (for example, an infectious disease that is caused by a specific known microorganism), there may be several other determinants, including predisposing factors. In the light of the many possibly clarifying but also possibly confounding factors, there is need for precision in definition and application if effective study is to be made. The terms and definitions used in epidemiology are similar to those used in other scientific areas of medicine, so that the principles of investigation may be more widely applied. However, it is important for the student to realize that potential differences can in certain circumstances become actual differences. Principles of statistical methods may be applied to both epidemiologic and clinical studies.

Before the types of study design can be understood, some basic methodology must be described. In studying health and the amount of health- or disease-related problems in a community, some basic demographic data are required. Vital and health statistics may be gathered from multiple sources. The accuracy of both collection and manipulation of these data may vary, and therefore it may not always be comparable in many respects.

The word *comparable* is of vital importance in these studies. Epidemiology frequently makes comparisons between one population and another. For this reason, the concept of rates is very important. The expression of a health problem in terms of a rate enables such a comparison. A rate may be defined as the number of events (such as death or disease diagnosis) in a specified period and multiplied by a number that is usually a factor of 10. This latter number is established by convention, the intention being to express the fraction as a manageable whole number. Thus rates are expressed per 1,000 or per 100,000 of the population at risk.

The population at risk is most frequently determined in relation to census figures. However, it may not be possible to collect the health data in such a way that they relate directly to census tracts. For this reason, a private rather than a government census is sometimes used; the population thus identified may then form the basis for a cohort study. This will be defined later.

Definitions of some rates

Mortality rate or **death rate** is the number of persons dying (due to a particular cause or from all causes) divided by the total number in the group, per unit of time. A mortality rate is really an incidence rate, but instead of referring to a specific disease it refers to the process of dying.

Crude death rate relates the number of deaths to the midyear population.

Age-specific death rate is the number of persons dying in a specific age-group divided by the total number of persons in the same group per unit of time.

Case fatality rate is the number of persons dying from a specified disease divided by the total number of patients having the disease.

Infant mortality rate is the number of live-born infants who die before age 1 year related to the total live births in the year.

Perinatal mortality rate relates the number of stillbirths (>28 weeks gestation) plus the number of deaths in the first 7 days of life to the total number of live births and stillbirths during the year.

Maternal mortality rate is the number of deaths from maternal causes (i.e., associated with pregnancy, childbirth, and the puerperium) within 42 days of delivery related to the number of live births in the year. Note that the true population of mothers at risk for maternal death should include those who have had stillbirths as well as live births. Although stillbirths are included in the calculation for perinatal mortality rate, classically they have not been included in the maternal mortality rate. The reason accepted is that there is greater difficulty in counting stillbirths, whereas live births have to be reported and registered.

Incidence rate is the number of persons developing a disease divided by the total number at risk per unit of time. This rate describes the continuing occurrence of new cases of the disease. The denominator for incidence rates may be the whole population or a segment of the population who are susceptible.

Prevalence rate is the number of persons with a disease related to the total number of persons in the group. It describes the total situation over a specified period of time. The point prevalence rate is the prevalence at a given point of time. Quite often the terms incidence and prevalence are used imprecisely in medical literature. One example of this might be, "the incidence of gallstones in middle-aged women is 20%." This misuse of incidence to describe prevalence or simple proportion should be avoided. The relationship between incidence, prevalence, and duration of disease may be simply expressed as follows:

$$\text{Prevalence} = \text{incidence} \times \text{mean duration.}$$

Attack rate is a cumulative incidence rate, often used to describe what is happening in populations observed for limited periods of time (e.g., during an epidemic). The secondary attack rate is used to describe familial aggregation of a contagious disease. The number of secondary cases divided by the number at risk, provided the latter can be identified, is used for this calculation.

This discussion of rates in a section on types of study design has been prompted for a very specific reason. The definitions of rates demonstrate some of the common problems relating to study design. It is relatively easy to count numbers of cases. Particularly in hospitals, with automated data systems that are now almost uniformly used, there is little problem in collecting data or in performing calculations based on the data. Many individual physicians' offices are also similarly equipped, so that data may be collected from ambulatory service areas also. These advances in technology have not yet led to a more precise definition of either the incidence or prevalence of disease. A recent visit to another country enabled a discussion on the incidence of myocardial infarction as a manifestation of coronary artery disease. The hospital being visited was reported to be serving a population of 5 million people. Yet the number of admissions to the hospital annually for myocardial infarction was reported to be only 15. It was impossible not to make a comparison with similar statistics from the author's own hospital, which serves a population of only 0.5 million. There the annual number of admissions for myocardial infarction approximates 250. Are these two reported figures for incidence truly comparable? What factors might account for the differences?

At first impression, it might be considered that the counting of cases in both institutions might be comparable and that the figures of 15 and 250 might be acceptable. Yet there might be differences in diagnostic criteria. If a study were seriously being made, the diagnostic criteria would first have to be defined.

The major problems in making comparisons are more likely to be related to identifying the denominator, or the population at risk. In the United States, where patients in general have freedom of choice in selecting health-care providers, they or the ambulance services that transport them in emergency to hospital may recognize a particular hospital as being either poor or a center of excellence in treating myocardial infarction. Thus, in respect to myocardial infarction, the hospital's catchment area may be either smaller or larger than its catchment area for patients in relation to treating other types of disease. The population at risk in this case may not be 0.5 million.

This particular possibility for comparison has been selected to demonstrate the need for a clear definition of the denominator. In other health-care systems, where there is less freedom of choice, the problems may not have such a degree of prominence. For example, in the United Kingdom, access to the health-care system, the British National Health Service, is restricted to consulting a general practitioner or in emergency through an accident department. Morbidity studies are much easier to perform in such a system. Incidence and prevalence are more readily calculated. In the United States, the National Ambulatory Care Study seeks to produce comparable results by collecting large amounts of data from a wide spectrum of health-care providers serving many communities. Here the

principles of biostatistics outlined earlier are being applied. The larger the size of the sample population being studied, the more likely it is to reflect the whole population in any particular characteristic.

Definitions of types of studies

In the realm of epidemiology, it is not always possible to set up experimental studies. Reliance must sometimes be placed on observational studies because an existing situation has to be investigated. This situation occurs particularly in the investigation of an epidemic, but it may exist in other circumstances also. Basically, in **observational studies** nature is allowed to take its course. The observer notes the changes in one variable and studies the relationships of differences in another variable. There may be two objectives of such studies: the first is to *describe* the occurrence of disease or disease-related phenomena in a particular population, using such measures as incidence, prevalence, or mortality rates and relating them to some basic characters of the group such as age, sex, race, and ethnic background. These are known as **descriptive studies**. The other objective may be to *explain* the observed patterns; if this is the objective, the procedure will be known as an **analytical study**. The difference between these two types of observational studies is not always distinct, but the terms do have some meaning.

In **experimental studies**, an active intervention is made to change one variable while measuring the effect on another. In this case, it is important to eliminate the possible effects of other variables. The two variables are classed as either the dependent variable, that on which the effect is to be measured, or the independent variable, that on which the change is to be induced. For example, if the question for study is whether the weather has any effect on the incidence of the common cold, the incidence of the common cold would be the dependent variable and observations of daily temperature might be one independent variable. The illustration demonstrates the fact that in observational studies, the same definition of types of variables may be applied, since the daily temperature cannot be changed by experimental intervention.

Cross-sectional studies are the simplest types of observational studies to design and perform. They are sometimes known as prevalence studies. In a specified population at a given point in time, the relationship between diseases and other characteristics or variables of interest is measured. A cross-sectional study may be aimed simply at fact finding, or a hypothesis may be tested. Sometimes a test is used to determine previous exposure to or infection by disease; examples might be tuberculin skin test sensitivity or hepatitis screening. On other occasions, a test may be used to detect current disease: throat swab for streptococcal throat infection, for example. Occasionally a questionnaire may be employed, as in the investigation of relationship between smoking and chronic bronchitis in the United Kingdom. Clinical records and other documentary resources may also be used.

The statistical methods used for analyzing findings in cross-sectional studies may include means, standard deviations, medians, percentiles, and other quantities and proportions.

Associations between variables may be measured by correlation and regression coefficients. The measure of the association is sometimes expressed as an **odds ratio**. For example, an odds ratio of three might mean that the odds in favor of developing a disease are three times higher in individuals exposed to a certain factor than in those who are not exposed. Alternatively, a **rate ratio** of three means that the prevalence rate of the disease is three times higher among people exposed to the factor in comparison than among those not exposed. The methods of calculation are shown in Table 6-1.

Cohort studies

Cohort studies have the characteristics of prospective studies. They are concerned with evaluating the development of disease rather than describing the characteristics of existing disease. First, a study population of individuals free of the disease is identified. Then the factors or attributes of interest are measured in this group or cohort. The cohort is divided into groups of those who either have or do not have the factor whose influence will be measured. The incidence of the disease in the whole cohort population is then recorded over a period of time, and comparisons are made. This is clearly a very convincing type of study, and its major disadvantage is that results are not quickly achieved. Occasionally such a study can be carried out retrospectively, but this depends on excellent recording of all relevant data in the past, which is not always available in the form required for study. One of the best known prospective cohort studies is the Framingham Heart Study. Such studies yield excellent results. Among the difficulties associated with such studies is the existence of confounding variables. These arise from confusion when the influence of a particular factor is being assessed. An underlying or initially hidden factor may be responsible for the differences being observed. An example is the investigation of the effect of heavy alcohol consumption on the development of heart disease. Heavy drinking may be accompanyied by cigarette smoking. Some of the increased incidence of heart disease among heavy drinkers is likely to be due to smoking cigarettes.

Complicated statistical calculations may be appropriate in determining the results of cohort studies. A discussion of these is beyond the scope of this chapter. Sophisticated statistical

Table 6-1. Methods of Calculating Odds Ratio and Rate Ratio

	Disease present	Disease absent	Total
Factor present	a	b	a+b
Factor absent	c	d	c+d
Total	a+c	b+d	N

Odds ratio = ad/bc

Rate ratio = $\dfrac{a/(a+b)}{c/(c+d)}$

analyses are inappropriate if bias exists in the conduct of the study. In evaluating study results, attention should be paid to the possibility of the existence of selection bias, follow-up bias, information bias, and post hoc bias.

Case-control studies

If records are inadequate for a retrospective cohort study or there is insufficient time available for a prospective study, a case-control study may be contemplated. After the initial identification of cases, a suitable control or comparison group of individuals without the disease is identified. The control group needs to be matched to the study group in as many ways as possible to enable valid comparisons to be made with regard to possible attributes affecting the incidence of disease. An observed exposure-disease association does not necessarily imply a causal relationship. In a strict sense, comparison groups in retrospective study are not controls: They are merely what the name implies. Controversy has surrounded the discussion of many case-control studies. As in the case of other types of studies, statistically valid conclusions may only be reached if the study design and observations are free from bias. For details of how these biases may be avoided or at least minimized in case-control studies, the reader is referred to standard epidemiology texts.

MEDICAL DECISION MAKING

The best medical decisions and the best advice to offer to patients depend on an unbiased understanding and interpretation of the facts related to a particular investigation. Here epidemiology as a science within medicine has skills to offer that are relevant to the practice of clinical medicine in all its disciplines. How may such decisions be reached in principle?

The first rules to be followed in medical decision making refer to the assessment of the exactitude of the test results. The first quality to be evaluated is the **validity** of the test. Validity is an expression of the degree to which an assessment measures what it aspires to measure. Validity has two components: **sensitivity** and **specificity**. Sensitivity refers to the ability to identify correctly the problem or disease. Specificity refers to the negative characteristic of not including those who do not have the problem or disease. An ideal test is both absolutely (100%) sensitive and specific. In reality, there is frequently error in both areas. Sometimes high levels of performance in one area are only achieved by sacrificing effectiveness in the other: High specificity can only be achieved at the expense of sensitivity or vice versa. To state the problem in more precise terms, both false-positives and false-negatives may be demonstrated by the test. It is frequently helpful to record these results in tabular form (Table 6-2).

Accuracy is the extent to which a measurement conforms to or agrees with the true value. A frequent error is to attribute a precise value to an investigation that is greater than the accuracy limit of the instrument performing the measurement. For example, a mean diastolic blood pressure for a particular patient may be reported as 92.5 mm Hg. Most observers cannot perform blood pressure readings to these levels of tolerance. The reported result appears to be the mean of several readings. A mean reading may very well be appropriate, but the

Table 6-2. Recording the Results of Screening Tests

Result of screening test	Disease state	
	Disease	No disease
Positive	True-positive (TP)	False-positive (FP)
Negative	False-negative (FN)	True-negative (TN)

Sensitivity may then be defined as $= \dfrac{TP}{TP + FN}$

Specificity $= \dfrac{TN}{TN + FP}$

result should not be reported to a greater level of accuracy than the technique of measurement allows. Of the alternative readings on the scale of most office sphygmomanometers, 92 or 94, the most appropriate reading to report would be 92 mm Hg.

Precision is the quality of being sharply defined. Height is very readily measured: linear measurements may be very accurately recorded. For example, it is relatively easy to record linear measurements to, say, one-tenth of a millimeter. Although such measurements are readily possible, most individuals adopt a different posture each time they stand to be measured. The measurement of linear height to such a degree of definition is therefore impractical and may introduce error into statistical calculations. Thus the precision of the measuring instrument has to be related to the practicality of biologic measurement. In other circumstances, the measuring instrument is insufficiently accurate for the observation to be reported with such precision; this is a problem of accuracy, which is defined above.

Reliability is the degree of agreement reached when a measurement is repeated under closely similar conditions. This may be influenced by faults in the instrument, by observer error, or by failure to standardize the conditions under which the measurement is made. An example of observer error that may occur in this category is digit preference, which arises as the result of personal idiosyncrasy.

Instrumental error includes all the sources of error that are inherent in the test itself. It has a wider meaning and application in statistics than would be applied if scientific standards alone were being considered.

Now it is possible to attempt an answer to the question, What is the possibility of disease in an individual with a positive test result? Referring back to the normal distribution curve, it is clear that at the end of each range of readings, high or low, a few normal individuals may be included. But for 95% of individuals, such high or low readings would be abnormal. So, in such a situation the risk of being abnormal, the probability, is 100:5, or 20:1. This is a practical application of **Bayes' theorem**. It relates the probabilities of a test's true-positive and false-positive rates. It can be expressed as the ratio of the number of individuals who have the disease and whose results are positive to the number of all those individuals whose tests are positive.

These considerations have formed the basis of one method of computerized diagnosis. In fact, modern technology is

being invoked to follow and possibly accelerate the diagnostic decision-making process that is followed by a wise physician in a clinical situation. Decision analysis has been an important part of management training for several years. Now it is becoming applied to medicine. There are some who would still maintain that it is impossible to automate the mysterious, creative, indescribable insights of the experienced practitioner. However, it is likely that this will form a more important part of undergraduate medical education in future years.

Physicians have at their disposal a great variety of clinical information to act as a guide in clinical decision making. The amount of material is sometimes overwhelming. To aid the process, it is important to separate the many factors into simple relationships. It is difficult, if not impossible, for them all to be considered at once. Formulating a decision-making tree, reducing each element of decision making into a simple choice between two alternatives, is a device that can help. This is the basis of automated systems, but the principle may be applied to other protocols.

Some pieces of information derive from diagnostic tests, which might be either expensive or dangerous or both. The justification for the test is whether it will aid in the process of arriving at a "correct" diagnosis and thereby selecting a best treatment. The test is proposed in order to obtain greater diagnostic certainty, to provide information that can be used to reassess the probabilities assigned to possible disease states. Almost no diagnostic test yields perfect information; rarely does a test identify with certainty which disease a patient has. In practice, choices among diagnoses are seldom made on the basis of consideration of the results of a single test. However, there are hazards that may be introduced into the process by the introduction of either repeated tests or multiple (different) tests. For a full discussion of this aspect of problems associated with probability, the reader is referred to more extensive discussions of clinical analysis.

Before this discussion is closed, however, one other aspect should be introduced. Medical care hopefully produces benefits for the individual and for society. The public is now very much aware that it also entails both risks and costs. In this case, the term *costs* is being applied in economic terms. Society is becoming painfully aware that "no man is an island" (John Donne). What may seem to be an individual cost frequently becomes a community responsibility. An operation costing $250,000 may be highly desirable for the individual, although even that individual may desire a second opinion regarding its necessity. But if the individual's health insurance is affected through an organization that also provides insurance under similar terms for only 1,000 others, the costs to each individual may be increased by $250. This may be significant to such an extent that others would want to be part of the decision-making process. On the other hand, if the insurance is provided under the same conditions for 1,000,000 others, there will not be the same disincentive to the expenditure of $0.25 per head. Society needs to know something of the risk-benefit analysis, and in the future physicians are likely to be required to explain this in measurable terms. The efficient allocation of limited resources can only be accomplished by a detailed mathematical approach. The wider implications will be further discussed toward the end of this section of the text.

EPIDEMIOLOGY OF HEALTH AND DISEASE: APPLICATIONS TO THE PATIENT AND COMMUNITY

PATTERNS OF DISEASE

The study of disease has characteristically been approached from two widely differing points of view. The physician usually asks the question, What is the cause of the patient's illness? The patient, on the other hand, asks, Why am I ill? The cause and the reason appear to be superficially similar questions, but there are major differences. The cause of the illness is sought because finding it leads to more effective curative measures. The reason for the illness may lead more to future prevention than to cure. The interest in prevention is now shared not only by individual patients but by the larger, and sometimes more powerful, groups that compose communities or even a whole society. Physicians and other health-care providers have recently begun to understand this and have as a result commenced studies that would lead to the adoption of more preventive measures. Such measures have in the past been directed toward the control of infectious disease, particularly as it occurs in epidemic form.

The following classification of disease relates more to the reasons for disease, etiologic factors, than it does to the causes of disease, pathophysiological factors. The two classes are clearly not unrelated, but the groupings of disease that result will be different from those noted elsewhere. These are **determinants of disease.**

Genetic and familial factors

Although it may be common for patients to believe that a particular disease afflicts their family, there is not always a scientific reason for determining that this is so. Initially we shall restrict our discussion to those conditions for which there is at present evidence of genetic origin. In these, the pattern of inheritance conforms with expectations for dominant genes, for recessive genes, or for sex-linked genes.

Some conditions have very clear genetic transmission. Included in this category are congenital abnormalities and some neurological abnormalities. For a fuller discussion of these, the reader is referred to descriptions of clinical conditions, either in this text or in more complete standard clinical reference works.

Abnormal hemoglobins are conveyed genetically. The prototype is sickle cell hemoglobin (HbS). Individuals who are heterozygous for the sickle cell gene possess both normal adult hemoglobin (HbA) and HbS, usually in the range of 25 to 40%. Sickling takes place under conditions of oxygen depletion. Most heterozygote individuals stay well except under extreme anoxic conditions, whereas homozygotes, possessing no HbA, may develop painful hemolytic and vascular occlusive symptoms in sickle cell crises, which may be provoked by relatively minor infections. It has been noted relatively recently that in some eastern African populations, the multiplication of malarial parasites is inhibited in patients who have beta-thalassemia, a variant of the HbS gene. The relationship between abnormal hemoglobins and malaria has provided some convincing evidence of the reasons for the natural control of disease in some populations.

A similar relationship has been observed between malaria and glucose-6-phosphate dehydrogenase (G6PD) deficiency. Since both G6PD deficiency and abnormal hemoglobins have some protective effect against malaria and individuals with both traits are not at a disadvantage, a positive correlation of their frequency in populations could be expected and has in fact been observed.

These examples have been included to illustrate the fact that other factors may impact on genetic factors, which together have a major effect on the incidence of disease. In some other situations, a familial or genetic association with disease seems to be clear, yet conclusive proof is not yet available. Such a condition is diabetes mellitus. Autoantibodies reacting with the cytoplasm of pancreatic islet cells (ICAb) are much more common in patients with diabetes controlled only with insulin injections than in those who may be controlled with oral hypoglycemic agents. Such observations and others provide strong evidence for the transmission of diabetes genetically, although attempts at genetic proof have so far failed.

Even more soft is the evidence for genetic transmission of some other conditions that are recognized to have familial incidence. This may be because the responsible underlying factors have not yet been identified. Many conditions of quite varied symptomatology may fall within this category. For example, low back pain and peptic ulcer disease might eventually be included.

Population and nutrition

At first sight, these two factors may appear to be unrelated. In fact there is an intimate relationship between food supply and the size of human populations. In some small population groups, kept small either voluntarily or involuntarily by food shortage, a relative lack of infectious disease, especially that caused by airborne infection, has been noted.

The study of these relationships is aided by the concept of ecosystems. This refers to the dynamic relationship that exists between communities, the plants and animals, and the local physical environment on which all depend. Three major ecosystems are frequently described.

In a hunter-gatherer ecosystem, individuals may have a lean, athletic body build and surprisingly a relatively good nutritional state. However, in times of food shortage, the order of preference for food distribution may determine which segment of the population begins to suffer first from malnutrition. The order might be women, dogs, children, hunting men, and old men. In such an ecosystem, atherosclerotic cardiovascular disease, obesity, and diseases related to sedentary occupations are likely to have a low incidence.

A peasant agricultural ecosystem may depend on a single crop such as a cereal or root vegetable, which leads to specific nutritional deficiencies. Crop failure may also result in general nutritional deficiency.

Perhaps fortunately, the major portion of the world's population lives in the affluent industrial ecosystem. In such a system there are frequent changes in food consumption. More recently, such changes have been induced by greater awareness of health issues relating to diet. This is not always the case, however, and temporary shortages or imbalance may exist through economic difficulty, through disasters caused by human agency, or through natural occurrences. These patterns are reflected in the patterns and incidence of disease. Undernutrition is not the only potential problem. Overnutrition is an actual problem in many communities.

Hazards in the physical environment

Environmental hazards may be either biologic or physical. Biologic hazards may range from microorganisms as small as viruses to much higher organisms such as poisonous plants or animals. Some of them occur naturally, whereas others may have been introduced as the result of human activity (anthropogenic). Chemical hazards in the environment have become the object of much attention in recent years.

Some substances are biodegradable: Their toxic effects are limited by the destruction of the toxic product occurring in the natural environment. Other substances are subject to bioaccumulation, in which compounds are retained in living organisms. Transport of toxic substances may occur naturally, either in solution in water supplies or in soil through leaching. Vaporization is yet another possibility.

Concern about adverse effects on public health has been expressed with regard to, among others, the following substances: asbestos, arsenic, cadmium, mercury, lead, nitrogen, sulfur, hydrocarbons, halogenated hydrocarbons, phenols and contaminants, organic acids and esters, bipyridils (especially those used in herbicides), and pesticides.

Infectious agents

Although the possibility of contagion was recognized in the 16th century or earlier, only relatively recently have the sources and agents been identified. This has been due to the combined efforts of epidemiologists and bacteriologists, with the former preceding the latter historically. Each infectious agent has, of course, its own characteristics, which include the method by which it is transmitted and the effects it has on humans when it invades. These are the main characteristics on which we will concentrate here, since these have chief interest in the field of public health.

An increasing number of viruses that are pathogenic to humans have been identified. All are obligate parasites, not replicating outside host cells. Of the DNA-containing viruses, there are five major groups of significance, listed in increasing order of the size of virus particles: parvoviruses (including adeno-associated viruses, and also possibly Norwalk and other similar viruses that cause gastroenteritis); papovaviruses (including the papilloma virus); adenoviruses, which may be involved in respiratory infections and other infections such as keratoconjunctivitis, cystitis and gastroenteritis; herpesviruses (including the viruses that cause herpes simplex and herpes genitalis, in addition to varicella-zoster, the Epstein-Barr virus, and cytomegalovirus); and the poxviruses, causing vaccinia, smallpox, cowpox, and monkeypox.

There are a greater number of RNA-containing viruses of public health importance. The picornaviruses are a large family of stable viruses containing no lipids. They cause a great many different diseases in humans. Of these, the enterovirus group is the largest, including the poliomyelitis virus, coxsackie A and B viruses, echoviruses (enteric cytopathic human orphan), and others. The family also includes the rhinoviruses and cardio-

virus. Another significant family is the paramyxoviruses: these include the parainfluenza viruses, mumps, Newcastle disease; the measles virus and those that cause canine distemper and rinderpest; and the respiratory syncytial virus.

Some viruses whose full identification is not yet complete are of considerable practical importance. These include the virus of hepatitis A, which is probably an RNA-containing enterovirus, and hepatitis B, which contains double-stranded DNA. The human immunodeficiency virus (HIV), responsible for the current epidemic of acquired immunodeficiency syndrome (AIDS), is attracting a great deal of attention.

In investigating outbreaks of illness that may be caused by any of these known and well-recognized viruses, the characteristics of the illness and the known methods of spread for each particular type are of great importance. However, it is quite likely that with the identification of presently unknown diseases in some of the world's populations, other viruses and disease configurations may become apparent. Vaccines will continue to be a principal means of prevention of most virus infections. Isolation of viruses is still difficult and does not yet provide a practical method of reaching a diagnosis in a timely fashion suitable for clinical use. The use of methods for detecting antibodies in active and convalescent serum is at present the most effective means of reaching a specific diagnosis.

Bacteria are autonomously replicating biologic entities that have many naturally occurring habitats that become reservoirs for potential host infection. The resultant diseases are usually based on the metabolic activities of the bacteria, and therefore on both the natural and host habitat. Diseases often occur, for example, as a result of toxic substances that are by-products of materials synthesized by the organisms to help obtain substrates necessary for growth and replication. Sometimes the end result is loss of life for the pathogen. In this relatively rare case, propagation occurs by direct passage from host to host.

Virulence normally depends on the method of conveyance of infection and the portal of entry. If a bacterium is to colonize and reproduce itself, it must have access to a suitable site for its growth. Thus an organism that is pathogenic in the lungs is conveyed through the respiratory tract. Enteric pathogens are not normally conveyed by this route. The principle applies in other locations also.

Sometimes bacterial infections are self-limiting. For example, the fever produced by the production of bacterial endotoxin may prevent the bacteria from effectively competing for vital iron stores from their host.

The diagnosis of bacterial disease is generally reached by cultivation and identification of the pathogen in the laboratory. This is generally desirable because it allows for appropriate antimicrobial therapy to be ordered. Occasionally, suitable specimens for culture are not available, or the laboratory facilities in order to culture not accessible. In such circumstances it may be justified to reach a diagnosis by a combination of clinical and epidemiologic methods.

Protozoa may also be pathogenic to humans. They have various portals of entry and colonize in various body locations. For example, the malarial parasite is transmitted by an arthropod vector and affects the blood and blood-forming organs; *Trichomonas vaginalis* is sexually transmitted and chronically infects the urogenital tract of men and women.

Finally, many helminths are invasive to human hosts. Modes of transmission are again varied, and frequently complex. All animal species harbor their own array of helminthic parasites; sometimes their larvae will penetrate the human integument, producing an assortment of symptoms.

The social milieu

The word *milieu* here is used to distinguish the social environment from the physical, chemical, or biologic environment, the effects of which have been discussed earlier. It relates to the interaction between what may be described as personal factors peculiar to the individual and the environment in which the individual is located. Examples of such interactions are family development and adolescence, each of which may be responsible for producing disease states.

Certain conditions are known to be more common in certain social classes. This is demonstrated in Table 6-3. In addition to these broad effects of social class on health, the association between social forces and life-styles also plays a part in the production of some diseases. Examples are smoking, diet, and exercise. Patterns of behavior in these areas, produced frequently by peer pressure, are significant in their influence on health and disease.

Culture, life-styles, and health are also related. Certain practices may lead to exposure to or protection from human hazards. Cultural barriers may exist to prevent change—for example, unwillingness to give up traditional diet. There may be similar unwillingness to change patterns of child rearing or working behavior, leading to adverse effects on mental and physical health.

Stress is frequently accused as a potent source of disease-producing factors. The relationship is properly established in

Table 6-3. Child Mortality: England and Wales

Social class*	1978–79 Perinatal mortality‡	Post-neonatal‡	1970–72 1–14 Years† Boys	Girls
I (4.8)§	11.2	3.1	74	89
II (20)	12.0	2.9	79	84
III N (16)	13.3	2.9	95	93
III M (33)	14.7	4.1	98	93
IV (19)	16.9	4.8	112	120
V (7.6)	19.4	7.6	162	156

*Of father.
I Leading professions, and managerial, business.
II Lesser professions, and managerial, business.
III Nonmanual skilled workers.
III Manual skilled workers.
IV Part-skilled workers.
V Unskilled workers.
†Rates per 1,000 relevant legitimate births.
‡Standardized mortality ratios; in England/Wales = 100.
§Percent of "heads of households" in the different social classes, census of 1971.
Sources: 1970–72 data from OPCS (1978). 1978–79 data from OPCS (weekly *Monitors*) and OPCS (personal communication).

some conditions. Traditionally, however, there has been scanty evidence that relates psychosomatic disorders to the social environment, in spite of the general acceptance that the psyche can affect the soma. Here the value of the terminology "determinants of disease" becomes very relevant. It is difficult to prove causal relationships.

Natural disasters and those caused by humans

Both natural disasters and those caused by humans have a major impact on the provision of health services, because of the human suffering that may be generated. Natural disasters have always occurred, probably with similar frequency over many centuries. The greater apparent rate of incidence recently is probably related only to improved communications. Natural disasters, especially if widespread, are likely to be followed by outbreaks or epidemics of infectious disease. Many medical teams responding to disasters have discovered that their services are frequently sought to provide assistance for seemingly nondisaster ailments such as ischemic heart disease, obstetrics, and renal failure.

Of the causes of morbidity and mortality attributed to humans, it is probable that the highest incidence worldwide may be due to road traffic accidents. The routine measures to be applied in order to prevent or minimize fatalities are not uniformly effective. These include appropriate engineering or other technological measures; early warning, so that avoidance measures may be instituted; and protection against human error. In spite of efforts at prevention, the hazards still exist.

There has been greater attention paid to the possibility of chemical and other environmental pollution. It seems impossible to eliminate risk. A cost-benefit analysis of risks is often further complicated by the fact that the advantages and disadvantages are often distributed unequally between population groups.

Much of the world's population regards the possibility of nuclear war as the ultimate man-made hazard. Certainly the possibility does exist for massive mortality and even greater subsequent morbidity from a nuclear encounter. Recent accidents such as the Chernoble disaster have made the possibility of this type of eventuality seem much more likely. The number of casualties caused in such an event would tax the limits of the most sophisticated medical resources.

Investigation of patterns of disease

Now that the possible determinants of disease have been listed, it is practicable to consider the investigation of an outbreak of disease. At this stage, the search for causal relationships may be commenced. In making a diagnosis, a selection must be made from the hundreds of known diseases to identify the one that most closely fits the clinical picture. In this process, a clinician is strongly influenced by an awareness of the diseases that are prevalent in the community at the time. This awareness may give rise to errors that are really erroneous clinical presuppositions. However, the awareness is important practically if cost-effective care is to be provided. A search for every possible disease cannot be made for every patient who presents.

Descriptive epidemiology is the science that is brought to bear on the study of such associations. To describe the occurrence of a disease clearly, three broad questions must be answered: Who is affected? Where do cases occur? When do cases occur? These questions are not only relevant in seeking an explanation for a sudden and unexplained outbreak of a disease (an epidemic), but also in the more routine work of a physician seeking to reach a diagnosis for an individual patient. Knowing that a patient is of a particular age, sex, or occupation and that he or she comes from a particular locality is very helpful in narrowing down the list of possible diseases that might be present.

Age and sex are obvious factors as determinants of disease. In the investigation of an outbreak of illness, these factors should be clearly recorded, as should ethnic background, race, and occupation. Marital status is frequently relevant, as are some factors relating to family status (e.g., family size, birth order, maternal age, parental deprivation).

Frequency of disease may be related to place of occurrence. This can be expressed in terms of natural barriers (e.g., mountain ranges, rivers, deserts) or by political boundaries (e.g., counties, states), or in terms of location in relation to a specific occurrence (e.g., eating in a particular restaurant, attending a certain school). A feature that has fairly recently assumed considerable significance is the association of some types of illness with particular occupations. This may be due to exposure to toxic substances. Such exposures may also occur as a result of geographical or environmental factors.

Occasionally, international comparisons become important. This was well demonstrated in the initial investigations of the occurrence of AIDS. Current geographic differences in the distribution of some diseases in the United States are demonstrated in Figures 6-3 through 6-6.

The study of disease occurrence by time is also a basic aspect of epidemiologic analysis. Short-term fluctuations are relevant in epidemics of infectious disease. Apart from infections, there are other observed causes of cyclic changes in the incidence of disease. Seasonal analysis has been of value in estimating the role of insect vectors in certain diseases, since temperature and humidity affect the activity and life of some insects.

When investigating the possibility of person-to-person spread of disease, the interval between cases is known as the **generation time**. This is the period between infection of the host and the moment of maximal communicability of that host. It is roughly equivalent to the incubation period, but the two periods may be different in that the time of maximal communicability may precede or follow the incubation period.

The influence of time on the incidence of disease may also be seen as the effect of the development of **herd immunity**. This has been defined as the "resistance of a group to invasion and spread of an infectious agent, based on the immunity of a high proportion of individual members of the group."

Natural history and prognosis. The natural history and prognosis may be addressed from two perspectives. For most clinicians, considerations turn immediately to the individual patient. Each disease process has its own natural history. The physician needs to be able to describe this to the patient in any case, whether or not a specific line of treatment will be advocated. If the patient is going to be able to give informed consent to a particular course of treatment, the likely course of

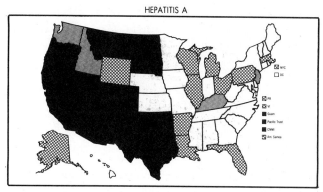

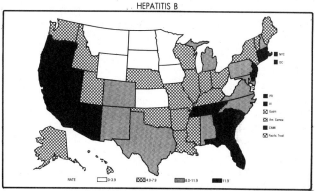

Figure 6-3. Rates of hepatitis A and B, by state, United States, 1984. (Rates are based on reported cases per 100,000 population). The states with the highest rates of hepatitis A in 1984 are concentrated in the West and Southwest. Half of these reported communitywide outbreaks, primarily involving person-to-person spread. The states with the highest rates of hepatitis B are clustered primarily on the east and west coasts, as in previous years. Hepatitis non-A/non-B remains a diagnosis of exclusion. The low reported rates for this disease are believed to be due to incomplete serological testing and underreporting.

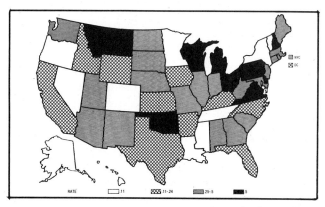

Figure 6-4. Legionellosis. Rates by state, United States, 1984. (Rates are based on reported cases per 100,000 population). A total of 750 cases of legionellosis were reported to CDC in 1984. Reported cases occurred more commonly in northern and midwestern states and less commonly in southern states. Legionellosis may be difficult to diagnose, and underreporting probably occurs. Thus, it is not known whether the reported incidence accurately reflects the true endemic incidence in this country.

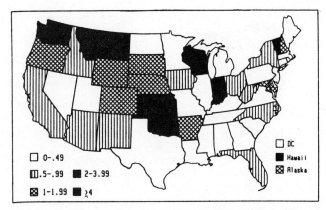

Figure 6-5. Pertussis (whooping cough). Rates by state, United States, 1984. (Rates are based on reported cases per 100,000 population). Only North Dakota and the District of Columbia did not report cases of pertussis in 1984. Seven states reported 100 or more cases — Washington (326), Indiana (259), Oklahoma (247), California (163), New York (129), Wisconsin (114), and Hawaii (102) — and accounted for 1,340 (59%) of the 2,276 cases.

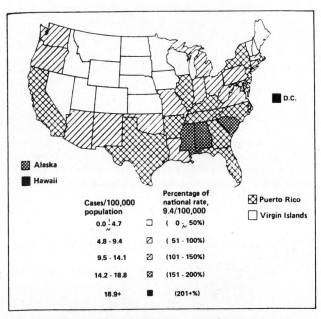

Figure 6-6. Tuberculosis. Rates by state, United States, 1984. In 1984, rates for the 50 states ranged from 21.0/100,000 population in Hawaii to 1.0/100,000 population in Wyoming. In general, the southeastern states and the states on the United States-Mexico border reported the highest case rates; rates were generally higher east of the Mississippi.

the disease both with and without treatment must be as clearly understood as possible. Both the risks and the benefits of action or inaction should be explained. An adequate explanation will depend on knowledge of recent medical literature, including studies that demonstrate the probability of survival. These studies must be interpreted in the light of how generalizable the results in the population studied were. On this basis, an attempt may be made to apply the published data to the individual circumstance.

The interpretation of these data is specific to each pathological condition. For specific applications, the reader is referred to descriptions of specific disease, some of which may be found in this text. In a great number of situations in practice, reference will need to be made to major texts or to more specific investigations reported in the general medical literature.

Some help may be derived from collected data in which communities or populations are studied. This is obviously a much more generalized approach, yet it has some relevance to the needs of an individual patient, in addition to shedding light on the problems of a community. This is the other applicable method of consideration of an understanding of the natural history and progress of disease.

The **cause-specific death rate,** which approximates the risk of death from a specific condition, is one of the most important epidemiologic indices available. This is defined as the number of deaths from a stated cause in a year and uses the midyear population as the denominator. It is usually expressed as a rate per 100,000 of the population. Confusion sometimes occurs with the **proportionate mortality ratio,** which should really only be used to describe the relative importance of a specific cause of death. This ratio is defined as the number of deaths in a given period of time from a specified cause, using the total number of deaths in that period as the denominator. It is usually expressed as a percentage.

However, as was stated earlier, mortality rates are inadequate for the study of the dynamics of diseases that either are not fatal or result in death only after a very protracted course. For such conditions, data on morbidity are required. The distinction between incidence and prevalence becomes very important.

Life expectancy is one way in which the phenomenon may be studied. It refers to the average number of years an individual is expected to live and in epidemiologic terms is generally calculated to refer to the expectation of life at birth, but it can be calculated for any age. In developed countries, the average life expectancy at birth has risen from 65.2 in the years 1950–1955 to 71.2 in 1970–1975. In developing counties, the rise has been equally dramatic, from 42.5 to 53.2. The average annual rate of increase in developed countries is now 0.16, but in developing countries where conditions relating to health and disease are still rapidly changing, the average increase is 0.38. In both cases, the biggest changes have come from improved conditions and services relating to infancy and early childhood. Further improvement in these figures may be more difficult to achieve, but concentration is now being made on conditions that affect adulthood and especially older age-groups.

More specific attempts are now being made to estimate disability, defined as "any temporary or long-term reduction of a person's activity as a result of an acute or chronic condition." This definition has enabled the collection of data regarding disability and the study of restricted activity days, work-loss days, and bed-disability days. In 1980, the World Health Organization published a classification of impairments, disabilities, and handicaps. This will presumably have a gradual effect in standardizing international literature in this area. Such descriptors as categories and degrees of handicaps have until now been difficult to compare.

Each of these parameters helps in determining the prognosis

for an individual but is more helpful for estimating the likely longevity and productivity of an individual who is representative of a "healthy" population. The prognostic capability for determining the likely outcome in a patient with a particular disease in many cases yet remains to be defined in clear scientific and statistical terms. These issues are studied in detail by insurance carriers who deal with three types of insurance: medical treatment, short- or long-term disability, and life. With the advent of much greater concern about the costs of health care, it is likely that these sources in the relatively near future will be able to produce statistical analyses that will enable physicians to answer patients' inquiries about prognosis more clearly and accurately.

Similar methods of study may be applied to clinical decision analysis. Many of the earlier attempts at application in this area have been directed toward medical training. While clinicians attempt to determine prognosis and course of action in each case on its individual characteristics, decision analysts seem to approach clinical decision making on an aggregate basis. This implies that there is one "best answer" that should apply over the whole population. These tools may be useful to physicians in training, but to many established physicians who prefer to rely on their own experience they seem to be unnecessary. The availability of computers in hospital settings and increasing relevance attributed to computing skills by those in training may ensure that this aspect of the application of statistical studies to medical prctice has a useful future.

A more detailed discussion of the natural history and prognosis of individual conditions will be given in the section dealing with primary and secondary prevention of specific conditions.

Risk factors. Factors whose presence is associated with an increased likelihood that disease will develop at a later stage are known as risk factors. At the beginning of such a study, the possibility of such an association may not be apparent. In the design of such studies, therefore, the most successful researchers will be those who are farsighted and who have the resources available to expand the scope of the study into areas where the assurance of relevant results is not immediately guaranteed. When such resources are available, the rewards can have great significance. Such a study has been the Framingham Heart Study, which has provided many landmarks in the application of epidemiology to the practice of medicine. Although the emphasis was initially on biologic variables (height, weight, blood pressure, serum lipids, etc.), biopsychosocial habits have also been included in studies. The association between heart disease and smoking has, for example, become increasingly clear as a result of the application of this type of study.

In some cases, it is not easy to establish that one particular is an independent risk factor. For example, major risk factors for coronary vessel disease are known to include cigarette smoking, elevated blood pressure and blood lipids, diabetes, and physical inactivity. These are often associated with obesity, but a debate continues as to whether overweight is an independent risk factor.

Because the study here is concerned with factors that are or may become determinants of disease, the associations may not be fully understood initially. At first, the relationship between

high levels of serum lipids and heart disease was noted. It was later discovered that relatively high levels of low-density lipoprotein (LDL) behave almost as a pathogen in atherosclerosis. Further investigation revealed, on the other hand, that high levels of high-density lipoprotein (HDL) have a protective effect against atherosclerotic disease. Although the initial observations did not lead fully to a correct conclusion, because the proportion of LDL in serum is normally higher than that of HDL, the observations lead correctly to the incrimination of cholesterol as a major risk factor.

The statement that cholesterol is a major risk factor in coronary heart disease still requires refining and qualification, however. When epidemiologic evidence is studied, the relationship between the usual or habitual diet, population levels of blood lipids, blood pressure, and coronary heart disease can be seen to be established more clearly. When weight is held constant, the largest dietary contributions to serum cholesterol level are saturated fat and dietary cholesterol, which tend to raise the serum cholesterol level, and polyunsaturated fat, which tends to lower it. Prediction of change in serum cholesterol levels is possible from known changes in diet. For how long must this kind of change be maintained before the risk of coronary heart disease is affected? Does this vary with the age of the individual being studied?

These considerations lead firmly to the conclusion that the assessment of the clinical relevance of risk factors cannot be considered in isolation from each other. In the situation discussed (the factors leading to increased risk of coronary heart disease), cholesterol cannot be considered as an isolated and sole risk factor. It plays a part in a complex scenario in which many other factors are involved. These include diet and exercise habits, weight, blood pressure, life-style, and stress, in addition to others. A risk factor is exactly what the title implies: an element of the individual's life or health that may not itself be causative of disease but that increases the risk of disease by a factor, large or small, which may sometimes be statistically determined. This definition may be applied to risk factors relating to diseases other than those from which it has been derived in the argument above.

There is thus a considerable difference between a risk factor and what may be regarded as a causative agent. Some of the criteria that are currently used to establish causality are as follows: (1) The cause is distributed in the population in the same manner as the disease. (2) The incidence of the disease is significantly higher in those exposed to the hypothesized cause than in those not so exposed. (3) Exposure to the supposed cause is more frequent among those with the disease than in controls without the disease, when all other risk factors are held constant. (4) Sequentially, the disease follows exposure to the supposed causative agent. (5) The greater the dose or length of exposure, the greater the likelihood of occurrence of the disease. (6) For some diseases, the spectrum of host responses following exposure to the supposed agent ranges from mild to severe. (7) The association between the supposed cause and the disease is found in different populations, even when different methods of study are used. (8) Other explanations for the association may be ruled out. (9) Elimination of the supposed cause from the environment, modification of it, or removal of its vector decreases the incidence of disease. (10) Prevention or modification of the host's response on exposure to the supposed cause by immunization, drug therapy, or other treatment decreases or eliminates the disease. (11) If experimental settings are possible, the disease will occur more frequently in animals or humans exposed to the supposed cause than in those not so exposed; this exposure may be deliberate in volunteers, experimentally induced in a laboratory, or demonstrated in a controlled regulation of natural exposure. (12). All of the findings and relationships so demonstrated should make epidemiologic and biologic sense.

Consideration of more examples of risk factors will be included in the following section, in which primary and secondary prevention of specific illnesses are discussed.

PRIMARY AND SECONDARY PREVENTION OF SPECIFIC ILLNESSES

Primary and secondary prevention of disease are frequently confused. In epidemiologic terms, primary prevention reduces the incidence of disease; secondary prevention reduces its prevalence. Primary prevention diminishes the occurrence of disease—for example, by immunization against infectious disease and by the use of safety equipment to protect workers in hazardous occupations. Secondary prevention means early detection and intervention, preferably before the condition is clinically apparent, and has the aim of reversing, halting, or at least retarding the progress of the condition. It is generally carried out in screening programs in which individuals with early and often asymptomatic manifestations of the disease are identified and offered help in prevention of its progression.

A third type of prevention of disease is also described, not surprisingly, as tertiary prevention. This is widely applied in clinical practice and implies minimizing the effects of disease and disability by surveillance and maintenance aimed at preventing complications and premature deterioration. This will not be further discussed here, since it is part of the routine clinical treatment, especially for chronic forms of disease.

INFECTIOUS DISEASES

Investigation and control of an epidemic

An epidemic is the occurrence in a community or region of cases of an illness, specific health-related behavior, or other health-related events clearly in excess of normal expectancy. The number of cases indicating the presence of an epidemic will vary according to the agent, size and type of population exposed, previous experience of or lack of exposure to the disease, and the time and place of the occurrence. Epidemicity is thus relative to usual frequency of the disease in the same area, among the specified population, at the same season of the year.

Because an epidemic is by definition an increase in the expected incidence of disease, investigation cannot be carried out prospectively. If the epidemic is already over, as is frequently the case, the investigation is fully retrospective. On rare occasions a contaminating source may be identified early, allowing the possibility of the investigation of exposed individuals prior to the development of the disease. For these reasons, case-control methods are normally applied to the investigation of epidemics.

It is important to realize that not all epidemics are caused by

outbreaks of infectious disease, although it is convenient to discuss them under this heading. The majority of epidemics are discovered to have infectious origins.

Of the many factors that may be responsible for the occurrence of an epidemic of disease, classification may be attempted under three headings. The first classification includes those affecting the agent of infection:

1. The introduction of a new agent.
2. Recent increase in dosage of the agent; multiplication.
3. Change in virulence of the pathogenic agent, possibly due to mutation or recombination of an old agent.
4. Old agents discovering a new portal of entry.
5. Invasive procedures.
6. New sexual practices.
7. Intravenous drug abuse.
8. Longer exposure to an old agent.
9. Migration of infected persons, birds, animals, or insects.
10. Multiple agents.

The second group includes those affecting the methods of transmission in the environment:

1. New growth media, either those produced by people (e.g., cooling towers or home humidifiers) or occurring naturally.
2. New methods of dispersion.
3. Exposure to new environments, either by individual or population movements or occasionally by the necessity for medical or other care in such places as intensive care units or day-care centers.

The third group includes those factors affecting host susceptibility:

1. Highly susceptible subgroups such as newborns and the nonimmunized.
2. Travel of susceptibles to an endemic area.
3. Increased susceptibility from immunosuppressive drugs or natural immunodeficiency.
4. Cultural or behavioral factors.

Not all these factors are as common as each other in the genesis of an epidemic, which makes the work of identifying the cause or causes easier. Using an understanding of these types of antecedents, it is possible to classify epidemics according to their patterns of onset. **Common-source outbreaks** develop after the exposure of a susceptible population or group to a common source of the pathogen. Sometimes an explosive outbreak occurs as a result, but occasionally the pattern is more prolonged—for example, because of the fact that although a single vehicle is contaminated, individual packs (prepacked foods, bottled beverages, drugs etc.) are not consumed simultaneously. **Point epidemics** are outbreaks occurring in a group of susceptibles exposed at the same time to a common source of the pathogen. **Propagative** or **progresive epidemics** involve the transfer of the epidemic agent from one host to another. This usually involves multiplication and release of the organisms from the host and may also involve carriers or vectors.

Mixed epidemics involve not only a single common exposure to an infectious agent but also secondary spread, most usually person-to-person transmission.

The pattern of onset may also be a direct reflection of the type of infectious agent. Some examples of classic intervals between time of exposure and onset of symptoms (the incubation period) are listed in Table 6-4.

An epidemic usually ceases when one or more of the following events occur:

1. The source of contamination is eradicated or modified or the pathogen becomes nonpathogenic.
2. The mode of transmission is interrupted or removed.
3. The number of susceptible persons is either exhausted or markedly reduced, possibly by conveyed immunity.
4. A cofactor or some other important risk factor is modified or removed.

In the investigation of the outbreak, therefore, the timing and sequence of events can be very important pieces of information that may lead to detection of the causative agent. The sequences may be recorded in the form of detailed log diaries or as epidemic curves or graphs. On the basis of such information, the first important question may be asked: Does an epidemic or outbreak exist? If so, what type of etiologic

Table 6-4. Examples of Epidemics According to the Incubation Period

Time frame	Examples
1. Hours	a. Acute food poisoning: toxins, staphylococci, *Clostridium perfringens*
	b. Heavy metal exposures: cadmium, copper, zinc
	c. Certain other poisonings: monosodium glutamate, mushrooms, shellfish toxins
2. Days	a. Some food poisonings: *Salmonella* (1–2 days), *Vibrio cholerae*, *Campylobacter jejuni*
	b. Bacterial infections: legionnaires' disease, *Mycoplasma pneumoniae*
	c. Viral infections: influenza (1–3 days), adenovirus (1–5 days), enteroviral infections (5–6 days
3. Weeks	a. Common childhood diseases: measles, mumps, rubella (2–3 weeks)
	b. Hepatitis A (2–5 weeks)
4. Months	a. Hepatitis B (2–6 months)
	b. Rabies (0.5–12 months)
5. Years	a. Radiation-induced leukemia after atomic bomb (peak after 6 years)
	b. Kuru (1–27 years)
	c. Bladder cancer in dyestuff workers (1–40 years)

Kelsey JL, Thompson WD, Evans AS: Methods in Observational Epidemiology. New York, Oxford University Press, 1986.

agent is likely to be involved? The answers to these questions become hypotheses that may be tested.

The next step in the investigation involves the appraisal of existing data. In addition to factors involving time, the following must be recorded: place, person, incidence data, clinical features, and some description of what may be relevant environmental factors. The hypotheses may now be expanded to the site of exposure and possible methods of transmission. Upon these, possible methods of control may also be suggested, and all the hypotheses may then be tested by laboratory investigation and by detailed analysis of all available data. If the hypotheses can be supported, the final step becomes the drawing of conclusions, with the devising of practical applications, which may be followed by long-term surveillance and prevention.

Active and passive immunization

The ultimate goal of immunization is eradication of disease. A more immediate goal is prevention of disease in individuals or groups. Infectious disease may be prevented by stimulating the individual to develop an active immunologic defense against a future exposure that might occur naturally or by supplying previously produced human or animal antibodies to individuals who may be or have been exposed to certain infectious agents. Not all infectious diseases are amenable to either or both methods of control.

Active immunization consists of the administration of all or part of a microorganism or a modified product of that organism—for example, a toxoid. Vaccines incorporating an intact infectious agent may be either live attenuated vaccines or killed inactivated. The vaccines and toxoids currently available in the United States and their route of administration are listed in Table 6-5.

Injectable vaccines should be administered in a site as free as possible from the opportunity for local neural, vascular, or tissue injury. For this reason, the upper outer aspect of the buttocks should not be used for immunization in infants because of the danger of damage to the sciatic nerve. All the benefits and potential risks of immunization should be explained to the individual being immunized or, if appropriate, to the parents. It is essential that informed consent be obtained.

Ideally, infants should be actively immunized against some infectious diseases during the first year of life. During this period, they are more susceptible to infection since their immune systems are not as fully able to cope with invading infectious organisms as are those of healthy adults. Immunization programs effectively introduced have significantly reduced neonatal and infant mortality. However, because the full effectiveness of the infant's immune system takes several months to develop, greater immunization effectiveness is achieved by a carefully prepared schedule of procedures, which in some cases includes the repetition of administration of immunizing agents. Table 6-6 is a recommended schedule currently in use.

One of the problems of the practice of preventive medicine is that not everyone is either willing or able to comply with recommended schedules. What modifications of these recommendations are in these circumstances most effective? Unfortunately, there are no simple answers to this question. The

Table 6-5. Vaccines (Including Toxoids) Available in the United States and Their Route of Administration

Vaccine*	Type	Route
BCG	Live bacteria	Intradermal (preferred) or SC
Cholera	Inactivated bacteria	SC, IM, or intradermal
DTP	Toxoids and inactivated bacteria	IM
Hepatitis B	Inactivated viral antigen	IM
Hemophilus b	Polysaccharide	SC, IM†
Influenza	Inactivated virus	IM (preferred) or SC
IPV	Inactivated virus	SC
Measles	Live virus	SC
Meningococcal	Polysaccharide	SC
MMR	Live viruses	SC
Mumps	Live virus	SC
OPV	Live virus	PO
Plague	Inactivated bacteria	IM
Pneumococcal	Polysaccharide	IM or SC
Rabies	Inactivated virus	IM
Rubella	Live virus	SC
Tetanus and Td, DT	Toxoids	IM
Typhoid	Inactivated bacteria	SC (boosters may be intradermal‡)
Yellow fever	Live virus	SC

*BCG = Bacillus of Calmette Guérin vaccine (tuberculosis); DTP = diphtheria and tetanus toxoids and pertussis vaccine, IPV = inactivated poliovirus vaccine; MMR = measles, mumps, and rubella vaccine; OPV = oral poliovirus vaccine; Td = tetanus and diphtheria toxoids for adult (≥ 7 years old) use; DT = diphtheria and tetanus toxoids.
† Preparations with adjuvants must be given IM.
‡ The interdermal dose is different.

Table 6-6. Recommended Schedule for Active Immunization of Normal Infants and Children

Recommended age	Immunization(s)	Comments
2 months	DTP,[1] OPV[2]	Can be initiated as early as 2 weeks of age in areas of high endemicity or during epidemics
4 months	DTP, OPV	2-month interval desired for OPV to avoid interference from previous dose
6 months	DTP (OPV)	OPV is optional (may be given in areas with increased risk of poliovirus exposure)
15 months	Measles, mumps, rubella (MMR)[3]	MMR preferred to individual vaccines; tuberculin testing may be done
18 months	DTP,[4,5] OPV[5]	
24 months	HBPV[6]	
4–6 years[7]	DTP, OPV	At or before school entry
14–16 years	Td[3]	Repeat every 10 years throughout life

[1]DTP—Diphtheria and tetanus toxoids with pertussis vaccine.
[2]OPV—Oral poliovirus vaccine contains attenuated poliovirus types 1, 2, and 3.
[3]MMR—Live measles, mumps, and rubella viruses in a combined vaccine.
[4]Should be given 6 to 12 months after the third dose.
[5]May be given simultaneously with MMR at 15 months of age.
[6]*Hemophilus* b polysaccharide vaccine.
[7]Up to the seventh birthday.
[8]Td—Adult tetanus toxoid (full dose) and diphtheria toxoid (reduced dose) in combination.

For all products used, consult manufacturer's package insert for instructions for storage, handling, and administration. Biologics prepared by different manufacturers may vary, and those of the same manufacturer may change from time to time. Therefore, the physician should be aware of the contents of the package insert.

situation is sufficiently common for some guidelines to be suggested. The recommendations for children over the age of 7 years may also be applied to those adults who have not been previously immunized or for whom no adequate documentation of immunologic state exists (Table 6-7).

Passive immunization may be appropriate in the following circumstances:

1. When no vaccine for a given disease is available and prevention or modification of the course of disease is possible by exposure to an antibody (e.g., hepatitis A).
2. When time does not permit adequate protection by active immunization alone (e.g., some postexposure situations involving measles, rabies, or tetanus).
3. When a specific toxic effect of venom is best managed by antibody administration (e.g., poisonous snake bite).
4. Therapeutically, when a disease already is present and the administration of antibody can ameliorate or aid in suppressing the effects of a toxin (e.g., botulism, diphtheria, or tetanus).

Table 6-7. Recommended Immunization Schedules for Children Not Immunized in First Year of Life

Recommended time	Immunization(s)	Comments
Less than 7 years old		
First visit	DPT, OPV, MMR	MMR if child ≥ 15 months old; tuberculin testing may be done
Interval after first visit		
1 month	HBPV*	For children 24–60 months
2 months	DPT, OPV	
4 months	DPT (OPV)	OPV is optional (may be given in areas with increased risk of poliovirus exposure
10–16 months	DPT, OPV	OPV is not given if third dose was given earlier
Age 4–6 years (at or before school entry)	DPT, OPV	DPT is not necessary if the fourth dose was given after the fourth birthday; OPV is not necessary if recommended OPV dose at 10–16 months following first visit was given after the fourth birthday
Age 14–16 years	Td	Repeat every 10 years throughout life
7 Years Old and Older		
First visit	Td, OPV, MMR	
Interval after first visit		
2 months	Td, OPV	
8–14 months	Td, OPV	
Age 14–16 years	Td	Repeat every 10 years throughout life

*Hemophilus b polysaccharide vaccine can be given, if necessary, simultaneously with DPT (at separate sites). The initial three doses of DPT can be given at 1- to 2-month intervals; so, for the child in whom immunization is initiated at 24 months old or older, one visit could be eliminated by giving DPT, OPV, MMR at the first visit; DPT and HBPV at the second visit (1 month later); and DPT and OPV at the third visit (2 months after the first visit). Subsequent DPT and OPV 10 to 16 months after the first visit are still indicated.

5. In individuals deficient in synthesis of antibody as a result of congenital or acquired B-lymphocyte cell defects, alone or in combination with other immunodeficiencies.

Passive immunization may be achieved by the use of immune globulin (human) or specific immune globulin (human). Immune globulin is derived from the pooled plasma of adults and contains specific antibodies in proportion to the infectious and immunization experience of the population from which it was derived. Large numbers of donors are used to ensure the inclusion of a broad spectrum of antibodies. Some indications for its use are listed below:

1. Replacement therapy in antibody-deficient disorders.
2. Hepatitis A prophylaxis.
3. Measles prophylaxis.

It has been also used in some other situations, for which at present the use must be regarded as not proven. These include hepatitis B prophylaxis, hepatitis non-A/non-B prophylaxis, asthma or severe allergic diathesis, burn patients, most acute infections, and occasionally in some other clinical situations such as septic, debilitated, or malnourished infants.

Specific immune globulins are produced from donors who are known to have high titers of the desired antibody. They include hepatitis B immune globulin (HBIG), tetanus immune globulin (TIG), rabies immune globulin (RIG), and varicella-zoster immune globulin (VZIG). Specific recommendations and dosages have been published for the United States by the Public Health Service Advisory Committee on Immunization Practices, in Morbidity and Mortality Weekly Reports.

The eradication of smallpox is a notable milestone in medical history. The last known indigenous case occurred in Merka, Somalia, on October 26, 1977. Two subsequent cases arose from an accidental laboratory infection in England in September, 1978. Final confirmation of eradication was certified by the World Health Organization (WHO) and confirmed in May, 1980. The eradication of this one major disease has become a challenge for workers in public health worldwide to attempt similar achievements with other infectious diseases. Some success has been achieved in the reduction of the incidence of poliomyelitis and some other communicable diseases.

CONTROL OF SOME SPECIFIC CONDITIONS

The method of classification adopted here is based on that of J.M. Last (1986).

Viral infections

Influenza remains one of the world's most important epidemic diseases. Control is difficult to achieve because it is caused by a highly mutable virus, in which a steady continuous drift in virus antigen configuration is occasionally interrupted by a sudden major antigen change. Clinically, the pattern of illness caused by a particular strain varies from exceedingly mild and insignificant to severe and fatal. Successful virus recovery depends on proper collection of specimens at optimum times, effective transport to the laboratory, and sensitive techniques. These combinations are not uniformly achieved, so accurate identification becomes a problem. Clinically, little purpose is served by identification of the type and strain in an individual case. From a public health perspective, such information is valuable in enabling preventive measures, especially the production of effective vaccines. Serological confirmation of influenza infection requires fourfold or greater increases in antibody titer from the early stage of the disease to that collected 2 or 3 weeks later. Rates of infection indicate that 10 to 25% of the population in the community succumb to infection during mild or moderately brisk epidemics. Of special concern are patients in nursing homes, where attack rates of up to 80% have been reported together with case-fatality rates of up to 30%. Commercially available vaccines are prepared annually based on formulation and potency regulations reviewed by WHO. Properly formulated inactivated and also live attenuated vaccines can provide good protection against influenza and its complications. Amantadine hydrochloride or an analogue is now available for prophylaxis and therapy of influenza A but has not been shown to be effective against B strains.

Acute respiratory tract infections are the most common illnesses suffered by humans. The Health Interview Survey has estimated that once a year at least half of the population of the United States suffers a respiratory tract infection forcing restricted activity. In developing countries, respiratory tract illnesses may be the second leading cause of death in children younger than 5 years. These infections are caused by a variety of agents, including members of the paramyxovirus subgroup, parainfluenza and respiratory syncytial viruses, rhinoviruses, coronaviruses, adenoviruses, and *Mycoplasma pneumoniae*. Other agents are less frequent or limited causes of acute illness. It is not in general possible to classify them etiologically on the basis of clinical characteristics. This is illustrated by Figure 6-7, a diagram of frequent symptoms. From this it is clear that there is considerable overlap of symptoms from one condition to

another and that similar symptoms also arise in other more serious diseases, for example hemolytic streptococcal sore throat. Such streptococci, which may be readily grown on plates in an office type of incubator, may also be isolated from asymptomatic individuals. Prevention and control of the whole main group of infections of the upper respiratory tract have proved very difficult to achieve.

Acute GI tract infections are the next most important group of conditions causing morbidity in the United States. A number of viral and bacterial pathogens have been identified as etiologic agents in recent years. Three groups of viruses have been incriminated: rotaviruses, Norwalk-like agents, and certain adenoviruses. The bacterial agents causing enteric illnesses are discussed elsewhere. For the viruses, the most likely method of spread is by the fecal-oral route. Any conclusions regarding control are tentative at present. The possibility of production of vaccines is being explored.

Measles has been under control in the United States since the early 1960s, with the production of a live attenuated measles vaccine. After an incubation period (8 to 16 days, mean 10 to 12 days), the first symptoms are generally fever and malaise, followed shortly by cough, coryza, conjunctivitis, Koplik's spots, and the exanthem. Viremia occurs toward the end of the incubation period. The period of communicability is from 4 days before to 4 days after the occurrence of the rash. Complications are frequent, the most common being pneumonia, which may be viral or secondary bacterial infection. Otitis media is also common. Measles encephalitis occurs typically 4 to 7 days after the rash. Passive immunity may be achieved in high-risk situations by the administration of immune globulin. Active immunization may be carried out using the vaccine and is now recommended at the age of 15 months. The vaccine is generally combined with that for mumps and rubella. In 5 to 15% of cases, measles vaccination is followed by fever of 39.4°C (103°F). The incidence of encephalitis following measles vaccination is lower than the incidence rate of encephalitis of unknown etiology in the community. Measles vaccine, by giving protection against measles, significantly lowers the possibility of developing subacute sclerosing panencephalitis, a rare degenerative nervous system disease.

Rubella, a usually mild and self-limited disease in children, is now recognized as important because of its ability to induce congenital defects in children of women who acquire the disease during pregnancy. Table 6-8 lists the manifestations of congenital rubella infection. As many as 50 to 70% of babies with congenital rubella infection may appear normal at birth, the defects only becoming obvious later. Control of rubella and the congenital rubella syndrome has almost been achieved in the United States by the introduction of the vaccination program. Much of the success in this may be attributed to the comprehensive school immunization laws.

Mumps has also dramatically declined in incidence since the introduction of an effective vaccine. Other viruses may also cause parotitis but infection with mumps virus, one of the myxovirus group, causes the epidemic variety of parotitis with which may be associated orchitis and meningitis or encephalitis.

Chicken pox is a mild childhood illness with few complications, affecting only 5% of individuals. In adults, the

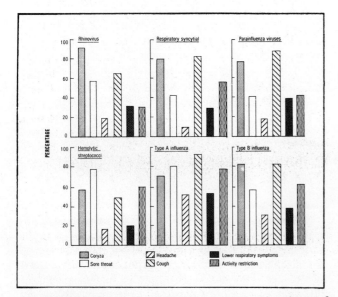

Figure 6-7. Characteristics of illnesses associated with isolation of viruses and hemolytic streptococci: percentage of those infected experiencing five symptoms and activity restriction.

Table 6-8. Manifestations of Congenital Rubella Infection

Bone lesions	
Cardiac defects	Patent ductus arteriosus
	Pulmonary stenosis and coarctation
	Myocardial necrosis
CNS defects	Encephalitis
	Mental retardation
	Microcephaly
	Progressive panencephalitis
	Psychomotor retardation
	Spastic quadriparesis
Deafness	
Eye defects	Cataracts
	Glaucoma
	Microphthalmia
	Retinopathy
Endocrinopathies	Adrenal disorders
	Diabetes mellitus
	Precocious puberty
	Growth retardation
	Growth hormone deficiency
GU tract defects	
Hematologic disorders	Anemia
	Thrombocytopenia
	Immunodeficiencies
Hepatitis	
Interstitial pneumonitis	
Psychiatric disorders	

course of primary varicella infection is usually more severe than in normal children. Primary infection with the varicella-zoster virus (VZV) is generally regarded as a prerequisite for developing shingles, zoster, in later life. The possibility of active immunization with a vaccine initially prepared in Japan is being investigated. At present, high-risk individuals may be protected passively by the use of VZIG.

Poliomyelitis, or infantile paralysis, became a noticeable epidemic phenomenon approximately 100 years ago. Three closely related poliovirus strains have been identified as causing the disease. The virus is conveyed by the fecal-oral route. Viremia occurs after intestinal absorption, leading to involvement of the lymph nodes, from where the virus obtains access to the CNS. The virus preferentially attacks the motor neurons of the spinal cord, and occasionally the bulbar area. Limited infections do not always cause flaccid paralysis, the likelihood of which seems to be provoked or increased by several factors. These include age of initial infection, stress, pregnancy, tonsillectomy, and adenoidectomy. Two types of vaccine have been produced, and their use has dramatically reduced the incidence of the disease in most developed countries. The first vaccine, prepared by Salk, was an inactivated poliovirus vaccine (IPV). Later, Sabin developed a mixture of three strains of attenuated live virus, and this vaccine is administered orally (OPV). OPV is now the vaccine of choice for the primary vaccination of children. Isolation of infected cases is no longer recommended, and quarantine is of no value.

Hepatitis is a general description for a collection of illnesses, the majority of which are caused by identifiable viruses whose common effect is jaundice resulting from liver inflammation. Hepatitis A virus (HAV) was identified in the stools of infected individuals in 1973. Hepatitis B virus (HBV) was first isolated earlier, in approximately 1965, at first being termed Australia antigen because it was identified in the serum of an Australian aborigine. Later it was linked to the causation of posttransfusion hepatitis. Some cases of posttransfusion hepatitis that are not caused by HBV are encountered. In these cases, hepatitis A cannot be incriminated either, leading to the rather cumbersome definition of non-A/non-B hepatitis. This emphasizes the fact that this latter diagnosis can at present only be made by exclusion: The causative agent is likely again to be a virus, but hepatitis C or any possible subsequent lettering has not yet been identified.

Many infections with HAV are asymptomatic. In clinical cases, the onset is often sudden, with fever, malaise, anorexia, nausea, and abdominal discomfort generally followed in a few days by jaundice. Most often the illness lasts only 1 to 2 weeks, but it is occasionally more severe and prolonged. The diagnosis is confirmed by the discovery of HAV in the patient's stool. The disease has a worldwide distribution, with seasonal peaks of incidence in temperate climates but none in the tropics. The most common route of infection is the fecal-oral route. Control measures are aimed at improving hygiene standards and habits. Passive immunity may be temporarily conveyed to those at special risk (e.g., travelers to tropical areas) by the administration of immune serum globulin (ISG).

The clinical onset of illness due to HBV is by contrast generally insidious. Anorexia, vague abdominal discomfort, and nausea and vomiting progressing to jaundice constitute a common sequence. Fever is only variably present and generally slight. However, although some cases are mild, others progress to severe fulminating disease, sometimes ending with fatal hepatic necrosis. HBV demonstrates heterogeneous morphological and immunologic characteristics. Complex antigenic components have been defined. One group of components is hepatitis B surface antigen (HBsAg), which includes HBV itself. An entirely separate antigen is associated with the internal component or core of the virus, known as hepatitis B core antigen (HBcAg). Hepatitis B is diagnosed by demonstrating HBsAg in the serum in the acute phase of the illness. However, jaundice from other causes can occur in individuals who are chronic carriers of HBsAg. The eventual identification of HBcAg in such individuals confirms the presence of HBV infection. This is made possible by the development of a test for IgM anti-HBc. The principal modes of transmission of hepatitis B virus are (1) direct percutaneous inoculation by needle of contaminated serum or plasma or transfusion of infected blood or blood products, (2) nonneedle percutaneous transfer of infective serum or plasma, (3) introduction of infective serum or plasma onto mucosal surfaces, (4) introduction of infective secretions other than serum or plasma onto mucosal surfaces, and (5) indirect transfer of infective serum or plasma via vectors or inanimate environmental surfaces. HBV carrier mothers have also been known to infect their infants at birth. Despite the occurrence of HBsAg in saliva, HBV-contaminated blood and saliva are not known to become significantly aerosolized.

Airborne transmission cannot be ruled out but seems unlikely. Measures for the control of the disease have centered around educating populations likely to be in contact with the illness. They are taught the need for caution in dealing with blood and blood products and in handling any materials or needles used for percutaneous injection. The production of HBV vaccine has permitted the active immunization of those at special risk, including members of the medical and nursing professions and others whose duties involve them in dealing with potentially infective groups.

Infectious mononucleosis results from primary infection with the Epstein-Barr virus (EBV), which is a member of the herpesvirus family. The characteristic feature is hematologic changes. Early there may be leukocytosis or leukopenia, followed by the appearance of atypical lymphocytes or T cells. The commonly used Monospot test is a slide variant of the Paul-Bunnell agglutination test. A positive test should not be relied on as the only diagnostic measure: In rare cases it may be a lingering response to a previous infection. A positive test, atypical lymphocytes, and a compatible illness all are necessary for positive identification. Knowledge concerning prevention and control of the disease is deficient.

Herpes simplex virus (HSV) infections are very common, but up to 95% may be asymptomatic. In humans, the virus may be detected in saliva, skin lesions, cervical secretions, and urine. The primary method of transmission is by transfer from one human to another, chiefly by close personal contact. Gingivostomatitis is the most common manifestation. In compromised hosts, the illness may be severe, but it is generally very mild. Most of these illnesses are caused by HSV type 1. Genital herpes, caused by HSV-2, is rapidly becoming one of the most important sexually transmitted diseases in the Western world. Latent HSV infections reactivate readily when cellular immunity is depressed. Progress in means of prophylaxis and treatment of HSV infections is rapid, and new drugs and newer formulations of older agents are being introduced. Both vidarabine and acyclovir have their place currently. As means of prevention and control, those who have active genital lesions should be discouraged from having sexual intercourse. Generalized HSV infections of the newborn may generally be prevented by cesarean section in women at term who have genital HSV infections. Such cesarean sections should be carried out before the membranes rupture.

Bacterial infections

Streptococcal disease has several manifestations, the importance of which relate not only to the immediate morbidity of the acute illness but also to the longer-term sequelae they produce. The latter follow infections with group A beta-hemolytic streptococci, which may be classified further into several serological types. In cases of streptococcal pharyngitis, physicians are encouraged to take and read their patients' throat cultures. This makes both diagnosis and control an economical possibility and also eliminates delay in commencing effective treatment. Recently, instant tests for the presence of group A beta-hemolytic streptococci have been introduced and show promise of much greater speed, with the sacrifice of only a very small proportion of false-negative and false-positive errors. In addition to causing pharyngitis, the organism can also give rise to pyoderma. Scarlet fever results from infection with strains of the same type of organism, which additionally produces erythrogenic toxin.

The principal aim of treatment, which also aids control of the spread of infection, is the elimination of the organisms from the nasopharynx. The organism is characteristically sensitive to penicillin. For practical reasons, it is generally administered orally, but it could be more effectively given by injection, thus eliminating problems associated with obtaining patient compliance. When patients are allergic to penicillin, erythromycin may be substituted. In spite of adequate treatment, some patients become chronic carriers, acting as a source of infection for others. In spite of this known tendency, the use of prophylactic antibiotics for family members of those who have the disease is not advisable. Prophylaxis with antibiotics should be reserved for those patients who have other conditions that make them especially vulnerable to complications following streptococcal infection. Subsequent development of rheumatic fever or nephritis is the major hazard.

Relatively recently, group B streptococci have also been shown to have epidemiologic significance, especially in causing neonatal sepsis and neonatal meningitis.

Diphtheria is most frequently transmitted by droplet infection containing the causative organism, *Corynebacterium diphtheriae*. Both respiratory tract and skin manifestations of the disease may appear after an incubation period of 1 to 7 days. The characteristic appearance in the pharynx is that of the membrane, initially white and readily removed but later blue and adherent. In severe cases, there is both submandibular edema and lymphadenopathy, giving rise to a characteristic "bull neck" appearance. The amount of toxin absorbed seems to be the determining factor in the development of the severe complications of the disease, namely myocarditis and neuritis. That the occurrence of the illness in the United States and elsewhere in the developed countries of the world has markedly diminished is attributed to well-established immunization programs. In recent years, more than 50% of the cases reported have occurred in persons over the age of 20 years. This has led to the performance of limited surveys, which suggest that 40% or more of adults lack protective levels of circulating antibodies against diphtheria. Active immunization is possible with diphtheria toxoid, which is generally combined with both pertussis and tetanus toxoids in the vaccine DPT, which is recommended for children under 7 years of age. Where there are contraindications to pertussis vaccine, DT should be used. In persons over the age of 7 years, the frequency and severity of local reactions increases with this regimen, so the substitution of Td, which contains less diphtheria toxoid per dose, is recommended. If this formulation is used, the primary series of inoculations is still three doses, but booster doses every 10 years are recommended.

Treatment of patients with respiratory tract diphtheria is by the administration of diphtheria antitoxin. This is an example of passive immunity being conveyed in order to be therapeutic, as it neutralizes the circulating toxin. Household members and other close contacts of the disease should be given a dose of diphtheria toxoid appropriate for their age unless they have completed a primary course of immunization or received a booster dose within 5 years. As an aid to control of the number of cases of infection with this severe disease, health-care providers should use every patient encounter as an opportunity to review immunization state and to administer booster doses if necessary.

Meningococcal meningitis has a high morbidity and epidemic potential. However, the most common type of infection caused by the meningococcus occurs in the oro- or nasopharynx. In an occasional person, the organisms penetrate repiratory tract epithelium and cause bacteremia. Overwhelming septicemia can be rapidly fatal. The most common systemic manifestation is meningitis, but arthritis, pericarditis, and pneumonia may occur. Carriers are a frequent source of infection. The proportion of carriers in the community varies depending on season, age, and living conditions and may be as low as 5% or as high as 70%. Carriage may persist for a long time; in one study the mean was 10 months. The organism classically has been sensitive to sulfonamides. More recently, resistant strains have appeared, but in 1980 only 12% of U.S. strains tested were resistant. Strains resistant to penicillin have not been documented. The usefulness of sulfadiazine in mass prophylaxis has been demonstrated, but rifampin has been introduced as an alternative because of the emergence of resistant strains. Vaccines for several serogroups have been prepared and tested in some outbreaks; some of these are available in the United States. Respiratory isolation of patients with meningococcal disease is widely practiced, but its value is not proven.

Pertussis is a highly communicable disease that may have serious sequelae, but it is also vaccine preventable. The onset of the illness is insidious: Initially a shallow, irritating, non-productive cough, it later becomes much worse with paroxysms of coughing, which may be accompanied by the characteristic inspiratory whoop and also vomiting. Major complications include hypoxia, pneumonia, malnutrition, hypoglycemia, seizures, and encephalopathy. Laboratory confirmation of the diagnosis is made by culture of the organism from posterior nasopharyngeal swabs. Active immunization is the only method of proven value in prevention of the illness. The vaccine is now generally combined with that for diphtheria and tetanus (DPT), which has already been discussed. Chemoprophylaxis has been attempted with erythromycin given for 14 days, but only anecdotal reports are available to support its effectiveness. The risks and benefits of pertussis vaccination have been extensively discussed following reports linking administration of the vaccine with the development of subsequent neurological deficits. The publication of these reports in the media led to a decline in acceptance of the vaccination, which opened the way for two large epidemics of the disease. In Japan, all vaccine was removed from the market when two deaths occurred shortly after administration of the vaccine. A subsequent epidemic claimed more lives and resulted in increased morbidity. These experiences have helped to prevent exaggerated public response but have not prevented the manufacturers of the vaccine from being sued for damages. As a result, the cost of available vaccine has increased. While a quest for a safer yet effective vaccine continues, analyses of the health and cost benefits of pertussis vaccine have confirmed the advantages of continuing to offer the program. Physicians need to explain the situation

and risks sufficiently clearly for parents or others responsible to give informed consent to the procedure.

Pneumococcal pneumonia is usually a sporadic disease, but epidemics have occasionally occurred. Infection frequently seems to follow some other, generally minor, upper respiratory tract infection. It has been estimated that normally not more than 1 in 500 persons who have been shown to harbor the organism in the course of a year actually develop pneumonia. Pneumococci are part of the indigenous flora of the upper respiratory tract. Nowadays it may not be assumed that a pneumonia associated with the pneumococcus will respond to treatment with penicillin, because resistance of the organisms to the antibiotic has developed widely, yet it remains effective presently in about 97% of cases. Polyvalent vaccines have recently been produced and are currently advised for administration to the following groups of individuals:

1. Adults with chronic illness, especially cardiovascular disease.
2. Adults with diseases known to be associated with increased risk of pneumonia (e.g., Hodgkin's disease, splenic dysfunction, cirrhosis, alcoholism, multiple myeloma, etc.).
3. Older adults, age 65 or over, who are otherwise healthy.
4. Children age 2 years or older with chronic illnesses similar to those in adults but also including such conditions as sickle cell disease, nephrotic syndrome, etc.

The availability of the vaccine is not, however, a complete solution to the problems of prevention and control of this disease.

Tuberculosis (TB) persists as a prominent cause of disability and death in spite of considerable advances in prevention and treatment. The infection is conveyed from humans to each other as droplets derived from respiratory tract secretions that then are inhaled. Since the mycobacteria are relatively resistant to chemical agents, they may remain viable for long periods in dried sputum and in dust. The organism has been conveyed through the alimentary tract, and therefore poor hand hygiene or exposure to infected discharges or urine can also be methods of transmission. The onset of TB is insidious. The incubation period is thought to be about 3 to 8 weeks. Early symptoms include lower respiratory tract disease, low-grade fever, night sweats, cough, weight loss, fatigue, and occasional minor hemoptysis. Confirmation of the diagnosis is obtained by radiology, bacteriologic studies, and tuberculin testing. The standard method for the latter is the Mantoux test, the intradermal injection of purified protein derivative (PPD) in carefully regulated quantity and dilution. Multiple puncture tests are now used less frequently but may still be employed for screening purposes because of their simplicity and acceptability, especially by children. Repeated injections of PPD have never been shown, in the doses used for skin testing, to provoke sensitivity.

Tuberculin testing of population groups on a wide scale over many years has yielded much information about the prevalence of TB. In most developed countries, there has been a sharp drop in prevalence throughout this century. This is attributed to improved socioeconomic conditions as well as to improved medical care and treatment. These trends are well illustrated in Figure 6-8, showing mortality rates for selected birth cohorts of males.

Some additional comments are necessary. The decline in mortality for the younger age-groups has not been matched completely in older people, in whom mortality is relatively higher. This poses problems for physicians who care for geriatric patients, in whom TB remains an important cause of morbidity. The marked decrease in prevalence has also been noted to be mainly among the pulmonary type of infection. The incidence of extrapulmonary TB in the United States has remained little altered and in 1980 accounted for 14.2% of all reported cases.

Prevention and control of TB are still important activities for workers in public health, who need the active help of physicians if their efforts are to be successful. Control of airborne droplet infection is a first major step. Ultraviolet radiation of the air or exhaust fans to extract infection from patient-care rooms have been employed. Case finding and treatment are clearly important and in developed countries are now more cost-effective than screening programs. Chemoprophylaxis using isoniazid reduces tuberculin conversions and TB morbidity. At present, the recommended regimen for preventive treatment is isoniazid, 5 to 10 mg/kg of body weight up to a maximum of 300 mg, taken as a single daily dose for 6 to 12 months. Patients should be seen monthly in order to detect manifest hepatitis while on the regimen. Tuberculin reactors should also be treated, especially if the conversion is known to be recent or if they are infants or young children. Those at special risk should also be treated in a similar manner (e.g., household contacts, diabetics with some contact, etc.). Vac-

cination as a means of protection against TB has so far been disappointing. The agent, baccille Calmette-Guérin (BCG), has been used worldwide, but in 12-year follow-up studies has not yielded positive information indicating an overall protective effect. Although human TB still remains a problem, a major achievement of preventive medicine has been the control of bovine TB through nationwide tuberculin testing of herds and slaughter of infected animals. To emulate the success in human medicine, unremitting vigilance for undetected cases must remain a priority.

Leprosy is an infection related to TB, the organism responsible being *Mycobacterium leprae*. There the similarity ends. A tuberculoid form of the infection is described, usually displaying well-demarcated skin lesions with early nerve involvement. In lepromatous leprosy, the skin lesions are diffuse and may ulcerate; mucous membranes, the upper respiratory tract, and the lymphoid system are later involved in these patients, who are immunologically incompetent and unable to offer effective resistance to the infection. The diagnosis can be made clinically if any two of the following criteria are present:

1. A skin lesion that is anaesthetic to touch.
2. Acid-fast bacilli detected from an incised smear or biopsy.
3. A palpably enlarged superficial nerve.

Confirmation of the diagnosis is by microscopy of skin biopsy. The lepromin test is not diagnostic; if negative in a clinically confirmed patient, it confirms the absence of full immunologic response and suggests that the type of infection is lepromatous. Infection is transmitted by close contact, especially with nasal secretions. Bed contact is more likely to spread the disease than room contact. No effective immunization procedure has yet been discovered. Control depends on preventive treatment during the incubation period, which may be 1 to 20 years, and active case finding. Improved socioeconomic conditions make the spread of disease far less likely. Worthy of considerable attention is the fact that the incidence of new cases is steadily falling, being zero in Hawaii in the past 20 years, near zero in Japan, and very low in China.

The **enteric infections** are grouped here for convenience. They include illnesses caused by infections with *Salmonella typhi*, the shigella group of organisms, cholera, and *Escherichia coli*. All the organisms are conveyed by the fecal-oral route, and humans are the source of infection. In the case of cholera generally, and typhoid occasionally, water supplies have become infected and are the point source of epidemics on a local basis. Flies contaminating food have become vectors in some situations. As a means of conveying infection, certain foods have attained notoriety. However, the responsibility lies more with the food handler, whose technique and hygiene need to be improved. Foods that are not cooked after handling may be particularly dangerous in such situations. These include such varied items as salad and ice cream. Shigellosis occurs particularly in children, and those in day-care centers have been found to be particularly susceptible. In each case, effective control begins with adequate treatment with appropriate antibiotics for all detected cases in such a dosage and for such a

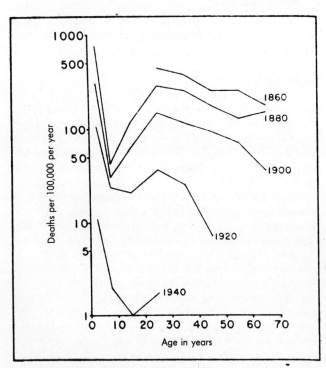

Figure 6-8. Tuberculosis mortality rates by age for selected birth cohorts of Massachusetts males.

duration as to minimize the risk of a chronic carrier state developing.

Vaccines are available to develop immunity to both typhoid and cholera. However, in the case of the former, the side effects of vaccination are so unpleasant and its effectiveness is so uncertain that its use is diminishing. Cholera vaccine, although without the unpleasant side effects of the typhoid vaccine, has nevertheless not been proved to be effective in control. New vaccines are being developed and may be an improvement. In either case, at present, since effective antibiotic treatment is now available, the most important step for the individual patient and for the community is for early cases to be adequately treated. Enterotoxic *E. coli* organisms cause diarrhea through both a heat-stable and a heat-labile toxin. This may be responsible for traveler's diarrhea, but other organisms may also be responsible (e.g., shigellae, salmonellae, vibrios, and certain viruses and parasites like giardiae and amoebas). Clean food and hygienic food handling are very good control measures, but the unfortunate traveler may not be able to locate them. Some have advocated the use of low-dosage prophylactic antibiotics in such situations, notably doxycycline and trimethoprim-sulfamethoxazole. Problems exist with this because some individuals are sensitive to the drugs and there is always the possibility of producing resistant strains of the organisms, perhaps more especially when low dosage is employed to minimize side effects.

Chlamydia trachomatis is an organism that has comparatively recently assumed greater importance. It has been recognized as being the causative agent of trachoma and inclusion conjunctivitis for some while, although the agent was earlier thought to be a virus. Now it is recognized that the same organism also causes lymphogranuloma venereum, nongonococcal urethritis, vaginitis, and cervicitis as a group of sexually transmitted diseases and that the infant born through an infected birth canal is at risk of contracting chlamydial pneumonia. At present, although the organism is susceptible to tetracyclines, at least in the more superficial types of infection it seems to respond more to good hygiene and sanitary precautions with improved socioeconomic conditions than to more specific measures.

Other bacterial infections that are common in medical practice have not been discussed here. The whole group of sexually transmitted diseases has not been fully discussed. In these and other situations, there are no specific preventive measures that are currently applicable from a purely medical point of view. There may be social implications in which the physician should become involved, but these are beyond the scope of this current work.

Parasitic infections

The most important member of this group is amebiasis. The organism is *Entamoeba histolytica*. Other amoebas infect human beings, but they are not pathogenic. The common site of amebiasis is the colon and rectum, but the organism does spread directly or by metastasis, especially to the liver. The cyst form of the parasite is the infective agent, and the portal of entry the alimentary canal. Cysts may remain viable in damp soil for at least 8 days and in clear cold water for as long as 90 days. Control of amebiasis can be a detailed epidemiologic exercise.

Studies of prevalence and of water and food supplies are necessary. The fecal-oral route clearly is implicated. Prophylactic medication is not recommended.

Nosocomial infections

Any infection that is neither incubating nor present at the time of admission but is acquired during the course of a hospital admission is defined as a nosocomial infection. During the mid-1970s, 5.7% of all admissions suffered nosocomial infections. Some were relatively minor, but most cause substantial morbidity, accounting for over 6 million excess hospital days per year, an average of three extra hospital days for each infected patient and an estimated additional cost of $2 billion annually at 1984 rates. Of infected patients, 1.5% die as a result of the infection, and nosocomial infection is a major contributing cause in the deaths of an additional 3 to 4% of infected patients.

Staphylococcus aureus used to be the organism that caused the majority of hospital infections. Although it remains a significant cause (10.8% of nosocomial infections), *E. coli* is now more common (19.7% of these infections). Now, all gram-positive bacteria cause 27.3% of these infections, gram-negative bacteria cause 47.6%, and all other organisms cause approximately 17%, the remainder not being identified as bacterial pathogens. In this group, about 6% are fungal infections.

To aid with the control of these infections, most hospitals now employ infection-control practitioners, the majority of whom are nurses, who assist with the collection and analysis of surveillance data. Much attention has been given to this problem by the Centers for Disease Control (CDC) on a national basis. As a result, an extensive literature has developed. Investigations have paid attention to microbiology laboratories, central services, housekeeping, food service operations, and laundries as potential sources of infection, in addition to physicians' behavior and nursing procedures in all areas of the hospital.

Foodborne disease

Foodborne diseases are a worldwide problem, occasionally referred to by the imprecise term "food poisoning." The latter description arose from those illnesses in which the multiplication of bacteria in food produces toxins that are injurious to humans. The wider description includes those diseases in which bacteria multiply and themselves invade the host, for example salmonellosis.

Three types of infection are included in a classification of foodborne diseases: Salmonellosis as has been stated is a notable example. In contrast to the toxin-producing diseases, fever is a common symptom. Of the viral infections, hepatitis A is a good example. The incubation period is frequently long, which makes identification of the food source very difficult. Parasitic infections include trichinosis and taeniasis.

The common forms of poisoning from toxins arise from staphylococcal or botulinal organisms. Certain chemicals, especially salts and oxides of arsenic, antimony, copper, and lead, can act as toxins producing GI upset. Poisons may also be of fungal or plant origins, including mushrooms, ergot-producing plants, and others such as hemlock. Of the animal-produced poisons, probably paralytic shellfish poisoning is the most common. Environmental pollution, for example from strontium 90, is no longer merely a theoretial risk of nuclear accidents or explosions.

The investigation of outbreaks is a very important epidemiologic activity. A careful history taken from every case of the disease, and later from all who have partaken of a suspected food source, is obviously important. Until the type of infection is known or at least suspected, the history of eating may need to vary from a meal eaten only 1 hour before the onset of symptoms to as much as 30 days. Once a source is suspected, a perfect match between all those who have eaten the particular item or meal may still not exist. There are several possible reasons for this: The implicated food may not be contaminated throughout; some individuals (hosts) may be more or less sensitive than others; the quantity of the item consumed varies; and there may be uncertainty or even attempts to deceive on the part of those who have given the health history. A further possibility is that some individual cases may have been infected from another source or that, although the symptoms are similar, there may be a different infection causing sporadic cases.

The history of the outbreak may give very clear clues to the infection. When a number of people develop acute, predominantly upper GI tract symptoms within a few hours of eating a meal, staphylococcal food poisoning may be suscepted. Rare outbreaks of botulism may be suspected when several individuals develop signs of cranial nerve weaknesses—for example, blurring of vision, double vision, or ptosis. Less than 30% of infected individuals are now likely to have a fatal outcome of this infection, the immediate cause of death being respiratory paralysis.

Arthropod-borne diseases

A full discussion of all the diseases conveyed to humans by arthropod vectors is beyond the scope of this present work. A textbook of tropical medicine or public health should be consulted.

There are numerous viruses that are pathogenic and conveyed by arthropods. They are frequently referred to as **arboviruses**, which is a contraction of "arthropod-borne viruses." These viruses may have little in common other than the means of transmission. Some are conveyed by mosquitoes, others by ticks, and one by the phlebotomus fly (phlebotomus fever). Of the 489 arboviruses listed in the *International Catalogue of Arboviruses,* about 100 are known to be pathogenic to humans. The most significant conditions are the various forms of encephalitis, yellow fever, several forms of hemorrhagic fever, and dengue fever. The latter is an endemic-epidemic disease with a worldwide distribution.

There are ten major rickettsial infections in humans: epidemic, murine, and scrub typhus; tick typhus, occurring in five forms (Rocky Mountain spotted fever, northern Asian tick typhus, boutonneuse fever, North Queensland tick typhus, and rickettsial pox); trench fever; and Q fever. All of these conditions are conveyed through a bite of the vector—various forms of ticks, fleas, mites, and lice. Prevention can clearly be achieved by improved personal hygiene and habits and control of the vectors.

Plague, caused by the organism now known as *Yersinia*

pestis, is conveyed by fleas. The disease has a wide spread but sporadic distribution. In 1983, 715 cases leading to death in 48 were reported to WHO. Streptomycin is the most commonly used antibiotic, but alternatives are available. Patients are nursed in strict respiratory isolation for at least 48 hours after the initiation of antibiotic therapy. Immunization with either killed or live vaccines has been reported to be successful, but clearly rodent control and avoidance of flea bites are important methods of control.

Relapsing fever is caused by several types of spirochetes. The disease is conveyed by lice and ticks. The louse-borne form can only be transmitted by crushing an infected louse. The animal reservoir, if any, for this form of the disease has not yet been clearly identified. The disease is prevented by avoiding its vectors. Measures include the elimination or reduction of the tick population in dwellings by rodent proofing and by the use of residual insecticides.

Several **parasitic infections** are conveyed by insects and other arthropods. Of these, **malaria** is the most important, infecting over 200 million worldwide annually and contributing to the death of at least 1 million, of whom most are infants and young children. It is caused by four different species of the parasite—*Plasmodium falciparum, Plasmodium malariae, Plasmodium vivax,* and *Plasmodium ovale.* Each of these cause a characteristic type of malaria with its own pattern of pathology and epidemiology. The life cycle of the malarial parasite is diagrammatically represented in Figure 6-9.

The incubation period of malaria varies from 10 to 28 days, depending on the type of malaria. Paroxysms of fever are associated with the completion of each asexual cycle of the parasite in the human subject. The treatment of the acute attack is dealt with elsewhere, but it is important from the preventive point of view to recognize that in certain areas in which malaria is endemic, chloroquine-resistant strains have been identified. Also, it is necessary to realize that when malaria is due to either *P. vivax* or *P. ovale,* a potential for relapse exists. The hypnozoites in the liver are generally treated with primaquine for 14 days, but caution in using the drug must be observed in patients who may have G6PD deficiency.

An effective way of controlling the spread of malaria has

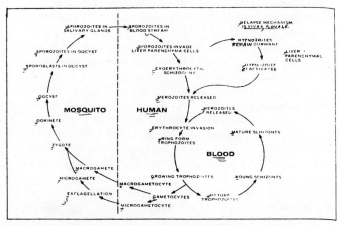

Figure 6-9. The life cycle of the malaria parasite.

been mosquito control. Various species of anopheles mosquito are known to transmit the disease, and each has its own habits and habitat. The elimination of breeding places of malaria-carrying mosquitoes by various methods is attempted. Substitution of alternative sources of blood meals for the mosquito other than the human host has also been attempted. Indoor house spraying with a residual insecticide containing chlorinated hydrocarbons retains an important role, in spite of concerns about the environmental effects of these substances. Pyrethrum extracts are still useful. Effective control may also be gained locally by the administration of drugs in preventive or suppressive dosages, but success here depends on the willingness of the population to support the project and comply with treatment regimens. Travelers are generally more willing to comply and may be effectively protected by this method.

Trypanosomiasis occurs in two forms: the African type causes sleeping sickness; the American type causes Chagas' disease. The former is conveyed to human subjects by the bites of *Glossina* flies, more commonly known as tsetse flies. A primary lesion or chancre occurs at this site, followed by parasitemia and CNS involvement. In the American form of the disease, infection is conveyed by various types of bugs. In this case, it is not the bug bites that convey the infection. When feeding, the bugs deposit infected feces, which may be rubbed into the skin, the parasites entering through the puncture wounds. A primary lesion or chancre is again formed, following which there is parasitemia. The form of the infection depends on the strain of the organism prevalent geographically: It may be neurotropic, viscerotropic, or cardiotropic. Several antiparasitic agents have been used in the treatment of the various forms of the disease, but effective therapy is difficult at present. This makes attempts at controlling the vectors and the amelioration of the social conditions that predispose toward the disease more important.

Other types of parasitic infections conveyed by arthropods include leishmaniasis, several filarial infections, and dracunculiasis (guinea worm disease). Full clinical descriptions are beyond the scope of the present work. The principles of prevention and control that have already been described apply in these conditions.

The zoonoses—diseases transmitted from animals

The lengthy list of zoonoses is perhaps surprising in view of the close relationship that appears to exist between humans and animals. Only those in which there are specific preventive measures will be considered here. Of these, perhaps one of the more important in view of the severity of the disease that may ensue and the possibility of contraction of the infection in the United States is **rabies**. This is a viral infection of the CNS conveyed by the bite of an infected animal. In the past 30 years, efforts to protect dogs from the disease by immunization have been largely successful, but the reservoir of the disease among wild animals seems to be increasing (Table 6-9).

The number of infected animals varies widely from state to state, in some the incidence of disease among animals being much higher. In such states it appears that there is an increasing risk of a higher incidence among the human population, but this has not yet been observed in fact. Table 6-9 does demonstrate the effectiveness of the canine immunization program that has been carried out, but it also demonstrates the need for continuing efforts in this area in view of the apparent increase of the reservoir of infection in wild animals, which, if not causing directly disease in humans, may once again increase the incidence in pets.

The incubation period of the disease in humans is quite variable. The more proximal the bite, the shorter the incubation period seems to be the rule. Extremes of 10 days to 1 year have been reported, with a mode of 6 weeks. Postexposure prophylactic treatment is made possible by this relatively long incubation period. The CDC recommends a five-dose regimen using a human diploid cell vaccine (HDCV), the vaccine being given on days 0, 3, 7, 14, and 28. Antirabies serum (ARS) or RIG should be given to all persons bitten by animals in which rabies cannot be ruled out and also for exposure to animals that are known to be rabid even if there is no history of a bite (Table 6-10).

In many parts of the world, rabies has been controlled or eradicated by quarantine measures applied to the dog population, but this is only effective where wild animals are not involved in the propagation of the disease. A permanent solution to the problem of the reservoir of disease in wild animals seems likely to prove exceedingly difficult.

Of the **bacterial diseases** communicated directly to humans from animals, several have important clinical importance. **Psittacosis** causes a pneumonitis spread directly from its reservoir in domestic pet birds, and sometimes from turkey processing plants. **Brucellosis** is contracted from mammals, especially those that are used to produce milk—cattle and

Table 6-9. Reported Rabies Cases in the United States (1938–1983)

Year	Dogs	Cats	Farm animals	Foxes	Skunks	Bats	Raccoons	Other animals	Humans	Total
1938	8,452	207	662	—	—	—	—	44	47	*
1946	8,384	455	1,055	—	—	—	—	956	33	10,883
1954	4,083	462	1,032	1,028	547	4	—	118	8	7,282
1962	565	232	614	594	1,449	157	62	52	2	3,727
1970	185	135	399	771	1,235	296	181	71	3[a]	3,276
1978	119	96	254	148	1,657	567	404	49	4	3,298
1983	132	169	282	111	2,285	909	1,906	45	2	5,841

*Lack of surveillance in earlier years yields incomplete totals.

Table 6-10. Postexposure Rabies Prophylaxis Guide

Animal species	Condition of animal at time of attack	Treatment of exposed person* (All bites and wounds should immediately be thoroughly cleansed with soap and water)
Domestic dog and cat	Healthy and available for 10 days of observation	None, unless animal develops rabies† RIG‡ and HDCV
	Rabid or suspected rabid	Consultation with public health officials. If treatment is indicated, give RIG‡ and HDCV
	Unknown (escaped)	
Wild: skunk, bat, fox, coyote, raccoon, bobcat, and other carnivores	Regard as rabid unless proved negative by laboratory test§	RIG‡ and HDCV
Other: livestock, rodents, and lagomorphs such as rabbits and hares	Consider individually. Local and state public health officials should be consulted about questions that arise about the need for rabies prophylaxis. Bites of squirrels, hamsters, guinea pigs, gerbils, chipmunks, rats, mice and other rodents, or rabbits and hares almost never call for antirabies prophylaxis.	

The above recommendations are only a guide. They should be applied in conjunction with knowledge of the animal species involved, circumstances of the bite or other exposure, immunization status of the animal, and presence of rabies in the region. Local or state public health officials should be consulted if questions arise about the need for rabies prophylaxis.

*If antirabies treatment is indicated, both rabies immune globulin (RIG) and human diploid cell vaccine (HDCV) should be given as soon as possible, regardless of the interval from exposure. Local reactions to vaccines are common and do not contraindicate continuing treatment. Discontinue vaccine if fluorescent antibody tests of animals are negative.

†Begin treatment with RIG and HDCV at first sign of rabies in biting dog or cat during the usual holding period of 10 days. The symptomatic animal should be killed immediately and tested.

‡If RIG is not available, use antirabies serum (ARS) of equine origin. Do not use more than the recommended dosage.

§The animal should be killed and tested as soon as possible. Holding for observation is not recommended.

goats. It is conveyed by direct contact with infected animals, especially after parturition or abortion, but the organisms may also be shed in milk. Worldwide, ingestion of unpasteurized dairy products is the most common source of infection. Pasteurization of these products and milk is an effective control method. **Anthrax** is also a disease affecting farm animals. The natural reservoir of the organism is in soil, from which animal outbreaks arise. Annual immunization of livestock helps to control the disease among humans. **Leptospirosis,** a type of spirochetal infection, occurs maainly though contact with the infected urine of animals. The animals infected may be dogs, cattle, swine, rats, and mice. Some types of *Salmonella* infection have reservoirs in animals, especially cattle, pigs, and poultry. In the early 1970s, a particular strain of *Salmonella* was introduced in poultry through infected fish meal. Later, this particular organism was isolated from many cases of salmonellosis in humans.

TOXICOLOGY, OCCUPATIONAL AND ENVIRONMENTAL MEDICINE

In the previous section, reference was made to the toxins produced by certain microorganisms. Other substances also have toxic effects in humans. Some of these occur naturally, and their study has given rise to the science of environmental toxicology. Many toxic substances encountered today do not occur naturally. Many are produced as products or by-products of industrial processes. The same industrial processes

and others may give rise to other morbidity and even cause significant mortality. It is convenient to consider all these industrially and environmentally related diseases together from the perspective of prevention.

THE EFFECTS OF TOXINS

The study of the harmful effects of chemicals on biologic systems is known as **toxicology**. It is built on the disciplines of biochemistry, physiology, pathology, physical chemistry, pharmacology, and public health. It describes and measures the biologic uptake, distribution, effects, metabolism, and excretion of toxic chemicals. A full description of all these processes is beyond the scope of this book. For additional details, the reader is referred to standard works on the subject, or for a more clinically related account of the topic in relation to occupational medicine to the text by Levy and Wegman.

Toxins may be ingested in various physical forms: as dusts, fumes, mists, and vapors as well as the common solids or liquid forms. Absorption may take place through the respiratory tract, the skin, and the GI tract. A variety of factors can influence the rate and amount of absorption through each of these routes. Some toxins exert their effects at the site of initial contact; others enter the body and are conveyed, usually by the bloodstream, to other parts of the body, eventually reaching an organ through which the toxic effects may become apparent and/or are stored to produce effects for a greater duration of time. Membranes are the main barriers to absorption. Toxins may pass through them in a manner that is governed by the physical chemistry of diffusion. Storage may involve binding to human proteins, thus prolonging toxic effects. Finally, metabolic transformation and excretion may affect the duration and severity of toxic effects.

The principles of the biologic effects produced depend also on a series of processes described as concepts. Exposure may be acute or chronic. Acute exposure is likely to produce acute effects, and chronic to produce chronic effects. The effects may be reversible or irreversible, and some toxins may produce both. For example, chronic lead poisoning may cause effects on the blood, renal system, CNS, GI tract, and reproductive system, but all but some late renal and possibly some nervous system effects are reversible. Generally, higher levels of exposure lead to more severe effects, but there may be a threshold for response and also a limit known as a **ceiling level**.

The potency of a toxin is frequently described in terms of the LD_{50}: the dose that is lethal to 50% of the population. Individual departures from the dose-response pattern may be determined by hypersusceptibility or hypersensitivity on the one hand or by tolerance on the other.

Some toxins, their routes of entry, and their effects are listed in Table 6-11.

THE MEDICAL OCCUPATIONAL HISTORY

With all the possibilities that exist for meeting toxic substances in the workplace, it becomes apparent that some form of occupational history is relevant for every patient. It is impracticable to take a detailed history of occupations for every patient, as this may take 20 minutes or longer. It is recommended that at least every history should include a note of the patient's two major previous jobs and current occupation. In cases where the complaints indicate the possibility of disease in the following categories, a more detailed occupational history is indicated because of the high probability that the disease may be occupationally related. Only if physicians follow this advice will it become possible to identify new possibilities of work-related disease in industries that are employing new technologies. The categories of disease of occupational significance are respiratory disease, skin disorders, hearing impairment, back and joint symptoms, cancer, coronary artery disease, liver disease, and neuropsychiatric disorders. Perhaps more importantly, the possibility of an occupationally related cause should be remembered in all cases of disease of unknown etiology.

Some industrial processes are reecognized to be particularly hazardous. Common processes and their recognized hazards and routes of entry are listed in Table 6-12.

The possibility of encountering carcinogens in the workplace has already been mentioned. These associations have frequently only been discovered by careful inquiry and documentation of cases by an individual physician. It is clearly important not to allow rumors to spread when a possible association is only being investigated. An injudicious comment to a patient under these conditions could lead to expensive legal actions and to harm to the patient, the employer, and/or the physician. Highest ethical standards of behavior and very careful observation and investigation are imperative if these unpleasant situations are to be avoided. Although it may be necessary to discuss with an employer and workers the possible association that is being investigated in an attempt to avoid

further possible loss or injury, extreme tact is needed. A strong, favorable interpersonal relationship between the physician and others involved prior to the investigation of the crisis is extremely valuable.

Table 6-13 lists the principal sites of well-recognized associations and contacts with carcinogens in the workplae.

OTHER HAZARDS IN THE WORKPLACE

In addition to exposing personnel to possible toxins, the workplace may harbor other hazards. Some of these are the result of inadequate or carelessly applied safety precautions, resulting in occupational accidents. In some of these, workers are struck by some of the tools, machinery, or materials that are being handled in the industrial process. This is one of the mechanisms of injury classified by the American National Standards Institute (ANSI). Other injuries may be caused by overexertion, falls from elevations or on the same level, being caught between materials or machinery, or motor vehicle accidents. Other trauma may result from the injurious nature of the working environment, such as ionizing radiation, or rather more mundanely by workplace noise, which may give rise to hearing impairment. It must not be forgotten also that infectious agents may be encountered in the workplace. Psychological and social factors may cause occupationally related stress. The responsibility for identifying the causes of these injuries is not solely that of the physician. Medically it is important for the sake of the individual patient, for the welfare and safety of his or her colleagues, and to enable the employer to identify possible and actual causes of injury that the possible relationship between work and these types of injury be recognized.

For further discussion of the specific conditions that are or may be occupationally related, the reader is referred to a later section dealing with specific types of preventable disease.

SCREENING FOR DISEASE

The early detection of disease is clearly an important function of any preventive medicine program. If disease can be detected at such an early stage that it is truly asymptomatic, this is recognized as secondary prevention. Since the 1920s, the practice of performing an annual physical examination was carried out in anticipation that this would confer long-term health benefits. Fifty years later, increasing cost consciousness, changing expectations of patients, and refined methods for studying the efficacy of diagnostic tests raised serious questions about the value of the annual checkup. The U.S. Preventive Services Task Force is now beginning to make its recommendations.

If a particular screening procedure is to be recommended for widespread adoption, it must meet some fairly rigid criteria. The impact of the disease on an individual for which a detection procedure is proposed must cause a current burden of suffering assessed by the years of life likely to be lost, the amount of disability, the pain and discomfort, the cost of treatment, and an effect on the individual's family that is significant. The impact on society in terms of mortality, morbidity, and the cost of treatment involved in dealing with

Table 6-11. Toxins—A Compendium

Agent	Exposure	Route of entry	System(s) affected	Primary manifestation	Aids in diagnosis*	Remarks
Metals and metallic compounds						
Arsenic	Alloyed with lead and copper for hardness; mfg. of pigments, glass, pharmaceuticals; by-product in copper smelting; intesecticides; fungicides; rodenticides; tanning	Inhalation and ingestion of dust and fumes	Neuromuscular	Peripheral neuropathy, sensory > motor	Arsenic in urine	
			GI	Nausea and vomiting, diarrhea, constipation		
			Skin	Dermatitis, finger and toenail striations, skin cancer, nasal septum perforation		
			Pulmonary	Lung cancer		
Arsine	Accidental by-product of reaction of arsenic with acid	Inhalation of gas	Hematopoietic	Intravascular hemolysis; hemoglobinuria, jaundice, oliguria or anuria		
Beryllium	Hardening agent in metal alloys; special use in nuclear energy production	Inhalation of fumes or dust	Pulmonary (and other organs)	Granulomatosis and fibrosis	Beryllium in urine (acute) Beryllium in tissue (chronic) Chest x-ray	Pulmonary changes virtually indistinguishable from sarcoid on chest x-ray.
Cadmium	Electroplating; solder for aluminum; metal alloys; process engraving; nickel-cadmium batteries	Inhalation or ingestion of fumes or dust	Pulmonary	Pulmonary edema (acute) Emphysema (chronic)		Also a urinary tract carcinogen.
			Renal	Nephrosis	Urinary protein	
Chromium	In stainless and heat resistant steel and alloy steel metal plating; chemical and pigment mfg.; photography	Percutaneous absorption, inhalation, ingestion	Pulmonary	Lung cancer	Urinary chromate (questionable value)	
			Skin	Dermatitis, skin ulcers, nasal septum perforation		
Lead	Storage batteries; mfg. of paint, enamel, ink, glass, rubber, ceramics; chemical industry	Ingestion of dust, inhalation of dust or fumes	Hematologic Renal GI	Anemia Nephropathy Abdominal pain ("colic")	Blood lead Urinary delta-aminolevulinic acid (ALA) Zinc protoporphyrin (ZPP); free erythrocyte protoporphyrin (FEP)	Lead toxicity, unlike that of mercury, is believed to be reversible, with the exception of late renal and some CNS effects.
			Neuromuscular	Palsy ("wrist drop")		
			CNS	Encephalopathy, behavioral abnormalities		
			Reproductive	Spontaneous abortions		

TABLE 6-11. (*Continued*)

Agent	Exposure	Route of entry	System(s) affected	Primary manifestation	Aids in diagnosis*	Remarks
Mercury (Hg) Elemental	Electronic equipment; paint; metal and textile production; catalyst in chemical mfg.; pharmaceutical production	Inhalation of vapor; slight percutaneous absorption	Pulmonary CNS	Acute pneumonitis Neuropsychiatric changes (erethism); tremor	Urinary Hg	Mercury illustrates several principles. The chemical form has profound effect on its toxicology, as is case for many metals. Effects of Hg highly variable. Though inorganic Hg poisoning is primarily renal, elemental and organic Hg poisoning are primarily neurological. These responses are difficult to quantify, so dose-response data are generally unavailable. Classic tetrad of gingivitis, sialorrhea, irritability, and tremor is associated with both elemental and inorganic Hg poisoning; the four signs not generally seen together. Many effects of Hg toxicity, especially those in CNS, are irreversible.
Inorganic		Some inhalation and GI and percutaneous absorption	Pulmonary Renal CNS	Acute pneumonitis Proteinuria Variable	Urinary Hg	
Organic	Agricultural and industrial poisons	Efficient GI absorption, percutaneous absorption, and inhalation	Skin CNS	Dermatitis Sensorimotor changes, visual field constriction, tremor	Blood and urine Hg, but ? sensitivity	
Nickel	Corrosion-resistant alloys; electroplating; catalyst production; nickel-cadmium batteries	Inhalation of dust or fumes	Skin	Sensitization dermatitis ("nickel itch")		
			Pulmonary	Lung and para-nasal sinus cancer		

TABLE 6-11. (*Continued*)

Agent	Exposure	Route of entry	System(s) affected	Primary manifestation	Aids in diagnosis*	Remarks
Nickel carbonyl	Intermediate in nickel refining; catalyst in petroleum, plastic, rubber industries	Inhalation of vapor, percutaneous absorption of liquid	Pulmonary	Severe irritation, pneumonitis Lung and paranasal sinus cancer	Urinary nickel (acute)	
Zinc oxide†	Welding by-product; rubber mfg.	Inhalation of dust or fumes that are freshly generated		"Metal fume fever" (fever, chills, and other symptoms)	Urinary zinc (useful as an indicator of exposure, not for acute diagnosis)	A self-limiting syndrome of 24–48 hours, with apparently no sequelae.
Hydrocarbons Benzene	Mfg. of organic chemicals, detergents, pesticides, solvents, paint removers; used as a solvent	Inhalation of vapor; slight percutaneous absorption	CNS Hematopoietic Skin	CNS depression Leukemia, aplastic anemia Dermatitis	Urinary phenol	Note that benzene, like toluene and other solvents, can be monitored via its principal metabolite.
Toluene	Organic chemical mfg.; solvent; fuel component	Inhalation of vapor, percutaneous absorption of liquid	CNS Skin	CNS depression Irritation, dermatitis	Urinary hippuric acid	Toluene lacks the leukemogenic effect of benzene, but commercial toluene is often contaminated with benzene.
Xylene	A wide variety of uses as a solvent; an ingredient of paints, lacquers, varnishes, inks, dyes, adhesives, cements; an intermediate in chemical mfg.	Inhalation of vapor; slight percutaneous absorption of liquid	Pulmonary Eyes, nose, throat CNS	Irriation, pneumonitis, acute pulmonary edema (at high doses) Irritation CNS depression	Methylhippuric acid in urine, xylene in expired air, xylene in blood	
Ketones Acetone Methyl ethyl ketone (MEK) Methyl n-propyl ketone (MPK) Methyl n-butyl ketone (MBK) Methyl isobutyl ketone (MIBK)	A wide variety of uses as solvents and intermediates in chemical mfg.	Inhalation of vapor, percutaneous absorption of liquid	CNS PNS Skin	Narcosis MBK has been linked with peripheral neuropathy Dermatitis	Acetone in blood, urine, expired air (used as an index of exposure, not for diagnosis)	The ketone family demonstrates how a pattern of toxic responses (i.e., CNS narcosis) may feature exceptions (i.e., MBK peripheral neuropathy).

TABLE 6-11. (*Continued*)

Agent	Exposure	Route of entry	System(s) affected	Primary manifestation	Aids in diagnosis*	Remarks
Trichloro-ethylene (TCE)	Solvent in metal degreasing, dry cleaning, food extraction; ingredient of paints, adhesives, varnishes, inks	Inhalation, percutaneous absorption	CNS PNS Skin Cardiovascular	CNS depression Peripheral and cranial neuropathy Irritation, dermatitis Arrhythmias	Breath analysis for TCE	TCE is involved in an important pharmacologic interaction. Within hours of ingesting alcoholic beverages, TCE workers experience flushing of the face, neck, shoulders, and back. Alcohol may also potentiate the CNS effects of TCE. The probable mechanism is competition for metabolic enzymes.
Carbon tetrachloride	Solvent for oils, fats, lacquers, resins, varnishes, etc.; used as a degreasing and cleaning agent	Inhalation of vapor	Hepatic Renal CNS Skin	Toxic hepatitis Oliguria or anuria CNS depression Dermatitis	Expired air and blood levels	Carbon tetrachloride is the prototype for a wide variety of solvents that cause hepatic and/or renal damage. This solvent, like trichlorethylene, acts synergistically with ethanol.
Carbon disulfide (CS$_2$)	Solvent for lipids, sulfur, halogens, rubber, phosphorus, oils, waxes, and resins; mfg. of organic chemicals, paints, fuels, explosives, viscose rayon	Inhalation of vapor, percutaneous absorption of liquid or vapor	CNS PNS Renal Cardiovascular Skin Reproductive	Parkinsonism, psychosis, suicide Peripheral neuropathies Chronic nephritic and nephrotic syndromes Acceleration or worsening of atherosclerosis; hypertension Irritation; dermatitis Menorrhagia and metrorrhagia	Iodine-azide reaction with urine (nonspecific since other bivalent sulfur compounds give a positive test); CS$_2$ in expired air, blood, and urine	A solvent with unusual multisystem effects, especially noted for its cardiovascular, renal, and nervous system actions.

TABLE 6-11. (*Continued*)

Agent	Exposure	Route of entry	System(s) affected	Primary manifestation	Aids in diagnosis*	Remarks
Methanol	Formaldehyde production; used in paints, varnishes, cements, inks, dyes	Inhalation of vapor, percutaneous absorption of liquid	Acid-base Ocular	Metabolic acidosis Optic nerve damage and blindness	Urinary formic acid; methanol in blood and urine; acidosis	Methanol acts through its metabolites formaldehyde and formic acid. Notable is its specific nerve toxicity.
Stoddard solvent	Degreasing, paint thinning	Inhalation of vapor, percutaneous absorption of liquid	Skin CNS	Dryness and scaling from defatting; dermatitis Dizziness, coma, collapse (at high levels)		A mixture of primarily aliphatic hydrocarbons, with some benzene derivatives and naphthenes.
Ethylene glycol ethers Ethylene glycol monoethyl ether (cellosolve) Ethylene glycol monoethyl ether acetate (cellosolve acetate) Methyl- and butyl- substituted compounds such as ethylene glycol monomethyl ether (methyl cellosolve)	The ethers are used as solvents for resins, paints, lacquers, gum, perfume, dyes, and inks; the acetate derivatives are widely used solvents and ingredients of lacquers, enamels, and adhesives. Exposure occurs in dry cleaning, plastic, ink, and lacquer manufacturing, and textile dying, among other places	Inhalation of vapor, percutaneous absorption of liquid	CNS Renal Liver Hematopoietic	Fatigue, lethargy, nausea, headaches, anorexia, tremor, stupor (due to encephalopathy) Renal failure following acute ingestion) Chemical hepatitis Pancytopenia	}	Effects associated with ethylene glycol ethers. Effects associated with ethylene glycol monomethyl ether (methyl cellosolve).
Dioxane	Used as a solvent for a variety of materials, including cellulose acetate, dyes, fats, greases, resins, polyvinyl polymers, varnishes, and waxes	Inhalation of vapor, percutaneous absorption of liquid	CNS Renal Liver	Drowsiness, dizziness, anorexia, headaches, nausea, vomiting, coma Nephritis Chemical hepatitis		Dioxane has caused a variety of neoplasms in animals. Dioxane should not be confused with "dioxin" (2,3,7,8-trichlorodibenzo-*p*-dioxin), a contaminant of the chlorphenoxy herbicide 2,4,5-T (2,4,5-trichlorophenoxyacetic acid) and a known teratogen.

TABLE 6-11. (*Continued*)

Agent	Exposure	Route of entry	System(s) affected	Primary manifestation	Aids in diagnosis*	Remarks
Irritant gases						

Note: The less water-soluble the gas, the deeper and more delayed its irritant effect.

Agent	Exposure	Route of entry	System(s) affected	Primary manifestation	Aids in diagnosis*	Remarks
Ammonia	Refrigeration; petroleum refining; mfg. of nitrogen-containing chemicals, synthetic fibers, dyes, and optics	Inhalation of gas	Upper respiratory tract	Upper respiratory irritation		Also irritant of eyes and moist skin.
Hydrochloric acid	Chemical mfg.; electroplating; tanning; metal pickling; petroleum extraction; in rubber, photographic, and textile industries	Inhalation of gas or mist	Upper respiratory tract	Upper respiratory irritation		Strong irritant of eyes, mucous membranes, and skin.
Hydrofluoric acid	Chemical and plastic mfg.; catalyst in petroleum refining; aqueous solution for frosting, etching, and polishing glass	Inhalation of gas or mist	Upper respiratory tract	Upper respiratory irrtation		In solution, causes severe and painful burns of skin.
Sulfur dioxide	Mfg. of sulfur-containing chemicals; as a food and textile bleach; tanning; metal casting	Inhalation of gas, direct contact of gas or liquid phase on skin or mucosa	Middle respiratory tract	Bronchospasm (pulmonary edema or chemical pneumonitis in high dose)	CXR, PFTs‡	Strong irritant of eyes, mucous membranes, and skin.
Chlorine	Paper and textile bleaching; water disinfection; chemical mfg.; metal fluxing; detinning and de-zincing iron	Inhalation of gas	Middle respiratory tract	Tracheobronchitis, pulmonary edema, pneumonitis	CXR, PFTs	Chlorine combines with body moisture to form acids, which irritate tissues from nose to alveoli.
Fluorine	Uranium processing; mfg. of fluorine-containing chemicals; oxidizer in rocket fuel systems	Inhalation of gas	Middle respiratory tract	Laryngeal spasm, bronchospasm, pulmonary edema	CXR, PFTs	Potent irritant of eyes, mucous membranes, and skin.

TABLE 6-11. (*Continued*)

Agent	Exposure	Route of entry	System(s) affected	Primary manifestation	Aids in diagnosis*	Remarks
Ozone	Inert-gas-shielded arc welding; food, water, and air purification; food and textile bleaching; emitted around high-voltage electrical equipment	Inhalation of gas	Lower respiratory tract	Delayed pulmonary edema (generally 6–8 hours following exposure)	CXR, PFTs	Ozone has a free radical structure and can produce experimental chromosome aberrations; it may thus have carcinogenic potential.
Nitrogen oxides	Mfg. of acids, nitrogen-containing chemicals, explosives, etc.; by-product of many industrial processes	Inhalation of gas	Lower respiratory tract	Pulmonary irritation, bronchiolitis fibrosa obliterans ("silo filler's disease"), mixed obstructive-restrictive changes	CXR, PFTs	
Phosgene	Mfg. and/or burning of isocyanates, and mfg. of dyes and other organic chemicals; in metallurgy for ore separation	Inhalation of gas	Lower respiratory tract	Delayed pulmonary edema (delay seldom longer than 12 hours)	CXR, PFTs	
Isocyanates TDI (toulene diisocyanate) MDI (methylene diisocyanate) Hexamethylene diisocyanate and others	Polyurethane manufacture	Inhalation of vapor	Predominantly lower respiratory tract	Asthmatic reaction and accelerated loss of pulmonary function	CXR, PFTs	Isocyanates are both respiratory tract "sensitizers" and irritants in the conventional sense.
Asphyxiant gases Simple asphyxiants: nitrogen, hydrogen, methane, and others	Enclosed spaces in a variety of industrial settings	Inhalation of gas	CNS	Anoxia	O_2 in environment	No specific toxic effect; act by displacing O_2
Chemical asphyxiants Carbon monoxide	Incomplete combustion in foundries, coke ovens, refineries, furnaces, etc.	Inhalation of gas	Blood (hemoglobin)	Headache, dizziness, double vision	Carboxyhemoglobin	

TABLE 6-11. (*Continued*)

Agent	Exposure	Route of entry	System(s) affected	Primary manifestation	Aids in diagnosis*	Remarks
Hydrogen sulfide	Used in mfg. of sulfur-containing chemicals: by-product of petroleum produce use; decay of organic matter	Inhalation of gas	CNS Pulmonary	Respiratory center paralysis, hypoventilation Respiratory tract irritation	PaO_2	
Cyanides	Metallurgy, electroplating	Inhalation of vapor, percutaneous absorption, ingestion	Cellular metabolic enzymes (especially cytochrome oxidase)	Enzyme inhibition with metabolic asphyxia and death	Thiocyanate (SCN^-) in urine	
Pesticides Organophosphates: malathion, parathion, and others		Inhalation, ingestion, percutaneous absorption	Neuromuscular	Cholinesterase inhibition, cholinergic symptoms: nausea and vomiting, salivation, diarrhea, headache, sweating, meiosis, muscle fasciculations, seizures, unconsciousness, death	Refractoriness to atropine; plasma or red cell cholinesterase	As with many acute toxins, rapid treatment of organophosphate toxicity is imperative. Thus, diagnosis is often made based on history and a high index of suspicion rather than on biochemical tests. Treatment is atropine, to block cholinergic effects and 2-pyridine-aldoxine methiodide (2-PAM) to reactivate cholinesterase.
Carbamates: carbaryl (Sevin) and others		Inhalation, ingestion, percutaneous absorption	Neuromuscular	Same as organophosphates	Plasma cholinesterase; urinary 1-naphthol (index of exposure)	Treatment of carbamate poisoning is the same as that of organophosphate poisoning except that 2-PAM is contraindicated.
Chlorinated hydrocarbons: chlordane, DDT, heptachlor, chlordecone (Kepone), aldrin, dieldrin, uridine		Ingestion, inhalation, percutaneous absorption	CNS	Stimulation or depression	Urinary organic chlorine, or *p*-chlorophenyl acetic acid	The chlorinated hydrocarbons may accumulate in body lipid stores in large amounts.

TABLE 6-11. (*Continued*)

Agent	Exposure	Route of entry	System(s) affected	Primary manifestation	Aids in diagnosis*	Remarks
Bipyridyls: paraquat, diquat		Inhalation, ingestion, percutaneous absorption	Pulmonary	Rapid massive fibrosis, only following paraquat ingestion		An interesting toxin in that the major toxicity, pulmonary fibrosis, apparently occurs only after ingestion.

*Occupational and medical histories are, in most instances, the most important aids in diagnosis.
†Zinc oxide is a prototype of agents that cause metal fume fever.
‡PFTs are useful aids in diagnosis of irritant effects if the patient is subacutely or chronically ill.
CXR = chest x-rays; PFTs = pulmonary function tests; PNS = peripheral nervous system.
Adapted from Levy BS, Wegman DH (eds): Occupational Health—Recognizing and Preventing Work-Related Disease. Little, Brown & Co., Boston, 1983.

Table 6-12. Common Unit Processes and Associated Hazards by Route of Entry

Unit process	Route of entry and hazard
Abrasive blasting (surface treatment with high-velocity sand, steel shot, pecan shells, glass, aluminum, oxide, etc.)	Inhalation: silica, metal, and paint dust Noise
Acid/alkali treatments (dipping metal parts in open baths to remove oxides, grease, oil, and dirt)	
Acid pickling (with HCl, HNO_3, H_2SO_4, H_2CrO_4, HNO_3/HF)	Inhalation: acid mist Skin contact: burns and corrosion
Acid bright dips (with HNO_3/H_2SO_4)	Inhalation: NO_2, acid mists
Molten caustic descaling	Inhalation: smoke and vapors
Bath (high temperature)	Skin contact: burns
Blending and mixing (powders and/or liquid are mixed to form products, undergo reactions, etc.)	Inhalation: dusts and mists of toxic materials Skin contact: toxic materials
Crushing and sizing (mechanically reducing the particle size of solids and sorting larger from smaller with screens or cyclones)	Inhalation: dust, free silica Noise
Degreasing (removing grease, oil, and dirt from metal and plastic with solvents and cleaners)	
Cold solvent washing (clean parts with ketones, cellosolves, and aliphatic, aromatic, and Stoddard solvents)	Inhalation: vapors Skin contact: dermatitis and absorption Fire and explosion (if flammable) Metabolic: carbon monoxide formed from methylene chloride
Vapor degreasers (with trichloroethylene, methyl chloroform, ethylene dichloride, and certain fluorocarbon compounds)	Inhalation: vapors; thermal degradation may form phosgene, hydrogen chloride, and chlorine gases Skin contact: dermatitis and absorption

TABLE 6-12. (*Continued*)

Unit process	Route of entry and hazard
Electroplating (coating metals, plastics and rubber with thin layers of metals) 　Copper 　Chromium 　Cadmium 　Gold 　Silver	Inhalation: acid mists, HCN, alkali mists, chromium mists Skin contact: acids, alkalis Ingestion: cyanide compounds
Forging (deforming hot or cold metal by presses or hammering)	Inhalation: hydrocarbons in smokes (hot processes), including polyaromatic hydrocarbons, SO_2, CO, NO_x, and other metals sprayed on dies (e.g., lead and molybdenum) Heat stress Noise
Furnace operations (melting and refining metals; boilers for steam generation)	Inhalation: metal fumes, combustion gases, e.g., SO_2 and CO Noise from burners Heat stress Infrared radiation, cataracts
Grinding, polishing, and buffing (an abrasive is used to remove or shape metal or other material)	Inhalation: toxic dusts from both metals and abrasives Noise
Industrial radiography (x-ray or gamma ray sources used to examine parts of equipment)	Radiation exposure
Machining (metals, plastics, or wood are worked or shaped with lathes, drills, planers, or milling machines)	Inhalation: airborne particles, cutting oil mists, toxic metals, nitrosamines formed in some water-based cutting oils Skin contact: cutting oils, solvents, sharp chips Noise
Materials handling and storage (conveyors, forklift trucks are used to move materials to/from storage)	Inhalation: CO, exhaust particulate, dusts from conveyors, emissions from spills or broken containers
Mining (drilling, blasting, mucking to remove loose material and materials transport)	Inhalation: silica dust, NO_2 from blasting, gases from the mine Heat stress Noise
Painting and spraying (applications of liquids to surfaces, e.g., paints, pesticides, coatings)	Inhalation: solvents as mists and vapors, toxic materials Skin contact: solvents, toxic materials
Soldering (joining metals with molten alloys of lead or silver)	Inhalation: lead and cadmium particulate ("fumes") and flux fumes
Welding and metal cutting (joining or cutting metals by heating them to molten or semimolten state) 　Arc welding 　Resistance welding 　Flame cutting and welding 　Brazing	Inhalation: metal fumes, toxic gases and materials, flux particulate, etc. Noise: from burner Eye and skin damage from infrared and ultraviolet radiation

The health hazards may also depend on the toxicity and physical form(s) (gas, liquid, solid, powder, etc.) of the materials used. For further information see Burgess WA: Recognition of Health Hazards in Industry: A Review of Materials and Processes. New York, Wiley, 1981.

Table 6-13. Principal Sites of Occupational Cancer

Site of cancer	Carcinogens	Occupations
Lung	Arsenic; asbestos; chromium; coal products; dusts; iron oxide; mustard gas; nickel; petroleum; ionizing radiation; bis-chloromethyl ether (BCME)	Vintners; miners; asbestos users; textile users; insulation workers; automobile brake and clutch mechanics; tanners; smelters; glass and pottery workers; coal tar and pitch workers; iron foundry workers; electrolysis workers; retort workers; exposed medical personnel; radium dial painters; chemical workers
Pleura and peritoneum	Asbestos	Asbestos users; textile users; insulation workers; automobile brake and clutch mechanics; construction workers; shipyard workers
Nasal cavity and sinuses	Chromium; isopropyl oils; nickel; wood and leather dusts	Glass, pottery, and linoleum workers; nickel smelters, mixers, and roasters; electrolysis workers; wood, leather, and shoe workers
Bladder	Coal products; aromatic amines; leather dusts	Asphalt, coal tar, and pitch workers; gas stokers; still cleaners; dyestuffs users; rubber workers; textile dyers; paint manufacturers; leather and shoe workers
Skin	Arsenic; sunlight; coal soot; coal tar and other products of coal combustion; petroleum and petroleum products	Insecticide makers and sprayers; oil refiners; vintners; smelters; farmers; gashouse workers; asphalt, coal tar, and pitch workers; coke-oven workers; miners; workers in contact with lubricating, cooling, or fuel oils
Liver	Arsenic; vinyl chloride	Tanners, smelters, vineyard workers; plastic workers
Bone marrow	Benzene; ionizing radiation	Benzene, explosives, and rubber cement workers; distillers; dye users; painters; exposed medical personnel

Adapted from Cole P, Merletti F: Chemical agents and occupational cancer. J Environ Pathol Toxicol 3:399, 1980.

the condition must also be significant. The greater the effect in these areas, the more likely is it that the procedure will be strongly recommended. Further, the test must have a sensitivity, specificity, and predictive value that are proven and must be safe, simple, not too costly, and acceptable to the patient.

Evidence for each of the above characteristics of an appropriate screening procedure is accepted based on the following criteria, the most significant being listed first:

1. Evidence obtained from at least one properly randomized controlled trial.
2. Evidence from controlled trials without randomization.
3. Evidence obtained from well-designed cohort or case-control analytic studies, preferably from more than one center or research group.
4. Evidence obtained from multiple time series studies with or without intervention. Dramatic results in uncontrolled experiments (such as the results of the introduction of penicillin treatment in the 1940s) could also be regarded as this type of evidence.
5. Opinions of respected authorities, based on clinical experience, descriptive studies, or reports of expert committees.

Based on these considerations, it is now possible to make recommendations about whether a specific test should be included in the periodic examination of an individual of a known age and sex. In some, there is good evidence to support the use of the test in the periodic examination. In others, the evidence is only fair or poor. Alternatively, there may be fair or good evidence that the test should be excluded from such examinations. These decisions are reached by calculations that include an assessment of cost-effectiveness as well as the more medical aspects of predictive value. For example, it was demonstrated that 47,207 routine proctosigmoidoscopies led to the discovery of 55 previously undiagnosed rectal cancers. From this has been derived the conclusion that it generally takes 4,000 of this kind of examination to find one cancer, at a cost of about $120,000 per discovery. This type of observation and comment has resulted in warnings that prevention may be so expensive that it could consume the whole of the health-care dollar. Thus the practice of good preventive medicine might be doomed in the infancy of the ability to perform reliable tests.

The value of a definitive test giving evidence of a treatable but potentially life-threatening condition to an asymptomatic individual cannot be readily assessed. The cost to those who undergo the test with negative results is more personally realized. The longevity of the predictive value of a negative test, and therefore its worth, is more difficult for the individual to assess. Expressed in more pragmatic terms, an individual who has effective treatment for a condition he or she recognizes as potentially life threatening will value very highly the performance of the test that led to its discovery. The larger proportion of the population similarly tested but with negative results may or may not think the expenditure in paying for the test is justified. Attempts of health economists to support or oppose such preventive procedures continue, but with inconclusive results from a scientific point of view.

To add two further dimensions to the problem of evaluating preventive strategies, both cultural norms and sociological perspectives must be considered. Most physicians understand very well the scientific system and its values, which express the current understanding of the etiology of health and disease. Most also begin to understand something of the economic system, which determines how health care is, or may be, financed. The cultural system, which defines the roles of and expectations for healers, is frequently less well understood. The sociological viewpoint describes the interaction between these three systems. Even if the fullness of this interaction cannot be appreciated by an individual whose basic training is in medicine, it may be possible to discern that these three systems and their interaction may so influence a particular locality at a given point in time that acceptable preventive procedures may not be those that are more generally acceptable.

As a result of some of these realizations, it has now been demonstrated that it is much more difficult to produce an "ideal" health-maintenance protocol than was formerly thought. Thus the content of an ideal periodic physical examination is less frequently described. Each physician should be encouraged to develop a protocol for regular physical examinations that are age and sex specific and that also take into account the cultural and economic backgrounds of the patients in the practice, the common local industries, local hazards that may lead to morbidity or mortality, and environmental and other stresses that are common in the community, in addition to reviewing continuously the descriptions in medical texts of new strategies and technologies. The prospect and its complexities may truly be described as daunting. The process is never complete and must be continuously revised and updated.

One such product is the collection of protocols for lifetime health maintenance developed by the Department of Family Medicine of Wayne State University. The assumptions made in defining the procedures including in the protocols are as follows:

1. The protocols are intended for asymptomatic people with no unusual risk factors yet identified.
2. A complete history and physical exam are considered to be an essential part of the intake process and form the initial data base.

3. The protocols are oriented to primary and early secondary prevention.
4. When a risk factor is identified, whether by the history, physical examination, laboratory, or x-ray results, the protocol no longer applies for that risk factor and person. For example, if a 45-year-old woman is evaluated and the history indicates that her maternal grandmother, her mother, and two sisters died of breast cancer, an accelerated schedule for breast examination and mammography should be implemented. However, for "healthy" elements in the person's profile, the protocol should be followed.
5. All the screening procedures, with the exception of mammography, should be feasible in a primary care physician's office.

The application of these principles is illustrated by Figures 6-10 through 6-14 from the Department of Family Medicine at Wayne State University. The procedures and visit frequency conform in general to those recommended widely but contain variations introduced for a population that includes many families of lower educational and socioeconomic levels. The Denver Prescreening Developmental Questionnaire is used four times during the first year of life and then less frequently up to the age of 8 years. The full Denver Development Scale is

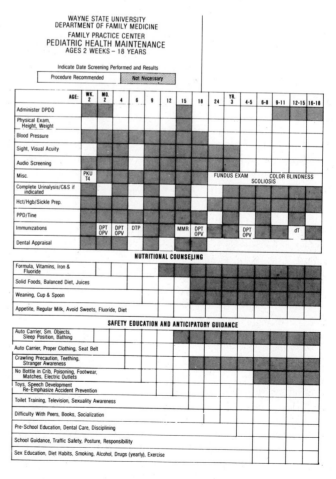

Figure 6-10. Protocol for pediatric health maintenance.

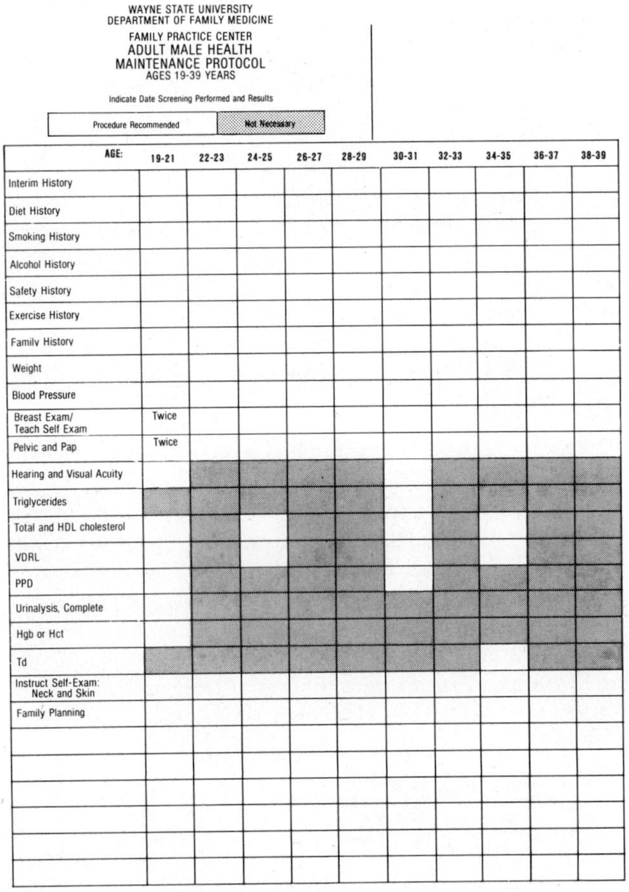

WAYNE STATE UNIVERSITY
DEPARTMENT OF FAMILY MEDICINE
FAMILY PRACTICE CENTER
ADULT MALE HEALTH
MAINTENANCE PROTOCOL
AGES 19-39 YEARS
Indicate Date Screening Performed and Results

Procedure Recommended | Not Necessary

AGE:	19-21	22-23	24-25	26-27	28-29	30-31	32-33	34-35	36-37	38-39
Interim History										
Diet History										
Smoking History										
Alcohol History										
Safety History										
Exercise History										
Family History										
Weight										
Blood Pressure										
Breast Exam/ Teach Self Exam	Twice									
Pelvic and Pap	Twice									
Hearing and Visual Acuity										
Triglycerides										
Total and HDL cholesterol										
VDRL										
PPD										
Urinalysis, Complete										
Hgb or Hct										
Td										
Instruct Self-Exam: Neck and Skin										
Family Planning										

Figure 6-11. Protocol for adult female health maintenance, ages 19–39 years.

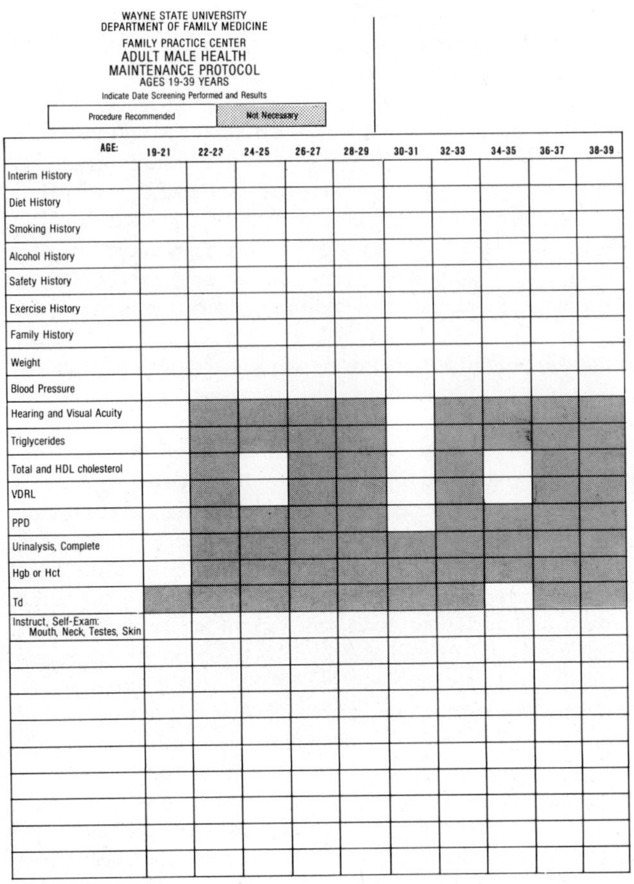

WAYNE STATE UNIVERSITY
DEPARTMENT OF FAMILY MEDICINE
FAMILY PRACTICE CENTER
ADULT MALE HEALTH
MAINTENANCE PROTOCOL
AGES 19-39 YEARS
Indicate Date Screening Performed and Results

Procedure Recommended | Not Necessary

AGE:	19-21	22-23	24-25	26-27	28-29	30-31	32-33	34-35	36-37	38-39
Interim History										
Diet History										
Smoking History										
Alcohol History										
Safety History										
Exercise History										
Family History										
Weight										
Blood Pressure										
Hearing and Visual Acuity										
Triglycerides										
Total and HDL cholesterol										
VDRL										
PPD										
Urinalysis, Complete										
Hgb or Hct										
Td										
Instruct, Self-Exam: Mouth, Neck, Testes, Skin										

Figure 6-12. Protocol for adult male health maintenance, ages 19–39 years.

used if the screening raises any questions about a child's developmental pattern.

Physical examination is constructed in accordance with the age and sex of the individual. Standard growth charts are also completed for children, who are examined for such physical findings as heart murmurs, otitis, undescended testicles, abdominal masses, and signs of Down's syndrome. Blood pressure monitoring is specifically included beginning at 24 months because of a higher-than-usual frequency in the population served. Examinations for funduscopic abnormalities and color blindness are performed at a suitable time during the period indicated when the child is cooperative. Nutritional anemia is relatively common in the population, so, although this is not generally recommended, routine hemoglobin tests are performed at ages 6 and 18 months.

At older ages, other variations are introduced to serve the particular needs of the population. A high proportion of women begin to have intercourse at an early age and have multiple partners, so the risk of carcinoma of the cervix is increased. Accordingly, Papanicolaou smears are recommended as part of the screening every 2 years after two negative smears 1 year apart. The city served has a TB mortality rate approaching 100 per 100,000, so reaction to PPD is tested every 10 years.

In the midadult years, ages 40 to 59, many agencies are now beginning to make recommendations for health-maintenance protocols. For example, the American Cancer Society recommends an annual digital rectal examination beginning at age 40, with occult blood testing annually beginning at age 50. Screening sigmoidoscopy is recommended at age 50, then annually for 2 years, then every 5 years after two negative examinations. However, on the protocol given as an example, sigmoidoscopy is not scheduled, but a discussion with a patient on this subject is recommended.

On the other hand, the protocol does include a recommendation for tonometry to be included, visualizing the fundus at approximately 6-year intervals. Although it can be of value in some asymptomatic individuals, tonometry as a screening procedure has been of questioned effectiveness. It does appear that the risk of field defects developing over a 5-year period in patients with moderate degrees of ocular hypertension is small.

For women in this age-group, mammography has been recommended by the protocol. This particular protocol does not include instruction in breast self-examination as a primary or supplemental screening test. The American Cancer Society recommends that this should be performed by all women at least monthly. However, it appears that at present, although the vast majority of women are aware of the need for breast self-

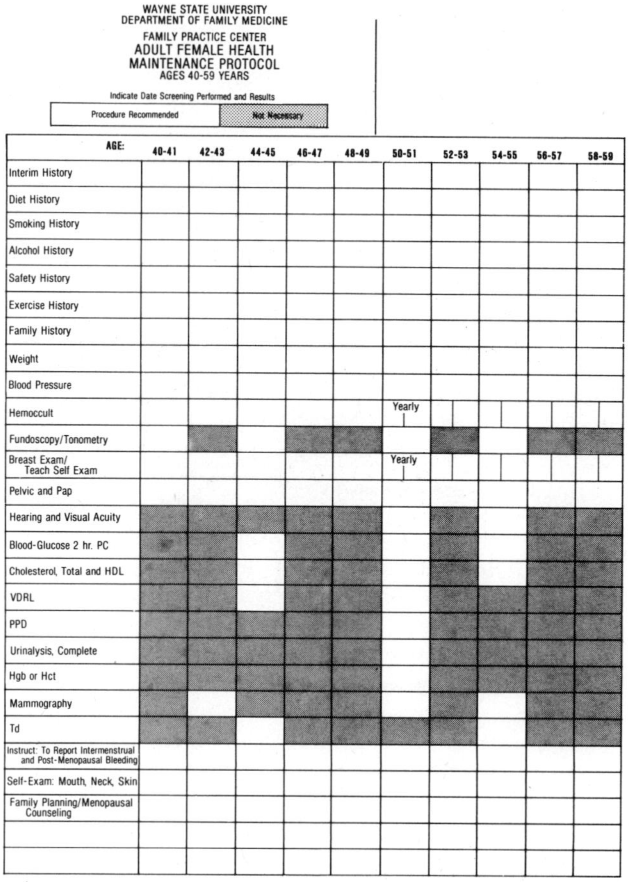

Figure 6-13 (Adult Female Health Maintenance Protocol, Ages 40-59 years)

WAYNE STATE UNIVERSITY
DEPARTMENT OF FAMILY MEDICINE
FAMILY PRACTICE CENTER
ADULT FEMALE HEALTH
MAINTENANCE PROTOCOL
AGES 40-59 YEARS

Indicate Date Screening Performed and Results
Procedure Recommended / Not Necessary

AGE:	40-41	42-43	44-45	46-47	48-49	50-51	52-53	54-55	56-57	58-59
Interim History										
Diet History										
Smoking History										
Alcohol History										
Safety History										
Exercise History										
Family History										
Weight										
Blood Pressure										
Hemoccult						Yearly				
Fundoscopy/Tonometry										
Breast Exam/Teach Self Exam						Yearly				
Pelvic and Pap										
Hearing and Visual Acuity										
Blood-Glucose 2 hr. PC										
Cholesterol, Total and HDL										
VDRL										
PPD										
Urinalysis, Complete										
Hgb or Hct										
Mammography										
Td										
Instruct: To Report Intermenstrual and Post-Menopausal Bleeding										
Self-Exam: Mouth, Neck, Skin										
Family Planning/Menopausal Counseling										

Figure 6-13. Protocol for adult female health maintenance, ages 40–59 years.

Figure 6-14 (Adult Male Health Maintenance Protocol, Ages 40-59 years)

WAYNE STATE UNIVERSITY
DEPARTMENT OF FAMILY MEDICINE
FAMILY PRACTICE CENTER
ADULT MALE HEALTH
MAINTENANCE PROTOCOL
AGES 40-59 YEARS

Indicate Date Screening Performed and Results
Procedure Recommended / Not Necessary

AGE:	40-41	42-43	44-45	46-47	48-49	50-51	52-53	54-55	56-57	58-59
Interim History										
Diet History										
Smoking History										
Alcohol History										
Safety History										
Exercise History										
Family History										
Weight										
Blood Pressure										
Hemoccult						Yearly				
Fundoscopy/Tonometry										
Rectal-Prostate										
Hearing and Visual Acuity										
Glucose 2 hr. PC										
Triglycerides										
Total and HDL cholesterol										
VDRL										
PPD										
Urinalysis Complete										
Hgb or Hct										
Td										
Instruct Self-Exam: Mouth, Neck, Skin										

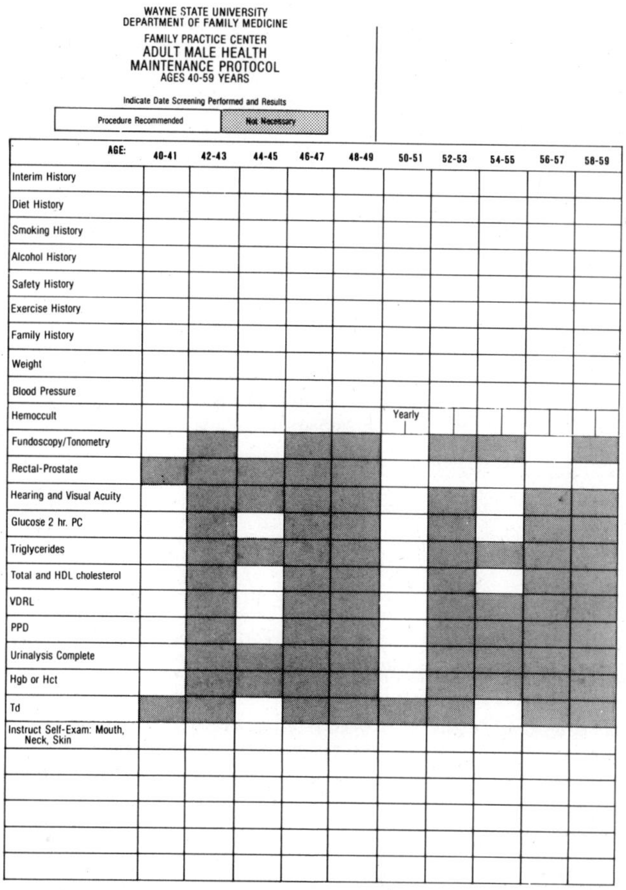

Figure 6-14. Protocol for adult male health maintenance, ages 40–59 years.

examination, only 15 to 40% perform it monthly. For an individual, breast self-examination is safe and relatively simple to perform, although the simplicity of performance may vary with breast size and/or the woman's weight. The individual performance of breast self-examination is inexpensive, and the procedure only takes a few minutes and requires no special equipment. Though not easily measured in dollars, the psychological costs of false-positive detections may be great and must be considered. The work done on breast self-examination to date indicates that this detection maneuver for breast cancer has potential, but many unanswered questions remain and require scientific investigation before this procedure can be advocated either as a supplemental or as a primary screening test for breast cancer. Breast cancer is the most common neoplasm of women and has shown no overall decline in the past 30 years. The mean age of diagnosis is in the mid to late 50s. The incidence is relatively low before age 40 and increases noticeably as women approach age 50 and move into the older adult period. The authors of the health-maintenance protocol used as illustration do not follow the American Cancer Society's guidelines. These recommendations are being continuously revised, and the protocol seems reasonable at present. The cost of mammography in a hospital radiology department now approximates $100. The standard recom-

mendations for mammograms to be performed more frequently, every 1 to 2 years until age 50, may be ideal but are not always practical.

In the late adult years, the emphasis of health-maintenance protocols is not so much on primary prevention but on secondary prevention and early detection of disease. In the illustration given, the only new procedure introduced is yearly administration of influenza vaccine after age 54. Many others would include advice that pneumococcal vaccine, given once in a lifetime at present, should also be included.

Before leaving the whole question of lifetime health-maintenance protocols, it is necessary to consider the costs of these procedures. The costs of the protocols used as illustration are given in Table 6-14.

FEATURES OF DISEASES THAT ARE PREVENTABLE

RESPIRATORY TRACT DISEASES

Only certain respiratory tract diseases are preventable. The major conditions for which preventive measures are applicable include two groups of diseases, which have been classified in many ways. In particular, the group of diseases recognized by

Table 6-14. Costs of Lifetime Health-Maintenance Protocols for Patient from Birth to Age

Pediatric/adolescent to age 18	$516.00	-or-	$28.67/year
Young adult period (19–39)			
Male	508.00	-or-	24.50/year
Female	595.00	-or-	30.00/year
Middle adult (40–59)			
Male	607.00	-or-	30.35/year
Female	1,033.00	-or-	51.65/year
Older adult (59–79)			
Male	878.00	-or-	43.90/year
Female	1,413.00	-or-	70.65/year
79-year total			
Male	2,509.00	-or-	31.75/year
Female	3,557.00	-or-	177.85/year

British physicians as "chronic bronchitis" is more likely to be described in this country as emphysema or more generally as **chronic obstructive pulmonary disease** (COPD). Although this difference in terminology may seem of little import, it becomes a necessary distinction if the international literature is consulted. The etiology of this group of conditions is related to some preventable causes. High among these is the habit of cigarette smoking. Air pollution, both urban and rural, is also a common etiologic factor. Atopy, allergy, or hypersensitivity also plays an important part. It has not yet been established whether repeated hospitalization for asthma in infancy or childhood and/or the presence of eczema plays an important role in the etiology of COPD. However, a history of "lung trouble" before the age of 16 years does seem to be associated with more severe pulmonary disease in the later years.

The upper respiratory tract is frequently associated with work-related symptoms. Workers frequently allege that nasal and paranasal sinus irritation, throat inflammation, and occasionally laryngeal inflammation are due to substances inhaled in the workplace. It is becoming increasingly common that bronchospasm, sometimes in the form of a straight allergic or irritant asthma, is also being recognized as an occupationally related disease. Precipitating agents include isocyanates, detergent enzymes, and some wood dust. More severe irritations of the lower respiratory tract may cause pulmonary edema and pneumonitis. These may later be followed by fibrotic changes in the lung. Within this group, cadmium poisoning, beryllium disease, silicosis, asbestosis, and byssinosis are frequently occupationally related.

Primary prevention of this group of diseases depends on removing the potential respiratory tract irritant or removing the individual from the irritant. As a result of repeated physician cautions, cigarette smoking is becoming far less common. However, in the past the efforts to discourage smoking have been directed largely to men, but women are now far more frequently beginning to suffer from respiratory tract diseases and lung cancer related to the smoking habit.

Secondary prevention is carried out by early detection of impairment of pulmonary function through the use of pulmonary function tests. Spirometry can be effectively performed in the physician's office with equipment that is not very expensive. Figure 6-15 illustrates the type of response that can be expected in normal individuals, in those with restrictive pulmonary diseases, and in those with obstructive diseases. It can be seen that the most discriminating test is the forced expiratory volume in 1 second (FEV_1) divided by the forced vital capacity (FVC). Calculating these two simple factors can

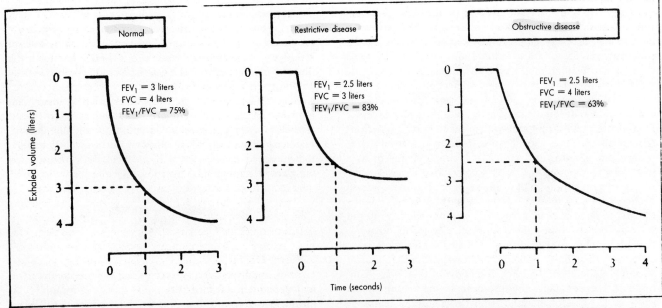

Figure 6-15. Spirographic results in normal and disease states. (Adapted from Nadel JA: Pulmonary function testing. Basics of RD. American Thoracic Society 1(4):2, 1973.

readily lead to a distinction between the types of disease and can also help monitor their progress.

The effect of smoking on the individual can also be demonstrated by spirometry (Fig. 6-16).

The present state of knowledge regarding the etiology of **asthma** does not help much in preventing the onset of the disease. We may be better placed to prevent attacks of asthma in those who have already developed the disease. Two basic approaches are possible: first, to prevent attacks by the effective use of drugs, and second, to control exposure to factors that may precipitate attacks. Apart from the respiratory irritants that have already been discussed, it is important to remember that aspirin has been shown to precipitate asthma in some individuals.

CARDIOVASCULAR DISEASE

In the United States, the complications of **arteriosclerosis** account for about one-half of all deaths and for about one-third of deaths in persons between the ages of 35 and 65 years (Fig. 6-17).

Seventy-five percent of arteriosclerosis-related deaths are the result of coronary artery disease, which is also the leading cause of permanent disability and accounts for more patient days in hospital than any other illness.

Atheromatous plaques are the lesions most usually observed at autopsy in fatal cases of coronary artery disease. Preventing the formation of *simple* plaques is widely regarded as the most promising long-term approach to coronary artery disease, but it appears that the formation of *complicated* plaques is irreversible.

The discovery that risk factors are associated with the development of atherosclerosis has turned many active clinicians into active participants in preventive medicine. It is widely recognized that atherosclerosis develops with increasing age. The observations that men are more frequently affected with the disease than women, that in males it develops at an earlier age, and that this condition is also associated with elevated plasma cholesterol levels, high arterial blood pressure, and cigarette smoking have led to active attempts to prevent these risk factors from being a powerful influence in the life of a particular patient.

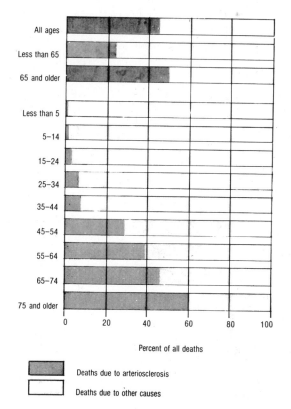

Figure 6-17. The proportion of deaths due to arteriosclerosis-related diseases is shown by age-group. The data are for the United States in 1978. Coronary artery disease accounts for about three-fourths of the arteriosclerosis-related diseases. (Hancock EW: Scientific American Medicine. I. Cardiology. Sci Am 8:2, 1987.)

The relation between the serum cholesterol level and the risk of death from coronary heart disease is statistically continuous and graded for all cholesterol levels greater than 100 mg/100 ml. Acceleration of atherosclerosis is principally correlated with elevation of the LDL, which is rich in cholesterol but poor in triglycerides. Elevation of the HDL fraction has a negative correlation with the development of atherosclerosis. The National Institutes of Health have announced a national cholesterol educational program based on the thesis that everyone should know his or her cholesterol level and should take steps to lower elevated levels. If individuals adhere to the dietary guidelines, it may be expected that plasma cholesterol levels will be decreased by 10 to 20%. Drug therapy for reduction of serum lipids is usually recommended only when 6 to 12 months of dietary therapy have proved ineffective.

Treatment of the conditions that are related to the development of coronary artery disease becomes a part of the practice of good preventive medicine. Clearly the two conditions that must receive most attention are hypertension and diabetes mellitus. Obesity, although associated with hypertension, diabetes, and hyperlipoproteinemia, has not been shown to be an independent risk factor.

Alcohol consumption in moderate amounts has been inversely correlated with cardiovascular disease in studies such as the Framingham study. Other investigators have criticized

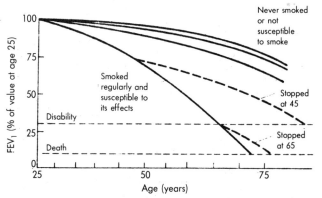

Figure 6-16. Smoking and loss of forced expiratory volume (FEV$_1$). (Holland WW, Detels R, Knox G (eds): Oxford Textbook of Public Health. Oxford University Press, New York, 1985.)

the accuracy of such correlations and point out that alcohol can impair glucose tolerance and increase body weight and blood pressure. At this point, the reason for the male/female differential in the incidence of coronary artery disease is not well understood.

Research into the risk factors and etiology of cardiovascular disease has led to a developing interest in nutrition as a means of practicing preventive medicine. The principle dietary goals that are recommended currently are as follows:

1. Avoid being overweight by balancing caloric intake with exercise-induced energy expenditure.
2. Reduce the overall fat intake from about 40% to about 30% of total calories.
3. Reduce the intake of saturated fat so that saturated fat and polyunsaturated fat each account for about 10% of caloric intake.
4. Reduce the cholesterol intake to about 300 mg/day.
5. Reduce the consumption of refined and processed sugars by about 45%, so that such sugars account for about 10% of the total calories; increase the consumption of complex and unrefined carbohydrates from about 28% to about 48% of caloric intake.
6. Limit the sodium intake to about 5 g/day.

GI TRACT DISEASE

The possibility of applying public health measures to reduce the risk of chronic GI tract illness gives rise to many problems at present. Reliable comparative epidemiologic data on which to base preventive measures is at present scarce.

A good example of this is evident in the study of **peptic ulcer disease**. Frequency varies greatly from time to time and from place to place, probably reflecting the interplay of environmental and genetic factors. In the past, gastric ulcer was more common in the poor than among the rich, whereas the reverse was true of duodenal ulcer. But now the social class patterns for both gastric and duodenal ulcer are much the same. Despite many attempts to relate the development of complications or exacerbations of ulcer disease to stress, no clear body of evidence has emerged to support the concept. However, there is clear evidence that smokers are more likely to die from peptic ulceration than nonsmokers, that ulcer is likely to be found more often in smokers than nonsmokers, and that duodenal ulcers are less likely to heal during cimetidine treatment if patients are smokers. Smoking is associated with the incidence of peptic ulcer at a young age. For example, in one study of college students, 10.7% of smokers had peptic ulcer disease but only 6.1% of nonsmokers had the same disease. Clinically, association between alcohol consumption and the use of various drugs has long been associated with the onset of peptic ulcer disease. Epidemiologically, it has been difficult to support these firmly held clinical impressions. However, a recent controlled clinical study has suggested that relapse of duodenal ulcer is less likely to occur in those taking dietary fiber supplements. In spite of conflicting evidence of this kind, alterations in disease patterns during the past hundred years indicate that environmental factors have been responsible for the decreasing incidence of gastric ulcer,

accompanied during the same period by an increasing incidence of duodenal ulcer.

The same problems exist when **inflammatory bowel disease** is considered. Both Crohn's disease and ulcerative colitis seem to be associated with Western cultural patterns, and their frequency contrasts with the relative rarity of infective dysenteric illness in these countries. It has been shown that smoking is associated with the incidence of ulcerative colitis but not of Crohn's disease.

The prevalence of **appendicitis** and **diverticulitis** has increased in Western countries during the 20th century. It has been suggested that diverticular disease is a disease of Western civilization related to a deficiency in dietary fiber. Diverticular disease has been shown to be associated with other diseases of Western civilization, such as ischemic heart disease, gallstones, hemorrhoids, varicose veins, and hiatal hernia. A deficiency of dietary fiber is probably not the sole etiologic factor, but at least one randomized control trial has shown the benefit of increasing dietary fiber intake in reducing symptomatic diverticular disease.

The incidence and prevalence of **gallstones** have been extensively studied. Formation of cholesterol-rich stones is believed to be a four-stage process involving (1) an individual with a genetic propensity or metabolic abnormality that allows (2) the production of bile saturated with cholesterol, (3) the initiation of stone formation, and (4) stone growth. At routine autopsy for other causes of death, great variations in gallstone prevalence worldwide have been demonstrated. In general, it is much lower in many African and third world nations. Obesity has long been recognized as a major risk factor in gallstone formation. Nutritional factors are undoubtedly important in gallstone formation, if only because obesity is a consequene of overnutrition. The deficiency or excess of no single dietary component has been shown to be associated with the development of gallstones. Efforts to reduce blood cholesterol levels by (1) giving Clofibrate and (2) administering estrogens, particularly in oral contraceptives, have been associated with an increased cholesterol excretion in bile, with the resulting formation of gallstones.

GU TRACT DISEASES

Many epidemiologic studies have undertaken investigating every form of urinary tract infection from asymptomatic bacteriuria to advanced pyelonephritis and glomerulonephritis. These have clearly indicated that screening for significant bacteriuria is of established cost benefit. In children, the presence of bacteriuria is a valuable marker for the existence of vesicoureteral reflux. Once a diagnosis of urinary tract infection has been unequivocally made in a child or infant, investigation is mandatory. The regional and national differences in the distribution of glomerulonephritis are not clearly understood. In temperate climates, the majority of glomerulonephritis cases have an unknown etiology. However, many cases in tropical climates have been associated with the coexistence of malaria. In third world countries, glomerulonephritis is seen as a common outcome of widespread infection and parasitemia in the presence of an immune system compromised by malnutrition. In a relatively few areas, glomerulonephritis is seen complicating schistosomiasis rather than malaria.

On the other hand, renal stones are a disease of rich nations, and rising incidence has been associated with the growth of industrialization and an increased net of domestic products. Urolithiasis is probably a multifactorial phenomenon that may sometimes result from inborn errors of metabolism. Infection also has some role in stone formation. Dietary and other factors may also be responsible. Although the incidence appears to be higher in Caucasians living in tropical areas, no simple correlation between stone incidence and climate has been demonstrated.

There are only a few instances of successful preventive measures in GU tract disease. Screening of women early in pregnancy for occult urinary tract infection reduces the incidence of pyelitis of pregnancy. Screening programs to detect occult urinary tract infection in young children do not appear to be cost-effective. Health education might heighten public awareness, which might in turn lead to the identification of high-risk children, among whom a higher yield of positive findings might be obtained. Routine medical examinations to detect proteinuria and hypertension may be pointers to important diseases of the urinary system. Care must be exercised in the prescription and use of drugs known to be nephrotoxic.

DISEASES OF THE BLOOD-FORMING SYSTEM

Many of the conditions that give rise to disorders of red blood cell formation arise external to the human organism. In other words, these are the direct results of environmental conditions, poor nutrition, or ingested toxins. Some of the conditions involving inadequate red cell production are listed in Table 6-15.

Iron deficiency anemia is the most common form of blood disease. The condition can exist without anemia if tissue iron stores are low but not depleted, but it is usually recognized clinically only when stores are fully depleted. Daily dietary requirements of iron are estimated at about 5 to 10 mg for men and 7 to 20 mg for women. Since an average diet may contain only about 5 to 6 mg of iron per thousand calories, a negative iron balance can easily occur. In many parts of the world, anemia results from dietary iron deficiency. Where diet is more adequate, iron deficiency is nearly always the result of blood loss. In addition to malnutrition and bleeding, iron deficiency may result from various conditions that result in impaired iron absorption, such as sprue. Public health programs play a vital role in prevention of iron deficiency. These include community programs designed to guarantee adequate nutrition as well as programs aimed at elimination of hookworm disease. Nutritional programs to prevent the development of anemia include special provision of iron supplements for young children and for women of childbearing age.

Public health programs in health education and in nutritional supplementation also have an important part to play in reducing the prevalence of folate deficiency anemias. The primary causes of vitamin B_{12} deficiency relate either to malabsorption or less commonly to decreased availability in the GI tract. In contrast to iron and folate deficiency, vitamin B_{12} deficiency only rarely results form dietary insufficiency.

Anemia may also result from excessive red cell destruction. Preventive measures in this area are linked more to genetic

Table 6-15. Conditions Involving Inadequate Red Cell Production

Deficiency of cell nutrients

Iron

Blood loss: GI lesions, menstruation, hookworm, blood donation, etc.

Inadequate diet: relative to need

Impaired absorption: gastric resection, achlorhydria, pica, sprue

Folic acid

Inadequate diet: relative to need (infancy, pregnancy, proliferative disease)

Impaired absorption: sprue, gluten-induced enteropathy

Drugs: phenytoin (? mechanism)

Vitamin B_{12}

Impaired absorption: pernicious anaemia (gastric atrophy and intrinsic factor deficiency), gastric resection, inherited defects, drugs

Decreased availability: intestinal loops, fish tapeworm

Inadequate diet: strict vegetarians

Other nutrients

Protein, ? trace materials

Impaired erythropoiesis

Aplastic anemia

Chemicals: benzene, drugs

Ionizing radiation

Infection

Idiopathic

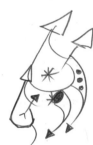

Sideroblastic anemias

Hereditary: often pyridoxine-responsive

Acquired: drugs, alcohol, lead

Idiopathic

Porphyrias

Acquired: chemicals

Inherited

Anaemias secondary to systemic illness

Cancer (marrow infiltration), endocrine disease, renal disease, cirrhosis, chronic inflammation

Holland WW, Detls R, Knox G (eds): Oxford Textbook of Public Health. Oxford University Press, New York, 1985.

considerations than to environmental or nutritional hazards. Among the more common of these conditions are the **hemoglobinopathies**, of which sickle cell disease is the most common. This is due to the presence of an abnormal hemoglobin known as sickle (S) hemoglobin. Genetic studies suggest that hemoglobin S may have arisen from a single gene mutation in Africa or the Middle East. When it exists in the homozygous state, it produces sickle cell anemia, whereas the heterozygous state produces sickle cell trait. Heterozygous individuals develop active hemolysis under conditions of physiological stress or hypoxia.

Abnormalities of globin synthesis are known as **thalassemia**.

Thalassemia major results from a homozygous state, and thalassemia minor results from the heterozygous state. Public health control of thalassemia and of the sickle cell diseases is restricted to health education programs and the provision of diagnostic and genetic counseling services, leading to intelligent use of health-care systems.

Populations in or derived from central Africa, the Mediterranean, the Middle East, India, and the Orient display both thalassemia and sickle cell diseases. In the same areas, a deficiency of G6PD is also noted. No specific public health measures exist at present to correct this deficiency.

Studies of many other blood-related disorders have also been directed toward the discovery of factors that might lead to active preventive measures. None of these investigations have so far proved very rewarding.

DIABETES

Diabetes has occupied the attention of many in the field of preventive medicine as well as those whose interest is mainly in the clinical care of patients. Understanding of the pathology and treatment of diabetes is rapidly advancing. Classically, diabetes mellitus is divided clinically into the following types:

Type I: Insulin-dependent (IDDM).
Type II: Noninsulin-dependent (NIDDM).
Type III: Other types (secondary to pancreatic, hormonal, drug-induced, insulin/receptor, genetic, and other identifiable abnormalities).
Type IV: Gestational (GDM).

There is another group of patients who display impaired glucose tolerance but in whom frank diabetes has not yet developed.

The newer knowledge of the etiology of the different forms of the diabetic syndrome has renewed interest in the potential for prevention. For both IDDM and NIDDM, the prevailing view is that diabetes often occurs in genetically predisposed persons subject to some environmental diabetogenic "load." A strong association exists between obesity and the development of NIDDM. However, obesity appears to play no role in IDDM development. Apart from genetic factors, virus infection has been the most accepted hypothesis; some strains of coxsackievirus B have been implicated, as has congenital rubella. The evidence has not yet been sufficient to justify contemplating protective actions against these viruses by such means as vaccine. It is recognized that noninfective agents such as food contaminants, additives, or fungal toxins may be initiating factors.

Secondary prevention of diabetes is carried out by population screening. When automated biochemistry made possible the processing of thousands of samples for glucose measurements, mass diagnostic screening drives were carried out in many populations. Enthusiasm for this early indiscriminate screening has diminished markedly in the past 10 years. This has been because it has been recognized that such screening mechanisms identify patients with lesser degrees of glucose intolerance, the vast majority of whom do not deteriorate in condition with the passage of time to produce an unequivocal diabetic diagnosis.

Although indiscriminate screening may be of limited value, screening during pregnancy is of immense value. Perinatal mortality is two to three times higher in a woman who is an established diabetic patient. Gestational diabetes is usually asymptomatic, suspected only because glycosuria is found on routine urine testing. The diagnosis is usually established by means of a formal oral glucose tolerance test (OGTT). This test is normally performed at the beginning of the third trimester. Prior to this, routine urine screening for glycosuria is regarded as adequate.

CANCER

Cancer represents a public health problem of major dimensions in economically well-developed countries. In economically developing countries, it is emerging as a growing problem. WHO has published in rank order an estimated number of cases of ten common cancers in 1975 (Table 6-16). These incidence figures are, of course, constantly changing. There has been a general tendency for the incidence of stomach cancer to regress, whereas the incidence of lung cancer continues to rise in most countries. It is likely that for both sexes the relative position of these two cancers is now reversed. Due largely to the success of presymptomatic detection and early diagnosis, the incidence of carcinoma of the cervix is decreasing in many populations and has already been displaced by breast cancer as the type of cancer with the highest incidence in women. A profile of the most common sites of cancer in men and women is somewhat graphically represented in Figure 6-18. It is to be noted that these figures do not include the nonmelanotic skin tumors, which are by far the most common cancers in white populations. They are readily diagnosed, rarely metastasized, and involve a case fatality of about 1%. It is important that such cancers should be excluded from most epidemiologic data at the present, because their inclusion may provide an overall unduly optimistic view of the current ability to control cancer once it has been detected. When considering statements about survival or "cures" for cancer, it is important to establish that nonmelanotic skin cancers have not been included in the data lest poor conclusions be drawn. Methods of treatment, surgical and otherwise, of cancer are continuously changing, but it is impossible at present to produce an overly optimistic review of improved survival rates. Overall figures do

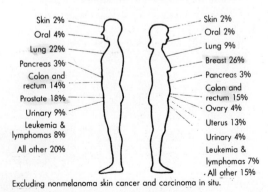

Excluding nonmelanoma skin cancer and carcinoma in situ.

Figure 6-18. Estimated percentage distribution of cancer incidence by site (United States, 1983). (Silverberg ES, Lubera JA: A review of American Cancer Society estimates of cancer cures and deaths. Cancer J Clinicians 33:2, 1983.)

Table 6-16. Rank Order and Estimated Number of Cases (in Thousands) of
Ten Common Cancers (1975)

Rank	Males		Females		Both sexes	
	Site	Cases	Site	Cases	Site	Cases
1	Lung	458	Breast	497	Stomach	698
2	Stomach	439	Cervix	422	Lung	588
3	Mouth-pharynx	254	Stomach	259	Breast	497
4	Colon-rectum	246	Colon-rectum	242	Colon-rectum	488
5	Esophagus	208	Lung	130	Cervix	422
6	Liver	183	Mouth-pharynx	122	Mouth-pharynx	376
7	Lymphatic tissue	129	Esophagus	108	Esophagus	316
8	Leukemia	88	Lymphatic tissue	89	Liver	257
9	—		Liver	74	Lymphatic tissue	218
10	—		Leukemia	67	Leukemia	155
Total:		2,005		2,010		4,015

Parkin DM, Stjernswa RDJ, Murrer CS: Estimates of the worldwide frequency of twelve major cancers. Bull WHO 62(3): 389–410, 1984.

not become quickly available, so most of the data that are published relate to periods ending several years ago. Although in no case may they be proved definitely statistically significant, Tables 6-17 and 6-18 illustrate in the main improved survival rates for many forms of cancer in both men and women over a 10-year period.

Two major determinants of malignant neoplasms have been identified: genetic (hereditary) and environmental (exogenous). Each of these determinants may exist singly or together, with either one predominating. Four broad categories of cancers distinguished by their determinants have been described:

1. Predominantly genetically determined cancers. These are characterized by familial aggregation, usually an earlier age-specific incidence pattern, a high frequency of bilateral involvement, or multifocal neoplasms. An example of this category is familial multiple polyposis coli.
2. Cancers produced by environmental agents; for example, lung cancer due to tobacco smoking.
3. Cancers produced by combined environmental and genetic variations. An example is xeroderma pigmentosum. In this group, familial predisposition may be demonstrated.
4. Cancers that are apparently independent of either genetic or environmental variation.

Some established environmental determinants of cancer include ultraviolet radiation; ionizing radiation, which may be due to background radiation of naturally occurring cosmic rays, medical exposure largely due to diagnostic x-ray procedures, exposure from occupations, nuclear power, and fallout; tobacco smoking; and other chemicals. Substances that have been established as chemical carcinogens in humans include the following:

4-Aminodiphenyl
Analgesic mixtures containing phenacetin
Arsenic and arsenic compounds
Asbestos
Azathioprine
Benzene
Benzidine
N,N-bis(2-chlorethyl)-2-naphthylamine (chlornaphazine)
Bis-chloromethyl ether and technical-grade chloromethyl methyl either
1,4-Butanediol dimethanesulphonate (Myleran)
Chlorambucil
Chromium and certain chromium compounds
Conjugated estrogens
Cyclophosphamide
Diethylstilbestrol
Melphalan
Methoxsalen with ultraviolet A therapy (PUVA)
Mustard gas
2-Naphthylamine
Soots, tars, and oils
Vinylchloride

In the section dealing with environmental hazards, several industrial processes and possible occupational exposures were also mentioned as being potentially carcinogenic.

Additionally, one or two biologic agents—for example, certain parasites invading the human organism—seem to be especially likely to provoke carcinomatous change. These include liver flukes and the organisms causing schistosomiasis. A number of epidemiologic investigations have shown that alcohol in the form of alcoholic beverages is responsible for the occurrence of cancers of the month, pharynx, larynx, and esophagus and that, in doses capable of causing cirrhosis, it can increase the risk of liver cancer.

Table 6-17. Trend in Survival by Site for
U.S. White Male Cancer Patients

Site	5-year relative survival rates (%)	
	1960–63	1970–73
Lip	84	87
Tongue	23	32
Salivary gland	(55)*	(53)
Mouth	42	40
Pharynx	21	27
Esophagus	4	4
Stomach	10	12
Colon	42	47
Rectum	36	43
Liver	1	2
Gallbladder and bile duct	6	7
Pancreas	1	2
Nose, nasal cavity, and middle ear	(39)	(48)
Larynx	54	63
Lung and bronchus	7	9
Bone	31	38
Soft tissue	41	52
Melanoma of the skin	51	62
Breast	(55)	(71)
Prostate gland	50	63
Testis	63	72
Penis	62	(56)
Urinary bladder	53	61
Kidney	36	44
Eye	(81)	78
Brain and CNS	16	18
Thyroid	75	82
Hodgkin's disease	34	66
Non-Hodgkin's lymphoma	31	39
Multiple myeloma	13	20
Lymphocytic leukemia		
Acute	4	27
Chronic	29	46
Granulocytic leukemia		
Acute	2	3
Chronic	13	18
Monocytic leukemia	1	3

*Rates in parentheses have standard errors between 5 and 10%. For other rates the standard errors are less than 5%.
Holland WW, Detels, R, Knox G (eds): Oxford Textbook of Public Health. Oxford University Press, New York, 1985.

Table 6-18. Trend in Survival by Site for
U.S. White Female Cancer Patients

Site	5-year relative survival rates (%)	
	1960–63	1970–73
Lip	(88)*	Too few cases
Tongue	44	46
Salivary gland	(82)	85
Mouth	50	51
Pharynx	35	31
Esophagus	6	4
Stomach	13	14
Colon	44	50
Rectum	41	48
Liver	3	6
Gallbladder and bile duct	9	9
Pancreas	2	2
Nose, nasal cavity, and middle ear	(44)	(50)
Larynx	(46)	56
Lung and bronchus	11	14
Bone	31	36
Soft tissue	54	54
Melanoma of the skin	68	75
Breast	63	68
Uterine cervix	58	64
Uterine corpus	73	81
Ovary	32	36
Vagina	(37)	(44)
Vulva	64	66
Urinary bladder	53	60
Kidney	39	50
Eye	74	77
Brain and CNS	21	22
Thyroid	87	87
Hodgkin's disease	48	69
Non-Hodgkin's lymphoma	31	43
Multiple myeloma	10	17
Lymphocytic leukemia		
Acute	3	29
Chronic	46	59
Granulocytic leukemia		
Acute	0	2
Chronic	11	19
Monocytic leukemia	1	4

*Rates in parentheses have standard errors between 5 and 10%. For other rates the standard errors are less than 5%.
Holland WW, Detels R, Knox G (eds): Oxford Textbook of Public Health. Oxford University Press, New York, 1985.

In addition to these established associations, there are other possible environmental determinants of cancer. Chemical pollution has been the focus of epidemiologic studies investigating cancer risk in relation to contamination of air, water, and food. Diet may considerably influence the development of cancer in a variety of ways. Research has been directed toward determining the causes of cancers of the stomach and large bowel, particularly in relation to dietary components. Epidemiologic and biochemical studies of diet and cancer are currently a high research priority. No association has yet been conclusively corroborated in humans.

Most of the early efforts in establishing preventive measures for the control of cancer in humans have depended on early detection and secondary prevention.

One of the best-known and longest-established screening

procedures has been the practice of taking cervical smears to detect carcinoma of the cervix in women. The following recommendations are generally adopted:

1. Initial smears should be obtained from all women over the age of 18 who are sexually active.
2. If the initial smear is satisfactory and without significant atypia, a second smear should be taken within 1 year.
3. Provided the initial two smears and all subsequent smears are satisfactory and without significant atypia, further smears should be taken at approximately 3-year intervals until the age of 35, and thereafter at 5-year intervals until the age of 60.
4. Women over the age of 60 who have repeated satisfactory smears without significant atypia may be dropped from the screening program for squamous carcinoma of the cervix.
5. Women who are not at high risk should be discouraged from having smears more frequently than is recommended above.
6. Women at continuing high risk should be screened annually.

To facilitate this, provision for taking cytological smears should be made at family planning clinics, student health clinics, youth clinics, venereal disease clinics, prenatal clinics, and medical facilities at which women are examined before admission to penal institutions.

Carcinoma of the breast and its early detection have already been discussed under the section dealing with health-maintenance protocols.

With regard to carcinoma of the colon and rectum, it is doubtful whether proctosigmoidoscopy, which has been advocated for yearly examination in all persons over 40 years of age, is a feasible screening approach, given its low acceptability. The guaiac test revealing occult bleeding (Hemoccult test) appears to be a feasible approach. The greatest specificity of the test is obtained by keeping subjects on a meat-free high-residue diet for at least 24 hours before the 3 days of stool collection.

PROVISION OF HEALTH SERVICES

Health services are provided through complex systems that in this country have arisen from a multitude of individual arrangements interacting with various social institutions. The nature of the social institutions providing health care is rapidly changing. Some of them are small and some are very large, organizing or owning institutions in many states and even purporting to be nationwide. These institutions are undertaking to provide health services of a personal nature and they therefore organize, finance, and control them. Health-care services of a personal nature are provided by physicians, dentists, nurses, pharmacists, and many other health personnel. These services are provided in a variety of locations and through different organizations, including the home, clinic, pharmacy, doctor's office, health center, hospital, and nursing home. The institutions providing health care and financing it may utilize personal, private, or public funding sources. They operate under a variety of controls on performance, which are imposed by their professions, the community, the payers that finance the services, and the government. Both state and federal agencies are involved.

This complex system of health care has arisen in a period of a little over 100 years. The whole health care industry is still involved in a period of rapid change. In Europe in the 19th century, hospitals were important places for the treatment of the sick poor. Later, the affluent were treated in separate sections of the hospital. Many of these hospitals became centers of medical education, associated with universities. As part of the same process, hospitals became places for clinical research, where large numbers of patients with similar diseases could be investigated and treated. This resulted in specialization within medicine, only those physicians with some specialized training being appointed to hospitals while the remainder without specialty qualifications practiced entirely in the community as general practitioners. In many European countries, this situation persists. The medical profession is divided between hospital physicians, either in training or already trained and established as "consultants," and general practitioners whose work and responsibilities rarely take them into the hospital.

In the United States, a similar pattern of development of medical care has occurred, but over a shorter period of time. Physicians, like many others, emigrated from Europe and began to set up their offices in villages and towns, much like other tradesmen. Seeing the need to train their successors, they developed training methods similar to apprenticeships. The first hospital was established in Philadelphia in 1750. In most towns, later including small towns, hospitals were built. Nearly all local doctors had access to them, eliminating the distinction between specialists and generalists. Fifteen years later, in 1765, the first medical school was established in Philadelphia. Medical schools multiplied, so that by the end of the 19th century there were 160. Many of these operated as commercial enterprises, not necessarily associated with any university. The curriculum could be as brief as 2 years.

In 1760, the first licensure law requiring examination prior to entering the practice of medicine was passed in New York City. At that stage, there was no requirement for graduation from a medical school. Because the early laws passed in New York City and elsewhere did not prohibit the practice of medicine by others not licensed, the public perceived licensure as a favor to those licensed, not as a demonstration of competence.

It was around the turn of the century that the supply of doctors had increased so that there was about one physician for every 700 persons in the population, a far greater proportion than in any European country at that time. However, their qualifications were not of even quality. In 1910, the Carnegie Foundation was responsible for a report on medical education, known now as the "Flexner Report" after its author, Abraham Flexner. As a result of this report, some control over the establishment and activities of medical schools was achieved. Higher admission standards and longer training periods and affiliations with universities became required. This led to the closure of some of the commercial operations so that by 1915, there were only 95 medical schools still operating. Fewer but better-trained physicians became available for the U.S. population.

In this nation, where equality of opportunity is a major goal, curable and preventable illness is viewed as limiting that opportunity and therefore unfair. Since 1983, when it was articulated by a presidential commission, it has been recognized that society has an ethical obligation to ensure equitable access to health care for all. The commission listed the following among its reasons for reaching this conclusion:

1. Scientific health care is a social product requiring the skills of many individuals; it is not something individuals can provide for themselves solely through their own efforts.
2. Because the need for health care is unevenly distributed among persons and is highly unpredictable and because the costs of health care may be great, few individuals could secure care without relying on some social mechanism to share the costs.
3. The need for health care is not wholly under the control of the individual; differences in health status and differences in need for health care are largely undeserved.

Society has recognized the principles that the commission enunciated by a demonstration of continued and growing interest in health-care issues. This interest and concern have increased as the size of the health-care industry has been realized. Health care is now the third or fourth largest industry in the United States. In 1982, the total expenditures on health services in the United States amounted to over $320 billion, or $1,365 per person. This amount represented 10.5% of the gross national product (GNP) in that year. For comparison, in 1929, health-care expenses totaled $3.6 billion, or 3.5% of GNP. There are now more than 7,000 hospitals, 14,000 nursing homes, 3,000 home health agencies, 3,000 local health departments, 1,500 companies underwriting health-insurance policies, and thousands of clinics, emergency rooms, surgicenters, mental health centers, prison health clinics, school health services, family planning clinics, pharmacies, laboratories, and optical shops. Each year, about 1 billion visits are made to and by physicians, an average of 4.7 visits per person per year. Each year there are about 40 million admissions to hospitals, with a mean length of stay of approximately 6.5 days, totaling over 270 million hospital days.

As these figures have been considered by the nation, there has been a growing sense that there is evidence that not all health services provided are effective or that they meet the levels of technical quality that modern medical practice should provide. Also, there is believed to be evidence that the way health care is organized, financed, and provided results in inefficiencies and higher costs than necessary.

As a result of these social concerns, government has increasingly played a major role in planning, regulation, and financing of health care. The major function of government policy to date has been to support services in the private sector, particularly those provided by physicians, hospitals, and nursing homes. The amount of government control has increased since the passing of Medicare and Medicaid legislation in 1965 as amendments to the Social Security Act. Since then, public support has risen from 21.6% of total personal health-care expenditure to almost 40%. Medicare and Medicaid

represent the largest, most important, and most expensive federal health programs. Most physicians and other health-care personnel are trained at least in part at public expense. Almost 65% of all health research and development funds are provided by the government. Most nonprofit community and university hospitals have been built or modernized with government subsidies. The bulk of government expenditure has been federal, with state and local governments contributing significant but much smaller amounts.

Ginzberg has identified four power centers in the health-care industry that influenced the nature of health care and the role of government: (1) physicians, (2) large insurance organizations, (3) hospitals, and (4) a highly diversified group of participants in profit-making activities within the health-care arena.

DETERMINANTS OF HEALTH-CARE UTILIZATION

It would be easy to suppose that the controlling factors in the organization of health care relate directly to the needs of the popoulation. However, personal use of health care is influenced by a number of factors, only one of which is illness. Certain characteristics of the population predetermine the utilization of health care. Outstanding among these characteristics is the age of the population. Persons age 65 and older currently constitute approximately 11% of the population but consume 29% of the cost of health care. By contrast, those under the age of 19 constitute 31% of the population but account for only 12% of the nation's health-care expenditures. Women use health services more frequently than men. This is not entirely due to their need for care during the reproductive phase of life. Although there is racial predisposition to certain diseases, a comparison of utilization of health care—for example, between white and black populations—has shown that the utilization is more closely related to income effects than to racial characteristics. Higher levels of education are associated with higher use of preventive health care of all types.

Other factors relating to the population have been demonstrated to enable or enhance the utilization of health-care services. The distinction between rich and poor in terms of their use of health care has been diminished by the introduction of public and private health-insurance programs. It is still true, however, that the poor make fewer visits to physicians than the nonpoor. Health-insurance coverage is one of the most powerful predictors of health-care use. Generally, persons living in rural areas use fewer health services than persons who live in metropolitan areas. This is one phenomenon of utilization related to accessibility of services. Conversely, the availability of the service greatly enhances the likelihood that it is perceived to be a necessary service. In this respect, provisions for health care do not behave in the same way economically as the remainder of the free-enterprise marketplace. It is quite common for services that are expensive to be regarded as more effective than those that are more modestly priced. This factor has allowed physicians who practice in areas where there are relatively more physicians than elsewhere to raise their fees. From the individual physician's point of view, this is economically sound, in that he or she determines the expected level of income and the number of services to be provided and prices each service accordingly. In other marketplaces, such an action might price the individual out of the market. This feature has made it extremely difficult to control escalating health-care costs, particularly as new and expensive technologies are developed. The assumption is made, on the part of the consumer population, that these new and expensive technologies are always better than the more moderately priced services that previously existed.

CHARACTERISTICS OF HEALTH PROFESSIONALS

It is frequently assumed that the availability of physicians determines the utilizaiton of the health service. In fact, physicians constitute only about 7% of all health personnel (Table 6-19). Although physicians constitute the minority of health-care personnel, it is true that they "order" the vast majority of services provided by other health-care personnel (Table 6-20).

The distribution of physicians by specialty and geographically has become a matter of some importance for study. Physicians prefer to locate in areas where they can practice their profession in a manner similar to that in which they were trained. This means that they need access to sophisticated hospital technology and suitable colleagues to whom to refer on a consultant basis, together with an appropriate work load, time off for leisure, and what are regarded as appropriate economic incentives. In rural areas, not all these factors are present. As a result, some localities may have one physician for

Table 6-19. Selected Health Personnel in the United States

Type of personnel	Total (1976–1980, various years, approximate)
Physicians	479,379
Registered nurses	1,250,000
Vocational nurses and aides	1,200,000
Pharmacists	142,500
Dentists	121,000
Medical technologists	112,000
Social workers	43,000
Dental hygienists	25,000
Physical therapists	24,000
Optometrists	22,000
Nurse practitioners	18,000
Chiropractors	18,000
Occupational therapists	11,500
Physician assistants	11,000
Podiatrists	8,800
Lay midwives	2,300

Last JM (ed): Maxcy-Rosenau Public Health and Preventive Medicine, 12th ed. Appleton & Lange, East Norwalk, 1986.

Table 6-20. Physicians (MDs) by Type of Activity (1981)

	No.	Total active (%)	No. of physicians in full-time care (%)
Professionally active:	425,568	100	
Nonfederal	407,125	96	
Patient care	370,096	87	100
Office-based practice	284,313	67	77
General/family practice	48,883		13
Internal medicine	43,629		12
Pediatrics	18,258		5
General surgery	22,513		6
Obstetrics/gynecology	20,640		6
Other specialties	130,390		35
Hospital-based practice	85,783	20	23
Residents	59,873		16
Full-time staff	25,910		7
Other activity	37,029	9	
Federal	18,443	4	
Patient care	14,543		
Other activity	3,900		
Inactive, not classified, and unknown	53,811		

Last JM (ed): Maxey-Rosenau Public Health and Preventive Medicine, 12th ed. Appleton & Lange, East Norwalk 1986.

every 500 people, whereas other areas have a proportion of only 1 to every 5,000 people.

There is an increasing trend toward specialization among physicians. Partly for economic reasons, the primary care specialties have proved less attractive than many other areas of medical practice. As a result, less than 40% of physicians practice in the primary care specialties of general and family practice, internal medicine, and pediatrics. On the other hand, in areas of excess specialization, because of inadequate demand for highly refined techniques and also because patients may believe that specialists are always able to offer a higher standard of medical care, many specialists provide primary care services to their patients.

Another factor that has led to what is now perceived as an imbalance between the numbers of physicians practicing in the primary care areas relates to the principles on which physician reimbursement has been based, especially since the Medicare and Medicaid legislation. Payments for procedurally based skills are at much higher levels than those for cognitive skills. In other words, treatment, especially when rendered by a physician personally, attracts higher payments than does the process of diagnosis, which leads to establishing the need for the treatment skill. Hence, 4 hours of patient care in an operating room attracts a higher fee than 4 hours of supervision of the patient in an intensive care unit. The supervision of care in the follow-up period is paid at even lower levels. There have been some indications that government is beginning to recognize these apparent inequities, but so far no regulations have been made to correct the trends.

These considerations have led to numerous studies, outstanding among which is the report of the Graduate Medical Education National Advisory Committee (GMENAC), as a result of which recommendations have been made about future training in the medical profession. The increasing supply of physicians is having major impacts on how physicians practice, their location, specialty, and the organization of practice. Following this report, reimbursement to hospitals for graduate medical education has been limited to physicians within 5 years of graduation from medical school. This may eventually have the effect of limiting the number of posts available for subspecialty training. Over a longer period, this may have an influence on the number of young physicians who elect this type of training, encouraging an increase in the number of those limiting the training to more general areas and eventually to an increase in those engaged in practice in the primary care areas.

The increasing competitiveness of the marketplace is not restricted only to the activities of physicians. With increasing realization of the need for cost containment, measures to control costs have been introduced by government and by third party health-care insurers. One of the aspects of this competition has been the advent of for-profit health-care corporations, some of which now own hospitals, alongside the development of other methods of providing health care through health maintenance organizations (HMOs) and preferred provider organizations (PPOs). Some of these types of institutions have sought to employ physicians directly. They have been aided in their efforts to recruit physicians by the increasing competition within the profession, persuading an increasing number of physicians to enter salaried employment.

Twenty years ago, independent solo practice attracted between 70 and 80% of all physicians. In the past 40 years, group medical practice has increased at an average rate of 8% per year. The association of physicians in prepaid group practices and in independent practice associations has increased. At present, the solo fee-for-service mode of practice attracts slightly more physicians than other systems of practice arrangement, 38.3% of all physicians. Of the remainder, 30.6% are in group fee-for-service, 9.4% in prepaid group practice, and 21.7% in independent practice associations.

HOSPITALS

Although the majority of the morbidity from illness arises from conditions that can be adequately treated in an ambulatory care setting, hospitals assume a major importance in the health-care system because most of the health-care personnel are employed by and work in hospitals. The facilities of high-technology medicine are required for patients whose treatment can be satisfactorily and safely carried out in an ambulatory setting. Such patients do not need the hotel or custodial type of care that characteristically has been carried out in a hospital setting. For both ambulatory and inpatient care, hospitals consume a considerable proportion of the national health-care expenditure. The perception of the American public is that the hospital, with its modern technology, is the pillar on which health-care services depend. Physicians frequently confirm this view, in that to them, the hospital is the place where most graduate medical education and clinical research take place.

Approximately half of the 7,000 hospitals existing in the United States are operated as voluntary nonprofit institutions. About 5% are owned and operated by the federal government; about 30% are owned and operated by state and local governments. The remainder, approximately 10%, are owned by investors and operate for profit. Most hospitals in the United States are designated as "short-term," with, by definition, an average length of stay in hospital of less than 30 days.

Because of the nature of their functions, hospitals are complex organizations with equally complex administrative structures. Most hospitals are legally controlled by a governing body, which may be the owner of the hospital, a community volunteer board of directors, a local government board of commissioners or supervisors, or university board of regents. The governing body holds the license to operate the hospital. It is also held legally responsible for all aspects of hospital government, including the quality of patient care. The administration of the hospital is under the supervision of the administrator or chief executive officer. This person is usually trained in health-care administration or general management. The administrator exercises supervision over associate and assistant administrators for managing such departments as personnel, finance, housekeeping, nutrition, nursing, laboratories, medical records, professional services, purchasing, emergency, and outpatient services. To the medical staff of the hospital is delegated the responsibility for the quality of patient care.

This division of responsibility within the organization of the hospital is complex and frequently creates some tension. However, like all tension, it can be productive, since hospitals need physicians to bring in patients and to care for those who are admitted. Physicians need the beds and equipment and support personnel offered by the hospital. This interdependence encourages a positive working atmosphere, although in an era of cost containment, competitiveness for scarce resources sometimes produces a degree of tension that may be disruptive.

LONG-TERM HEALTH-CARE FACILITIES

Long-term care in the United States has developed around nursing homes, which are responsible for 90% of the expenditures on long-term care. It is estimated that 20% of the population over age 85 are in nursing homes. The average age of nursing home residents is over 80 years. Most nursing homes are operated as proprietary institutions, of which 14,000 are registered with more than 25 beds. Licensure is essential in order to be qualified to participate in Medicare or Medicaid reimbursement. In addition, intermediate care facilities are certified under Medicaid. These facilities are not required to have full-time professional nurse staffing.

AMBULATORY CARE

Traditionally, ambulatory care has not been organized in the United States. More recently, various types of organizations have been applied to this setting. Most hospitals offer ambulatory care through emergency rooms. Some also offer organized outpatient clinics available generally to poor patients or to those who do not have a personal physician.

As a result of a federal initiative during the 1960s and through a variety of agencies, neighborhood and community health centers, community mental health centers, migrant health programs, maternal and child health centers, and children and youth projects were established. Young health professionals were recruited and paid through the National Health Service Corps to practice in medically underserved areas. As the economic needs of communities have altered, so has the structure of these health-care centers. Federal funds are now considerably diminished, and the centers have increasingly looked to third party payers such as health insurance and Medicaid for reimbursement.

The major and fastest-growing segment of organized ambulatory care is private medical group practice. Such practices are defined generally to include groups of three or more physicians who practice under a formal agreement and jointly use equipment and personnel, distributing income in accordance with mutually determined methods. Such groups can be based on a single specialty discipline or be multidisciplinary. Many of the multidisciplinary groups are quite large, including more than 15 physicians. For the most part, groups function on a fee-for-service basis, although prepayment modes such as those organized by HMOs are increasing in number. However, physicians in group fee-for-service practice tend to have higher incomes than physicians in prepaid group arrangements and also higher incomes than those in solo practice. Group-practice physicians tend to be younger than solo practitioners, and those in prepaid group practice have the shortest working year, on average about 47 weeks, and spend less time in patient care than physicians in other practice settings.

All of these organized ambulatory care settings have some disadvantages for physicians, including less professional freedom, the possibility of limiting the number of referrals from outside the group, less individual incentive, and the possibility of interpersonal difficulties. However, there are advantages, among which is the fact that physicians can avoid much administrative responsibility by using the clinic, hospital, or group management to undertake these responsibilities. There is also more opportunity for interaction with professional colleagues and a greater ease of referral to specialists who are well known. There is more sharing of responsibility for patient care, including coverage on call and on vacations, and a broad array of ancillary services is frequently available. The individual joining the organized ambulatory care setting is less likely to be involved in capital expenditure on facilities and equipment, but is likely to have more time available for continuing education and vacation.

THE FINANCING OF HEALTH SERVICES

Reference has already been made to the fact that most physician services are charged on a fee-for-service basis. Hospitals similarly base their charges on items of service. The responsibility for payment for these services lies with the patient. At present, almost 80% of the civilian population of the United States has some form of private health insurance in the hope that the anticipated costs of personal health care may be spread out. Most of the current methods available to provide this coverage had their origins in the times of financial crisis during the Great Depression of the 1930s. During this period, it was recognized that health care, particularly hospital care, was a very much needed service but one that was increasingly expensive as well as effective. During this period, several private practice clinics offered, in cooperation with consumer groups, services on a prepayment basis. At that same time, Keiser invited a group of physicians to provide prepaid medical care to the workers at the Grand Coolee Dam. Thus the Keiser Permanente Medical Plans came into being. Later, but during the same period, physicians began to recognize the need to protect their incomes. With AMA approval, they organized a Blue Shield plan, which enabled patients to have free choice of a physician and yet to receive some health-care coverage. Blue Shield was generally limited to physician services, and later Blue Cross was developed to provide similar coverage for hospital care.

Commercial insurance carriers were initially reluctant to offer health insurance. Their concept of insurance was that "hazards" should be relatively rare, unpredictable, undesirable, and uncontrollable. Thus, death or accident policies were frequently available but health care was not attractive to these commercial enterprises. Low-cost events such as doctor visits are presumed to be under the control of, and therefore within the ability to budget by, the individual. Insurable hazards should be measured in terms of clear and unambiguous losses that can be independently estimated by the insurer. The principle of health-care insurance violated these principles because the availability of health-insurance coverage increased the probability of the occurrence of the "loss." Thus, it was not until the 1940s that insurance companies began to offer health-care policies, recognizing the potential for an increasing market but offering specific indemnity-type insurance, with stated dollar limits on coverage and also with deductibles and coinsurance required.

Thus it is that now almost 80% of the civilian population has some form of this insurance. Yet, private health insurance pays for only about 27% of national expenditures on personal health care. As a result, in 1982, private health insurance paid $76.6 billion in health-care costs. The cost of operating this insurance amounted to about 10%, or an additional $7.7 billion. Many patients imagine that when they have health-care insurance, all their costs will be covered. In reality, this is limited by limiting the extent of the services covered and also by the frequency of use.

From an insurance point of view, the most catastrophic event is for the patient to be admitted to the hospital for an extended period. This is the event for which most insurance provides most cover. More people have coverage for physician services in hospital than out of hospital. The incentives to provide care in the hospital under these circumstances are obvious and have been a major influence in increasing the use of hospital care.

It would seem logical, therefore, to assume that health-insurance carriers would be willing to contemplate payment for preventive health services. The reason that they frequently do not seems to be related to an actuarial assessment that a cost-benefit analysis of preventive services has not been positive. From the individual patient's perspective, prevention is frequently better than cure, but, in total, preventive measures taken for a population can be very expensive.

Blue Cross and Blue Shield are nonprofit organizations that tend to be controlled by hospitals and physicians. They operate exclusively to provide health benefits and may be the only plan in a geographic area. They frequently offer service benefits to the provider, providing a guarantee of payment directly for covered services. They offer free choice of participating providers, but the percentage of fees reimbursed can be greater for those providers who are "participating" than for those who do not participate in the plan. Participating providers have somewhat less flexibility in assessing their charges than those who do not participate. The assumption is that direct patient billing, with its attendant risks of collection, may provide greater rewards for the nonparticipating physician.

Commercial insurance is provided by profit-making organizations, whose primary function is general insurance with health insurance as only part of their business activity. They generally offer reimbursement to the subscriber rather than to the provider, and this reimbursement is frequently for a specified dollar amount not necessarily related to the full charge for the service. Most provide for some deductibles to be paid by the patient for coinsurance. In general they place no limits on the choice of providers, since the dealing is directly between the subscriber and the company.

Independent plans include some that are arranged by profit organizations and others by nonprofit. Some of these have evolved from the earlier prepaid group practice plans, and others have grown out of a movement to provide consumer cooperatives, now frequently appearing as HMOs. HMOs contract to serve an enrolled popoulation for prepaid services. They generally provide a comprehensive range of services

directly through contracted providers, thus limiting the choice of provider in return for a guarantee of service rather than just for payment. Some of these plans have been set up specifically to provide preventive as well as curative services. Such independent plans currently provide cover for 15 to 20% of patients. Many and very varied estimates have been provided for the potential growth of this type of plan. Some have estimated that 50% of patient swill have this type of cover sometime during the 1990s, but others have challenged this projection. This more gloomy view has been supported by the financial failure of several HMOS.

Most health insurances are offered to groups of employees and their dependents. In most cases, the employer pays the full amount of the premium. There is some evidence that employees will increasingly be paying more of the premiums, especially as they wish to control the range of services provided. However, group coverage offers some advantages, particularly in low marketing or selling costs and also avoiding for the insurer the sense that the insurance may be purchased by a patient with a specific possible need already in view. This clearly increases the risk to the third party.

Medicare was introduced through amendments to the Social Security Act in 1965. Part A provides hospital insurance, a compulsory insurance program for the aged to cover the cost of hospitalizations and financed by payroll taxes. Part B of the program provides supplementary medical insurance and is a voluntary program for the aged to cover physician services in and out of hospital, paid for with monthly premiums by the elderly aided by subsidies from the federal general revenue. This part of the Medicare program provides for deductibles and coinsurance. Medicaid, on the other hand, is a means-tested, welfare-oriented, state-administered health-care program primarily for the poor, with eligibility levels and the scope of benefits dependent on state decisions within federal guidelines.

Details of each of these federally mandated provisions are included in Tables 6-21 through 6-23.

In these descriptions, certain technical terms have been used in relation to health insurance. Deductibles are a specific stated amount to be paid by the consumer before health insurance begins. For example, under Medicare Part A the patient is required to pay an amount that is roughly equivalent to the cost of a day in the hospital before additional costs are covered. Coinsurance requires a patient to pay a specified proportion of the bill, irrespective of the total amount charged, this amount usually being paid after the service is provided. Copayment is the charging of a set amount per service item, for example, $5 per office visit. All these measures have been introduced largely with the aim of reducing overuse of health services for which third-party carriers may be financially responsible. Curbing utilization has been demonstrated to be an effective means of cost containment in health care.

Cost containment has been a very popular topic nationally in response to the ever increasing costs of health care. Each new technology introduced, while potentially saving lives, potentially also increases total health-care costs. Until recently, utilization depended primarily on the physician's knowledge of available resources. Now there is increasing awareness of a public responsibility to monitor health-care costs.

Several methods of controlling utilization have been in-

Table 6-21. Medicare (Part A)

Who is covered	Originally, all persons over 65 who are entitled to Social Security or Railroad Retirement benefits, with a grandfathering of virtually all persons over 65 at the beginning of the program; 1972 amendments added persons with end-stage renal disease and persons under 65 who are entitled to monthly disability benefits under SSA or Railroad Retirement; voluntary enrollment is possible for persons over 65, enrolled in Part B and not otherwise eligible for Part A, subject to payment of a premium, amounting to $113 per month in 1983.
What is covered	Inpatient hospital services, for 90 days in a benefit period with an annual deductible roughly equivalent to a day of hospital care and copayment of roughly 25% of a day of care for days 61 to 90; outpatient hospital diagnostic services; 100 days of posthospital skilled nursing services, with copayments after the 21st day; 100 days of posthospital home health services, in 1981 the limit was removed; hospice benefits were added in 1982.
How financed	Payroll tax, placed in the Health Insurance Trust fund.
How are providers paid	Reasonable costs; changed in 1983 to a prospective payment system, based on regional costs per case for diagnosis-related groups (DRGs) for hospitals.
Which providers participate	Hospitals that meet standards for accreditation by the Joint Commission on Accreditation for Hospitals and have utilization review procedures; nursing homes and home health agencies that meet conditions of participation as determined by state health agencies.
How administered	By the Health Care Financing Administration of the Department of Health and Human Services with use of private agents: providers select a fiscal intermediary, usually the Blue Cross Plan, which determines that the provider is a participant and processes the claims and conducts other administrative functions.

Last JM (ed): Maxcy-Rosenau Public Health and Preventive Medicine, 12th ed. Appleton & Lange, East Norwalk, 1986.

troduced. In certain circumstances, utilization review requires a provider to receive prior authorization before initiating a course of treatment or hospitalization. Exceptions are only made for those cases that are subsequently deemed to be urgent or emergency cases. Other attempts have been introduced to control utilization at the same time as delivery of the service. An example of this is, on admission to hospital, making an estimate of expected length of stay, with the necessity for the provider to obtain approval of any plans to lengthen the stay. Other steps are taken after the delivery of service, though not

Table 6-22. Medicare (Part B)

Who is covered	Voluntary for any U.S. citizen over age 65 or any person eligible for Part A on payment of a premium.
What is covered	Physicians' services in and out of hospital, home health visits, other outpatient medical services such as laboratory diagnostic tests and rental of durable medical equipment; subsequent additions included physical therapy services, limited optometric and chiropractic services; speech pathology, rural clinic services; all services subject to an annual deductible, originally $50 per year, by 1983 $75 per year and pegged to 25% of program costs, plus 20% coinsurance for the remainder.
How financed	Premiums of subscribers, originally $3 per month, and in 1983 amounting to $12.20 per month.
How are providers paid	Physicians may decide in each instance whether to accept "assignment," in which case payment is made directly to the physician of 80% of the usual, customary, or reasonable (UCR) charges, and the physician bills the patient for the remaining 20% coinsurance; if the physician does not accept assignment, the patient is paid the 80% UCR directly by the carrier, and the physician may bill the patient directly for usual charges. In 1984, a freeze on fees was imposed, with incentives for physicians to accept assignment and requirement for laboratories to accept assignment with a national fee schedule.
Which providers participate	Any licensed physician may choose to participate; independent laboratories must be certified as meeting conditions of participation by the state health agency.
How administered	As under Part A, but providers may select carriers who perform functions similar to intermediaries under Part A.

Last JM (ed): Maxcy-Rosenau Public Health and Preventive Medicine, 12th ed. Appleton & Lange, East Norwalk, 1986.

necessarily related to payment. The providers are subject to in-hospital medical audit and may be denied payment for services that do not conform to certain criteria or that are unrelated to the established diagnosis. After payment, investigations of fraud and abuse may be carried out.

Specific controls that apply particularly to Medicare patients have been introduced. One such control that has had a profound effect is the introduction of payment for hospital care on a prospective basis by case, classified by diagnostic related group (DRG). Other regulations have frozen physician fee increases and provided incentives to accept assignment for claims. Control of capital expenditures, preventing the investment of funds for unneeded expensive equipment and facilities,

Table 6-23. Medicaid

Who is covered	Determined largely by the states, but most include recipients of cash assistance under the welfare programs of Aid to Families with Dependent Children (AFDC), Aid to the Aged, Aid to the Blind, and Aid to the Disabled. (These latter three categories have been merged into the federal Supplemental Security Income [SSI] programs.) States have the option to cover persons eligible for but not receiving cash assistance and persons with incomes above the welfare levels, called the medically needy. States determine income levels for all groups. In 1984, states were required to cover women pregnant for the first time, and pregnant women in two-parent families with unemployed breadwinner, and children up to age 5 in the same families, subject to general state welfare income levels.
What is covered	States must provide inpatient hospital care, physicians' services, outpatient hospital care, laboratory and x-ray, skilled nursing services. Later added requirements included early and periodic screening, diagnosis, and treatment for children, family planning, rural clinics. States may also include home health care, dental, drugs, therapies, dentures, eyeglasses, intermediate care facilities, inpatient psychiatric care, clinic services. Copayments may be imposed for the medically needy and for optional services, and for all services subject to prior approval by the federal government.
How financed	Federal general revenue funds in the form of grants to the states, matched by state and sometimes local tax funds, with varying percentages of 23 to 50% state share.
How are providers paid	Originally according to Medicare methods for hospitals, later at state option subject to federal approval. Other providers' payment methods left to the states. UCR, fee schedules, and other methods are used.
Which providers participate	Determined by states with original federal requirement for freedom of choice. This requirement may be waived on application to the federal agency, as of 1983.
How administered	By the states, subject to federal regulations.

Last JM (ed): Maxcy-Rosenau Public Health and Preventive Medicine, 12th ed. Appleton & Lange, East Norwalk, 1986.

especially where these are already available in other institutions, has been introduced.

All of these measures have had a profound effect on the practice of medicine. Although the desirability of economic control is clear in an age of escalating costs, many physicians have been concerned about the impact of these controls on their care of the individual patient. Some of these issues pose major ethical dilemmas.

BIBLIOGRAPHY

American Academy of Pediatrics: Report of the Committee on Infectious Disease, 20th ed. American Academy of Pediatrics, Chicago, Illinois, 1986.

Armitage P: Statistical Methods in Medical Research. Blackwell Scientific Publications, Oxford, 1977.

Berge TO (ed): International Catalogue of Arboviruses, 2nd ed. U.S. Dept. of Health, Education and Welfare, Publ. No. (CDC) 75-8301, 1975.

Bourke GJ, Daly LE, McGilvray J: Interpretation and Uses of Medical Statistics, 3rd ed. Blackwell Scientific Publications, Oxford, 1985.

Centers for Disease Control: Annual Summary 1984: Reported morbidity and mortality in the United States. MMWR 33:54, 1986.

Colton T: Statistics in Medicine. Little, Brown & Co., Boston, 1974.

Dawber TR: The Framingham Heart Study: The Epidemiology of Atherosclerotic Disease. Harvard University Press, Cambridge, 1980.

Fox JP, Hall CE, et al: Epidemiology: Man and Disease. Macmillan, New York, 1970.

Frame PS, Carlson SJ: A critical review of periodic health screening using specific screening criteria (four parts). J Fam Pract 2:29, 1975.

Ginzberg E (ed): Regionalization and Health Policy. U.S. Government Printing Office, Washington, DC, 1977.

Hess JW, Liepman MR, Ruane TJ (eds): Family Practice and Preventive Medicine. Human Sciences Press, New York, 1983.

Holland WW, Detels R, Knox G (eds): Oxford Textbook of Public Health. Oxford University Press, New York, 1985.

Last JM (ed): Maxcy-Rosenau Public Health and Preventive Medicine, 12th ed. Appleton & Lange, East Norwalk, 1986.

Levy BS, Wegman DH (eds): Occupational Health—Recognizing and Preventing Work-Related Disease. Little, Brown & Co., Boston, 1983.

National Center for Health Statistics: Catalog of Publications of the National Center for Health Statistics. DHHS pub. no. (PHS) 81-1301. Public Health Service, Washington, DC, 1981.

O'Malley MS, Fletcher SW: Screening for breast cancer with breast self-examination: U.S. Preventative Services Task Force Report. JAMA 257:16:2197, 1987.

Pipkin FP: Medical Statistics Made Easy. Churchill Livingstone, New York, 1984.

Schefler WC: Statistics for Health Professionals. Addison-Wesley, Reading, Mass., 1984.

World Health Organization: International Classification of impairments, disabilities and handicaps. WHO, Geneva, 1980.

SAMPLE QUESTIONS

DIRECTIONS: Each question below contains five suggested answers. Choose the one best response to each question.

1. Meningococcal meningitis is not a very common disease, but it may occur in epidemics. The proportion of carriers in the community may be

   A. less than 5%
   B. no more than 10%
   C. no more than 30%
   D. no more than 50%
   E. up to 70%

2. Which of the following statements regarding tuberculosis is true?

   A. Case fatality rates in children and the elderly are steadily declining
   B. Bacille Calmette Guérin (BCG) used worldwide has proved to produce an effective active immunization
   C. Both pulmonary and extrapulmonary disease are occurring with lower prevalence
   D. The most effective preventive treatment is isoniazid, 5 to 10 mg/kg body weight for 6 to 12 months

3. Chagas' disease, the American form of trypanosomiasis, is conveyed to humans by

   A. the bites of *Glossina* flies
   B. flea bites
   C. bug bites
   D. rat bites
   E. fecal contamination by arthropod vector

4. All of the following are classic clinical signs of mercury poisoning EXCEPT

   A. gingivitis
   B. erythema
   C. sialorrhea
   D. tremor
   E. irritability

5. Which of the following statements is correct?

   A. Blue Cross and Blue Shield provide identical coverage
   B. The costs of the majority of health care are covered by insurance
   C. The most catastrophic event from an insurer's point of view is myocardial infarction
   D. Participating providers have less flexibility in assessing their charges
   E. Most third-party insurance carriers pay for preventive or health maintenance services

6. Which of the following statements is correct?

   A. Co-insurance means the necessity for the individual to have alternate medical insurance
   B. Deductibles are a percentage by which all insurance reimbursement of medical bills is reduced
   C. Copayment is the charging of a set fee for each item of service
   D. Cost containment is a device used by third-party carriers to control their losses
   E. Utilization review is an audit system applied by third-party carriers to hospital utilization

7. The standard error of the mean is

   A. the difference between the measured mean of a large population and the estimation of what it should be
   B. the difference between the means of two samples of populations that should be identical
   C. the deviation between a small sample mean and the average of means of other small samples
   D. a factor in calculating variance
   E. a factor in calculating standard deviation

8. The chi-square test may be used

   A. to compare ratios of paired results
   B. to assess whether the observed frequency departs significantly from expected frequency
   C. to compare expected numbers less than 5
   D. for all of the above
   E. for none of the above

9. The mortality rate is an example of

   A. prevalence rate
   B. incidence rate
   C. attack rate
   D. an average
   E. none of the above

10. A prevalence study is

    A. a descriptive study
    B. an experimental study
    C. a cross-sectional study
    D. a cohort study
    E. a case-control study

11. All of the following may be called determinants of disease EXCEPT

    A. genetic factors
    B. nutritional factors
    C. physical hazards
    D. stress factors
    E. natural disasters

12. Which of the following statements is true?

    A. An epidemic is an outbreak of infectious disease
    B. The number of cases of illness in an epidemic is not directly related to previous exposure
    C. An epidemic generally results from the introduction of a new agent in the community
    D. The development of an epidemic most often results from a new method of dispersion in the community
    E. The development of an epidemic is conditioned by factors affecting host susceptibility

13. The current epidemic of acquired immunodeficiency syndrome (AIDS) is most likely to be

    A. a point epidemic
    B. a propagative epidemic
    C. a progressive epidemic
    D. a mixed epidemic
    E. none of the above

14. Passive immunization is appropriate in all of the following circumstances EXCEPT when

    A. the vaccine is cheaper than an active agent
    B. no active vaccine is available
    C. a toxin is best managed by antibody administration
    D. time does not permit adequate protection by active immunization
    E. the individual is unable to synthesize antibody

15. Which of the following virus infections is most likely to give rise to sore throat?

    A. Rhinovirus
    B. Respiratory syncytial virus
    C. Parainfluenza virus
    D. Type A influenza
    E. Type B influenza

16. All of the following are possible manifestations of congenital rubella infection EXCEPT

    A. hydrocephaly
    B. patent ductus arteriosus
    C. mental retardation
    D. diabetes mellitus
    E. immunodeficiencies

17. Which of the following statements about infectious mononucleosis is true?

    A. The causative virus is a member of the coxsackievirus family
    B. The disease may be diagnosed by a Monospot test (variant of the Paul-Bunnell test) alone
    C. The disease may be prevented by avoiding kissing
    D. The characteristic feature is lymphadenopathy
    E. The characteristic feature is hematologic changes

18. Which of the following statements about diphtheria is true?

    A. The incubation period is 7 to 14 days
    B. The severity of the disease is dependent on the amount of toxin absorbed
    C. The severity of the disease depends on the development of bacteremia
    D. The administration of the toxoid produces passive immunization
    E. DPT or DT should be used for immunization before age 14

19. Which of the following statements about leprosy is true?

    A. The infection is caused by a mycobacterium that behaves similarly to tuberculosis
    B. Confirmation of the disease is by the identification of acid-fast bacilli in sputum
    C. The disease can only be confirmed by biopsy
    D. The lepromin test is confirmatory and is sensitive
    E. The infectious route is droplet infection

20. All of the following conditions may be caused by *Chlamydia trachomatis* EXCEPT

    A. trachoma
    B. vaginitis
    C. lymphogranuloma venereum
    D. Reiter's syndrome
    E. nongonococcal urethritis

21. The majority of nosocomial infections are now caused by

    A. *Staphylococcus aureus*
    B. *Escherichia coli*
    C. gram-positive bacteria
    D. gram-negative bacteria
    E. none of the above

22. Of the following parasitic infections, which is most common worldwide?

    A. Intestinal helminthiasis
    B. Amebiasis
    C. Malaria
    D. Trypanosomiasis
    E. Schistosomiasis

DIRECTIONS: The groups of questions below consist of lettered choices followed by several numbered items. For each numbered item, select the **one** lettered choice with which it is **most** closely associated. Each lettered choice may be used once, more than once, or not at all.

Questions 23–26. For each of the following metals that produce toxic affects, choose the body system that is frequently affected.

    A. Skin
    B. Neuromuscular
    C. Hematopoietic
    D. Renal
    E. None of the above

23. Arsenic

24. Chromium

25. Lead

26. Zinc

Questions 27–32. Match the following:

    A. Death rate
    B. Crude death rate
    C. Case fatality rate
    D. Infant mortality rate
    E. None of the above

27. Number of deaths related to midyear population

28. Number of deaths related to the total number in group

29. Number of persons dying from a disease related to total number in the group

30. Number of persons dying from a disease related to the total number of affected individuals

31. Number of live-born infants who die before age 1 year related to the total number of births

32. Number of stillbirths over 20 weeks gestation and numbers of deaths before age 1 related to total number of live births and stillbirths in 1 year

ANSWERS

1. E		17. E	
2. D		18. B	
3. E		19. C	
4. B		20. D	
5. D		21. D	
6. C		22. A	
7. C		23. B	
8. B		24. A	
9. B		25. C	
10. C		26. E	
11. D		27. B	
12. E		28. A	
13. D		29. E	
14. A		30. C	
15. D		31. D	
16. A		32. E	

INDEX

Cyomegalovirus (*see also* TORCH syndrome), 222

D

Deafness, 104
Dehydration in children, 272–273
Delirium, 296–297
Dementia, 297–299
Dependent personality disorder, 316
Depression, 303–307
Diabetes insipidus, 38, 78
Diabetes mellitus, 83–86
   juvenile, 274–275
   in pregnancy, 202–205
   prevention, 372
   renal disease and, 39–40
Diagnostic radiology (*see* Radiology, diagnostic)
Diarrhea, 55–57, 282–283
Diffuse pulmonary fibrosis, 48–49
Diphtheria, 346–347
Disease prevention, 367–375
Disk, herniated intervertebral, 107
Disseminated intravascular coagulation, 77
Dissociative disorders, 318–319
Diverticular disease, 58
Down's syndrome, 269
Dressler's syndrome, 20
Drowning, 50, 266
Drug abuse, 100–101, 158, 300–302
Dysfunctional uterine bleeding, 239
Dysphagia, 80, 119

E

Eaton-Lambert syndrome, 106
Eclampsia, 200–201
Ecthyma gangrenosum, 12
Electroconvulsive therapy, 307, 322
Electrolytes (*see* Fluid and electrolyte disturbances)
Embolism:
   arterial, 29
   pulmonary, 207
   venous, 30
Embryo, 150–151
Emphysema, 47
Encephalitis, 12
Endocarditis, 13, 207
Endocrine and metabolic disorders, 77 ff.
   in childhood, 274–275
   leading to cirrhosis, 285
   in gynecology, 224–226
   in pregnancy, 213–215
Endometriosis, 237–238
Enteric infections, 4–5
Environmental hazards, 335, 353
Epidemiology, 334–340
Epilepsy, 102–103
   in pregnancy, 216–217

Erysipelas, 12
Esophageal diseases, 53–54
   in pregnancy, 215
Estrogen, 148, 153, 225–226

F

Family planning, 223–224
Fanconi's syndrome, 37, 40
Fetal alcohol syndrome, 267–268
Fetus, 151–153, 161–168
Fever, 2, 4, 5, 100, 122
Fluid and electrolyte disturbances, 127–129
   in children, 271–273
Folate, 66
Food poisoning, 56, 349–350
Forceps delivery, 178
Frostbite, 30

G

Galactorrhea, 78
Gangrene, 135
Gardnerella, 230
Gastritis, 55
Gastroesophageal reflux, 53
Gastrointestinal tract:
   acute infection, 344
   bleeding, 124–125
   diseases, 52 ff.
   disease prevention, 370
   disorders in childhood, 282–283
   pregnancy and, 215
Gay bowel syndrome, 11
Generalized anxiety disorder, 314
Genetic disorders, 267–269, 334
Genitals (*see* Pelvic organs *and* Genitourinary tract)
Genitourinary tract (*see also* Sexually transmitted diseases)
   diseases, 32–41
   disease prevention, 370–371
Giant cell arteritis, 95–96
Giardiasis, 8, 57
Gigantism, 78
Gilbert's disease, 61
Glaucoma, 104
Glomerulonephritis, 33
   in pregnancy, 212
Goiter, 80–81
Gonorrhea, 9–10, 229
   in pregnancy, 219
Goodpasture's syndrome, 33
Gout, 88–89
Graft-versus-host disease, 228
Granuloma inguinale, 11, 222, 230
Graves' disease, 79, 121
Guillain-Barré syndrome, 107